Color Atlas
and
Synopsis of
Clinical Dermatology

Thomas B. Fitzpatrick, M.D., Ph.D., D.Sc.(Hon.)
Wigglesworth Professor of Dermatology, Emeritus
Chairman, Emeritus
Department of Dermatology, Harvard Medical School
Dermatologist
Massachusetts General Hospital
Consultant in Dermatology
Brigham and Women's Hospital, The Children's Hospital, and Beth Israel Hospital
Boston, Massachusetts

Richard Allen Johnson, M.D.C.M.
Clinical Instructor in Dermatology
Harvard Medical School
Clinical Associate in Dermatology
Massachusetts General Hospital
Associate in Dermatology
Beth Israel Hospital
Associate Physician (Dermatology)
Brigham and Women's Hospital
Dermatologist
New England Deaconess Hospital
Boston, Massachusetts

Machiel K. Polano, M.D.
Professor Emeritus and Chairman
Department of Dermatology, University Hospital
Leiden, The Netherlands

Dick Suurmond, M.D.
Professor Emeritus and Chairman
Department of Dermatology, University Hospital
Leiden, The Netherlands

Klaus Wolff, M.D.
Professor and Chairman
Department of Dermatology I
University of Vienna Medical School
Chief, Dermatology Service I
General Hospital of Vienna
Vienna, Austria

Color Atlas and Synopsis of Clinical Dermatology

Common and Serious Diseases

Second Edition

Thomas B. Fitzpatrick, M.D.

Richard Allen Johnson, M.D.

Machiel K. Polano, M.D.

Dick Suurmond, M.D.

Klaus Wolff, M.D.

McGRAW-HILL, INC
Health Professions Division

New York St. Louis San Francisco Auckland Bogotá Caracas
Lisbon London Madrid Mexico Milan Montreal New Delhi
Paris San Juan Singapore Sydney Tokyo Toronto

Color Atlas and Synopsis of Clinical Dermatology

345678910 KPKP 998765432

ISBN 0-07-021209-0

This book was set in Times Roman by York Graphic Services, Inc.; the editors were J. Dereck Jeffers and Mariapaz Ramos Englis; the production supervisor was Roger Kasunic.

Areata Graphics/Kingsport was printer and binder.

Library of Congress Cataloging-in-Publication Data

Color atlas and synopsis of clinical dermatology : common and serious
  diseases / Thomas B. Fitzpatrick . . . [et al.].—2d ed.
      p.   cm.
  Rev. ed. of: Color atlas and synopsis of clinical dermatology /
Thomas B. Fitzpatrick, Machiel K. Polano, Dick Suurmond. c1983.
  Includes bibliographical references and indexes.
  ISBN 0-07-021209-0
  1. Dermatology—Atlases. I. Fitzpatrick, Thomas B. (Thomas
Bernard)
  [DNLM: 1. Skin Diseases. 2. Skin Diseases—atlases. 3. Skin
Manifestations.   4. Skin Manifestations—atlases. WR 17 C718]
RL81.C65   1991
616.5—dc20
DNLM/DLC
for Library of Congress   91-20833
                                                                      CIP

The color photographs herein are from the collections of the Departments of Dermatology at the University Medical Center, Leiden; the University of Vienna Medical School, Vienna; and Harvard Medical School, Massachusetts General Hospital, Boston.

The following companies are gratefully acknowledged for making educational grants that helped make possible the publication of this Atlas:

BURROUGHS WELLCOME CO.
ROCHE DERMATOLOGICS
STIEFEL LABORATORIES, INC.
SYNTEX LABORATORIES, INC.
ZYMA, SA

Contents

ix

xiii

xiv

PREFACE
Second Edition

For an increasing number of physicians who are not dermatologists, the management of skin disorders has recently become a major challenge. This is because of changes in the practice of medicine in which referral to specialists is being seriously restricted by third-party insurance carriers. Familiarity with dermatology is now necessary because of the large number of patients presenting with skin lesions as incidental findings or as major complaints that are being seen first by the primary care physician, pediatrician, and certain types of internists (allergists, rheumatologists, infectious disease consultants). The prevalence of skin lesions and skin disorders now extant has stimulated general physicians to become "paraspecialists" in dermatology. Just as a chest physician must look at and interpret the chest films or the orthopedist the bone films, so the nondermatologist must now be able to "read" skin lesions, as he or she should be able to interpret a blood smear.

This atlas-text has a single and specific goal: to acquaint members of the health professions with the principal lesions of the skin in order to facilitate dermatologic diagnosis. As skin lesions are visually recognized, a logical approach to learn how to make a dermatologic diagnosis is first and foremost to carefully study a color photograph of typical lesions, and simultaneously, while viewing the lesions, to consult across the page a succinct summary of the major features of the disease. With this aim in mind, we have placed large color photographs of skin lesions opposite a synopsis of the essential facts of diagnosis and treatment of the common skin disorders; in addition, in this second edition the skin signs of many of the serious systemic diseases are depicted and summarized in the same style.

To keep pace with the much expanded role of dermatology in general medical practice, we have assembled this new practical clinical tool; the second edition contains 250 more photographs and 86 more précis than the first edition of *Color Atlas and Synopsis of Clinical Dermatology* by T.B. Fitzpatrick, M.K. Polano, D. Suurmond, and R.A. Johnson, which went through nine reprintings in seven years. However, even in this expanded version, the Atlas serves only to supplement the complete presentations of dermatology provided in the several available current textbooks of dermatology. The text has been a cooperative effort of three dermatology departments: Leiden (The Netherlands), Boston (United States), and Vienna (Austria).

The color plates are from the collections of the Department of Dermatology, University Hospital, Leiden, the Department of Dermatology, University of Vienna, and the Massachusetts General Hospital, Boston. Some of the color plates were prepared in the lithographic institute Sturm of Basel, Switzerland, on appointment by CIBA-Geigy. We are grateful to CIBA-Geigy for their permission to use certain photographs in this book.

The line drawings and halftones were prepared by Gail Burroughs except for the three half-tones depicting primary melanoma, which were done by Gail Cooper, M.D.

The authors are grateful to Patricia K. Novak for her diligence and her experienced hand in helping to prepare the manuscript and the illustrations. Finally, we would like to acknowledge the cooperation of J. Dereck Jeffers, Mariapaz Ramos Englis, and Roger Kasunic of the Health Professions Division of McGraw-Hill, Inc.

Thomas B. Fitzpatrick
Richard Allen Johnson
Machiel K. Polano
Dick Suurmond
Klaus Wolff

Introduction
Approach to Dermatologic Diagnosis[1]

"The art of being wise is the art of knowing what to overlook"
WILLIAM JAMES

Too often, it seems, many health professionals make no serious attempt to identify skin lesions promptly, although accurate recognition is usually possible; asymptomatic skin lesions are considered trivial and are overlooked. Undiagnosed asymptomatic lesions are treated for months with topical and oral corticosteroids and/or antibiotics; this postponement of appropriate treatment prolongs discomfort, aids and abets disfigurement, not uncommonly leads to an irreversible generalization of the disorder, or, most critically, to a delay in diagnosis, which can result in multisystem illness or death.

One must be aware that robust *well* people can have asymptomatic skin lesions that are signs of serious multisystem diseases, and these lesions cannot be overlooked without endangering the patient's health. Certain skin changes that may be encountered during a routine physical examination are just as important to detect as are enlarged lymph nodes, such as, for example, early malignant melanoma in a curable stage of evolution, or the small yellow papules of hyperlipoproteinemic xanthomas, a treatable potentially fatal disease.

Similarly, for acute and chronically *ill* patients, ambulatory or in hospital, identification of skin lesions[2] and frequently a skin biopsy[2] is necessary. Of all the organs, the skin is the easiest to obtain material for study of the pathologic changes that are the basis of the clinical lesion. In this manner puzzling multisystem disorders can be diagnosed, such as sarcoidosis, deep fungal infections, cutaneous infarcts in septicemia, or the characteristic tender nodules on the leg that occur in acute pancreatitis.

"What's the use of a book," thought Alice, "without pictures or conversations?"
LEWIS CARROLL

As the identification of skin lesions is a visual exercise, a logical approach to dermatologic diagnosis is, first to study a color photograph and simultaneously, while viewing the lesions, to look across the page for the major features of the disease. With this aim in mind, we have placed color photographs of skin lesions opposite a synopsis presented in a readily accessible outline format summarizing essential facts of diagnosis and treatment of the common skin disorders and of the skin signs of multisystem diseases.

This atlas + text is proposed as a "field guide" to the recognition of skin disorders. The skin is a treasury of important lesions that can usually be clinically recognized. At present gross morphology in the form of skin lesions remains the hard core of dermatologic diagnosis. Skin lesions are visible (1 : 1) to the unaided eye just as pulmonary and brain lesions are gross pathology but visible only with imaging. Both require a differential diagnosis and both can often lead the clinician to the correct diagnosis—and thus the proper management of the patient.

---

1. See page xviii for *Outline of an Approach to Diagnosis*
2. See Appendices A and B for illustrations of *Types of Skin Lesions* and *Special Clinical and Laboratory Aids to Dermatologic Diagnosis*

Outline of an Approach to Dermatologic Diagnosis

I. Epidemiology and Etiology   Age, race, sex, occupation

II. History

    A. Duration of onset of skin lesions: days, weeks, months, years
    B. Relationship of skin lesions to season, travel history, heat, cold, previous treat-
        ment, drug ingestion, occupation, hobbies; effects of menses, pregnancy
    C. Skin symptoms: pruritus, pain, paresthesia
    D. Constitutional symptoms
        1. "Acute illness" syndrome: headache, chills, feverishness, weakness
        2. "Chronic illness" syndrome: fatigue, weakness, anorexia, weight loss, malaise
    E. Systems review

III. Physical Examination

    A. Appearance of patient: uncomfortable, "toxic," well
    B. Vital signs: pulse, respiration, temperature
    C. Skin—four major skin signs: (1) type, (2) shape, (3) arrangement, (4) distribu-
        tion of lesions
        1. **Type** of lesion (see Appendix A)

Basic lesions	*Sequential lesions*
Macule	Scale
Papule-plaque	Exudation: dry (crust)
Wheal	wet (weeping)
Nodule	Erosion
Cyst	Scar
Vesicle-bulla	Lichenification
Pustule	
Ulcer (also sequential)	
Hyperkeratosis (also sequential)	
Sclerosis	
Atrophy (also sequential)	
Telangiectasia	
Infarct	
Purpura	

          Color of lesions or of the skin if diffuse involvement: *"skin color"; white:*
          leukoderma, hypomelanosis; *red:* erythema; *pink; violaceous; brown:* hyper-
          melanosis or hemosiderin; *black; blue; gray; orange; yellow.* Red or purple
          purpuric lesions do not blanch with pressure (diascopy).
          Palpation
              Consistency (soft, firm, hard, fluctuant, boardlike)
              Deviation in temperature (hot, cold)
              Mobility of lesion or of skin
              Presence of tenderness
              Estimate of the depth of lesion (i.e., dermal or subcutaneous)
        2. **Shape** of individual lesions
          Round, oval, polygonal, polycyclic, annular (ring-shaped), iris, serpiginous
          (snakelike), umbilicated

3. **Arrangement** of multiple lesions

Grouped: herpetiform, zosteriform, arciform, annular, reticulated (net-shaped), linear, serpiginous (snakelike)

Disseminated: scattered discrete lesions or diffuse involvement (i.e., without identifiable borders)

4. **Distribution** of lesions

Extent: isolated (single lesion), localized, regional, generalized, universal

Pattern: symmetrical, exposed areas, sites of pressure, intertriginous areas, follicular localization, random

Characteristic patterns: secondary syphilis, atopic dermatitis, acne, erythema multiforme, candidiasis, lupus erythematosus, pemphigus, pemphigoid, porphyria cutanea tarda, xanthoma, necrotizing angiitis (vasculitis), Rocky Mountain spotted fever, Lyme disease, rubella, rubeola, AIDS, scarlet fever, toxic shock syndrome, typhoid, Kawasaki's disease, herpes zoster, varicella, scalded-skin syndrome, toxic epidermal necrolysis, Kaposi's sarcoma (epidemic)

D. Hair and nails

E. Mucous membranes

F. General medical examination

IV. **Diagnosis and Differential Diagnosis**

V. **Laboratory and Special Examinations**

A. Dermatopathology

1. Light microscopy: site, process, cell types
2. Immunofluorescence
3. Special techniques: stains, transmission electron microscopy, etc.

B. Microbiologic examination of skin material: scales, crusts, exudate, or tissue

1. Direct microscopic examination of skin (see Appendix B)

For yeast and fungus: 10% potassium hydroxide preparation (see pages 99 and 773, Figures 51 and 69)

For bacteria: Gram's stain

For virus: Tzanck smear (see pages 71 and 773)

For spirochetes: dark-field examination

For parasites: scabies mite from a burrow (see page 774)

2. Culture

Bacterial ⎫
Viral   ⎬ For granulomas, culture of minced tissue
Parasitic ⎪
Mycologic ⎭

C. Laboratory examinations of blood

Bacteriologic: culture

Serologic: ANA, STS, serology

Hematologic: hematocrit or hemoglobin, cells, differential smear

Chemistry: fasting blood sugar, blood urea nitrogen, creatinine, liver function and thyroid function tests (if indicated)

D. Imaging (x-ray, CT scan, MRI, ultrasound)

E. Urinalysis

F. Stool examination (for occult blood, e.g., in vasculitis syndromes; for ova and parasites; for porphyrins)

G. Wood's lamp examination (see page 772)

Urine: pink-orange fluorescence in porphyria cutanea tarda (add 1.0 ml of 5.0% hydrochloric acid)

Hair (in vivo): green fluorescence in tinea capitis (hair shaft)
Skin (in vivo)
    Erythrasma: coral-red fluorescence
    Hypomelanosis: decrease in intensity
    Brown hypermelanosis: increase in intensity
    Blue hypermelanosis: no change in intensity
  H. Patch testing (see page 773)
  I. Acetowhitening—whitening of subclinical penile warts after application of 5% acetic acid (see page 773)

VI. Pathophysiology

VII. Course and Prognosis

VIII. Treatment

IX. General References

Arndt KA: *Manual of Dermatologic Therapeutics with Essentials of Diagnosis,* 4th ed, Little, Brown, Boston, 1989

Demis DJ et al (eds): *Clinical Dermatology,* 4 vol, Harper & Row, New York, 1979

Fitzpatrick TB et al (eds): *Dermatology in General Medicine,* 3d ed, 2 vol, McGraw-Hill, New York, 1987

Lever WF, Schaumburg-Lever G: *Histopathology of the Skin,* 7th ed, Lippincott, Philadelphia, 1990

Moschella SL, Hurley HJ Jr: *Dermatology,* 2d ed, 2 vol, Saunders, Philadelphia, 1985

Polano MK: *Topical Skin Therapeutics,* Churchill-Livingston, Edinburgh, 1984

Rook A et al (eds): *Textbook of Dermatology,* 4th ed, 3 vol, Blackwell, Oxford, 1986

Color Atlas
and
Synopsis of
Clinical Dermatology

Disorders of Sebaceous and Apocrine Glands

Acne Vulgaris (Common Acne) and Acne Cystica

Acne is a chronic inflammation of the pilosebaceous units of certain areas (face and trunk) that occurs in adolescence and manifests as comedones, papules, nodules, cysts, or papulopustules, often, but not always, followed by pitted or hypertrophic scars.

EPIDEMIOLOGY AND ETIOLOGY

Age   10 to 17 years in females; 14 to 19 in males; may appear first at 25 years

Sex   More severe in males than females

Race   Lower incidence in Orientals and blacks; rare in China

Occupation   Exposure to acnegenic mineral oils, dioxin

Drugs   Lithium, hydantoin, systemic corticosteroids may cause exacerbation

Genetic Aspects   Multifactorial; severe acne associated with XYY syndrome

Other Factors   Endocrine factors (see Pathophysiology). Emotional stress (school, social problems) can definitely cause exacerbations. Pressure on skin by leaning face on hands is a very important exacerbating factor. Acne is not caused by chocolate or fatty foods, or, in fact, by any kind of food.

HISTORY

Duration of Lesions   Months

Season   Worse in fall and winter

Symptoms   Pain in lesions (especially nodulocystic type)

PHYSICAL EXAMINATION

Skin Lesions
TYPE:
   Comedone—open (blackheads, Figure 1) or closed (whiteheads)

   Papules (Figure 2)—with (red) or without inflammation

   Nodules, noduloulcerative lesions, or cysts—2 to 5 cm in diameter (Figure 3)

   Scars—atrophic depressed (often pitted) or hypertrophic (keloid) scars

   Seborrhea of the face and scalp is often present

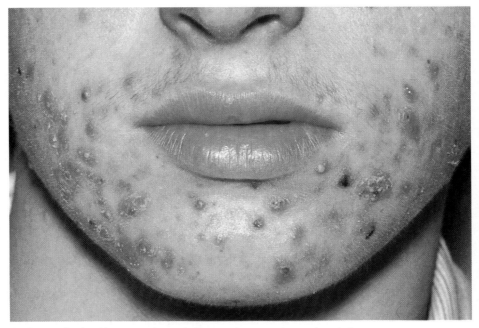

1   Acne vulgaris   *Note comedones, inflammation, papules, and pustules.*

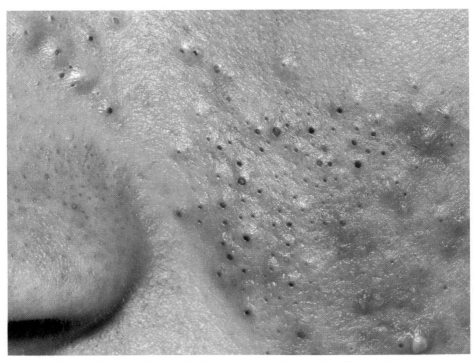

2   Acne vulgaris   *Note the closed (white) comedones and open (black) comedones.*

ACNE VULGARIS (COMMON ACNE) AND ACNE CYSTICA   3

SHAPE   Round; nodules may coalesce to form linear mounds

ARRANGEMENT   Isolated single lesion (e.g., nodule) or scattered discrete lesions (papules, cysts, nodules)

SITES OF PREDILECTION   Face, neck, upper arms, trunk

SPECIAL FORMS

Acne Conglobata   Severe cystic acne with coalescing nodules, cysts, and abscesses

Acne Fulminans   *Acute,* severe cystic acne with concomitant suppuration of most of the lesions, fever, and generalized arthritis

DIFFERENTIAL DIAGNOSIS

Persistent acne in a hirsute female with irregular or no menses is an indication for a search for hypersecretion of androgens, plasma testosterone, and/or dehydroepiandrosterone (e.g., polycystic ovarian syndrome). Also, recalcitrant acne can be related to partial 11- or 12-hydroxylase block.

PATHOPHYSIOLOGY

The lesions of acne (comedones) are the result of complex effects of hormones (androgens) and bacteria (*Propionibacterium acnes*) in the pilosebaceous unit. Androgens stimulate sebaceous glands to produce larger amounts of sebum; bacteria contain lipase that converts lipid into fatty acids. Both sebum and fatty acids cause a sterile inflammatory response in the pilosebaceous unit; this results in hyperkeratinization of the lining of the follicle with resultant plugging. The enlarged follicular lumen contains this inspissated keratin and lipid debris (the whitehead). When the follicle has a portal of entry at the skin, the semisolid mass protrudes, forming a plug (the blackhead). The black color is due to oxidation of tyrosine to melanin by tyrosinase contained in the follicular orifice. The distended follicle

walls may break and the contents (sebum, lipid, fatty acids, keratin, etc.) may enter the dermis, provoking a foreign-body response (papule, pustule, nodule). Rupture plus intense inflammation leads to scars.

COURSE

Acne may persist in women to age 35

TREATMENT

Mild
Topical antibiotics (clindamycin, erythromycin)

Benzoyl peroxide gels (2%, 5%, or 10%)

Topical retinoids (vitamin A acid) are effective but require detailed instructions and gradual increases in concentration. Improvement occurs over a period of months (2 to 5) and may take even longer for noninflamed comedones. For most patients, start with tretinoin 0.01% gel and increase after 1 month to 0.025% applied nightly after washing with a mild soap. Topical antibiotics are applied during the day.

Severe
Oral tetracyclines added to the above—minocycline, 50 to 100 mg b.i.d., for instance; can be tapered to 50 mg/day.

In females only, severe acne can be controlled with high doses of oral estrogens combined with progesterone. Cerebrovascular disorders are a serious risk, however.

Oral 13-*cis*-retinoic acid (Accutane) is highly effective for cystic acne. This treatment requires experience. As retinoids are teratogenic in pregnant females, it is necessary that female patients have a pretreatment pregnancy test and they must be on oral contraceptives at least 1 month prior to beginning treatment, throughout treatment, and for 2 months after treatment is discontinued.

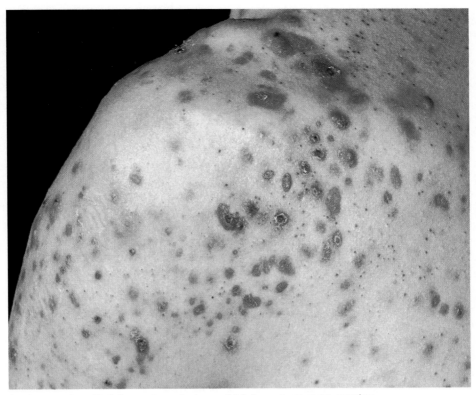

3 Acne cystica *Nodules, cysts, and ulcers which leave permanent scarring.*

Furthermore, a patient must have a negative serum pregnancy test within the 2 weeks prior to beginning treatment. *Dosage:* 0.5 to 1 mg/kg/day with meals for a 15- to 20-week course, which is usually adequate. About 30% of patients require two 4-month courses with a 2-month rest period in between. Careful monitoring of the blood is necessary during therapy, especially in patients with elevated blood triglycerides before therapy is begun.

Hidradenitis suppurativa is a chronic, suppurative, cicatricial disease of aprocrine gland–bearing skin of the axillae and anogenital region. Sometimes associated with severe cystic acne.

Synonyms: Apocrinitis, hidradenitis axillaris, abscess of the apocrine sweat glands.

EPIDEMIOLOGY AND ETIOLOGY

Age From puberty to climacteric

Sex Males more often have anogenital involvement; females, axillary

Etiology Predisposing factors: obesity, genetic predisposition to acne. Apocrine duct obstruction, secondary bacterial infection

HISTORY

Intermittent pain, abscess formation in axilla(e) and/or anogenital area; severe cystic acne

PHYSICAL EXAMINATION

Skin Findings

TYPE OF LESION Inflammatory nodule/abscess (Figure 4) which may resolve or point to surface and drain purulent/seropurulent material; relationship to hair follicle usually not apparent. Eventually sinus tracts form. Fibrosis, "bridge" scars, hypertrophic and keloidal scars, contractures. Subsequently, open comedones, at times double, form. Rarely, lymphedema of associated limb. Comedones that are "double" may be present, even when active nodules are absent.

COLOR Erythematous nodules

PALPATION Lesions moderately to exquisitely tender. Pus emitted from opening of abscess and sinus tracts.

DISTRIBUTION OF LESIONS Axillae, breasts, anogenitalia, groins. Often bilateral in axillae and/or anogenital area; may extend over entire back and buttocks.

General Examination Often obesity. Severe cystic acne (acne conglobata).

DIAGNOSIS AND DIFFERENTIAL DIAGNOSIS

Diagnosis Clinical diagnosis

Differential Diagnosis *Early:* furuncle, carbuncle, lymphadenitis, ruptured tricholemmal cyst, cat-scratch disease, tularemia. *Late:* lymphogranuloma venereum, donovanosis, scrofuloderma, actinomycosis, sinus tracts and fistulae associated with ulcerative colitis and regional enteritis.

LABORATORY AND SPECIAL EXAMINATIONS

Bacteriology *Staphylococcus aureus,* streptococci, *Escherichia coli, Proteus mirabilis, Pseudomonas aeruginosa* commonly cultured from drainage.

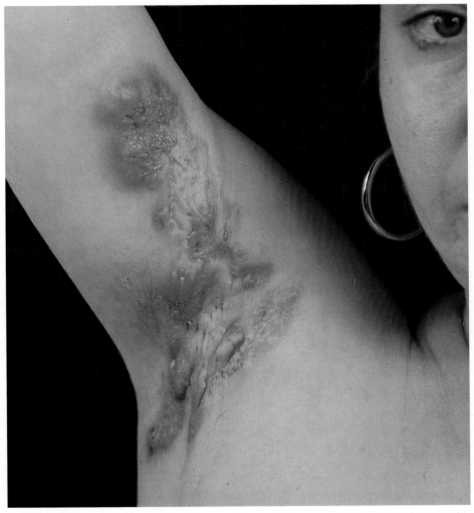

4 Hidradenitis suppurativa *Inflammatory nodules and abscesses, sinus tracts, and hypertrophic and keloidal scars.*

Dermatopathology *Early:* keratin occlusion of apocrine duct and hair follicle, ductal/tubular dilatation, inflammatory changes limited to single apocrine gland. *Late:* destruction of apocrine/eccrine/pilosebaceous apparatus, fibrosis; pseudoepitheliomatous hyperplasia in sinuses.

PATHOPHYSIOLOGY

Sequence of changes: keratinous plugging of the apocrine duct → dilatation of apocrine duct and hair follicle → severe inflammatory changes limited to a simple apocrine gland → bacterial growth in dilated duct → ruptured duct/gland results in extension of inflammation/infection → extension of suppuration/tissue destruction → ulceration and fibrosis, sinus tract formation.

COURSE AND PROGNOSIS

Spectrum of disease is very broad. Many patients have mild involvement and do not seek therapy. The disease usually undergoes a spontaneous remission with age (over 35 years). In some individuals, the course can be relentlessly progressive, with marked morbidity related to chronic pain, draining sinuses, and scarring. Complications (rare): fistulas to urethra, bladder, and/or rectum; anemia, amyloidosis.

TREATMENT

Early: erythromycin (250 to 500 mg q.i.d.), or tetracycline (250 to 500 mg q.i.d.), or minocycline (100 mg b.i.d.) until lesions resolved. Intralesional triamcinolone (3 to 5 mg/mL) into early inflammatory lesions.

Late: maintenance therapy with these antibiotics. Prednisone may be given concurrently if pain and inflammation are severe, 70 mg, tapered over 14 days.

Role for oral 13-*cis*-retinoic acid in advanced disease is not established, but it appears to be useful in early disease and when combined with surgical excision of individual lesions.

With extensive, chronic disease: complete excision of axilla or involved anogenital area may be required. Excision should extend down to fascia and requires split skin grafting.

Rosacea (Latin, "like roses") is a chronic acneform inflammation of the pilosebaceous units of the face, coupled with a peculiar increased reactivity of capillaries to heat, leading to flushing and telangiectasia.

EPIDEMIOLOGY AND ETIOLOGY

Age   30 to 50 years

Sex   Females predominantly

Race   Celtic peoples (skin phototypes I and II); less frequent in pigmented (brown and black) peoples

Other Factors   Patients have periodic reddening of the face (flushing) with increase in skin temperature in response to heat stimuli in the mouth (hot liquids); alcohol is a factor in rosacea, possibly by its "flushing" effect.

HISTORY

Duration of Lesions   Days, weeks

Skin Symptoms   Flushing; papular and papulopustular lesions may be tender

PHYSICAL EXAMINATION

Skin Lesions
TYPE
   Telangiectasia (Figure 5)

   Papules (2 to 3 mm), papulopustules [the pustule (Figure 5) is often *minute* on the "crest" of the papule]

   Nodules (Figure 6)

   No comedones
COLOR   Rose-red facies, papules and nodules (Figures 5 and 6)

SHAPE   Papules and nodules are round, dome-shaped
ARRANGEMENT   Scattered discrete lesions
DISTRIBUTION   Characteristic is a symmetrical localization on the face (cheeks, chin, forehead, nose) and, rarely, neck

Eye Lesions   Blepharitis, conjunctivitis, and episcleritis. Rosacea keratitis is a serious problem because corneal ulcers may develop. An ophthalmologist should follow the patient with eye involvement.

DIFFERENTIAL DIAGNOSIS

The differential diagnosis of flushing will include carcinoid syndrome and SLE, but the *sine qua non* of the diagnosis of rosacea are the small papules and papulopustules.

COURSE

Prolonged. Recurrences are common. After a few years the disease tends to disappear spontaneously. Men may develop rhinophyma, which is successfully treated by surgery.

TREATMENT

   Marked reduction or elimination of alcoholic and hot beverages

   Topical 0.75% metronidazole is effective treatment.

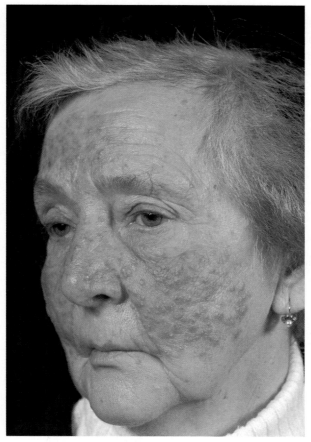

5   Rosacea   *Clusters of papulopustules on the cheek and forehead. Note that many of the erythematous papules have a tiny pustule at the crest.*

Tetracycline or erythromycin, 250 mg t.i.d. for 1 week, then b.i.d., then gradually reduced to daily doses, should be used if metronidazole fails.

Topical antibiotics are somewhat effective.

Systemic 13-*cis*-retinoic acid is an alternative in severe cases not responding to antibiotics.

Emotional stress may be a factor, and this should be emphasized to the patient.

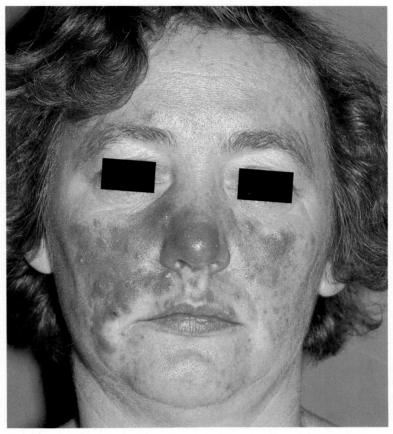

6   Rosacea   *A striking erythema is noted with large, almost cystic, lesions.*

Perioral dermatitis is a facial dermatosis occurring mainly in young women, characterized by discrete erythematous micropapules which often become confluent forming inflammatory plaques, on the perioral and periorbital skin.

Synonym: rosacea-like dermatitis.

EPIDEMIOLOGY AND ETIOLOGY

Age   15 to 40 years; can occur in children

Sex   Females predominantly

Etiology   Unknown

Other Factors   May be markedly aggravated by potent topical (fluorinated) corticosteroids

HISTORY

Duration of Lesions   Weeks to months

Skin Symptoms   Cosmetic disfigurement, occasional itching or burning

PHYSICAL EXAMINATION

Skin Lesions
TYPE   Initial lesions are erythematous micropapules. Papules increase in number with central confluence and satellite lesions, including papules, vesicles, and/or pustules (Figure 7). Confluent plaques may appear eczematous with erythema and scale.
COLOR   Pink to red
ARRANGEMENT   Papules are irregularly grouped.
DISTRIBUTION   Initial lesions usually in nasolabial fold. Symmetry is common. Rim of sparing around the vermilion border of lips. At times, micropapules also occur on the lower and upper eyelids. Uncommonly, only periorbital involvement is present. Uncommonly, glabella and forehead involved.

DIAGNOSIS AND DIFFERENTIAL DIAGNOSIS

Diagnosis   Clinical

Differential Diagnosis   Allergic contact dermatitis, atopic dermatitis, seborrheic dermatitis, rosacea, acne vulgaris, steroid acne, sarcoidosis, lymphocytic infiltrate

COURSE

Appearance of lesions is usually subacute over weeks to months. Perioral dermatitis is, at times, misdiagnosed as an eczematous or a seborrheic dermatitis and treated with a potent topical corticosteroid preparation, aggravating perioral dermatitis or inducing steroid acne. Untreated, perioral dermatitis fluctuates in activity over months to years but is not nearly as chronic as rosacea. With adequate treatment for several months, mild recurrences do occur but are usually controlled with topical metronidazole gel or a low-dose tetracycline.

TREATMENT

Topical: metronidazole 0.75% gel or erythromycin 2.0% gel applied to involved areas b.i.d.

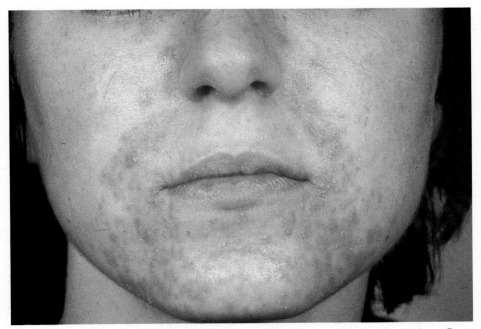

7   Perioral dermatitis *Individual erythematous papules and papulopustules and confluent plaques, which appear eczematous with scaling.*

Systemic: tetracycline 500 mg b.i.d. until clear, then 500 mg daily for 1 month, then 250 mg daily for 1 additional month **or** minocycline 50 mg b.i.d. until clear, then 100 mg daily for 1 month, then 50 mg on alternating days for 1 additional month **or** doxycycline 100 mg b.i.d. until clear, then 100 mg daily for 1 month, then 50 mg daily for 1 additional month

Eczematous Dermatitis

Contact Dermatitis

Contact dermatitis is an acute, subacute, or chronic inflammation of the epidermis and dermis caused by external agents, toxicity, or an allergic reaction and characterized by pruritus or burning of the skin.

EPIDEMIOLOGY AND ETIOLOGY

Age   No influence on capacity for sensitization

Race   Black skin is less susceptible.

Occupation   This is the important cause of disability in industry.

Etiology   Clinical syndrome usually *delayed-hypersensitivity reaction* (type IV) with a latent period of a few days or years between the first exposure and the reexposure that precipitates the allergic contact dermatitis or due to a *primary* irritant that produces inflammation on first or repeated contact

HISTORY

Duration of Lesion(s)   Acute contact—days, weeks; chronic contact—months, years

Skin Symptoms   Pruritus

Constitutional Symptoms   "Acute illness" syndrome (see page xviii) (including fever) in severe allergic contact dermatitis (e.g., poison ivy)

PHYSICAL EXAMINATION

Skin Lesions
TYPE *Acute*   Irregular, poorly demarcated patches of erythema and edema on which are superimposed closely spaced, nonumbilicated vesicles, punctate erosions exuding serum, and crusts (Figure 8)

Subacute   Patches of mild erythema showing small, dry scales or superficial desquamation, sometimes associated with small, red, pointed or rounded, firm papules

Chronic   Patches of lichenification (thickening of the epidermis with deepening of the skin lines in parallel or rhomboidal pattern), with satellite, small, firm, rounded or flat-topped papules, excoriations, and pigmentation of mild erythema

ARRANGEMENT   Often linear, with artificial patterns, an "outside job" (Figure 9). Plant contact often results in linear lesions.

DISTRIBUTION *Extent*   Isolated, localized to one region (e.g., shoe dermatitis) (Figure 10), or generalized (e.g., plant dermatitis)

Pattern   Random or on exposed areas (as in airborne allergic contact or photocontact dermatitis)

Characteristic Patterns   See Figures I and II.

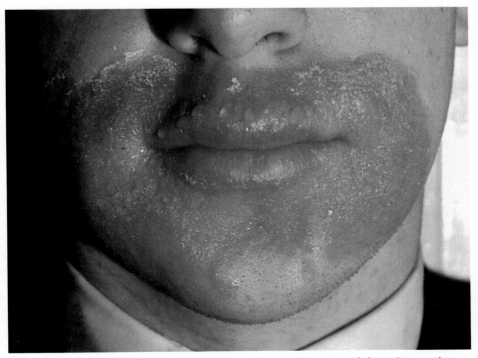

8 Contact eczematous dermatitis caused by balsam of Peru *Note areas of sharp demarcation.*

LABORATORY AND SPECIAL EXAMINATIONS

Dermatopathology

SITE   Epidermis and dermis

PROCESS   Inflammation with intraepidermal intercellular edema (spongiosis) and monocyte and histiocyte infiltration in the dermis suggest allergic contact dermatitis, while more superficial vesicles containing polymorphonuclear leukocytes suggest a primary irritant dermatitis. In chronic contact dermatitis there is lichenification (hyperkeratosis, acanthosis, elongation of rete ridges, and elongation and broadening of papillae).

Patch Tests   Sensitization is present on every part of the skin; therefore application of the allergen to any area of normal skin will provoke inflammation. A positive patch test shows erythema *and* papules, possibly vesicles confined to the test site. Patch tests should be delayed until the dermatitis has subsided at the selected site of application for at least 2 weeks. See page 772.

PATHOPHYSIOLOGY

Allergic contact dermatitis is the classic example of type IV hypersensitivity reaction (cellular, cell-mediated, delayed, or tuberculin type) caused by sensitized lymphocytes (T cells) after contact with antigen. The antigen processing occurs via Langerhans cells. The tissue damage results from cytotoxicity by T cells and from release of lymphokines.

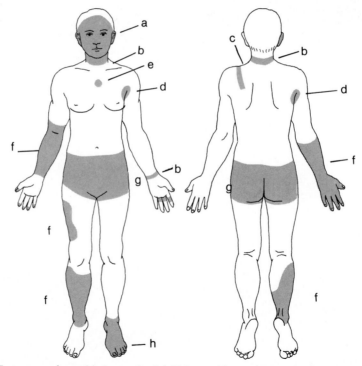

Figure I   Eczematous dermatitis (contact)   *(a) Airborne allergens (plants, pollens, sprays; (b) jewelry, clothing, furs; (c) clothing straps; (d) deodorant, antiperspirant; (e) metal tags; (f) plants; (g) trunks and panties; (h) shoes or hose.*

ECZEMATOUS DERMATITIS

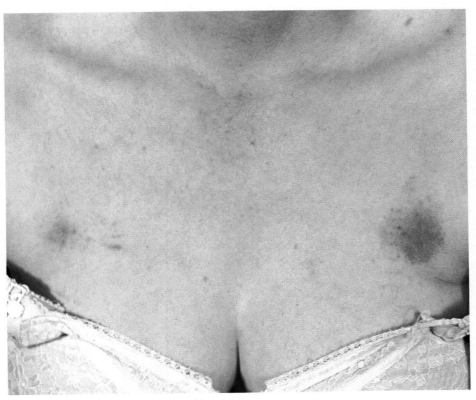

9   Contact eczematous dermatitis caused by nickel

TREATMENT

Acute

Identify and remove the etiologic agent.

Larger vesicles may be drained but tops should not be removed.

Wet dressings using cloths soaked in Burow's solution changed every 2 to 3 hours. Topical corticosteroid creams. In severe cases systemic corticosteroids may be indicated.

Prednisone: 1 mg/kg (40–60 mg/day) reduced over 2 to 3 weeks, divide daily doses into 3 doses at mealtime).

Subacute and Chronic If the lesions are not bullous it is possible to use short course of one of the potent topical corticosteroid preparations, betamethasone dipropionate or clobetasol propionate.

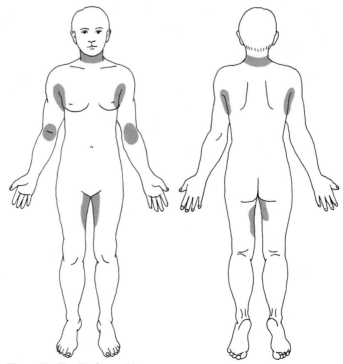

Figure II Textile dermatitis

ECZEMATOUS DERMATITIS

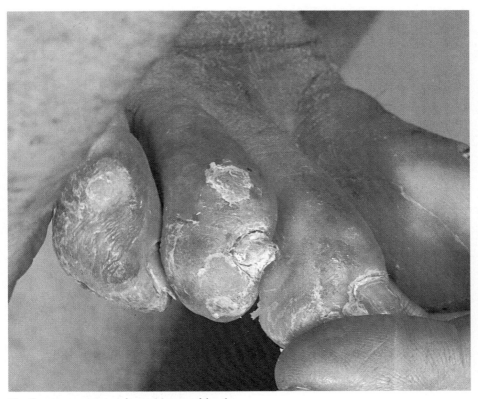

10 Contact eczematous dermatitis caused by shoes

Atopic dermatitis is an acute, subacute, but usually chronic, pruritic inflammation of the epidermis and dermis, often occurring in association with a personal or family history of hay fever, asthma, allergic rhinitis, or atopic dermatitis.

EPIDEMIOLOGY AND ETIOLOGY

Age Onset in first 2 months of life and by first year in 60% of patients

Sex Slightly more common in boys than girls

Hereditary Predisposition Over two-thirds have personal or family history of allergic rhinitis, hay fever, or asthma. An allergic work-up is rarely helpful in uncovering an allergen.

HISTORY

Duration of Lesions Most patients become afflicted between infancy and age 12, with 60% by first year; 30% seen for the first time by age 5, with only 10% developing atopic dermatitis between 6 and 20 years of age.

Skin Symptoms Pruritus is the *sine qua non* of atopic dermatitis. The constant scratching leads to a vicious cycle of itch-scratch-rash-itch—the rash being lichenification of the skin. Itching is precipitated by wool, detergents, soaps, a change in room temperature, and mental and/or physical stress.

SKIN LESIONS

Erythema, papules, scaling, excoriations, and crusting.

Lichenification. Lesions usually confluent and ill defined. See Figures 11 to 13; Figure III.

SPECIAL CLINICAL FEATURES

Tendency to develop generalized infections, especially herpes simplex

White dermographism on stroking involved skin and/or delayed blanch to cholinergic agents

Bilateral cataracts occur in up to 10% in the more severe cases; the peak incidence is between 15 and 25 years of age

Ichthyosis vulgaris and keratosis pilaris in 10% of patients

Nonspecific: periorbital pigmentation, infraorbital fold in eyelids (Dennie-Morgan sign), loss of lateral portions of eyebrows

DIFFERENTIAL DIAGNOSIS

Certain rare metabolic disorders mimic atopic dermatitis and these should be considered: acrodermatitis enteropathica, gluten-sensitive enteropathy, glucagonoma syndrome, histidinemia, phenylketonuria; also, some immunologic disorders, including Wiskott-Aldrich syndrome, sex-linked agammaglobulinemia, hyper-IgE syndrome, Letterer-Siwe disease, selective IgA deficiency.

DERMATOPATHOLOGY

Site Epidermis and dermis

Process Varying degrees of acanthosis with rare intraepidermal intercellular edema (spongiosis). The dermal infiltrate is comprised of lymphocytes, monocytes, and mast cells with few or no eosinophils.

LABORATORY EXAMINATION

Increased IgE in serum

Culture and sensitivity for bacterial infection

Culture for HSV if indicated

PATHOPHYSIOLOGY

Type I (IgE-mediated) hypersensitivity reaction occurring as a result of the release of vasoactive substances from both mast cells and basophils that have been sensitized by the interaction of the antigen with IgE (reaginic or skin-sensitizing antibody); however, the role of IgE in atopic dermatitis is still not clarified.

COURSE AND PROGNOSIS

Spontaneous more or less complete remission during childhood is the rule with occasional, more severe recurrences during adolescence. In most patients the disease persists for 15 to 20 years. From 30 to 50% of patients develop asthma and/or hay fever.

TREATMENT AND MANAGEMENT

Atopic dermatitis is considered by many to be related, at least in part, to emotional stress. Education of the patient to avoid rubbing and scratching is most important. Topical preparations are valuable but are useless if the patient continues to scratch and rub the plaques. Topical antipruritic (menthol/camphor) lotions are helpful in controlling the pruritus.

Warn patients of their special problems with herpes simplex and frequency of superimposed staphylococcal infection, for which oral erythromycin or dicloxacillin is indicated. Acyclovir is indicated if HSV is suspected.

Acute See page 20.

Subacute and Chronic

1. H$_1$ antihistamines are probably useful in reducing itching.

2. Hydration (oilated baths) followed by application of unscented emollients (e.g., hydrated petrolatum) is a basic daily treatment needed to prevent xerosis. Soap showers are permissible in order to wash the body folds, but soap should not be used on the other parts of the skin surface.

3. Topical anti-inflammatory agents such as corticosteroids, hydroxyquinoline preparations and tar are the mainstays of treatment. Of these, corticosteroids are the most readily accepted by the patient.

4. Systemic corticosteroids should be avoided, except in rare instances for only short courses.

5. Patients should learn and use stress management techniques.

Infantile atopic dermatitis is one of the most troublesome skin eruptions in children. There is an "atopic" background without a clearly defined immunologic pattern. Skin lesions seem to be a reaction to itching and rubbing. Since the advent of topical corticosteroids, the problem has lost much of its seriousness.

PHYSICAL EXAMINATION

Skin Lesions

TYPE   Red skin, tiny vesicles on "puffy" surface, scaling, exudation with wet crusts, and cracks (fissures)

DISTRIBUTION   Regional, especially the face (sparing the mouth) (Figure 11), the antecu-bital and popliteal fossae, wrists, and lateral aspects of the legs

CHARACTERISTIC PATTERN   See Figure III

TREATMENT

Influence of dietary measures at best uncertain. Prompt response to potent corticoste-

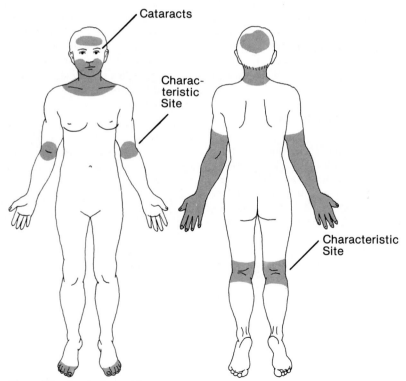

Figure III   Atopic dermatitis

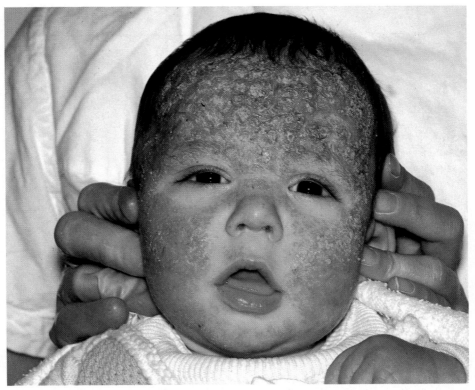

11   Infantile atopic eczema   *The face is characteristically involved but the perioral skin is spared.*

roids; after improvement, use low-potency corticosteroids or emollients. For recurrence, return for a short period to the stronger corticosteroids. Beware of skin atrophy. With sensible use, no danger of suppression of pituitary-adrenal axis. For extra security, monitor growth curve. Tars (ointments, pastes, and gels) also effective. Reassurance of mother. (See Treatment, page 23).

Childhood-Type Atopic Dermatitis

PHYSICAL EXAMINATION

Skin Lesions

TYPE Papular, lichenified plaques, erosions, crusts

DISTRIBUTION Especially on the antecubital and politeal fossae (Figure 12). See Figure III.

TREATMENT

See pages 20 and 23.

Adult-Type Atopic Dermatitis

Adult-type atopic dermatitis is a chronic recurrent disease in patients who have or have not had infantile or childhood atopic dermatitis or asthma. Exacerbations are often related to mental stress.

PHYSICAL EXAMINATION

Skin Lesions

TYPE Papular and lichenified plaques, excoriations, pustules, erosions, dry and wet crusts, and cracks (fissures) (see page 762)

DISTRIBUTION Often generalized with predilection for the flexures, front and sides of the neck, eyelids, forehead, face, wrists, and dorsa of feet and hands

TREATMENT

See page 23.

Secondary staphylococcal infection is quite common and, in acute flare-ups, oral antibiotics are indicated, given over a period of weeks.

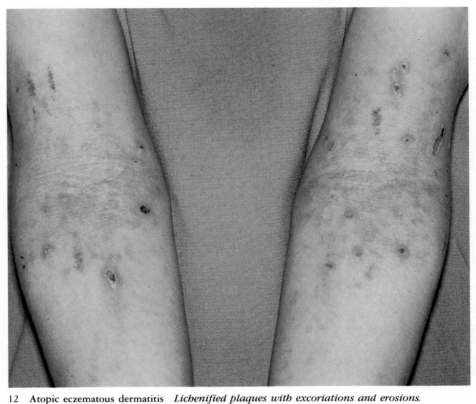

12   Atopic eczematous dermatitis   *Lichenified plaques with excoriations and erosions.*

Lichen simplex is a circumscribed area of lichenification resulting from repeated physical trauma (rubbing and scratching), occurring especially in women on the nuchal areas, arms, legs, and ankles, and in both sexes in the anogenital area.

EPIDEMIOLOGY

Age Over 20 years

Sex More frequent in women

Race A possible higher incidence in Asians

Factors Emotional stress in some cases

HISTORY

Duration of Lesion(s) Weeks to months

Skin Symptoms Pruritus, often in paroxysms. The lichenified skin becomes like an erogenous zone—it becomes a pleasure (orgiastic) to scratch. Often the areas on the feet are rubbed at night with the heel. The rubbing becomes automatic and reflexive and an unconscious habit.

PHYSICAL EXAMINATION

Skin Lesions
TYPE A solid plaque of lichenification; scaling is minimal except in nuchal lichen simplex (Figure 13).
COLOR Brown or black hyperpigmentation, especially in skin phototypes IV, V, and VI
SHAPE Round, oval, linear (following path of scratching)
DISTRIBUTION Isolated single lesion or several scattered plaques (see Figure IV)
CHARACTERISTIC SITES Nuchal area (female), scalp, ankles, lower legs, upper thighs, exterior forearms, vulva, pubis, anal area, scrotum

DIFFERENTIAL DIAGNOSIS

Lichenification also occurs in psoriasis, mycosis fungoides, and contact dermatitis (chronic) (see page 16)

DERMATOPATHOLOGY

Hyperplasia of all components of epidermis: hyperkeratosis, acanthosis, and elongated and broad rete ridges. Spongiosis is infrequent. In the dermis there is a chronic inflammatory infiltrate.

PATHOPHYSIOLOGY

A special predilection of the skin to respond to physical trauma by epidermal hyperplasia; skin becomes highly sensitive to touch, a fact probably related to proliferation of nerves in the epidermis.

TREATMENT

Difficult! The rubbing and scratching must be stopped, and hospital treatment is sometimes necessary to completely suppress the scratching with anti-inflammatory agents (topical corticosteroids and crude coal tar) covered by continuous dry occlusive gauze dressings. For small localized areas, intralesional corticosteroids are often highly effective. It is important to apply occlusive bandages at night to prevent rubbing and to facilitate penetration of topical corticosteroids; new occlusive hydrocolloid dressings are very effective used with corticosteroids.

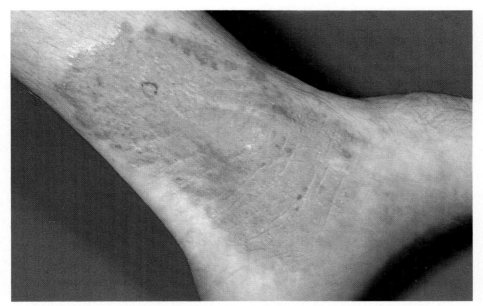

13 Lichen simplex chronicus (localized lichenified dermatitis) *Isolated single plaque of thick lichenified skin resulting from repeated rubbing with the heel of the other foot.*

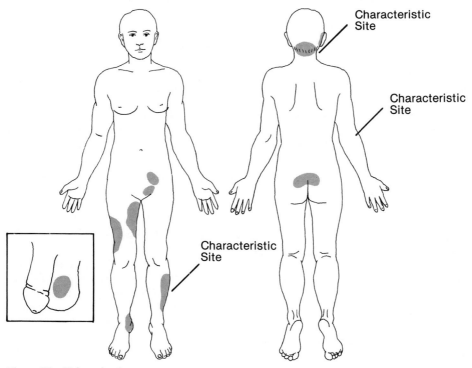

Characteristic Site

Characteristic Site

Characteristic Site

Figure IV   Lichen simplex

LICHEN SIMPLEX CHRONICUS   29

Nummular eczema is a chronic, pruritic, inflammatory dermatitis occurring in the form of coin-shaped plaques composed of grouped small papules and vesicles on an erythematous base, especially common on the lower legs of older males during winter months; often seen in atopic individuals.

EPIDEMIOLOGY

Age and Sex 50 to 80 years in males; 20 to 40 years in females

HISTORY

Duration of Lesions Weeks, with remissions and recurrences

Skin Symptoms Pruritus, often intense

PHYSICAL EXAMINATION

Skin Lesions
TYPE
  Closely grouped, small vesicles and papules that coalesce into plaques, often more than 4 to 5 cm in diameter, with an erythematous base with indistinct borders, crusts, and excoriations (Figure 14)

  Dry scaly plaques that may be lichenified (see page 762)
COLOR Dull red
SHAPE Round or coin-shaped, hence the adjective nummular (Latin *nummularis,* "like a coin")
DISTRIBUTION *Extent* Regional clusters of lesions (e.g., legs) or generalized
Pattern Random
Sites of Predilection Lower legs (older men), trunk, hands and fingers (younger females)

DIFFERENTIAL DIAGNOSIS

In a single plaque, *dermatophytosis* must be excluded by a KOH examination of crusts or scales. *Contact dermatitis* must be excluded by history and localization. *Psoriasis* and *mycosis fungoides* may simulate nummular eczema—a biopsy is helpful. *Impetigo. Familial pemphigus.*

LABORATORY AND SPECIAL EXAMINATIONS

Dermatopathology
SITE Predominantly epidermal
PROCESS Acute inflammation with acanthosis, intraepidermal vesicles, and spongiosis

Microbiologic Examination
DIRECT MICROSCOPIC EXAMINATION OF CRUSTS AND EXUDATE Gram's stain often reveals intracellular gram-positive cocci.
CULTURE *Staphylococcus aureus* in some patients

PATHOPHYSIOLOGY

A curious variety of the eczematous reaction pattern, often with heavy colonization of staphylococci, frequently occurring in the asteatotic (dry) skin of older men during winter and starting under woolen stockings

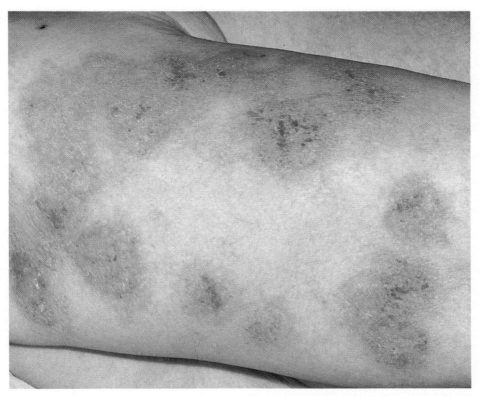

14   Nummular eczematous dermatitis   *Coin-shaped plaques composed of papules and vesicles on an erythematous base with some excoriations also present.*

COURSE AND PROGNOSIS

Remissions with treatment but frequent recurrences unless the skin is kept hydrated and lubricated

TREATMENT

Oral dicloxacillin or erythromycin

Topical corticosteroids

Crude coal tar pastes combined with corticosteroids are very effective

Hydration of skin with oil water baths followed by application of water-in-oil ointments (hydrated petroleum)

See Treatment, page 23.

This is a special vesicular type of hand and foot eczema. It is an acute, chronic, or recurrent dermatosis of the fingers, palms, and soles characterized by a sudden onset of deep-seated pruritic, clear "sago-like" vesicles; later, scaling, fissures, lichenification occur. Secondary bacterial infection is very often a complication. The bullous form is called *pompholyx*.

EPIDEMIOLOGY

Age Majority under 40 years (range, 12 to 40 years)

Sex Equal ratio

HISTORY

Duration of Lesions Onset rapid (1 to 3 days); duration limited to a few days or may extend to several weeks

Skin Symptoms Pruritus and especially painful fissures that are incapacitating. Summer exacerbations are not infrequent.

PHYSICAL EXAMINATION

Skin Lesions
TYPE *Early* Vesicles, usually small (1.0 mm), deep-seated, appearing like "tapioca" in clusters (Figure 15), occasionally bullae, especially on the feet
Late Scaling, lichenification, painful fissures, and erosions (Figure 16)
ARRANGEMENT Vesicles grouped in clusters
DISTRIBUTION Regional [hands (80%) and feet] with sites of predilection bilaterally on the sides of fingers, palms, and soles
NAILS Dystrophic changes (transverse ridging, pitting, and thickening)

Hyperhidrosis is present in some patients.

DIFFERENTIAL DIAGNOSIS

Vesicular reaction to active dermatophytosis on the feet; acute contact dermatitis.

DERMATOPATHOLOGY

Site Epidermis

Process Eczematous inflammation (spongiosis and intraepidermal edema) with subcorneal vesicles usually unrelated to sweat ducts

PATHOPHYSIOLOGY

Despite the name *dyshidrotic eczema*, there is no evidence that sweating plays a role in the pathogenesis. About half the patients have an atopic background. Emotional stress is possibly a precipitating factor. The role of nickel ingestion in the diet is unsettled. Lesions can be induced by ingestion of high doses of nickel.

COURSE AND PROGNOSIS

Recurrent attacks with intervals of weeks to months with spontaneous remissions in 2 to 3 weeks.

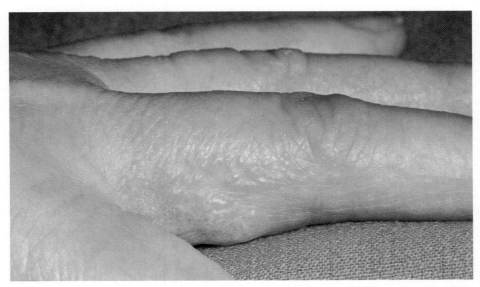

15　Dyshidrotic eczematous dermatitis　*Note tapioca-like, deep-seated vesicles on the sides of the fingers.*

TREATMENT

A frustrating experience. Avoid systemic corticosteroids except in rare, short-term flare-ups; patients can become dependent on low-dose corticosteroids and serious complications can occur.

Vesicular stage (early): Burow's wet dressings; large bullae should be drained but not unroofed. Small vesicles respond dramatically but unpredictably to "black cat" applied once daily. Black cat is 10% crude coal tar in equal parts of acetone and flexible collodion. *Eczematous stage* (later), with fissures, scaling, lichenification. Topical corticosteroids are unpredictably successful in a few patients but should be tried. High-potency corticosteroids (e.g., clobetasol-17-propionate) should be tried with proper warning about cutaneous and systemic side effects.

Bacterial infection may be present even without obvious signs (crusts, tenderness, etc.) and erythromycin or dicloxacillin, 250 mg q.i.d. should be started in most patients with moderate or severe disease.

Diet restriction of certain metals (nickel, cobalt, or chromium) has been suggested to be successful in two-thirds of patients in one series.

PUVA (oral, or topical as "soaks") is successful in most patients if given over prolonged periods of time and is worth trying, especially in severe cases.

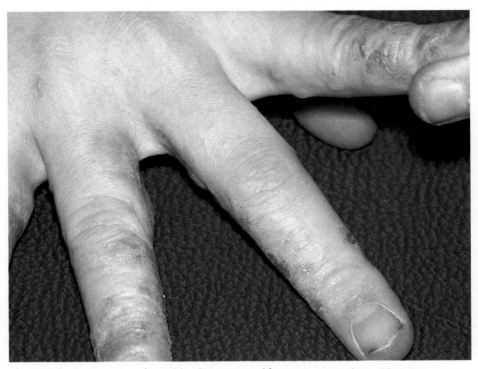

16 Dyshidrotic eczematous dermatitis *Later stage with a more eczematous appearance.*

Stasis dermatitis is a recalcitrant chronic dermatitis of the lower legs in persons with chronic venous insufficiency; ulceration occurs frequently.

EPIDEMIOLOGY

Age   Over 50 years

Sex   More common in women

HISTORY

Duration of Lesions   Months

Skin Symptoms   Mild pruritus, pain (if ulcer present)

Other Features   Aching discomfort in the limb, swelling of the ankle, nocturnal cramps

PHYSICAL EXAMINATION

Skin Lesions
TYPE
   Erythematous scaling plaque with exudation, crusts, and superficial ulcers (see Figure 17)

   Brown reticulated hemosiderin hyperpigmentation (on ankles and lower legs)
SHAPE   Round or oval
DISTRIBUTION   *Extent*   Localized
Site of Predilection   Medial aspect of ankle (Figure 17)

TYPES OF STASIS

Primary varicose veins are hereditary, often unilateral. The *postphlebitic limb* is associated with the most severe venous stasis, and the ulcers are usually larger. Fibrosing panniculitis with firm tender induration may be observed.

DIFFERENTIAL DIAGNOSIS

In the absence of the typical pigmentation and small-vein enlargement of venous stasis, the diagnosis of stasis dermatitis is suspect and other causes for ulcers should be considered, such as *organic disease of arteries, carcinoma, cryoglobulinemia, sickle cell anemia, necrobiosis lipoidica, and pyoderma gangrenosum.*

LABORATORY AND SPECIAL EXAMINATIONS

Culture ulcer base or purulent, crusted areas to determine whether secondary infection is present.

TREATMENT

Stasis Dermatitis
ACUTE   Burow's wet dressings and cooling pastes and, later, topical corticosteroids; systemic antibiotics if cellulitis is present.
CHRONIC   Elevation of the leg

Ulcer   Wet-to-dry dressings using normal saline or Dakin's solution. Silver sulfadiazine applied between wet-to-dry dressings. Eleva-

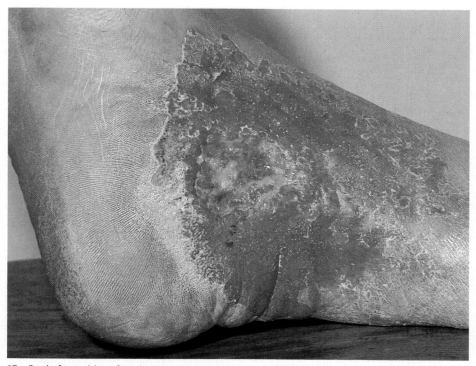

17 Stasis dermatitis and stasis ulcer *Exudation, crusts, and superficial ulcers on the medial aspect of the ankle. These may be very painful.*

tion of the leg, compressive bandages with adequate counterpressure and full use of the leg muscle pump followed by specially measured supportive stockings, and surgery are necessary adjuncts to topical therapy. For larger persistent ulcers, special techniques are now available.

Asteatotic Dermatitis (Eczema Craquelatum[1])

Asteatotic dermatitis is a relatively common dermatitis that occurs in the winter and in older persons on the legs, arms, and hands and is characterized by dry, "cracked," fissured skin.

EPIDEMIOLOGY

Age Over 40 years

Sex More common in males

HISTORY

Duration of Lesions Weeks, months

Skin Symptoms Pruritus

Other Factors Often a history of too frequent bathing in hot, soapy baths or showers

PHYSICAL EXAMINATION

Skin Lesions
TYPE Dry "cracked" skin (see Figures 18 and 19) with red fissures and slight scaling, and sometimes lichenification [see Nummular (Discoid) Eczema]
ARRANGEMENT Diffuse skin involvement (without identifiable borders), irregular reticulation
DISTRIBUTION *Extent* Generalized
Sites of Predilection Lower legs, dorsa of hands and forearms

DERMATOPATHOLOGY

Site Epidermis

Process Eczema with spongiosis and mild dermal infiltrate

PATHOPHYSIOLOGY

Asteatosis (loss of lipids) can occur with over-bathing, old age, a genetic tendency for dry skin (not necessarily ichthyosis), and high environmental temperature with low relative humidity (as in heated rooms).

TREATMENT

Increase ambient humidity, preferably above 50%; room humidifiers (in the bedroom) are very helpful

Tepid water baths containing bath oils with immediate liberal application of emollient ointments

Medium-potency corticosteroid ointment applied b.i.d. until the eczematous component has resolved

---

[1] A word meaning "marred with cracks," as in old china or ceramic tile.

ECZEMATOUS DERMATITIS

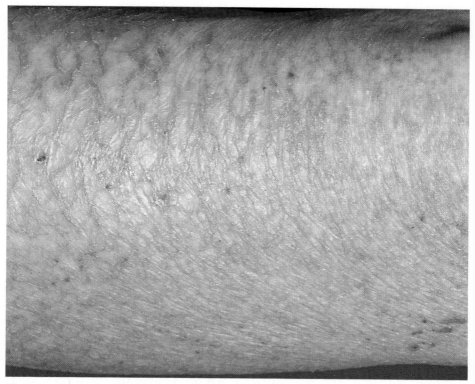

18 Asteatotic eczema *This common skin alteration occurs in the winter. The skin appears dry and cracked.*

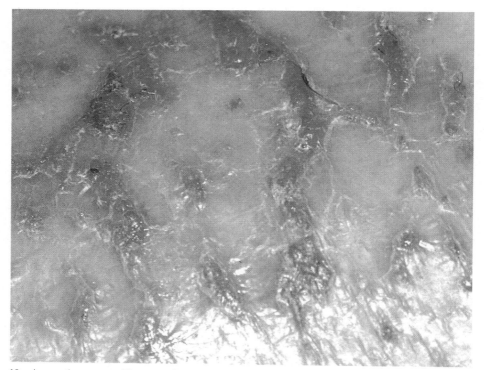

19 Asteatotic eczema *There are fissures with erythema.*

Psoriasis

Psoriasis

Psoriasis, which affects 1.5 to 2.0% of the population in western countries, is an hereditary disorder of skin with several clinical expressions—but most typically chronic scaling papules and plaques in a characteristic distribution, largely at sites of repeated minor trauma. The HLA types most frequently associated with psoriasis are HLA-B13, -B16, -B17, -B37, -DR7, and -Cw6.

EPIDEMIOLOGY AND ETIOLOGY

Age One-third of patients before 20 years of age, especially in females

Sex Equal in males and females

Race Low incidence in West Africans, American Indians, and Asiatics

Other Features Multifactorial inheritance. Minor trauma (Koebner's phenomenon) is a major factor (45% of patients) in eliciting lesions. Certain drugs (systemic corticosteroids, lithium, alcohol, chloroquine), sunlight, stress, and obesity are believed to cause exacerbation of preexisting psoriasis. HIV infection must be considered in patients at risk.

HISTORY

Duration of Lesions Usually months but may be sudden as in acute guttate psoriasis and generalized pustular psoriasis (von Zumbusch)

Skin Symptoms Pruritus is reasonably common, especially in scalp and anogenital psoriasis; most often occurs in patients with atopic diathesis.

Constitutional Symptoms Arthritis, fever, and "acute illness" syndrome (weakness, chills, fever) with generalized pustular psoriasis (von Zumbusch)

PHYSICAL EXAMINATION

Skin Lesions
TYPE
  Papules and plaques, sharply marginated with marked silvery-white scale (see Figures 20 to 23 and 25); removal of scale results in the appearance of miniscule blood droplets (Auspitz phenomenon).

  Pustules (see Figure 26)

  Erythroderma
COLOR "Salmon pink"
SHAPE Round, oval, polycyclic, annular
ARRANGEMENT Zosteriform, arciform, serpiginous, scattered discrete lesions, or erythroderma (diffuse involvement without identifiable borders)
DISTRIBUTION *Extent* Single lesion or lesions localized to one area (e.g., penis, nails), regional involvement (scalp), generalized or universal (entire skin)

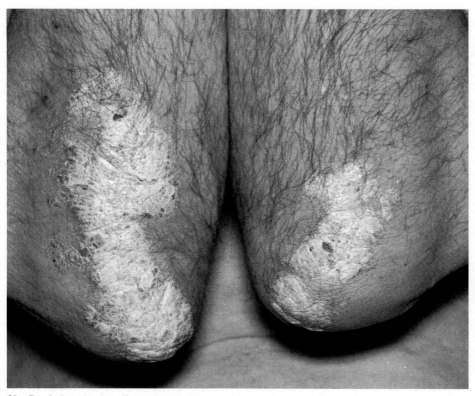

20   Psoriasis vulgaris   *Characteristic silvery-white, scaling plaques in sites of repeated trauma.*

Pattern (1) Bilateral, rarely symmetrical; most often spares exposed areas; favors elbows, knees, facial region, scalp, and intertriginous areas. For characteristic pattern of distribution, see Figure V. (2) Disseminated small lesions without predilection of site (guttate psoriasis) (see page 44 and Figure 21).

Hair and Nails

Hair loss (alopecia) is not a common feature even with severe scalp involvement.

Fingernails and toenails frequently (25%) involved, especially with concomitant arthritis. Nail changes include: pitting (Figure 24) (frequent but nonspecific), subungual hyperkeratosis, onycholysis (also nonspecific), and yellowish-brown spots under the nail plate—the "oil spot" (pathognomonic!).

Arthritis

Incidence is uncommon (3 to 4%). The skin lesions and the arthritis may occur together, or the arthritis may precede the onset of the skin lesions.

Two types: (1) "distal"—seronegative and without subcutaneous nodules, involving terminal interphalangeal joints of hands and feet; often associated with severe nail involvement; (2) mutilating psoriatic arthritis with bone erosion and osteolysis and, ultimately, ankylosis; especially involving the sacroiliac, hip, and cervical areas with ankylosing spondylitis; seen especially in erythrodermic and pustular psoriasis; also seronegative.

Type 2 associated with HLA-B28.

DIFFERENTIAL DIAGNOSIS

Seborrheic dermatitis—may be indistinguishable in sites involved and morphology; *lichen simplex chronicus*—may complicate psoriasis due to pruritus; *candidiasis*—confused especially with intertriginous psoriasis; *psoriasiform drug eruptions*—especially β blockers, gold, and methyldopa; *glucagonoma syndrome*—important differential as this is a serious disease (malignant tumor of pancreatic islet cells). Its psoriasiform lesions are atypical—annular lesions but with vesicles and erosions. Distinguishing features of glucagonoma syndrome include lesions in groin and on face (rare in psoriasis), marked weight loss, unexplained anemia, intermittent diarrhea, stomatitis; the histology is quite specific.

LABORATORY AND SPECIAL EXAMINATIONS

Dermatopathology

SITE   Epidermis and dermis

PROCESS   Inflammation plus alteration of the cell cycle. There is (1) marked thickening and also thinning of the epidermis with elongation of the rete ridges; (2) increased mitosis of keratinocytes, fibroblasts, and endothelial cells; (3) parakeratotic hyperkeratosis (nuclei retained in the stratum corneum); and (4) inflammatory cells in the dermis (usually lymphocytes and monocytes) and in the epidermis (polymorphonuclear cells), forming microabscesses of Munro in the stratum corneum.

Serology   Sudden onset of psoriasis may be associated with HIV infection. Determination of HIV serostatus indicated in at-risk individuals.

PATHOPHYSIOLOGY

Psoriasis probably refers to a cluster of diseases of differing pathogenesis. The principal abnormality in psoriasis is an alteration of the cell kinetics of keratinocytes. The major change is a shortening of the cell cycle from 311 to 36 hours; this results in production of 35,000 epidermal cells per day, 28 times the normal production. The etiologic basis for this increased production is not known. The epidermis and dermis appear to respond as an integrated system: the changes in the germinative zone of the epidermis and the inflammatory changes in the dermis, which may "trigger" the epidermal changes. There are changes in the level of cyclic nucleotides, arachidonic acid metabolism, the production of cytokines, and expression of adhesion molecules in psoriatic lesions, but it is not known whether these are primary events or secondary control mechanisms for keratinocyte proliferation. Immunologic phenomena also play a role.

FACTORS INFLUENCING SELECTION OF TREATMENT

1. Age: children, adolescence, young adults, middle age, >60 years

2. Type: guttate, plaque, palmar and pustular pustulosis, generalized pustular psoriasis, von Zumbush's syndrome, erythrodermic psoriasis.

3. Site and extent of involvement: *localized* to palms and soles, scalp, anogenital area, scattered plaques but <5% involvement; *generalized and >30%*

4. Previous treatment: ionizing radiation, systemic corticosteroids, PUVA

5. Associated medical disorders (e.g., AIDS)

TREATMENT

Instruct the patient that he or she should never rub or scratch the lesions as this trauma stimulates the psoriatic proliferative process (Koebner's phenomenon).

Treatment only with topically administrated agents.

1. Topical fluorinated corticosteroids (betamethasone valerate, fluocinolone acetonide, betamethasone propionate, clobetasol propionate) in ointment base applied after removing the scales by soaking in water. The ointment is applied to the wet skin, covered with plastic wrap, and left on overnight.

2. Use of hydrocolloid dressing left on for 24 to 48 hours is helpful and effective and prevents scratching. During the day fluorinated corticosteroid creams can be used without occlusion. Patients will develop tolerance after long periods. *Caveat*: Prolonged application of the fluorinated corticosteroids leads to atrophy of the skin, striae, and unsightly telangiectasia. Clobetasol-17-propionate is stronger and active even without occlusion. To avoid systemic effects: maximum 50 g ointment a week.

3. For very small plaques (4.0 cm or less) triamcinolone acetonide, aqueous suspension, 3.3 mg/mL is injected into the lesion 0.1 mg/mm. The injection should be intradermal rather than subcutaneous; *if the injection does not require some pressure to inject, it is not going into the dermis. Warning:* Atrophic, hypopigmented macules can result.

4. Topical anthralin preparations are excellent when used properly. Follow directions on the package insert with attention to details.

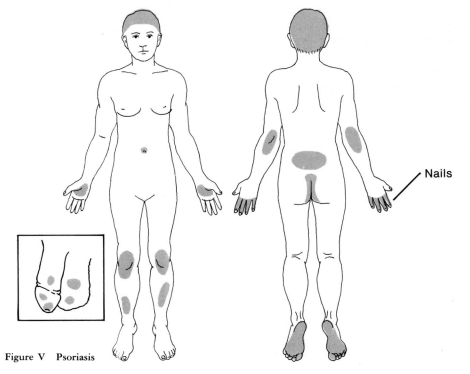

Nails

Figure V   Psoriasis

Psoriasis Vulgaris: Guttate Type

This type of psoriasis, which is relatively rare (less than 2.0% of all psoriasis), is like an exanthem: a shower of lesions appears rather rapidly in young adults, often following streptococcal pharyngitis. Guttate psoriasis may, however, be chronic and unrelated to streptococcal infection.

PHYSICAL EXAMINATION

Skin Lesions (Figure 21)
TYPE   Papules 2.0 mm to 1.0 cm
COLOR   "Salmon pink"
SHAPE   Guttate (Latin, "spots that resemble drops")
ARRANGEMENT   Scattered discrete lesions
DISTRIBUTION   Generalized, usually sparing the palms and soles and concentrating on the trunk, less on the face, scalp, and nails

DIFFERENTIAL DIAGNOSIS

Psoriasiform drug eruption, secondary syphilis, pityriasis rosea

LABORATORY EXAMINATION

Serologic: an increased antistreptolysin titer in those patients with antecedent streptococcal infection.

Culture: throat culture for group A β-hemolytic streptococcus.

COURSE AND PROGNOSIS

Sometimes this type of psoriasis spontaneously disappears in a few weeks without treatment.

TREATMENT

The resolution of lesions can be accelerated by UVB phototherapy or judicious exposure to sunlight. For persistent lesions, treatment same as for generalized plaque psoriasis (see page 48).

Penicillin VK or erythromycin if group A β-hemolytic streptococcus on throat culture.

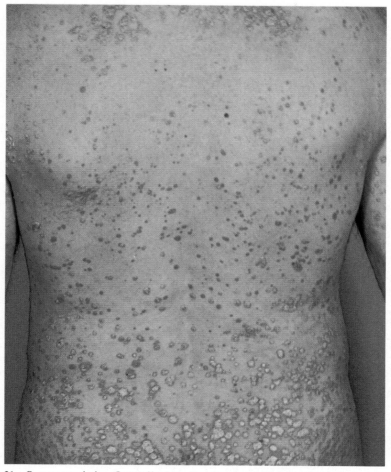

21 Guttate psoriasis *Generalized, scattered, salmon-pink, scaling papules.*

Psoriasis of the scalp presents a special therapeutic problem, similar to that of anogenital psoriasis. Both areas are inaccessible for phototherapy and are usually pruritic, which results in lichenification and koebnerization.[1] Psoriasis of the scalp may be part of generalized plaque psoriasis, may coexist with isolated plaques, or may be the only site involved. It usually does not lead to hair loss.

HISTORY

Duration   Months to years

Relationship to Season   Does not go into remission with sunlight exposure as does the exposed psoriatic skin

Skin Symptoms   Mild to severe pruritus, which often causes compulsive and subconscious scratching

PHYSICAL EXAMINATION

Type
> Plaques, often with thick adherent scales (Figure 22)
>
> Lichenification (often superimposed on the basic psoriatic lesions and resulting from rubbing and scratching)
>
> Exudation and fissures, especially behind the ears

Arrangement   Scattered discrete plaques or diffuse involvement of the entire scalp.

(*Note:* Paradoxically, alopecia is an uncommon complication of psoriasis of the scalp, even after years of thick, plaque-type involvement. Thus the condition is not exposed to public view, and this may be one reason why patients learn to live with it and do not seek treatment.)

DIFFERENTIAL DIAGNOSIS

Seborrheic dermatitis of the scalp may be almost indistinguishable from psoriasis. Some have called this ''seborrhiasis.''

PATHOPHYSIOLOGY

There may be a subset of psoriasis of the scalp that could be related to the colonization of pityrosporal yeasts inasmuch as one controlled study showed a beneficial effect of oral and topical ketoconazole.

TREATMENT

Mild   (superficial scaling and lacking thick plaques):

- Tar shampoos *followed by*
- Betamethasone valerate 0.1% lotion 2 times weekly; if refractory, clobetasol propionate 0.05% scalp application

Severe   (thick adherent plaques):

- Removal of plaques before active treatment. Topical applications are virtually useless unless the thick scale is removed. This is accomplished by applications of 2 to 10% salicylic acid in mineral oil, covered with a plastic cap, left on overnight.

---

[1] The phenomenon of induction of new lesions on ''normal'' skin by physical trauma, including rubbing and scratching.

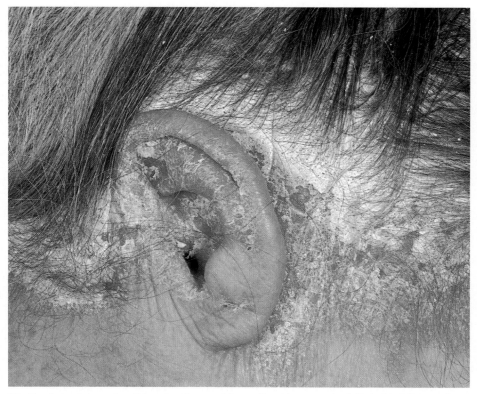

22　Psoriasis of the scalp　*Discrete, silvery-white, scaling plaques, especially behind the ears in an area of easy accessibility to rubbing. Scratching and rubbing must be avoided.*

- After scales have been removed (in 1 to 3 treatments), fluocinolone cream or lotion is applied and the scalp is covered with plastic sheets or a shower cap, which is left on overnight.
- When the thickness of the plaques is reduced, clobetasol propionate 0.05% scalp application can be used for maintenance. *Compulsive subconscious scratching and rubbing will negate all attempts for maintenance treatment.* Hands off!

COURSE AND PROGNOSIS

The prognosis for control is good; following treatment as outlined above, the scalp lesions may undergo a remission for several months to years. Scratching and rubbing must be avoided in order to maintain the remission.

Psoriasis vulgaris is a challenge for the physician, as chronic generalized psoriasis is one of the "miseries that beset mankind," causing shame and embarrassment and a compromised life-style. The "heartbreak of psoriasis" is no joke. As the writer John Updike so poignantly said about a person with psoriasis, "Lusty, though we are loathsome to love. Keen-sighted, though we hate to look upon ourselves. The name of the disease, spiritually speaking, is Humiliation."

TREATMENT

The management of generalized plaque-type psoriasis is the province of the dermatologist or of a psoriasis center where these major options are available: (1) UVB phototherapy with emollients, (2) PUVA photochemotherapy, (3) methotrexate (given weekly), (4) combination therapy using etretinate (or other retinoids such as acitretin or isotretinoin) or methotrexate with PUVA is perhaps the ideal treatment available at the present time. Up to 50% respond well to UVB plus emollients when given according to a published protocol. Those who do not respond are treated with oral PUVA photochemotherapy. Methothrexate is used only if UVB or PUVA treatment fails. For males, combination etretinate and oral PUVA photochemotherapy is the most effective therapy. For females, isotretinoin can be used if appropriate contraception during and 2 months after treatment is preformed.

Oral PUVA Photochemotherapy Treatment consists of oral ingestion of 8-methoxy-psoralen (8-MOP) (0.3 to 0.6 mg 8-MOP per kg body weight) and exposure to varying doses of UVA, depending on the sensitivity of the patient. Approximately 1 hour after ingestion of the psoralen, UVA is given, starting at a dose of 1 J/cm^2, adjusted upward for skin phototype. Alternatively, phototoxicity testing can be done which permits a better adjustment of the UVA dose to the individual's sensitivity to PUVA. The UVA dose is increased by 0.5 to 1.0 J/cm^2 each dose. Treatments are per-

formed 2 or 3 times a week or, if employing a more intensive protocol, 4 times a week. The majority of patients clear after 19 to 25 treatments, and the amount of UVA needed ranges from 100 to 245 J/cm^2. In patients with recalcitrant, plaque-type psoriasis, etretinate may be combined with other antipsoriatic therapy, e.g., PUVA, UVB, topical corticosteroids, anthralin, or methotrexate. These combination modalities have been shown to reduce the length of treatment as well as the total amount of an antipsoriatic drug necessary for clearing. Topical corticosteroids, anthralin, methotrexate, and etretinate, combined with either PUVA or UVB, have all been shown to be effective in reducing the dose of one another.

Psoriasis Day-Care Centers or Inpatient Services These facilities have available UVB + emollients *or* UVB + tar (Goeckerman regimen) and PUVA.

Methotrexate Therapy Oral methotrexate (MTX) is one of the most effective treatments and certainly the most convenient treatment for generalized psoriasis of the plaque type. Nevertheless, MTX is a potentially dangerous drug, principally because of liver toxicity that can occur following prolonged therapy. Hepatic toxicity occurs after cumulative doses in normal persons, but other risk factors include a history of: alcohol intake, abnormal liver chemistries, IV drug use; obesity is also a risk factor for hepatic toxicity. Inasmuch as hepatic toxicity is related to total life dose, this therapy should, in general, not be given to

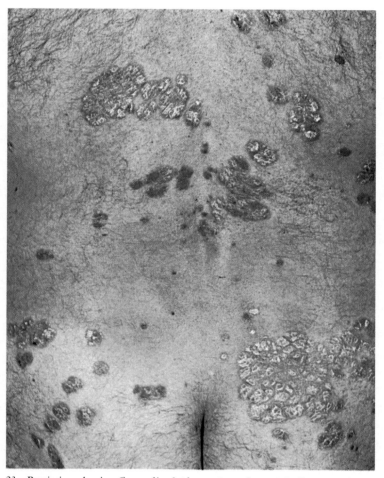

23 Psoriasis vulgaris *Generalized plaque type. Scattered, discrete, silvery-white, scaling plaques of varying sizes.*

young patients. Furthermore, there is some evidence that older patients require lower doses of MTX for control.

A pretreatment liver biopsy is required on all patients with a history of liver disease or in patients with abnormal liver chemistries. In patients with normal liver chemistries and in whom no risk factors are present, a liver bi-opsy should be done after a cumulative dose of approximately 1500 mg of MTX; if the post-MTX liver biopsy is normal, repeat liver bi-opsy should be done after further therapy following an additional 1000 to 1500 mg of MTX. (For details regarding MTX therapy of psoriasis, see: Roenigk HH Jr et al: Metho-trexate in psoriasis: revised guidelines. *J Am Acad Dermatol* 19:145, 1988.)

Psoriasis Vulgaris: Nails (Figure 24)

Psoriasis of the nails is quite common (25% of patients with psoriasis), varies in severity of involvement, and often disappears spontaneously or with treatment of psoriasis of the skin, especially with the three major treatments: UVB phototherapy, PUVA photochemotherapy, and methotrexate.

TREATMENT

Specially directed treatments of the fingernails (inasmuch as the nails are disfiguring and a nuisance) are unsatisfactory. Injection of the nail fold with intradermal triamcinolone acetonide (5 mg/mL) is quite effective but almost invariably produces atrophy.

PUVA photochemotherapy is somewhat effective; the ultraviolet A is administered in special hand and foot lighting units providing high-intensity UVA.

Psoriasis Vulgaris: Palms and Soles (Figure 25)

This disease is a major therapeutic challenge. The palms and soles may be the only areas involved. Topical corticosteroids with plastic occlusion are quite ineffective. UVB phototherapy is not often effective. Intralesional triamcinolone acetonide is hazardous because of risks of bacterial infection in the hand.

TREATMENT

Two quite effective treatments available are:

1. PUVA photochemotherapy, administered in specially designed hand and foot lighting cabinets that deliver UVA.

2. Retinoids (etretinate) given alone orally are sometimes effective in clearing psoriasis vulgaris of the palms and soles. However, combinations of oral retinoids and PUVA improve the efficacy of each and permit a reduction of the dose and duration of each (see page 48).

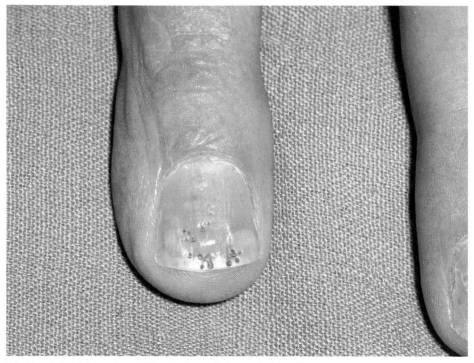

24 Psoriasis of the nails *Pitting and onycholysis of the nail.*

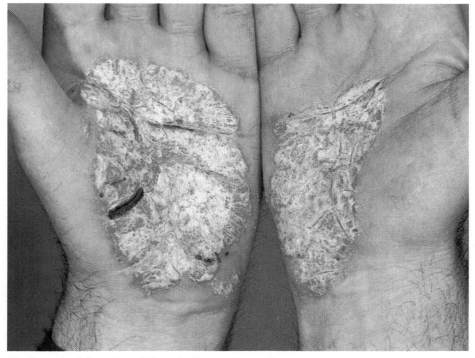

25 Psoriasis of the palms *Bilateral, silvery-white, scaling plaques with some fissures.*

Palmoplantar pustulosis is a chronic, relapsing eruption limited to the palms and soles and characterized by numerous sterile, yellow, deep-seated, small pustules that evolve into dusky-red macules.

EPIDEMIOLOGY AND ETIOLOGY

Incidence Low

Age 50 to 60 years

Sex More common in females (4:1)

Other Features Patient may or may not have psoriasis or may develop it in other sites (scalp, trunk, etc.). This disorder may or may not be a variant of psoriasis—studies of a large series of patients showed no increase in the HLA-B13 or -Bw17, two antigens that have been found to be associated with psoriasis vulgaris. Stopping smoking may or may not improve the condition.

HISTORY

Duration of Lesions Months

Skin Symptoms Tenderness and burning as new lesions appear and when fissures are present; may interfere with walking or using the hands.

PHYSICAL EXAMINATION

Skin Lesions

TYPE Vesicles and pustules (Figure 26) in varying stages of evolution, 2.0 to 5.0 mm, deep-seated, develop into dusky-red macules; present in areas of erythema and scaling.

DISTRIBUTION Localized to palms and soles

SITES OF PREDILECTION Thenar and hypothenar, flexor aspects of fingers, heels, and insteps; acral portions of the fingers and toes usually spared.

DIFFERENTIAL DIAGNOSIS

A quite characteristic clinical presentation, but tinea manus, tinea pedis, and pustular psoriasis should always be excluded by examination of scales; dyshidrotic eczematous dermatitis is always pruritic, vesicles are more numerous than pustules, and fissures and secondary infection often occur.

DERMATOPATHOLOGY

SITE Epidermis and dermis

PROCESS Edema and exocytosis of mononuclear cells forming a vesicle and later many neutrophils, which form a unilocular pustule that usually extends into the dermis and slightly above the plane of the skin; small spongiform pustules and some acanthosis

CELL TYPES Mononuclear cells at first and later myriads of neutrophils

PATHOPHYSIOLOGY

A leukotactic factor similar to that found in psoriasis vulgaris has been isolated from the stratum corneum in palmoplantar pustulosis. This could elicit migration to the target tissue of myriads of neutrophils that carry leukotriene B_4, a potent neutrophil chemoattractant.

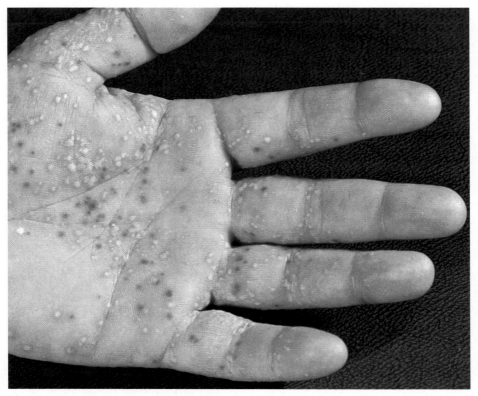

26 Palmar pustulosis *Deep-seated, dusky-red macules and creamy-yellow pustules (2.0 to 3.0 mm in diameter).*

TREATMENT

The condition is recalcitrant to treatment, but PUVA and etretinate, alone or in combination, and methotrexate are effective but not curative (see page 48 for details). Topical corticosteroids, dithranol, and coal tar are ineffective. Strong corticosteroids under plastic occlusion (e.g., for the night) are often effective, but skin atrophy may limit prolonged use.

PROGNOSIS

Persistent for years and characterized by unexplained remissions and exacerbations.

Common Scaling Eruptions of Unknown Etiology

Seborrheic Dermatitis

This is a common chronic dermatosis characterized by redness and scaling. It occurs in the areas of the skin in which the sebaceous glands are most active, such as the face and scalp, and in the body folds, and presternal region.

EPIDEMIOLOGY

Age Infancy (within the first months), puberty, majority between 20 and 50 years or older

Sex More common in males

Incidence Very common

Predisposing Factors Often a genetic diathesis, the "seborrheic state," with marked seborrhea and marginal blepharitis. HIV-infected individuals have an increased incidence.

HISTORY

Duration of Lesions Gradual onset

Skin Symptoms Pruritus is variable, often increased by perspiration, worse during winter months

PHYSICAL EXAMINATION

Skin Lesions

TYPE Yellowish-red, often greasy, or white dry scaling macules and papules of varying size (5 to 20 mm), rather sharply marginated (Figure 27). Sticky crusts and fissures ("weeping") are common when external ears, scalp, axillae, groins, and submammary areas are involved.

SHAPE Nummular, polycyclic, and even annular on the trunk

ARRANGEMENT Scattered, discrete on the face and trunk; diffuse involvement of scalp (see Figure VI)

Distribution and Major Types of Lesions (based on localization and age)

HAIRY AREAS OF HEAD Scalp, eyebrows, eyelashes (blepharitis), beard (follicular orifices); "cradle cap" (Figure 28)

FACE The flush areas ("butterfly"), behind ears, on the forehead ("corona seborrhoica")

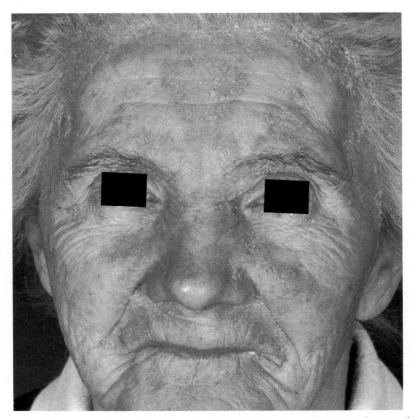

27   Seborrheic dermatitis   *Yellowish-red, often greasy or white, dry, scaling macules, papules, and plaques.*

TRUNK   Simulating lesions of pityriasis rosea, tinea versicolor, or tinea faciale; yellowish-brown patches over the sternum

BODY FOLDS   Axillae, groins, anogenital area, submammary areas, umbilicus—presents as a diffuse, exudative, sharply marginated, brightly erythematous eruption; fissures are common.

GENITALIA   Often with yellow crusts and psoriasiform lesions

DIFFERENTIAL DIAGNOSIS

Psoriasis—the two diseases may be indistinguishable and some recognize a ''sebor-rhiasis''; *tinea faciale,* a tricky presentation simulating seborrheic dermatitis. *Dermatophytosis* and *candidiasis,* in intertriginous skin (KOH examination and cultures must be done); *histiocytosis X* (occurs in infants, usually associated with perifollicular purpura); *acrodermatitis enteropathica* and *zinc deficiency*—dietary or in patients receiving hyper-alimentation; *lupus erythematosus*—especially facial-paranasal lesions, biopsy is sometimes necessary; *pemphigus foliaceus*—may be difficult diagnosis and biopsy is essential; *glucagonoma syndrome*—often regarded on first impression as an atypical psoriasis, severe seborrheic dermatitis, or mucocutane-ous candidiasis.

DERMATOPATHOLOGY

Site Epidermis

Process Focal parakeratosis, with few pyknotic neutrophils, moderate acanthosis, spongiosis (intercellular edema), nonspecific inflammation of the dermis. The most characteristic feature is neutrophils at the tips of the dilated follicular openings, which appear as crusts/scales.

PATHOPHYSIOLOGY

No etiologic organism has been proved, yet pyogenic infection is often present. Experimental inoculations have not been successful in producing seborrheic dermatitis. *Pityrosporum ovale* is said to play a role in the pathogenesis. High-fat diet and alcohol ingestion appear to play some role. Rosacea is not uncommonly associated with seborrheic dermatitis of the face and scalp. Lesions simulating seborrheic dermatitis develop during experimental niacin deficiency and are seen in nutritional deficiencies such as zinc deficiency (as a result of IV alimentation) and in Parkinson's disease (including drug-induced).

COURSE AND PROGNOSIS

The course is variable and facial lesions may disappear for days and then return. There are also recurrences and remissions on the scalp, sometimes associated with alopecia. Infantile and adolescent seborrheic dermatitis disappear with age. In children, seborrheic erythroderma may occur. Seborrheic erythroderma associated with diarrhea and failure to thrive and to generate C5a chemotactic factor is called *Leiner's disease*.

TREATMENT

Topical
SCALP Removal of crusts with 2 to 3% salicylic acid in olive oil is very helpful, especially in infants and children; shampoos containing selenium sulfide or zinc pyrithione or tar, and more recently, ketoconazole-containing shampoos, which when used intermittently control the eruption; topical vioform-hydrocortisone lotion or betamethasone valerate lotion following one of these medicated shampoos, for more severe cases. In very severe involvement, for short periods only, clobetasol propionate 0.05% scalp application is excellent.

FACE This is a difficult therapeutic problem; topical nonsteroidal creams such as ketoconazole have been largely disappointing. Our European colleagues who have used ketoconazole shampoos for a few years tell us that using the "foam" from the shampoo on the paranasal areas is very effective. We have relied on hydrocortisone acetate cream, 1 or 2.5% b.i.d. with or without vioform. Avoid prolonged fluorinated corticosteroids because of side effects (telangiectasia, erythema, and perioral dermatitis) that can occur, even with hydrocortisone acetate. Ketoconazole creams and 3% sulfur and 2% salicylic acid in oil-in-water emulsion-type base are alternatives to topical corticosteroids or can be used in combination for chronic resistant lesions, especially on the face and chest.

INTERTRIGINOUS AREAS Castellani's paint in oozing dermatitis of the body folds is very often effective, although staining is a problem.

Oral
Controlled, randomized, double-blind studies have established oral ketoconazole as an effective treatment for seborrheic dermatitis. Seborrheic dermatitis is not an approved indication for oral ketoconazole and it is rarely used in this disease for prolonged periods, largely because of the potential side effects, especially hepatotoxicity—an incidence of 1:10,000 exposed patients. Also, oral ketoconazole in high doses (800 mg) has been shown to lower serum testosterone levels.

SEBORRHEIC DERMATITIS

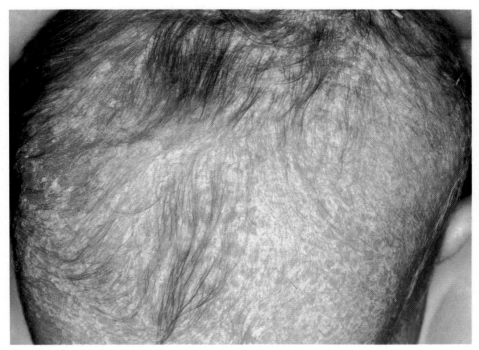

28 Seborrheic dermatitis of infants ("cradle cap")

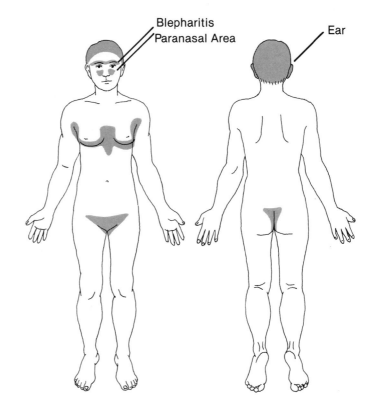

Figure VI Seborrheic
dermatitis

This exanthematous, maculopapular, red, scaling (Greek *pityron,* "bran") eruption occurs largely on the trunk and is probably caused by an infectious agent.

EPIDEMIOLOGY

Age   10 to 35 years

Incidence   2% of dermatologic outpatients

HISTORY

Duration of Lesions   Days. A "herald" patch (see Figure 29, 2 o'clock position) precedes the exanthematous phase. The exanthematous phase develops over a period of 1 to 2 weeks (Figure 29).

Skin Symptoms   Pruritus—absent, mild, or severe

PHYSICAL EXAMINATION

Skin Lesions
TYPE   *Herald plaque*   (80% of patients) 2 to 5 cm, bright red, fine scale
Exanthem   Fine scaling macules and papules with typical marginal collarette (Figure 30)
COLOR   Dull pink or tawny (exanthem)
SHAPE   Oval
ARRANGEMENT   Scattered discrete lesions
DISTRIBUTION   Characteristic pattern of lesions—the long axes of the lesions follow the lines of cleavage in a "Christmas tree" distribution (see Figure VII). Lesions usually confined to trunk and proximal aspects of the arms and legs.

DIFFERENTIAL DIAGNOSIS

Drug eruptions (e.g., captopril), *secondary syphilis* (obtain serology and it is always positive), *guttate psoriasis* (no marginal collarette), *erythema migrans* with secondary lesions

DERMATOPATHOLOGY

Nonspecific

COURSE

Spontaneous remission in 6 to 12 weeks or less. If the eruption persists for over 6 weeks, a skin biopsy should be done to rule out parapsoriasis.

TREATMENT

Pruritus may be controlled by UVB treatment if this is begun in the first week of the eruption. The protocol is 5 consecutive exposures starting with 80% of the minimum erythema dose and increasing 20% each exposure.

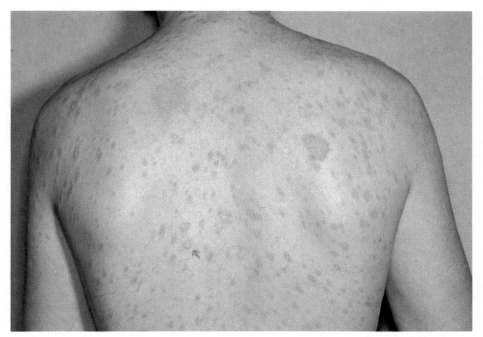

29   Pityriasis rosea   *Scattered over the back and the shoulders are ovoid erythematous lesions (arrow) with somewhat elevated borders, on the inner margin of which fine scaling is seen. Their long axes are in the lines of cleavage of the skin. On the right scapula is the primary lesion (larger than the others).*

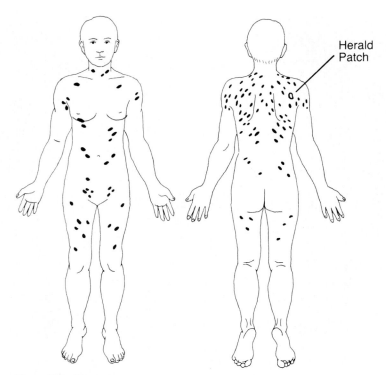

Figure VII   Pityriasis rosea

COMMON SCALING ERUPTIONS OF UNKNOWN ETIOLOGY

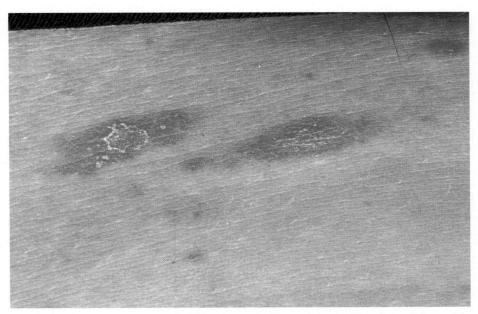

30 Pityriasis rosea *On the left is a typical marginal collarette of scales. Note the oval shape of the lesions.*

Section 5

Viral Skin Infections

Human Papilloma Virus Infections

The common wart, a discrete benign epithelial hyperplasia, is manifested as papules and plaques caused by the human wart virus of the papova group, human papilloma virus (HPV). Different papovaviruses are more or less specific for different clinical manifestations.

Verruca Vulgaris (See Figure 31)

EPIDEMIOLOGY AND ETIOLOGY

Age School children; incidence decreases after age 25

Sex Girls more than boys

Etiology HPV. Those that infect the general population (HPV 1, 2, 3, 4). Those that predominantly infect patients with epidermodysplasia verruciformis (HPV 5, 8— oncogenic potential).

Other Factors Contagion occurs in groups—small (home) or large (school gymnasium). Verruca vulgaris and condyloma acuminatum viruses are antigenically distinct. Verruca vulgaris, however, rarely occurs on the penile shaft. More common and widespread in immunosuppressed patients.

PHYSICAL EXAMINATION

Skin Lesions
TYPE Firm papules, 1 to 10 mm or rarely larger, hyperkeratotic, clefted surface, with vegetations

COLOR Skin colored, characteristic "reddish-brown dots" (thrombosed capillary loops) seen with hand lens (Figure 31, look at 11 to 12 o'clock position)
SHAPE Round, polycyclic
ARRANGEMENT Isolated lesion, scattered discrete lesions
SITES OF PREDILECTION Sites of trauma— hands, fingers, knees

DIFFERENTIAL DIAGNOSIS

The reddish-brown dots are a diagnostic marker; they are pathognomonic and best seen with a 7 × to 10 × hand lens after application of a drop of mineral oil. Seborrheic keratosis. Molluscum contagiosum.

TREATMENT

For small lesions: salicylic acid and lactic acid in collodion

For large lesions: 40% salicylic acid plaster for 1 week, then application of salicylic acid–lactic acid in collodion

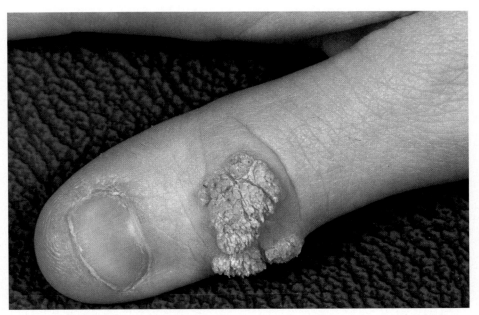

31   Verruca vulgaris (common wart)   *Large verrucous nodule exhibiting vegetations (multiple conical projections). Note the thrombosed capillary loops at 11 o'clock; these are highly characteristic.*

Removal by curettage with local anesthesia

Liquid nitrogen (10 to 30 seconds) for flat lesions or electrocautery, but never surgery

Laser surgery

EPIDEMIOLOGY

Age 5 to 25, but can occur at any age

Sex Females more than males

Other Factors Trauma is a factor as the lesions often occur on sites of pressure.

PHYSICAL EXAMINATION

Skin Lesions

TYPE Early small, shiny, sharply marginated papule → plaque with rough hyperkeratotic surface, often covered by a calluslike hyperkeratosis.

COLOR Skin-colored. To identify diagnostic reddish-brown dots, many plantar warts must be pared with a scalpel to remove the overlying hyperkeratosis.

PALPATION Tenderness may be marked, especially in certain acute types

DISTRIBUTION *Extent* Usually 1 but may be 3 or 6 or more

Sites Pressure points, heads of metatarsals, heels, toes

DIFFERENTIAL DIAGNOSIS

Clavus, callus, foreign body

TREATMENT

If asymptomatic, no treatment, as 50% disappear in 6 months

Do not excise (recur with painful scars)

40% salicylic acid plaster for 1 week, then liquid nitrogen or salicylic acid–lactic acid in collodion

Hyperthermia using hot water (113°F) immersion for 1/2 to 3/4 hour 2 or 3 times weekly for 16 treatments is often effective, as the wart virus is thermolabile.

Relieve pressure with metatarsal bar (on the outside of the shoes)

Cryosurgery (painful)

Laser surgery

Electrosurgery

Radiation therapy is contraindicated

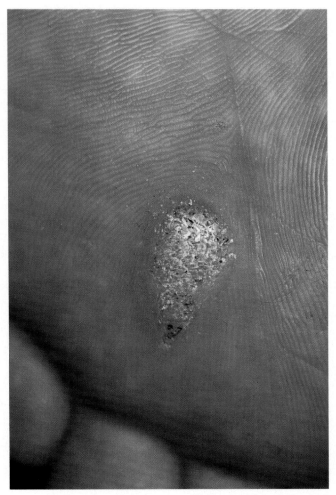

32 Verruca vulgaris (plantar) *Note thrombosed capillaries in this hyperkeratotic plaque. These differentiate this lesion from a clavus (corn), which has a central hyperkeratotic core, and from a callus, which has normal skin markings.*

Verruca Plana ("Flat Wart")

EPIDEMIOLOGY

Age Young children of both sexes, but also adults

Sex Women

PHYSICAL EXAMINATION

Skin Lesions

TYPE Papules (1 to 5 mm), ''flat'' surface; the thickness of the lesion is 1 to 2 mm (Figure 33)

COLOR Skin colored or light brown

SHAPE Round, oval, polygonal, linear lesions (inoculation of virus by scratching)

DISTRIBUTION Always numerous discrete lesions, closely set

SITES OF PREDILECTION Face, dorsa of hands, shins

TREATMENT

Avoid drastic destructive treatments as the lesions tend to spontaneously disappear, often after suggestion alone.

Retinoic acid cream 0.5% once daily over several weeks

Gentle cryosurgery or electrosurgery

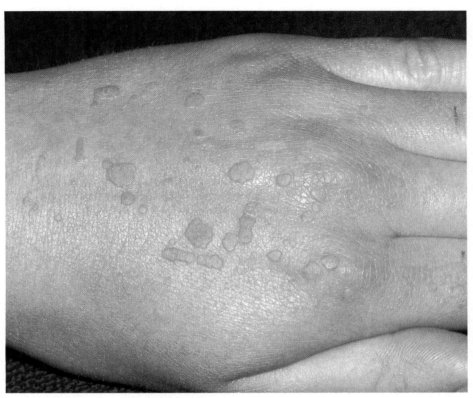

33 Verruca plana (flat warts) *Mesalike flat-topped papules. The linear configuration in the lower part of the picture is due to autoinoculation.*

These are discrete, umbilicated, pearly-white papules caused by a poxvirus and occur in both children and adults.

EPIDEMIOLOGY

Age Children; adults (often sexually transmitted)

Sex Males more than females

Risk Factors HIV-infected individuals may have hundreds of small or giant lesions on the face.

HISTORY

Duration of Lesions Develop in 2 to 3 months

Skin Symptoms None, pruritic if secondarily infected, or with spontaneous regression

PHYSICAL EXAMINATION

Skin Lesions
TYPE Papules (1 to 2 mm), nodules (5 to 10 mm) (rarely giant) (see Figure 34). Hundreds of lesions occur in HIV-infected patients (see Figure 232).
COLOR Pearly-white or skin-colored
SHAPE Round, oval, hemispherical, umbilicated (see Figure 35)

ARRANGEMENT May be linear
DISTRIBUTION Isolated single lesion or multiple scattered discrete lesions
SITES OF PREDILECTION Neck, trunk, anogenital area, eyelids. Multiple facial mollusca suggest HIV infection.

DIFFERENTIAL DIAGNOSIS

Keratoacanthoma (central keratotic plug); *basal cell carcinoma* (hard, telangiectasia). In HIV-infected individuals, cutaneous dissemination of *Histoplasma capsulatum* or *Cryptococcus neoformans* may be present with molluscum-like facial papules.

LABORATORY EXAMINATION

Direct microscopic examination of Giemsa-stained central semisolid core (obtained by pointed scalpel without local anesthesia) reveals "molluscum bodies" (inclusion bodies).

TREATMENT

Liquid nitrogen (10 to 15 seconds)

Light electrocautery

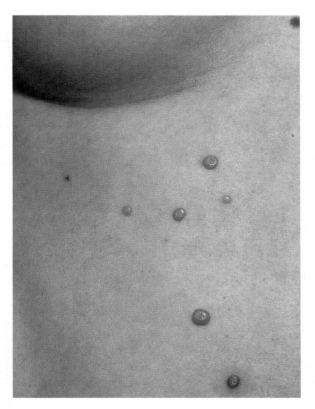

34 Molluscum contagiosum *Discrete, solid, skin-colored papules, 1.0 to 2.0 mm in diameter with central umbilication.*

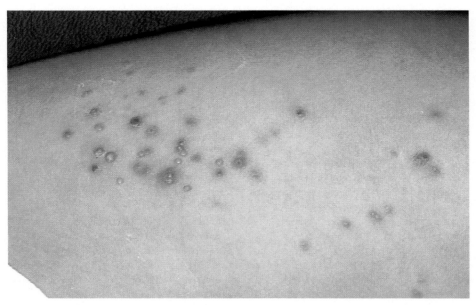

35 Molluscum contagiosum *Multiple, scattered, and discrete lesions, some of which are inflamed.*

MOLLUSCUM CONTAGIOSUM

Nongenital herpes simplex virus (HSV) infection, whether primary or recurrent, is characterized clinically by grouped vesicles arising on an erythematous plaque on keratinized skin or mucous membrane.

Synonyms: herpes, herpes simplex, cold sore, fever blister, herpes febrilis, herpes labialis, herpetic whitlow.

EPIDEMIOLOGY AND ETIOLOGY

Age   Most commonly young adults; range, infancy to senescence

Etiology   HSV type 1 far more common than type 2. Herpetic whitlow in patients <20 years usually HSV-1; >20 years, usually HSV-2.

Transmission   Usually skin/skin, skin/mucosa, mucosa/skin contact. Herpes ''gladiatorum'' transmitted by skin-to-skin contact in wrestlers.

Precipitating Factors for Recurrence Usual factors for herpes labialis: UV radiation, menstruation, fever, ''cold,'' ''stress''

HISTORY

Incubation Period   2- to 20-days (average 6) incubation period for primary infection

Systems Review
PRIMARY HERPES   Many individuals with primary HSV infection are either asymptomatic or have only trivial symptoms. Symptomatic primary herpes, which is uncommon, is characterized by vesicles at the site of inoculation associated with regional lymphadenopathy, at times accompanied by fever, headache, malaise, myalgia, peaking within the first 3 to 4 days after onset of lesions, resolving during the subsequent 3 to 4 days. Primary herpetic gingivo- stomatitis is the most common symptom complex accompanying primary HSV infection in children. It is a severe, painful, ulcerative stomatitis with hypersalivation, lymphadenopathy, and fever.
RECURRENT HERPES   Prodrome of tingling, itching, or burning sensation usually precedes any visible skin changes by 24 hours. Systemic symptoms are usually absent.

PHYSICAL EXAMINATION

Skin Findings
TYPE   *Primary herpes*   An erythematous plaque is often noted initially, followed soon by grouped, often umbilicated, vesicles, which may evolve to pustules (Figure 36). These become eroded as the overlying epidermis sloughs. Erosions may enlarge to ulcerations, which may be crusted or moist. These epithelial defects heal in 2 to 4 weeks, often with resultant postinflammatory hypo- or hyperpigmentation, uncommonly with scarring. The area of involvement may be circumferential around the mouth.
Recurrent herpes   Lesions similar to primary infection but on a reduced scale. Often a 1- to 2-cm plaque of erythema surmounted with vesicles. Heals in 1 to 2 weeks.
Eczema herpeticum   (See Section 14)
Chronic herpetic ulcer   Relentlessly progressive ulcerative form of herpes in immunosuppressed individuals or patients with HIV infection (see Section 17).

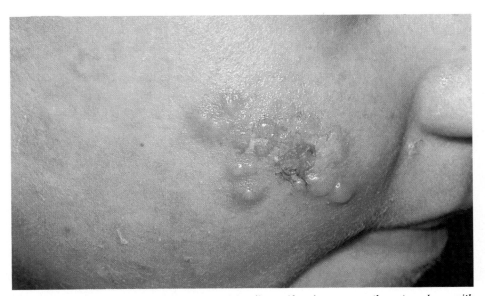

36 Herpes simplex, recurrent *Grouped vesicles (herpetiform) on an erythematous base with some crusting*

ARRANGEMENT Herpetiform, i.e., grouped vesicles (Figure 36)

DISTRIBUTION May occur at any mucocutaneous site. Most common sites are perioral, cheek, nose tip, distal finger (herpetic whitlow). Periocular localization requires examination of the cornea. Herpes gladiatorum occurs on the head, neck, or shoulder.

MUCOUS MEMBRANES Oral mucosa usually involved only in primary HSV infection with vesicles which quickly slough to form erosions at any site in oropharynx, scanty to numerous; gingivitis with gingival tenderness, edema, violaceous color. Documented recurrent intraoral HSV is uncommon.

General Findings Fever is often present during symptomatic primary herpetic gingivostomatitis. Fever in recurrent herpes not usual.

PRIMARY HERPES Regional lymph nodes enlarged, firm, nonfluctuant, tender; usually unilateral. Signs of aseptic meningitis: headache, fever, nuchal rigidity, CSF pleocytosis with normal sugar content, and positive HSV CSF culture.

RECURRENT HERPES May be associated with regional lymphadenitis

DIAGNOSIS AND DIFFERENTIAL DIAGNOSIS

Diagnosis Clinical suspicion confirmed by Tzanck smear (acantholytic giant cells)

Differential Diagnosis *Primary intraoral HSV infection:* aphthous stomatitis, hand-foot-and-mouth disease, herpangina, erythema multiforme. *Recurrent lesion:* fixed drug eruption.

LABORATORY AND SPECIAL EXAMINATIONS

Tzanck Smear (Figure 37) Optimally, fluid from intact vesicle is smeared thinly on a microscope slide, dried, and stained with either Wright's or Giemsa's stain. Positive if giant acanthocytes or multinucleated giant keratinocytes are detected. Positive in 75% of early cases, either primary or recurrent.

Dermatopathology Ballooning and reticular epidermal degeneration,, acanthosis and intraepidermal vesicles; intranuclear inclusion bodies, multinucleate giant keratinocytes; multilocular vesicles.

Electron Microscopy (where available) Negative stain of smear reveals HSV particles.

Viral Culture Cultures are readily available and helpful. HSV can be cultured from vesicle fluid or scraping from base of erosion; must be done early in the course of the outbreak and prior to acyclovir treatment. Documents the presence of HSV in 1 to 10 days.

Serology Primary HSV infection can be documented by demonstration of seroconversion. Recurring herpes can be ruled out if seronegative for HSV antibodies.

PATHOPHYSIOLOGY

Transmission and primary infection of HSV occurs through close contact with a person shedding virus at a peripheral site, mucosal surface, or secretion. HSV is inactivated promptly at room temperature; aerosol or fomitic spread unlikely. Infection occurs via inoculation onto susceptible mucosal surface or break in skin. Subsequent to primary infection at inoculation site, HSV ascends peripheral sensory nerves and enters sensory or autonomic nerve root ganglia, where latency is established. Latency can occur after both symptomatic and asymptomatic primary infection. Recrudescences may be clinically symptomatic or asymptomatic.

COURSE AND PROGNOSIS

Recurrences of HSV tend to become less frequent with the passage of time. Eczema herpeticum (see Section 14) may complicate atopic dermatitis, keratosis follicularis (Darier's disease), and second and third degree thermal burns. Patients with immunodeficiency may experience cutaneous and systemic dissemination of HSV (see Section 17), and chronic herpetic ulcers (see Section 17). Erythema multiforme may complicate herpes, occurring 1 to 2 weeks after an outbreak.

TREATMENT

First Clinical Episode of Herpes Simplex
Acyclovir 200 mg p.o. 5 times a day for 7 to 10 days or until clinical resolution occurs.

Inpatient Therapy
For patients with severe disease or complications necessitating hospitalization. Acyclovir 5 mg/kg body weight IV every 8 hours for 5 to 7 days or until clinical resolution occurs.

Recurrent Episodes
Most episodes of recurrent herpes do not benefit from therapy with oral acyclovir. In severe recurrent disease, patients who start therapy at the beginning of the prodrome or within 2 days after onset of lesions benefit from therapy.

Acyclovir 200 mg p.o. 5 times a day for 5 days *or*

Acyclovir 800 mg p.o. b.i.d. for 5 days

Daily Suppressive Therapy
Daily treatment reduces frequency of recurrences by at least 75% among patients with frequent (more than 6 per year) recurrences. After 1 year of continuous daily suppressive therapy, acyclovir should be discontinued so that the patient's recurrence rate may be reassessed.

Acyclovir 200 mg p.o. 2 to 3 times a day *or*

Acyclovir 400 mg p.o. b.i.d.

Herpes Among HIV-Infected Patients
Neither the need for nor the proper increased dosage of acyclovir has been conclusively established. Patients with genital herpes who do not respond to the recommended dose of acyclovir may require a higher oral dose of acyclovir, IV acyclovir, or be infected with a resistant HSV strain, requiring IV foscarnet (side-effects: genital ulcerations).

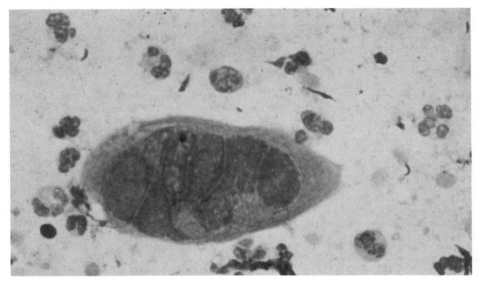

37 Tzanck preparation showing multinucleate giant epidermal cell (Giemsa's stain) *(Courtesy of Arthur R. Rhodes, M.D.)*

Herpes zoster is an acute localized infection caused by varicella-zoster virus (VZV) and is characterized by unilateral pain and a vesicular or bullous eruption limited to a dermatome innervated by a corresponding sensor ganglion.

EPIDEMIOLOGY AND ETIOLOGY

Age Majority of cases occur in individuals over 50 years of age, while less than 10% are under 20 years

Sex and Race No differences

Incidence 300,000 (1.4 to 3.4/100,000) annually (United States)

Other Factors Immunosuppression, especially from lymphoproliferative disorders and chemotherapy, and local trauma to the sensory ganglia are predisposing factors for herpes zoster. Also old age is a risk factor. Zoster is about one-third as contagious as varicella, and susceptible contacts can contract varicella. HIV-infected individuals have an eight-fold increased incidence of zoster.

HISTORY

Duration of Lesions Days to 2 to 3 weeks

Skin Symptoms Pain, tenderness, paresthesia (itching, tingling, burning) in the involved dermatome precedes the eruption by 3 to 5 days. Pain usually persists throughout the eruption, but lessens with time. Nerve involvement can occur without cutaneous zoster.

Constitutional Symptoms Headache, malaise, fever occur in about 5% of patients.

PHYSICAL EXAMINATION

Skin Lesions
TYPE Papules (24 hours) → vesicle-bullae (Figure 38) (48 hours) → pustules (96 hours) → crusts (7 to 10 days). New lesions continue to appear for up to 1 week. Necrotic and gangrenous lesions sometimes occur.
COLOR Erythematous edematous base with superimposed clear vesicles (Figure 38), sometimes hemorrhagic (Figure 39)
SHAPE The vesicle-bulla is oval or round, sometimes umbilicated
ARRANGEMENT Zosteriform (dermatomal), with herpetiform clusters of lesions (Figures 38 and 39)
DISTRIBUTION Unilateral
SITES OF PREDILECTION Thoracic (>50%), trigeminal (10 to 20%) (Figure 40), lumbosacral and cervical (10 to 20%). In HIV-infected individuals, may be multidermatomal (contiguous or noncontiguous) and/or recurrent.

Mucous Membranes Vesicles and erosions occur in mouth, vagina, and bladder depending on dermatome involved.

Lymphadenopathy Regional nodes draining the area are often enlarged and tender.

Sensory or Motor Nerve Changes Detectable by neurologic examination.

Ramsay Hunt Syndrome Zoster involving facial and auditory nerves associated with

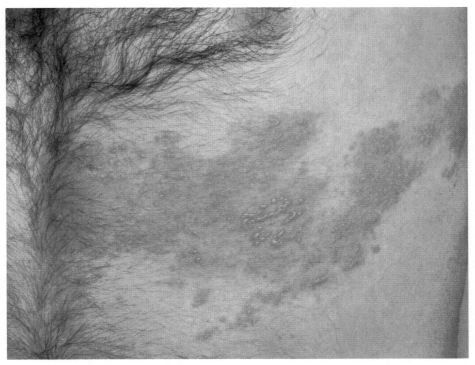

38 Herpes zoster involving T6 dermatome *Note erythematous base with superimposed, grouped, herpetiform vesicles.*

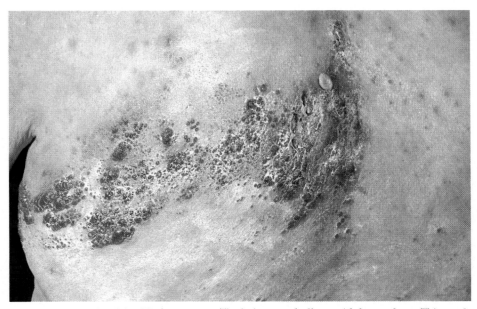

39 Herpes zoster involving T5 dermatome *The lesions are bullous with hemorrhage. This rarely occurs now with the use of acyclovir, if the medication is begun within the first few days.*

ipsilateral facial paralysis and herpetic vesicles on the external ear or tympanic membrane

Eye In ophthalmic zoster, nasociliary branch involvement occurs in about one-third of cases and is heralded by vesicles on the side and tip of the nose (Figure 40). There is usually associated conjunctivitis and occasionally keratitis, scleritis, or iritis. An ophthalmologist should always be consulted.

DIFFERENTIAL DIAGNOSIS

The prodromal pain of herpes zoster can mimic cardiac or pleural disease, and acute abdomen, or vertebral disease. The rash must be distinguished from zosteriform herpes simplex virus eruption which has a different course and prognosis. These can be distinguished by viral culture but not by Tzanck smears or negative stain. Contact dermatitis or localized bacterial infection should also be excluded.

PATHOPHYSIOLOGY

Varicella-zoster virus, during the course of varicella, passes from the skin lesions to the sensory nerves and travels to the sensory ganglia and establishes latent infection. It is postulated that humoral and cellular immunity to VZV established with primary infection persists at low levels, and, when this immunity ebbs, viral replication within the ganglia occurs. The virus then travels down the sensory nerve, resulting in the dermatomal pain and skin lesions. As the neuritis precedes the skin involvement, pain appears before the skin lesions are visible.

COURSE AND PROGNOSIS

The risk of postherpetic neuralgia is around 20% in patients over 60 years of age, but it has been quoted to occur in as high as 40%. In one large follow-up study, postherpetic neuralgia was present 1 month after the onset of the rash in 60%, by 3 months there was some pain in 24%, and by 6 months 13% of the patients still had pain. The highest incidence of postherpetic neuralgia is in ophthalmic zoster. In HIV-infected individuals, zoster may be multidermatomal, recurrent, or chronic.

Dissemination of zoster—20 or more lesions outside the affected or adjacent dermatomes— occurs in up to 10% of patients, usually in immunosuppressed patients. Motor paralysis occurs in 5% of patients, especially when the virus involves the cranial nerves.

TREATMENT

In immunocompetent patients, high-dose oral acyclovir, 800 mg 5 times daily for 7 days, has been shown to hasten healing and lessen *acute* pain if given within 48 hours of the onset of the rash. Large controlled studies in patients over 60 years of age have not, however, demonstrated any effect on the incidence and severity of *chronic* postherpetic neuralgia of high-dose oral acyclovir. A recent preliminary study of older patients (age 60) demonstrated a reduced frequency of persistent pain when IV acyclovir, 10 mg/kg every 8 hours for 5 days was given within 4 days of the onset of the pain or within 48 hours after the onset of the rash.

In immunosuppressed patients, IV acyclovir or recombinant interferon alpha-2a to prevent dissemination of herpes zoster is indicated.

In patients older than 50 years in whom the chance of developing postherpetic neuralgia is high, systemic corticosteroids have been recommended, starting with the onset of the eruption, if no contraindications exist: 60 mg of prednisone per day, tapered to zero over a course of 4 weeks. Possibly this treatment prevents postherpetic neuralgia but it has not been proved.

VIRAL SKIN INFECTIONS

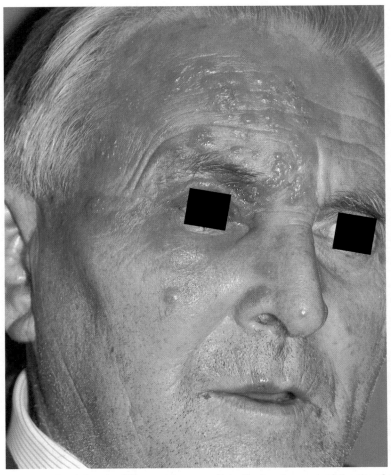

40　Herpes zoster involving the fifth cranial nerve *Note the involvement of the tip of the nose, which may be a signal of eye involvement because the virus travels along the nasociliary branch.*

Milker's nodules (MN) and human orf (HO) are cutaneous infections caused by parapoxviruses, which normally infect animals and accidentally cause infection in humans, and are characterized clinically by nodular lesions on exposed cutaneous sites.

Synonyms: MN: pseudocowpox, paravaccinia; HO: ecthyma contagiosum, contagious pustular dermatitis.

ETIOLOGY AND EPIDEMIOLOGY

Age Usually second and third decades, but a wide range

Sex More common in males

Etiology Members of the *Parapoxvirus* genus of the Poxvirus family

Occupation
MN Dairy farmers
HO Farmers, veterinarians, sheep shearers

Animal Hosts
MN Cattle
HO Ungulates (sheep, goats, yaks, etc.)

Season
MN Spring and autumn
HO Springtime (when lambs are born); season of slaughter of lambs and sheep.

Geography Worldwide. HO epidemics have occurred in Norway, New Zealand, Europe; rare in North America.

Epidemiology
MN Bovine lesions occur on muzzles of calves and teats of cows.
HO The virus survives for many months on fences, feeding basins, and on surfaces within the barn. Only newborn lambs lacking viral immunity are susceptible. In lambs, orf is manifested by erythematous, exudative nodules occurring about the mouth which heal spontaneously in about a month, producing permanent immunity.

Transmission
MN Humans can be infected from contact with lesions on teats or the teat cups of milking machines.
HO Humans become infected either by inoculation of the virus by direct contact with lambs, i.e., during bottle feeding, or indirectly from knives, barbed wire, towels, or other contaminated surfaces. Human-to-human infection does not occur.

Incubation Period 5 to 7 days

HISTORY

Contact with cows, lambs, sheep, etc.

Skin Symptoms Initial lesions may be pruritic; as lesions enlarge and become eroded, may be painful and purulent.

Systems Review May be febrile

PHYSICAL EXAMINATION

Skin Lesions
TYPE *MN* Hemispherical, cherry-red papules; enlarge gradually into firm, elastic, purple, smooth hemispherical nodules varying up to 2 cm in diameter (Figure 41); may become umbilicated.

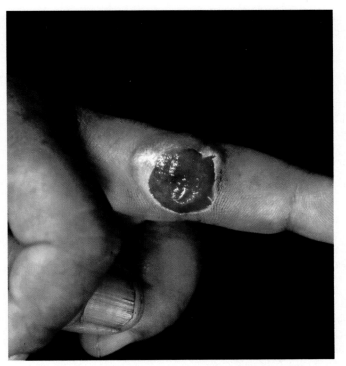

41 Milker's nodule   *Firm, purple, eroded nodule occurred following milking a cow.*

HO Six clinical stages are described, each lasting approximately 6 days: papular stage, target stage, nodular stage, acute weeping stage, regenerative stage, regressive stage. Initially, papule(s) to nodule(s) to plaque(s) at site of inoculation; may appear very edematous to vesicular to bullous. Older nodules have central crusting with purulent discharge. Ascending lymphangitis may occur. Lesions average 1.6 cm in diameter; most commonly only one lesion is present, but can be 10 or more (Figure 42). Healing without scarring.

COLOR *MN* Bright red to purple

HO Pink to erythematous to violaceous. Older lesions may have a target configuration with central crusting, middle ring of pallor, and outer ring of violaceous erythema.

PALPATION Older nodules may be tender.

ARRANGEMENT Initially, papule(s) at site of inoculation.

DISTRIBUTION Exposed skin sites, i.e., hand(s); also arms, legs, face. Most common site: dorsum of right index finger.

Systemic Findings May have regional lymphadenopathy.

DIAGNOSIS AND DIFFERENTIAL DIAGNOSIS

Diagnosis Clinical diagnosis on history of bovine or ungulate exposure

Differential Diagnosis Furunculosis, cat-scratch disease, cellulitis, erysipelas, erysipeloid, insect bite, swimming pool granuloma, leishmaniasis, pyogenic granuloma, bacillary angiomatosis

LABORATORY AND SPECIAL EXAMINATIONS

Dermatopathology During target stage, acanthosis with intranuclear and intracytoplasmic inclusions in superficial vacuolated keratinocytes; in time epidermis ulcerates and then regenerates. *Dermis:* dense mononuclear cell infiltrate, inclusions in endothelial cells.

Electron Microscopy Aspirate of lesion shows a *Parapoxvirus* in epidermal cells.

Viral Culture *Parapoxvirus* can be cultured on human embryonic lung cells.

COURSE AND PROGNOSIS

The highest risk of HO is in workers slaughtering sheep, infecting approximately 4% of workers. Spontaneous resolution occurs within 4 to 6 weeks. Occasionally may be complicated by erythema multiforme. Subsequent reinfection can occur.

TREATMENT

No effective veterinary vaccine for MN or HO is available for animals.

Symptomatic treatment of pain. Antibiotics for treatment of secondary bacterial infection.

VIRAL SKIN INFECTIONS

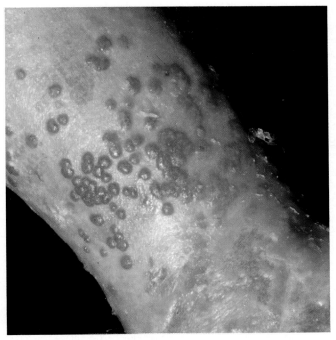

42 Milker's nodule *Multiple, purple papules and nodules occurred in a second degree scalding burn sustained in a milking barn.*

Section 6

Bacterial Infections

This is an acute purulent infection which is at first vesicular and later crusted—a very superficial infection of the skin due either to *Staphylococcus aureus,* group A β-hemolytic streptococci, or a mixed infection.

EPIDEMIOLOGY AND ETIOLOGY

Age Preschool children and young adults

Predisposing Factors Crowded living conditions, poor hygiene, and neglected minor trauma. "Impetiginization" also occurs on lesions of eczema and scabies. It is important to obtain cultures of household and other close contacts, and those who are positive should be treated.

HISTORY

Duration of Lesions Days

Skin Symptoms Variable pruritus

PHYSICAL EXAMINATION

Skin Lesions
TYPE
   Transient thin-roofed vesicles → crusts
   Erosions
COLOR Golden-yellow "stuck on" crusts
   (see Figure 43)
SIZE AND SHAPE 1.0 to 3.0 cm; round or
   oval; central healing

ARRANGEMENT Scattered discrete lesions, some large confluent lesions; satellite lesions occur by autoinoculation
DISTRIBUTION Face (Figure 43), arms, legs, buttocks

Miscellaneous Physical Findings Regional lymphadenopathy

DIFFERENTIAL DIAGNOSIS

In the early vesicular stage impetigo may simulate *varicella* and *herpes simplex. Tinea corporis* with central clearing and pustules shows mycelia in scrapings and culture.

LABORATORY AND SPECIAL EXAMINATIONS

Gram's Stain of Early Vesicle Gram-positive intracellular cocci, in chains or clusters, may be present.

Culture Currently most commonly caused by *Staph. aureus.* Use of a moistened culture swab to dissolve crusts may be necessary to isolate the pathogens.

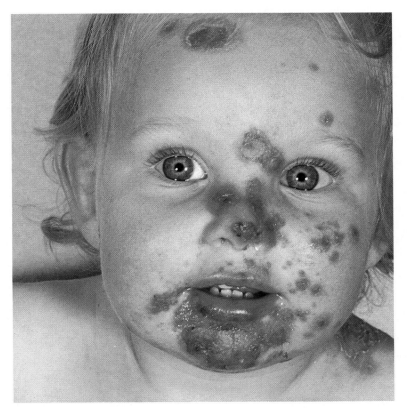

43 Impetigo *Extensive involvement of the face with scattered, discrete lesions and large conflu-ent lesions; there are golden-yellow "stuck-on" crusts.*

Biopsy Usually not necessary. Acantholytic cleft in the stratum granulosum with leukocytes and cocci.

TREATMENT

Mupirocin (pseudomonic acid) is a new topical antibiotic ointment which is highly effective in eliminating both group A streptococci as well as *Staph. aureus* and is an effective treatment of impetigo. Systemic antibiotic therapy is still considered the standard treatment for most patients with impetigo, at least when extensive lesions are present.

1. Dicloxacillin (1 to 2 g per day in 4 divided doses for 10 days).
2. Erythromycin administered for 10 days. This is used if patient cannot take penicillins and if *Staph. aureus* is erythromycin sensitive.

COMPLICATIONS

Glomerulonephritis with certain streptococcal strains

Bullous (Staphylococcal) Impetigo

This form of impetigo occurs as scattered thin-walled bullae arising in normal skin and containing clear yellow or slightly turbid fluid without surrounding erythema.

EPIDEMIOLOGY AND ETIOLOGY

Age Neonates or older children, may occur in adults

Predisposing Factors This may occur in epidemic form in infant nurseries.

Etiology Phage II staphylococci, which produce an extracellular exotoxin and which also produce, besides bullous impetigo, rarely, exfoliative disease (staphylococcal scalded-skin syndrome, see page 294). *Staph. aureus* can usually be recovered from nasal swabs.

PHYSICAL EXAMINATION

Skin Lesions
TYPE   Vesicles and bullae (see Figure 44): thin-walled, easily ruptured, without surrounding erythema which contain clear light- to dark-yellow fluid; later crusts and erosions
ARRANGEMENT   Scattered discrete lesions
DISTRIBUTION   Trunk, face, intertriginous sites

DIFFERENTIAL DIAGNOSIS

Bullous varicella (which probably represents superinfection of varicella with phage II staphylococci), candidal intertrigo

LABORATORY EXAMINATION

Gram's Stain of Early Vesicle Gram-positive cocci, extracellular and within PMN

Culture *Staph. aureus*

TREATMENT

Mupirocin ointment 2% is effective treatment for some cases of bullous impetigo and should be applied to the lesions and to the nostrils. Standard treatment, however, is the administration of systemic antibiotic:

Dicloxacillin (adult dose, 1 to 2 g per day in 4 divided doses for 10 days)

Alternatively, and if *Staph. aureus* is sensitive, erythromycin (adult dose, 1 to 2 g per day in 4 divided doses for 10 days).

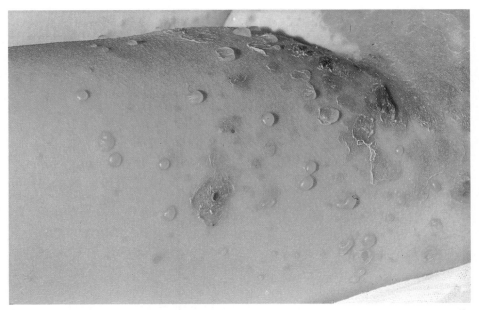

44 Bullous impetigo *Scattered, discrete vesicles and bullae; the bullae are thin-walled and easily ruptured. They leave erosions, such as can be seen especially in the upper left portion of this picture.*

Ulcerative Impetigo (Ecthyma)

This is a confusing term that usually refers to an ulcerative bacterial infection caused most frequently by group A streptococci or staphylococci, or both.

EPIDEMIOLOGY AND ETIOLOGY

Age Children, adolescents, elderly

Predisposing Factors Lesion of neglect—develops in excoriations; insect bites; minor trauma in elderly patients, soldiers, sewage workers, alcoholics, homeless people

HISTORY

Duration of Lesions Weeks

Skin Symptoms Pruritic and tender

PHYSICAL EXAMINATION

Skin Lesions
TYPE Vesicle or pustule → ulcer: raised border, violaceous
COLOR Dirty yellowish-gray crust (see Figure 45)
SHAPE AND SIZE Round or oval, 0.5 to 3.0 cm
PALPATION Indurated and tender
ARRANGEMENT Scattered, discrete
SITES OF PREDILECTION Ankles, dorsa of feet, thighs, buttocks

DIAGNOSIS AND DIFFERENTIAL DIAGNOSIS

Diagnosis Confirmed by Gram's stain and bacterial culture

Differential Diagnosis Cutaneous diphtheria (rare), cutaneous leishmaniasis

LABORATORY AND SPECIAL EXAMINATIONS

Culture *Staph. aureus,* GABHS

COURSE AND PROGNOSIS

Lesions often heal with a scar.

TREATMENT

Systemic antibiotic treatment is usually indicated.

Dicloxacillin (adult dose, 1 to 2 g per day in 4 divided doses for 10 days)

Alternatively, and if *Staph. aureus* is sensitive, erythromycin (adult dose, 1 to 2 g per day in 4 divided doses for 10 days)

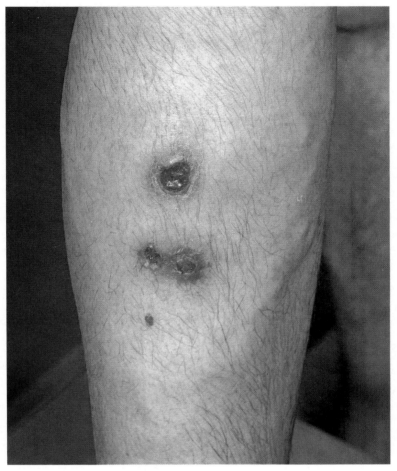

45 Ecthyma *Multiple ulcers with a raised border.*

This superficial inflammation of hair follicles, often bacterial, heals without scarring.

EPIDEMIOLOGY AND ETIOLOGY

Occupation Contact with mineral oils

Predisposing Factors Exposure to tar, adhesive plaster, plastic occlusive dressings. *Staph. aureus* folliculitis aggravated by shaving, i.e., beard area, axillae, legs

HISTORY

Duration of Lesions Days

Skin Symptoms Usually nontender or slightly tender; may be pruritic

Constitutional Symptoms None

PHYSICAL EXAMINATION

Skin Lesions
TYPE Pustule confined to the ostium of the hair follicle
COLOR Dirty yellow or gray with erythema
ARRANGEMENT Scattered discrete or more frequently grouped
DISTRIBUTION *Face* Folliculitis (sycosis) barbae due to staphylococcal infection (see Figure 46). Papulopustules may coalesce to deeply infiltrated plaques similar to kerion-like tinea barbae (see page 114).
Scalp or legs Follicular impetigo of Bockhart
Trunk *Pseudomonas aeruginosa* (''hot tub'') folliculitis
Back *Candida albicans* in febrile hospitalized patients; in ill-kept babies often furuncle-like (''periporitis suppurativa'')

DIFFERENTIAL DIAGNOSIS

Beard area: acne, flat warts, molluscum contagiosum, tinea barbae, eczema herpeticum
Trunk: tinea corporis (presence of mycelia in direct preparation); pustular miliaria is not perifollicular, occurring in hot, humid weather.

LABORATORY FINDINGS

Gram's Stain Look for gram-positive cocci in clusters within PMN

Culture *Staph. aureus, Candida albicans, Pseudomonas aeruginosa*

TREATMENT

Exciting agents (e.g., tar, mineral oils) should be removed. Mupirocin ointment may be effective for *Staph. aureus* folliculitis and is applied to the hairy area involved and to the nostrils.

Systemic antibiotic treatment is usually indicated for *Staph. aureus* folliculitis.

Dicloxacillin (adult dose, 1 to 2 g per day in 4 divided doses for 10 days)

Alternatively, and if *Staph. aureus* is sensitive, erythromycin (adult dose, 1 to 2 g per day in 4 divided doses for 10 days)

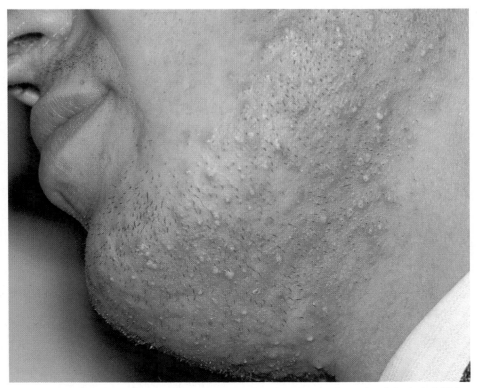

46 Superficial folliculitis *Scattered, discrete pustules occurring in the ostia of the hair follicles. There are also erythematous follicular papules.*

A furuncle is an acute, deep-seated, red, hot, very tender, inflammatory nodule that evolves from a staphylococcal folliculitis. A carbuncle is a conglomerate of multiple coalescing furuncles.

EPIDEMIOLOGY AND ETIOLOGY

Age Children, adolescents, and young adults

Sex More common in boys

Predisposing Factors Chronic staphylococcal carrier state in nares or perineum, friction of collars or belts, obesity, bactericidal defects (e.g., in chronic granulomatosis, defects in chemotaxis, hyper-IgE syndrome). May complicate scabies, pediculosis, or abrasions.

HISTORY

Duration of Lesions Days

Skin Symptoms Throbbing pain and invariably exquisite tenderness

Constitutional Symptoms Not infrequently low-grade fever and malaise

PHYSICAL EXAMINATION

Skin Lesions
TYPE Hard nodule, then fluctuant abscess with central necrotic plug; then ruptures into an ulcer, with erythematous halo (see Figures 47 and 48)
COLOR Bright red
PALPATION Indurated
SHAPE Round
DISTRIBUTION Isolated single lesions or a few multiple lesions

ARRANGEMENT Scattered, discrete
SITES OF PREDILECTION Occur only where there are hair follicles and in areas subject to friction and sweating: nose, neck, face, axillae, buttocks
CARBUNCLE A conglomerate of multiple coalescing furuncles

SPECIAL STUDIES

Culture of blood in cases with fever and/or constitutional symptoms before beginning treatment; if blood culture is positive, IV antibiotics are necessary.

Incision and drainage of abscess for Gram's stain, culture, and antibiotic sensitivity studies.

DIFFERENTIAL DIAGNOSIS

Necrotic herpes simplex, hidradenitis suppurativa (in axillae, groin, vulva; presence of double comedones), *ecthyma gangrenosum*

COURSE AND PROGNOSIS

Most cases resolve with incision and drainage and systemic antibiotic treatment. At times, however, furunculosis is complicated by bacteremia and possible hematogenous seeding of heart valves, joints, spine, long bones, and viscera (especially kidneys). Some patients are subject to recurrent furunculosis.

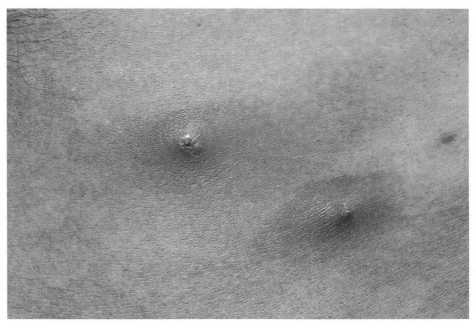

47   Furuncle   *These are exquisitely tender, discrete, hard nodules which become fluctuant; the lesion is surrounded by a broad erythematous flare.*

TREATMENT

Simple furunculosis is treated by local application of heat. Incision and drainage is commonly required, particularly for carbuncles. No systemic antibiotics are needed except in patients at risk for bacteremia (e.g., immunosuppressed patients).

Furunculosis with surrounding cellulitis or with fever should be treated with systemic antibiotics such as dicloxacillin or with erythromycin. Treatment should continue for 1 to 2 weeks.

Recurrent furunculosis may be difficult to control. This may be related to persistent staphylococci in the nares, perineum, and body folds. Effective control can sometimes be obtained with frequent showers (not baths) with povidone-iodine soap and antibacterial ointments (mupirocin) applied daily to the inside of the nares. Appropriate antibiotic treatment is continued until all lesions have resolved and then may be given as a once-a-day prophylactic dose for many months. Alternatively, rifampin (600 mg PO for 7 to 10 days) is effective.

BACTERIAL INFECTIONS

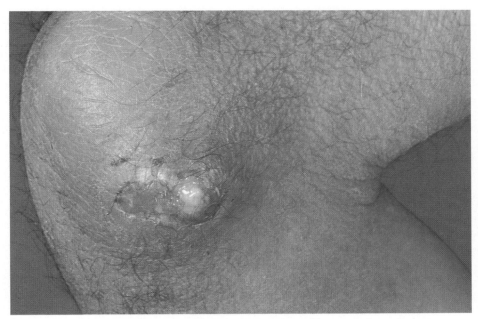

48 Furuncle *This lesion has ruptured, producing an ulcer with a central purulent core.*

Erythrasma (Greek, "red spot") is a chronic bacterial infection caused by *Corynebacterium minutissimum* affecting the intertriginous areas of the toes, groins, and axillae.

EPIDEMIOLOGY AND ETIOLOGY

Age Adults

Race Higher incidence in obese middle-aged blacks

Predisposing Factors Diabetes; warm, humid climate

HISTORY

Duration of Lesions Months, years

Skin Symptoms Irritation

PHYSICAL EXAMINATION

Skin Lesions
TYPE Scaling (fine) macules, sharply marginated (see Figure 49)
COLOR Red or brownish red (see Figure 49)
ARRANGEMENT Scattered discrete lesions, confluent patches
SITES OF PREDILECTION Groin, axilla, intergluteal, submammary

DIFFERENTIAL DIAGNOSIS

Tinea cruris (positive skin scrapings for hyphae), *seborrheic dermatitis* (negative preparations for organisms and absence of fluorescence), *inverse pattern psoriasis*

LABORATORY AND SPECIAL EXAMINATIONS

Direct Microscopic Examination of Scales with KOH (5%) Rods and filaments

Wood's Lamp Characteristic coral-red fluorescence

TREATMENT

Econazole cream applied b.i.d. Showers with povidone-iodine soap usually sufficient for minor cases. Good clearing occurs with erythromycin, 250 mg q.i.d. for 14 days. Relapses usually occur within 6 months to a year. Topical antibacterial agents are less effective.

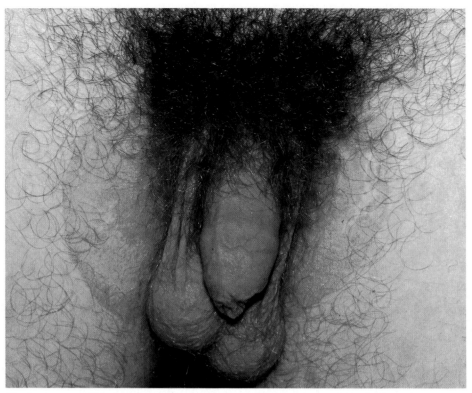

49   Erythrasma   *This sharply marginated, brownish-red, scaling eruption exhibits a characteristic "coral-red" fluorescence when viewed with a Wood's lamp.*

Erysipeloid is an acute but slowly evolving cellulitis occurring at sites of inoculation, most commonly the hands, and is often occupational, associated with handling fish, shellfish, meat, poultry, hides, bones.

Synonym: crab dermatitis

EPIDEMIOLOGY AND ETIOLOGY

Age, Sex   Adults; males > females

Occupation   Fishermen, fish handlers, butchers, meat processing workers, poultry workers, farmers, veterinarians, abattoir workers, housewives

Etiology   *Erysipelothrix rhusiopathiae,* a gram-positive rod

Transmission   Organism is primarily saprophytic. Human infection restricted to persons who handle dead animal matter, either edible (meat, poultry, fish, shellfish, crustaceans) or nonedible (bones, shells). No vectors. Not contagious.

Season   Summer and early fall

Geography   Worldwide

HISTORY

Incubation Period   1 to 4 days

History   Occupational exposure

Skin Symptoms   Itching, burning, throbbing, pain

Systems Review   Systemic symptoms uncommon

PHYSICAL EXAMINATION

Skin Findings
TYPE   Painful, swollen plaque with sharply defined irregular raised border, occurring at the site of inoculation. Enlarges peripherally with central fading. Vesiculation uncommon. Nonsuppurative, nonpitting.
COLOR   Purplish-red acutely (Figure 50). Brownish with resolution
DISTRIBUTION   Finger or hand, spreading to wrist and forearm but not beyond

General Findings
LYMPH NODES   Occasional lymphangitis or lymphadenitis

DIAGNOSIS AND DIFFERENTIAL DIAGNOSIS

Diagnosis   Clinical diagnosis by history and unique clinical appearance

Differential Diagnosis   Other types of bacterial cellulitis, including *Vibrio* cellulitis, allergic contact dermatitis

LABORATORY AND SPECIAL EXAMINATIONS

Dermatopathology   Acute inflammation

Culture   Difficult; most successful from bi-

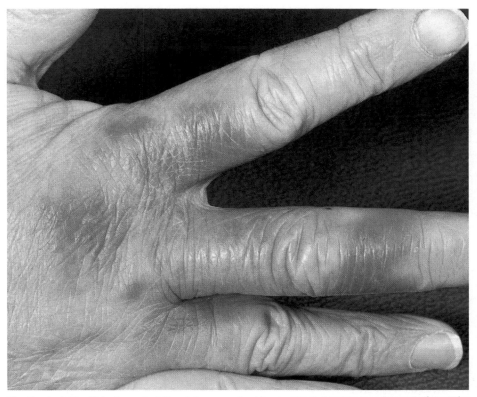

50 Erysipeloid *This characteristic, violaceous, sharply marginated lesion is composed of macules and plaques. The lesions are slightly tender and warm but not hot.*

opsied tissue. May also inject nonbacteriostatic saline into advancing edge of lesion and culture the aspirate.

PATHOPHYSIOLOGY

Infection follows an abrasion, scratch, puncture wound while handling organic material containing the organism.

COURSE AND PROGNOSIS

Usually self-limited, subsiding spontaneously in about 3 weeks. Relapses may occur. Endocarditis or septic arthritis may rarely complicate bacteremia.

TREATMENT

Drug of choice: penicillin VK, 250 mg p.o. q.i.d. for 10 days. Alternative: erythromycin 250 mg q.i.d. for 7 days.

Superficial Fungal Infections

GENERAL REMARKS

These are superficial infections caused by dermatophytes, i.e., fungi that thrive only in nonviable keratinized tissue of the skin (stratum corneum, nails, hair). The three principal genera are *Microsporum, Trichophyton,* and *Epidermophyton;* they cause dermatophytosis, or *"tinea"* (used generically for dermatophytoses, e.g., tinea capitis).

EPIDEMIOLOGY AND ETIOLOGY

Age Children have scalp infections (*Microsporum* and *Trichophyton*) and young adults have intertriginous infections.

Sex No profound differences

Race Adult blacks are said to have a lower incidence of dermatophytosis.

Transmission Dermatophyte infections can be acquired from three sources: from another person by fomites, from animals such as puppies or kittens, and least commonly from soil.

Classification of the Dermatophytoses Dermatophytes grow only on or within keratinized structures and, as such, infect keratinized epidermis, nails (tinea unguium or onychomycosis), and hair (trichomycoses such as tinea capitis, tinea barbae, and Majocchi's [trichophytic] granuloma). Dermatophytic infection of the epidermis includes tinea pedis, tinea manus, tinea cruris, tinea corporis, and tinea faciale.

Other Predisposing Factors *Immunosuppressed patients* have a higher incidence and more intractable dermatophytoses. With topical immunosuppression (i.e., with prolonged application of topical corticosteroids) there can be marked modification in the usual banal character of dermatophytosis; this is especially true of the face, groin, and hands.

Topical Antifungal Agents Effective for Treatment of Cutaneous Dermatophytosis	
AGENT	PREPARATION
Imidazoles:	
Clotrimazole	Cream, lotion, solution
	Cream, solution
Econazole nitrate	Cream
Ketoconazole	Cream, shampoo
Miconazole nitrate	Cream, lotion
	Cream
Ciclopirox olamine	Cream

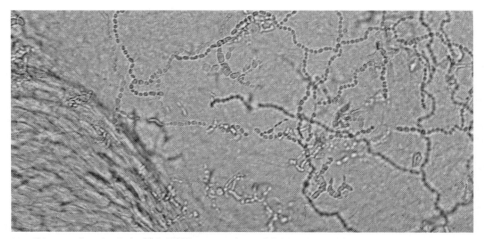

51 Skin scrapings (scales) *This KOH preparation exhibits septate hyphae.*

Potassium Hydroxide Mount

HAIR

Epilated hairs should be studied immediately. Several hairs are placed on a slide, 10 or 30% KOH and a coverslip are added, and the slide is warmed without boiling. After 15 to 30 minutes, the slide may be examined for the presence of fungi. For this and most other microscopic examinations, the substage or condenser diaphragm should be closed to approximately one-half its normal opening area and the condenser lowered until best contrast with the specimen is obtained.

SKIN SCRAPINGS (SCALES)

Specimens can be obtained by scraping scale from the lesional margin with either another glass slide or a #15 scalpel onto a collection slide held at right angles to the skin or several tiny pieces of the scrapings should be placed on a glass slide without overlapping. KOH (10 to 30%)[1] and a coverslip are used; the specimen is gently heated and then allowed to stand for about 5 minutes. The specimen may then be studied for hyphae, arthrospores, or, occasionally, budding cells (see Figure 51). One cannot identify specific organisms but only note the presence or absence of hyphae.[2]

NAIL SCRAPINGS

Several thin pieces of the specimen should be placed on a glass slide without overlapping. A few drops of KOH (10 to 30%)[1] and a coverslip are used. The slide is gently heated to near-boiling and then allowed to sit for approximately *one-half hour*. Avoid boiling, which causes bubbles that both disrupt the fungus and produce artifacts. The specimen may then be studied for hyphae and budding cells.

---

[1] Specially prepared 10% KOH with ink and detergent (Swartz-Lamkins stain) may be used as an alternative to higher concentrations of KOH and is less likely to damage microscope lenses.

[2] Obtain fungal cultures for species identification.

Tinea Pedis (Athlete's Foot)

ETIOLOGY

Predisposing Factors Hot and humid weather; occlusive footwear

PHYSICAL EXAMINATION

Skin Lesions

TYPE Scaling, plus maceration (Figure 52), and vesicles or bullae

COLOR Red; opaque white scales

DISTRIBUTION Usually localized in third and fourth interdigital spaces and later the sole, especially in the arch (most often *Trichophyton mentagrophytes*); scaling and hyperkeratosis of the soles extending to the foot in the area covered by a ballet shoe (Figure 53) most often caused by *Trichophyton rubrum* (also called moccasin-type tinea).

LABORATORY AND SPECIAL EXAMINATIONS

Direct microscopic examination (see Figure 51) and culture

COURSE AND PROGNOSIS

Tends to be chronic with exacerbations in hot weather. May provide portal of entry for streptococcal infection, producing lymphangitis or cellulitis, especially in patients whose leg veins have been removed for coronary artery bypass surgery and who have chronic low-grade edema of leg.

TREATMENT

Acute Vesicular Stages Burow's wet dressings, followed by clotrimazole 1% or other topical antifungals (see under "Dermatophyte Infections," page 98)

Subacute (Maceration, Scaling)

Topical preparations (see under "Dermatophyte Infections")

Liberal use of powder between the toes and in the shoes

Chronic

1. Same as treatment of subacute

2. Shoes should be treated with antifungal powder.

3. Griseofulvin (ultramicrosize), 250 mg orally b.i.d. with food for several weeks. If toenails are involved, treatment may require 6 or more months. Griseofulvin alone is not always effective in chronic tinea of the feet unless combined with topical treatment.

4. Ketoconazole, 200 mg orally daily, is an effective alternative to griseofulvin. There is some risk of hepatic injury with oral ketoconazole; liver function tests should be monitored.

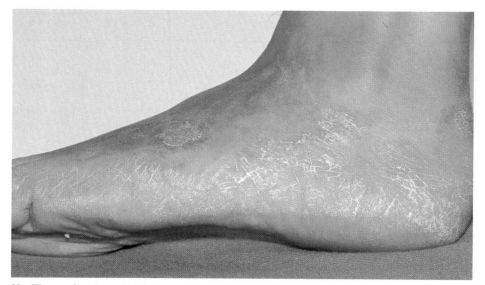

52   Tinea pedis   *Superficial white scales in a moccasin-type distribution. Note arciform pattern of the scales, which is characteristic.*

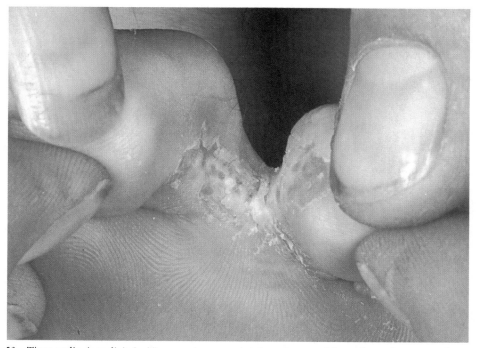

53   Tinea pedis, interdigital   *The area is macerated, has opaque white scales and some erosions.*

TINEA PEDIS (ATHLETE'S FOOT)

Tinea manus is a chronic dermatophytosis of the hand(s), often unilateral, and most commonly on the dominant hand, in which there is almost invariably a preexisting tinea pedis, usually nails and interdigital skin, and often fingernail dermatophytosis (onychomycosis).

ETIOLOGY

Most often *Trichophyton rubrum*

PHYSICAL EXAMINATION

Skin Lesions

TYPE   Hyperkeratosis, scaling papules and vesicles in clusters

COLOR   Erythematous

SHAPE   Annular, polycyclic (see Figure 54), especially on the dorsum of the hand

DISTRIBUTION   Diffuse hyperkeratosis of the palms or patchy scaling on the dorsa and sides of fingers; 50% of patients have *unilateral* involvement

LABORATORY AND SPECIAL EXAMINATIONS

Direct microscopic examination of scales (see Figure 51) taken from the advancing crescentic edge

TREATMENT

As outlined for tinea pedis

SIGNIFICANCE

When combined with onychomycosis, tinea manus may recur following treatment, and this can be a frustrating problem, particularly in patients who use their hands for fine skills or who are exposed to the public.

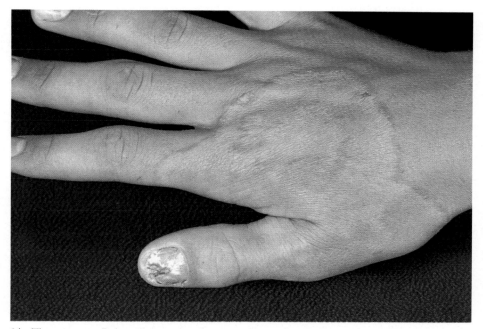

54 Tinea manus *Polycyclic pattern of an eruption composed of scaling papules with involvement of the thumb nail; the nail exhibits destruction of the nail plate.*

Tinea unguium defines dermatophyte infection of the nail plate; *onychomycosis* comprises infection of nails by any fungus, including yeasts.

EPIDEMIOLOGY

Common; dermatophytosis of the toenails is very common, particularly with advancing age.

ETIOLOGY

Most common causes of tinea unguium are *Trichophyton rubrum* (most frequent), *T. mentagrophytes,* and *Epidermophyton floccosum.* Onychomycosis due to nondermatophytes is usually caused by *Candida* species.

PREDISPOSING FACTORS

Reduction in blood flow as occurs with age and peripheral nerve injury contribute to the susceptibility of nail keratin to dermatophyte infections, as does mechanical pressure by footwear. *Candida* invades nail plates only in chronic mucocutaneous candidiasis, but other *Candida* species and dermatophytes may also affect antecedently diseased nails, as in psoriasis.

NAIL LESIONS

Distal Subungual Onychomycosis A whitish-brownish-yellow discoloration of the free edge of the nail. Subungual hyperkeratosis leads to separation of nail plate and nail bed with subungual accumulation of friable keratinous debris (Figure 55).

White Superficial Onychomycosis Appears as white, sharply outlined area on the nail plate (of toenails). Surface of nail friable, rough. This presentation occurs relatively commonly in HIV-infected patients in both toe- and fingernails.

Proximal Subungual Onychomycosis This is rare. Starts as whitish-brown area on the proximal part of the nail plate. May enlarge to affect the whole nail plate.

***Candida* Infection** Thickening of nail plate which is rough, furrowed, and eventually disintegrates into a hyperkeratotic, brittle, and fissured horny mass.

DISTRIBUTION

Characteristically, infected nails coexist with normal-appearing nails. Toenails more frequently involved than fingernails; the latter often unilaterally after vertebral or other injury. In chronic immunosuppression, tendency of involvement of all nails, also in chronic mucocutaneous candidiasis or acrodermatitis enteropathica *(Candida).*

DIFFERENTIAL DIAGNOSIS

Psoriasis of nails, onychogryphosis

LABORATORY AND SPECIAL EXAMINATIONS

Direct microscopic examination of scrapings and culture

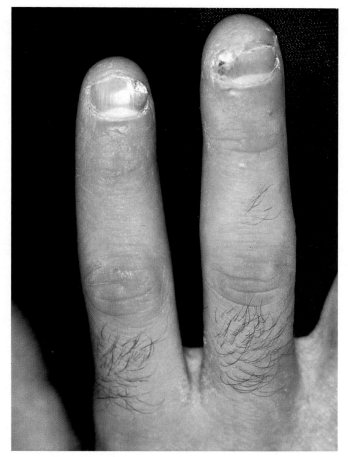

55 Tinea unguium *The nails of the index and middle fingers are deformed as a result of an infection by the dermatophyte. There is onycholysis and subungual keratosis.*

TREATMENT

Dermatophytosis Unguium

Griseofulvin (ultramicrosize) 500 mg b.i.d. for up to 10 or more months plus topical antifungals. Fingernails respond better than toenails, and if there is a predisposing lesion the rate of recurrence is extremely high. This also holds for tinea unguium of the toes, particularly in the elderly, which may not respond in the first place. The failure and recurrance rates are high and treatment of dermatophytosis of nails is thus a frustrating problem.

Ketoconazole, 200 mg orally daily, is an effective alternative to griseofulvin; liver function tests should be monitored.

Onychomycosis Due to Nondermatophytes Treatment of underlying disease. Ketoconazole 200 mg b.i.d. and topical preparation (see under "Dermatophyte Infections").

Tinea cruris is a subacute or chronic dermatophytosis of the upper thigh in males, usually caused by *Epidermophyton floccosum* or *Trichophyton rubrum*.

EPIDEMIOLOGY AND ETIOLOGY

Age   Young adults (''jock itch'')

Sex   Male

Predisposing Factors   Warm, humid environment; tight clothing worn by men; obesity

HISTORY

Skin Lesions
TYPE   Plaques with papular, scaling, sharp margins with occasional pustules and central clearing
COLOR   Dull red
ARRANGEMENT   Arciform, polycyclic
DISTRIBUTION   Intertriginous areas (Figure 56) and adjacent upper thigh and buttock. Scrotum is rarely involved, in contrast to candidiasis
SYMPTOMS   Pruritus

DIFFERENTIAL DIAGNOSIS

The coral-red fluorescence seen in erythrasma with Wood's lamp is not observed.

LABORATORY AND SPECIAL EXAMINATIONS

Direct microscopic examination of scrapings for mycelia (see Figure 51)

TREATMENT

For acute and subacute tinea cruris, use topical preparation (see under ''Dermatophyte Infections'').

If there is no response, or there is irritation from topical antifungals, then griseofulvin (ultramicrosize) 500 mg b.i.d. with food for 3 to 4 weeks, or ketoconazole 200 mg q.d. for 2 to 3 months.

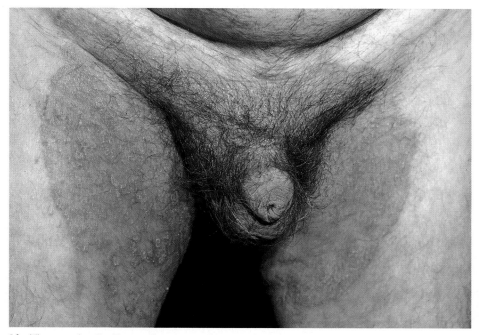

56　Tinea cruris　*Scaling erythematous plaque with sharp margins.*

These scaling papular lesions occur in an annular arrangement with peripheral enlargement and central clearing on the trunk, limbs, or face ("ringworm").

EPIDEMIOLOGY AND ETIOLOGY

Age   All ages

Occupation   Animal (large and small) workers

Predisposing Factors   Infection is acquired from an active lesion of an animal *(Trichophyton verrucosum, Microsporum canis),* by direct human contact *(T. rubrum),* or, rarely, from soil.

PHYSICAL EXAMINATION

Skin Lesions

TYPE   Small-to-large, scaling, sharply marginated plaques (Figure 57) with or without pustules or vesicles

SHAPE AND ARRANGEMENT   Peripheral enlargement and central clearing, producing an annular configuration

DISTRIBUTION   Single and occasionally scattered multiple lesions

SITES OF PREDILECTION   Exposed skin of forearm, neck

DIFFERENTIAL DIAGNOSIS

Erythema annulare centrifugum, psoriasis, erythema migrans.

LABORATORY AND SPECIAL EXAMINATIONS

Direct microscopic examination of scales from the advancing border

TREATMENT

Topical antifungal creams (see under "Dermatophyte Infections") b.i.d. for 7 to 10 days. If extensive or resistant to topical treatment, griseofulvin or ketoconazole is indicated, combined with topical antifungal preparations.

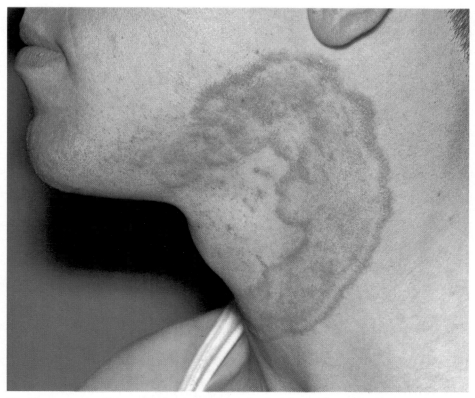

57　Tinea corporis　*This neck lesion is composed of a sharply marginated, arciform, erythematous plaque with central clearing.*

Tinea faciale is dermatophytosis of the glabrous facial skin, characterized by a well-circumscribed erythematous patch, and is more commonly misdiagnosed than any other dermatophytosis.

Synonyms: tinea faciei, ringworm of the face.

EPIDEMIOLOGY AND ETIOLOGY

Age   More common in children

Etiology   *Trichophyton mentagrophytes, T. rubrum* most commonly; also *Microsporum audouini, M. canis*

Predisposing Factors   Animal exposure

HISTORY

Skin Symptoms   Most commonly asymptomatic. At times, pruritus.

PHYSICAL EXAMINATION

Skin Lesions
TYPE   Well-circumscribed macule to plaque of variable size; elevated border and central regression (Figure 58). Scaling often is minimal.
COLOR   Pink to red. In black patients, hyperpigmentation.

DISTRIBUTION   Any area of face but usually not symmetric

DIFFERENTIAL DIAGNOSIS

Seborrheic dermatitis, contact dermatitis, erythema chronicum migrans, lupus erythematosus, polymorphic light eruption, photodrug eruption, lymphocytic infiltrate

LABORATORY AND SPECIAL EXAMINATIONS

Direct microscopic examination of scraping shows hyphae. Scrapings from patients who have used topical corticosteroids show massive numbers of hyphae.

TREATMENT

Topical antifungal preparations are usually effective.

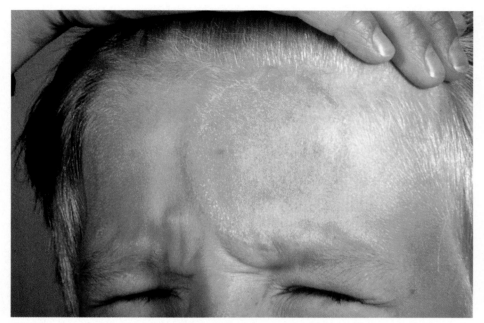

58 Tinea faciale   *Sharply marginated, erythematous, annular plaque with central clearing and a peripheral scaling in a young child.*

Tinea capitis is a dermatophytic trichomycosis of the scalp, the acute infection being characterized by follicular inflammation with painful, boggy nodules which drain pus and result in scarring alopecia, and the subacute to chronic infection, by scaling patches.

EPIDEMIOLOGY AND ETIOLOGY

Age Children or, rarely, adults

Pathogenesis *Noninflammatory lesions:* invasion of hair shaft by the dermatophytes, principally *Microsporum audouini* (child to child, via barber, hats, theater seats), *M. canis* (young pets to child and then child to child), or *Trichophyton tonsurans. Inflammatory lesions: M. canis, T. tonsurans, T. verrucosum,* and others.

HISTORY

Duration of Lesions Weeks to months

Skin Symptoms Loss of hair; pain and tenderness in inflammatory type

PHYSICAL EXAMINATION

Skin Lesions and Hair Changes

FOUR TYPES *"Gray patch" ringworm* Brittle hair; shafts break off close to scalp surface. Caused by *M. audouini* and *M. canis* (see Figure 59)

"Black dot" ringworm Broken-off hairs near surface give appearance of "dots." Tends to be diffuse and poorly circumscribed. Caused by *T. tonsurans* and *T. violaceum.*

"Kerion" (Greek, "honeycomb") Boggy, elevated, purulent, inflamed nodules and plaques (see Figure 62) which are extremely painful and drain pus. Hairs do not break off but fall out and can be pulled without pain. Heals with scarring alopecia.

Favus Cutaneous atrophy, scar formation, and scarring alopecia are typical of favus, due to infection with *Trichophyton schoenleinii.* So-called scutula, i.e., yellowish adherent crusts, are present on the scalp. Only in the marginal zones does the hair still grow normally. Favus has now become very uncommon in Western Europe and North America. In some parts of the world (Middle East, South Africa), however, it is still endemic. See Figure 60.

Systemic Findings Regional lymphadenopathy, especially if of long duration and if superinfected.

LABORATORY AND SPECIAL EXAMINATIONS

Fluorescence Examination with Wood's Lamp Examination of scalp with filtered ultraviolet (Wood's lamp) reveals *bright green* hair shafts in scalp infections caused by *M. audouini* and *M. canis. T. schoenleinii* fluorescence is grayish green. *T. tonsurans,* however, does not exhibit fluorescence.

Direct Microscopic Examination with 10% KOH Spores can be seen invading the hair shaft (*T. tonsurans* and *T. violaceum*).

TREATMENT

Griseofulvin (ultramicrosize), adult dose: (1) "gray patch" ringworm, 250 mg b.i.d. for 1 or 2 months (or 5 mg/kg for children); (2) "black dot" ringworm, longer treatment and higher doses—continued 2 weeks after Wood's lamp, KOH, and cultures are negative. (3) Kerion: 250 mg b.i.d. for about 4 weeks; antibiotics for accompanying staphylococcal infection. Alternative: ketoconazole.

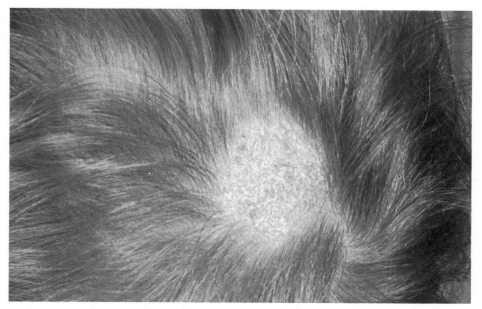

59   Tinea capitis from *Microsporum canis*   *An area of hair loss in a circular pattern can be observed; this results from the fracture of hair shafts, close to the scalp surface. The hair shafts exhibit a green fluorescence when viewed with a Wood's lamp.*

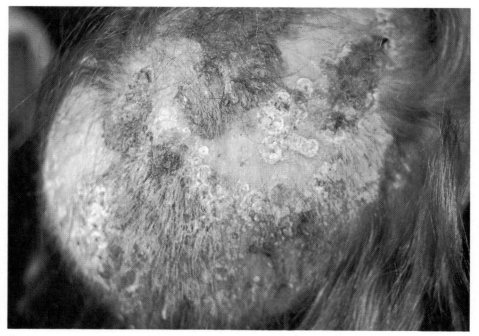

60   Tinea capitis from *Trichophyton schoenleinii* (favus)   *Yellowish, adherent crusts and scales, known as* scutula. *May be complicated by atrophy, scarring, and permanent hair loss.*

TINEA CAPITIS   113

Tinea barbae is a dermatophytic trichomycosis involving the beard and moustache areas, closely resembling tinea capitis with invasion of the hair shaft.

Synonym: ringworm of the beard.

EPIDEMIOLOGY

Age Adult

Sex Males only

Etiology *Trichophyton verrucosum, T. mentagrophytes* most commonly. May be acquired through animal exposure.

Predisposing Factors More common in farmers

HISTORY

Skin Symptoms Pruritus, tenderness, pain

PHYSICAL EXAMINATION

Skin Lesions

TYPE Pustular folliculitis (Figure 61), i.e., hair follicles surrounded by red inflammatory papules or pustules, often with exudation and crusting. Involved hairs are loose and easily removed. With less follicular involvement, there are scaling, circular, reddish patches in which hair is broken off at the surface. As with tinea capitis, kerion formation may occur (Figure 62).

COLOR Red

DISTRIBUTION Beard and moustache areas, rarely eyelashes, eyebrows

Systemic Findings Regional lymphadenopathy, especially if of long duration and if superinfected

DIFFERENTIAL DIAGNOSIS

Staphylococcus aureus folliculitis, furuncle, carbuncle, acne vulgaris, rosacea, pseudofolliculitis, HSV infection (recurrent or eczema herpeticum)

LABORATORY AND SPECIAL EXAMINATIONS

Direct Microscopic Examination of Plucked Hair Shows hyphae invading hair sheath and/or shaft.

Culture Tinea barbae is not uncommonly superinfected with *Staph. aureus* and its detection does not rule out tinea barbae.

TREATMENT

Topical antifungal preparations are ineffective.

Griseofulvin 500 mg b.i.d. or ketoconazole 200 mg q.d. given for 4 to 6 weeks.

SUPERFICIAL FUNGAL INFECTIONS

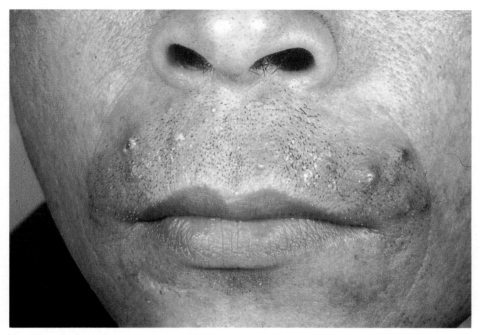

61 Tinea barbae *Scattered, discrete, follicular pustules.*

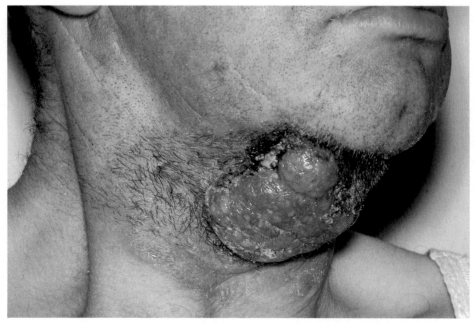

62 Tinea barbae, kerion *Sharply demarcated red nodule (4.0 × 6.0 cm). The surface is moist and studded with multiple yellowish pustules. Regional lymph nodes are not enlarged.*

TINEA BARBAE   115

Mucocutaneous candidiasis is a superficial mycotic infection occurring on moist cutaneous sites and mucosal surfaces; many patients have predisposing factors that alter local immunity, such as increased moisture at the site of infection, diabetes, antibiotic therapy, or alteration in systemic immunity.

Synonym: moniliasis.

EPIDEMIOLOGY AND ETIOLOGY

Age   Any age. Infants (diaper area, mouth)

Sex   Both. Women (vulvovaginitis), males (balanitis)

Occupation   Persons who immerse their hands in water; housewives; bartenders; florists; HIV-infected individuals; prolonged use of steroid inhalants; bakers develop paronychia.

Other Predisposing Factors   Diabetes, obesity, hyperhidrosis, heat, maceration, immunologic defects (depressed T-cell function), polyendocrinopathies, pregnancy, oral contraceptives, systemic antibacterial agents,

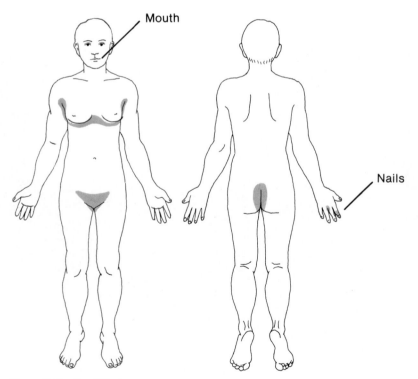

Mouth

Nails

Figure VIII   Candidiasis

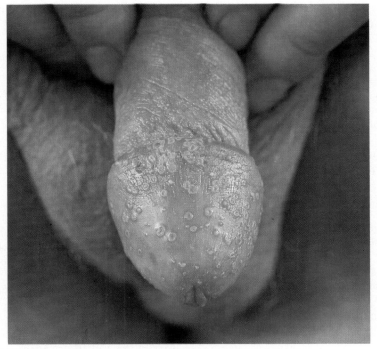

63 Balanoposthitis *Numerous discrete pustules are present.*

systemic and topical corticosteroids, chronic debilitation (carcinoma, leukemia), chemotherapy

COMMON CLINICAL TYPES
(See Figure VIII)

Mucosal Candidiasis See page 422.

Vulvovaginitis Pruritus; thick creamy-white, curdy discharge; meaty-red erythema of vaginal skin and mucous membrane. Spreads to perineum and groin. Satellite pustules.

Balanoposthitis Erosions, flat pustules, edema, delicate scaling (Figure 63)

Diaper Candidiasis Erythema, edema with papular and pustular lesions; erosions, oozing, colarette-like scaling at the margins of lesions involving perigenital and perianal skin, inner aspects of thighs and buttocks (Figure 64).

Interdigital and Intertriginous Candidiasis Fairly sharply demarcated, polycyclic erythematous, erosive lesions with colarette-like scales and small pustular lesions at the periphery. Interdigital (usually between third and fourth fingers) (Figure 65), submammary (Figure 66), groin, and scrotum (Figure 67).

Paronychial Candidiasis Redness and swelling of nail folds. Pressure releases purulent, creamy material from nail fold. Painful. Nails may show distal onycholysis, discoloration, and ridging. See Figure 68.

Follicular Candidiasis Small, discrete pustules, cigarette paper-like scaling

LABORATORY AND SPECIAL EXAMINATIONS

Direct microscopic examination of skin or mucosal scraping, or of pus using Gram's stain or 5% KOH preparation (see Figure 69).

Culture is essential for specific identification of *C. albicans*.

TREATMENT

Mucosal Candidiasis (See Section 17)

Vulvovaginitis
Vaginal tablets or suppositories used once daily at bedtime (for 3 to 7 nights): clotrimazole, miconazole, other imidazoles, allylamines

Male partners should also be treated to prevent conjugal candidiasis

Balanitis Imidazole cream followed by nystatin powder. Keep foreskin retracted.

Diaper Candidiasis Topical nystatin ointment plus liberal use of powder. Avoid rubber or plastic diaper pants.

Interdigital and Intertriginous Candidiasis For interdigital involvement, use nystatin or imidazole or allylamine creams. For intertriginous involvement, air-dry frequently; loose clothing; topical nystatin ointment followed by nystatin powder or miconazole; oral ketoconazole. Castellani's paint is very effective.

Paronychial Candidiasis Application of gentian violet in water, 2%, deeply under nail fold once daily. Eliminate immersion in water. Topical miconazole. Oral ketoconazole is sometimes indicated if gentian violet fails.

SUPERFICIAL FUNGAL INFECTIONS

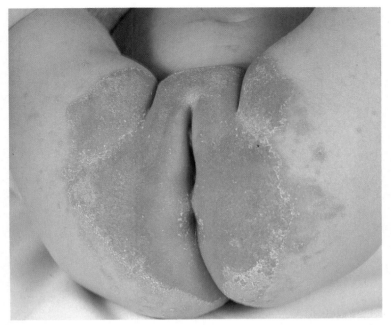

64 Candidal intertrigo   *The infant shows red macular areas on the vulva surrounded by a delicate collar. Outside the main lesions are a few satellite lesions.*

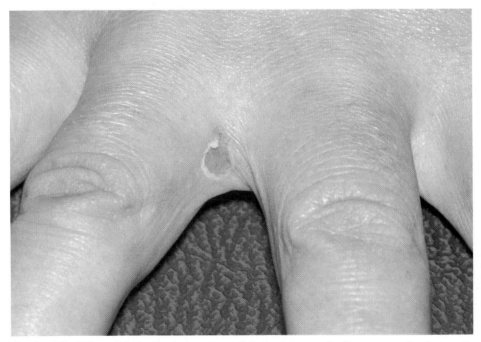

65 Candidiasis (interdigital)   *Erythematous eroded area between the fingers occurring in a waitress.*

MUCOCUTANEOUS CANDIDIASIS   119

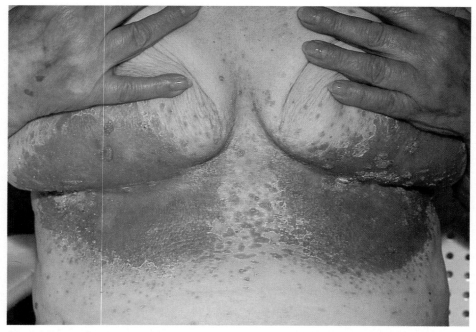

66 Intertrigo *Confluent and discrete, erythematous, eroded areas with pustular and erosive satellite lesions.*

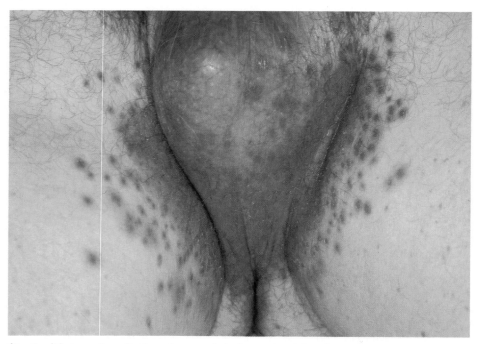

67 *Candida* intertrigo *Erythematous, eroded plaques involving the scrotum and inguinal area with satellite lesions.*

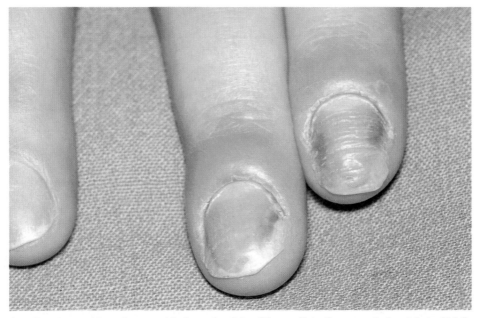

68 Chronic onychia and paronychia from *Candida albicans* Note the warm but not hot, slightly tender, edematous nail fold with some onycholysis. This is very often misdiagnosed as staphylococcal paronychia.

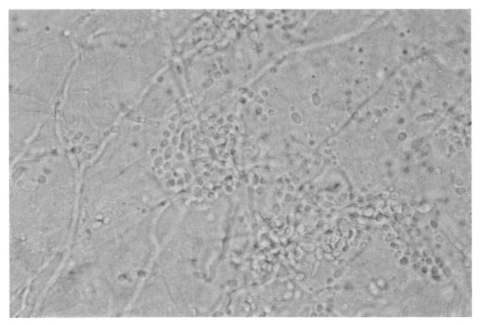

69 *Candida* in potassium hydroxide preparation *Pseudomycelia and clusters of grapelike yeast cells.*

MUCOCUTANEOUS CANDIDIASIS

Tinea versicolor is a chronic asymptomatic superficial fungal infection of the trunk, characterized by white or brown scaling macules.

Synonym: pityriasis versicolor.

EPIDEMIOLOGY AND ETIOLOGY

Age Young adults

Etiology *Pityrosporum orbiculare (ovale)*

Predisposing Factors Climatic factors appear to be important as the disease is far more common in the tropics and in the summer in temperate climates. High levels of cortisol appear to increase susceptibility—both in Cushing's syndrome and with prolonged administration of corticosteroids (topical or systemic).

HISTORY

Duration of Lesions Months to years

Skin Symptoms None

PHYSICAL EXAMINATION

Skin Lesions
TYPE Macule, sharply marginated, with fine scaling that is easily scraped off with the edge of a glass microscope slide
COLOR Brown of varying intensities and hues (Figure 70); off-white macules (Figure 71)
SIZE AND SHAPE Round or oval macules varying in size from 1.0 cm to very large (>30.0 cm)
DISTRIBUTION Scattered discrete lesions
SITES OF PREDILECTION Upper trunk (Figure 70), upper arms, neck, abdomen, axillae, groins, thighs, genitalia. Rarely on the face.

DIFFERENTIAL DIAGNOSIS

Tinea versicolor is recognized by the distribution and shape of the lesions and is easily identified by examination of the scales for fungus. The hypopigmented type may be confused with vitiligo, but careful examination of all the lesions for small areas of focal fine scaling and with Wood's lamp reveals scales with a pale yellow-green fluorescence, and these will contain the fungus.

LABORATORY AND SPECIAL EXAMINATIONS

Direct Microscopic Examination of Scales Prepared with KOH Hyphae and spores referred to as "spaghetti and meatballs"

Wood's Lamp Examination Faint yellow-green fluorescence of scales

PATHOPHYSIOLOGY

Dicarboxylic acids formed by enzymatic oxidation of fatty acids in skin surface lipids inhibit pigment synthesis in epidermal melanocytes and thereby lead to hypomelanosis. The enzyme is present in the organism.

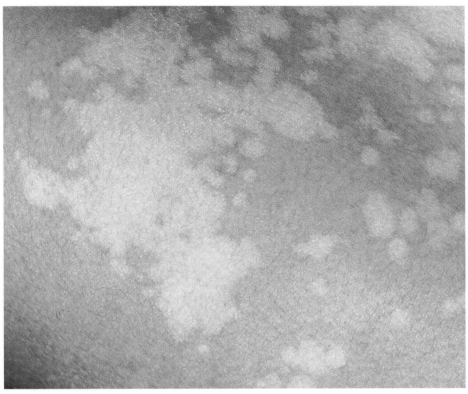

70 Tinea versicolor *There are sharply marginated, uniformly hypopigmented macules with a fine, sometimes barely perceptible scale, but they are easily scraped off with a microscopic slide. When the lesions are very large, as on the left, they can be confused with vitiligo.*

TREATMENT

Topical agents:

- Short applications of selenium sulfide (2.5%) for 12 nights, wash off in 30 minutes. Repeat every 2 weeks.
- Miconazole cream.

- Topical ketoconazole (2%) either as shampoo or cream

Systemic therapy:

- Ketoconazole 200 mg orally daily for 10 days taken with a glass of orange juice on empty stomach

SUPERFICIAL FUNGAL INFECTIONS

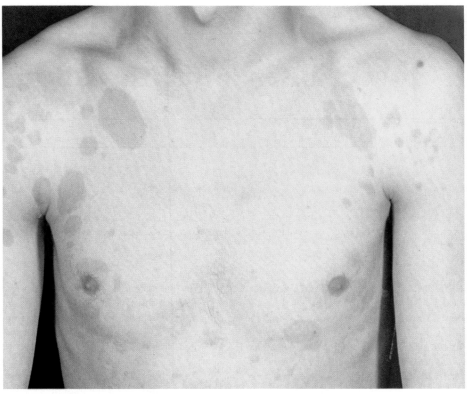

71   Tinea versicolor   *These are hyperpigmented macules which have a fine scale.*

Insect Bites and Infestations

Pediculosis Capitis

Pediculosis capitis is an infestation of the scalp by the head louse, which feeds on the scalp and neck and deposits its eggs on the hair, whose presence is associated with few symptoms but much consternation.

EPIDEMIOLOGY AND ETIOLOGY

Age More common in children, but all ages

Etiology The subspecies of *Pediculus humanus* var. *capitis*. Unlike *P. humanus corporis,* the head louse is not a vector of infectious diseases.

Race More common in whites than blacks

Transmission Shared hats, caps, brushes, combs; head-to-head contact. Epidemics in schools.

HISTORY

Skin Symptoms Pruritus of the back and sides of scalp. Scratching and secondary infection associated with occipital and/or cervical lymphadenopathy.

PHYSICAL EXAMINATION

Skin Lesions
TYPE
> *Head lice* identified with eye or with hand lens. The majority of patients have a population of <10 head lice.

"Nits" (Figure 72), or oval grayish-white egg capsules (1 mm long) firmly cemented to the hairs; vary in number from only a few to thousands. Nits are deposited by head lice on the hair shaft as it emerges from the follicle. With recent infestation, nits are near the scalp; with infestation of long standing, nits may be 10 to 15 cm from scalp. In that scalp hair grows 0.5 mm daily, the presence of nits 15 cm from the scalp indicates that the infestation is approximately 9 months old. New viable eggs have a creamy-yellow color; empty eggshells are white.

Excoriations, crusts, and secondary impetiginized lesions are commonly seen and mask the presence of lice and nits; may extend onto neck, forehead, face, ears. In the extreme, scalp becomes a confluent, purulent mass of matted hair, lice, nits, crusts, and purulent discharge, so-called plica polonica.

Papular urticaria, i.e., site of the louse bite, is sometimes apparent on the neck.

SITES OF PREDILECTION Head lice nearly always confined to scalp, especially occipital and postauricular regions. Head lice may rarely infest beard or other hairy sites.

INSECT BITES AND INFESTATIONS

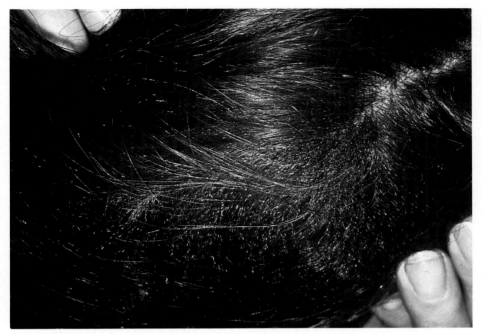

72　Pediculosis capitis　*Myriads of nits (oval, grayish-white egg capsules) are firmly attached to the hair shafts. On close examination these have a bottle shape.*

DIAGNOSIS AND DIFFERENTIAL DIAGNOSIS

Diagnosis　Clinical findings confirmed by detection of nits and/or lice

Differential Diagnosis　Hair casts, hair lacquer, hair gels, dandruff (epidermal scales), impetigo, lichen simplex chronicus

LABORATORY AND SPECIAL EXAMINATIONS

Culture　If impetiginization is suspected, bacterial cultures should be obtained

TREATMENT

Recommended Regimen　Permethrin (1%) rinse applied to scalp and washed off after 10 minutes *or* 0.5% malathion

Alternatives　Pyrethrins with piperonyl butoxide applied to scalp and washed off after 10 minutes *or* 0.5% malathion lotion. Patients should be reevaluated after 1 week if symptoms persist. Re-treatment may be necessary if lice are found or eggs are observed at the hair-skin junction.

Secondary Bacterial Infection　Should be treated with appropriate doses of erythromycin *or* dicloxacillin.

Pediculosis pubis is an infestation of hairy regions, most commonly the pubic area but at times the hairy parts of the chest and axillae and the upper eyelashes; it is manifested clinically by mild to moderate pruritus.

Synonyms: crabs, crab lice, pubic lice.

ETIOLOGY AND EPIDEMIOLOGY

Age   Most common in young adults; range from childhood to senescence

Sex   More extensive infestation in males

Etiology   *Pthirus* or *Phthirus pubis,* the crab or pubic louse. The life cycle from egg to adult is 22 to 27 days: the incubation period for the egg is 7 to 8 days; the rest of the life cycle is taken up with larval and nymphal development. The average life span is 17 days for the female and 22 days for males. Lives exclusively on humans. Prefers a humid environment; does not tend to wander.

Transmission   Close physical contact, such as sexual intercourse; sleeping in same bed; possibly exchange of towels.

HISTORY

Skin Symptoms   May be asymptomatic. Mild to moderate pruritus for months. Patient may note a nodularity to hairs which is detected while scratching. With excoriation and secondary infection, lesions may become tender and be associated with enlarged regional, e.g., inguinal, lymph node.

PHYSICAL EXAMINATION

Skin Lesions
TYPE
> *Lice* appear as 1- to 2-mm, brownish-gray specks (see Figures 73 and 75) in the hairy areas involved. Remain stationary for days; mouth parts embedded in skin; claws grasping a hair on either side. Usually few in number.

> *Eggs (nits)* attached to hair (Figures 73 and 74) appear as tiny white-gray specks. Few to numerous.

> *Papular urticaria* (small erythematous papules) noted at sites of feeding, especially periumbilical; feeding sites may rarely become bullous.

> Secondary changes of *lichenification, excoriations,* and *impetiginized excoriations* detected in patients with significant pruritus. Serous crusts may be present along with lice and nits when eyelids are infested; occasionally edema of eyelids with severe infestation.

> *Maculae caeruleae* (taches bleues) are slate-gray or bluish-gray macules (Figure 76), 0.5 to 1.0 cm in diameter, irregular in shape, nonblanching. Pigment thought to be breakdown product of heme affected by louse saliva.

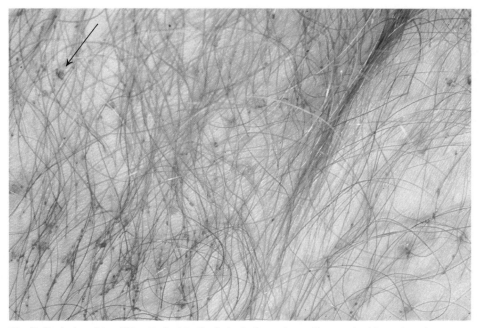

73   Pediculosis pubis   *Nits attached to the hair shaft can be easily seen in this patient, but sometimes only a few are present. There are several crab lice present.*

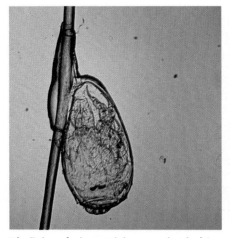

74   Enlarged nit containing an unhatched louse

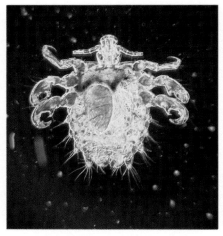

75   *Phthirius pubis*, the crab or pubic louse

DISTRIBUTION   Most commonly found in pubic and axillary areas; also perineum, thighs, lower legs, and trunk, especially periumbilically. In hairy males: nipple areas, upper arms, rarely to wrists; rarely beard and moustache area. In children, eyelashes and eyebrows may be infested without pubic involvement. Maculae caeruleae (see Figure 76) most common on lower abdominal wall, buttocks, upper thighs.

General Findings   With secondary impetiginization, regional lymphadenopathy

DIAGNOSIS AND DIFFERENTIAL DIAGNOSIS

Diagnosis   Clinical diagnosis

Differential Diagnosis   Eczema, tinea, folliculitis; taches bleues: ashy dermatosis

LABORATORY AND SPECIAL EXAMINATIONS

Microscopy   Lice and nits may be identified with hand lens or microscope. See Figures 74 and 75.

Cultures   Bacterial cultures if excoriation impetiginized.

Serology   Patients should be screened with blood tests for syphilis and HIV infection.

TREATMENT

Same as for pediculosis capitis (see p. 127).

Secondary bacterial infection should be treated with appropriate antibiotics.

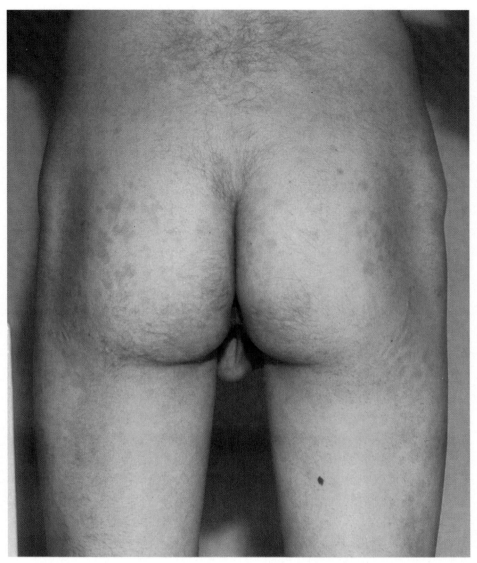

76   Pediculosis pubis   *Maculae cerulae. These are slate-gray or blue-gray macules on the buttocks.*

PEDICULOSIS (PHTHIRIASIS) PUBIS   131

Scabies is a skin infestation by a mite, *Sarcoptes scabiei,* which is usually spread by skin-to-skin contact and causes a generalized intractable pruritus, with frequent secondary bacterial infection. The diagnosis may be easily missed and should be considered in a patient of any age with persistent generalized severe pruritus. Chronic undiagnosed scabies is the basis for the colloquial term "the seven year itch."

EPIDEMIOLOGY AND ETIOLOGY

Age Young adults (often acquired by sexual contact); contact with mite-infested sheets in elderly and bedridden patients in the hospital; children (often 5 years or under).

Other Factors Epidemics of scabies occur in cycles every 15 years, the latest epidemic began in the late 1960s but curiously has continued to the present.

Transmission Scabies is associated with personal skin-to-skin contact, as with sexual promiscuity, crowding, poverty, or as a nosocomial outbreak. The scabies mite can remain alive for over 2 days on clothing or in bedding, and, therefore, scabies can be acquired without skin-to-skin contact.

HISTORY

Duration of Lesions Primary (first) infection has an incubation period of 1 month. In primary infection the itching begins a month after the infection. In this period the patient becomes sensitized against the mite and its products. After a second infection the itching begins immediately because the patient is already sensitized.

Skin Symptoms Intense generalized intractable pruritus, a *sine qua non*. For reasons that are not clear, generalized intense nocturnal pruritus may occur with a minimal number of skin lesions.

PHYSICAL EXAMINATION

Skin Lesions
TYPE *Primary lesions*
"Burrows"—gray or skin-colored ridges, 0.5 to 1.0 cm in length (see Figures 77 and 78), either linear or wavy with a minute vesicle or papule at the end of the burrow

Vesicles—independent of burrows

Nodules—brownish-red, 1 to 2 cm, indurated, indolent (months)

Secondary lesions Small urticarial papules, eczematous plaques, excoriations (Figure 78), and crusts of superimposed bacterial infection
SITES OF PREDILECTION (See Figure IX)
Primary lesions In adults, the scalp, face, and upper back are usually spared, but in infants the scalp, face, palms, and soles are involved.

Burrows—hands (digital webs, palms) (90%) (Figure 77), wrists (flexor), penis, vulva, nipples, natal cleft and buttocks, axillae, toes

Vesicles—sides of fingers

Nodules—scrotum, penis, buttocks, groin, axillary folds (Figure 79), upper back, lateral edge of foot (infants). These lesions, which may be few or many, are firm, red, and 0.5 cm or slightly larger.

Secondary lesions Abdomen, buttocks, thighs

INSECT BITES AND INFESTATIONS

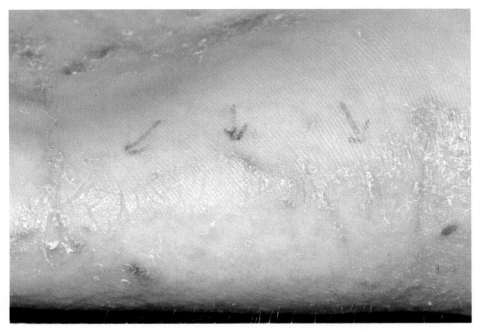

77   Burrows   *There are several, slightly scaling, threadlike burrows (see arrows); these are gray or skin-colored ridges, either linear or wavy, with a minute vesicle or papule at the end of the burrow.*

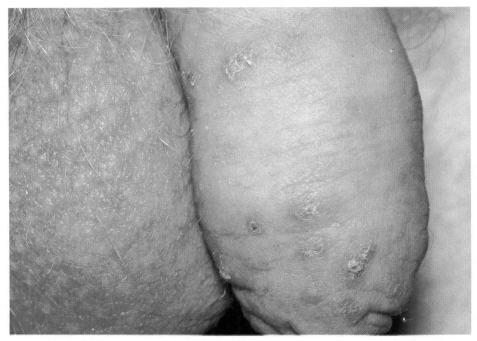

78   Scabies involving the penile shaft   *This is a typical site; there are crusted, excoriated papules.*

SPECIAL FORMS OF SCABIES

1. *Geriatric scabies* Lesions may occur on the back and appear as excoriations.

2. *Nodular scabies* Exclusively on the covered parts of the body: scrotum, penis, buttocks, groin, axillary folds (Figure 79), upper back, lateral edge of foot (infants). These lesions, which may be few or many, are firm, red, 0.5 cm or slightly larger, very pruritic, and may be present for weeks. Nodules do not respond to antiscabetic treatments. Intralesional corticosteroids may be helpful. In refractory lesions, oral PUVA photochemotherapy is said to be effective.

3. *"Crusted" scabies (Norwegian scabies)* Psoriasiform lesions of the palms and soles. Occur in debilitated persons, in persons with Down's syndrome, and immunosuppressed patients (e.g., AIDS).

4. *Animal scabies (dogs)* No burrows, distribution is atypical.

DIFFERENTIAL DIAGNOSIS

Assiduous search for burrows should be made in every patient with severe generalized pruritus. Sometimes when the mite cannot be demonstrated, a "therapeutic test" will clinch the diagnosis.

SPECIAL EXAMINATION TO DETECT MITE

Look with lens for typical burrows on the finger webs, flexor aspects of wrists, and penis.

Look for "dark point" at the end of the burrow—this is the mite (Figure 80).

Open this part of the burrow slowly and the

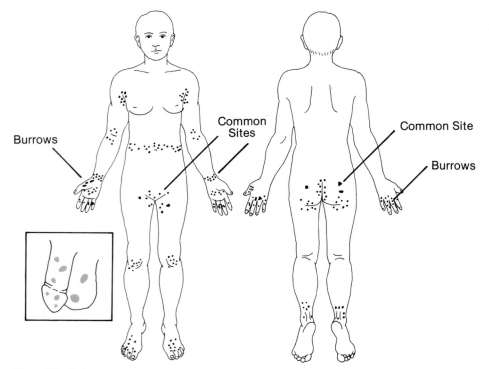

Figure IX   Scabies

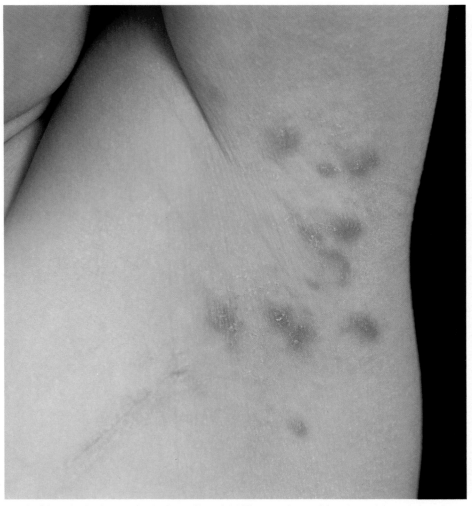

79 Scabies *Scabetic nodules in the axillary fold. These are brownish red, pruritic nodules, almost pathognomonic for scabies.*

mite will stick to the needle and can be easily transferred to the slide.

If there is a nodule, biopsy may reveal portions of the body of the mite in the corneal layer.

TREATMENT

Specific instructions must be given by the physician—and followed by the patient:

1. Bath or shower
2. Apply to the *entire* skin (neck down); in infants the total body is treated. Permethrin 5% cream is applied to the skin for 8 to 12 hours. A second application may be indicated a week later if symptoms are not improved.
3. Change underwear and bed sheets.
4. Take systemic antipruritics (hydroxyzine hydrochloride).
5. Generalized itching that persists a week or more is probably caused by hypersensitivity to remaining dead mites and mite products. Nevertheless, a second treatment 7 days after the first is recommended by some physicians.
6. Treat close family and personal contacts.
7. Secondary infection is quite common and antibiotics may be indicated if there are honey-colored crusts or tender erythema surrounding the lesions.
8. Nodular lesions may persist for weeks following treatment and need special attention, usually with intralesional corticosteroid suspensions or PUVA photochemotherapy.

INSECT BITES AND INFESTATIONS

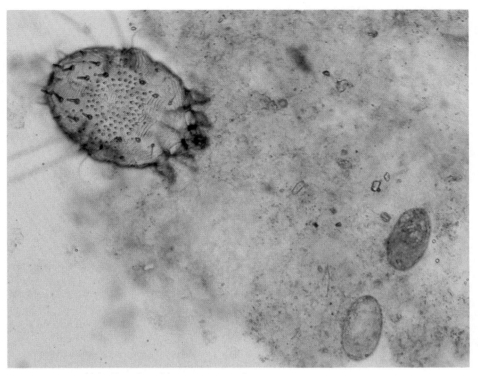

80   *Sarcoptes scabiei   Female, with two eggs nearby.*

Cutaneous reaction to flea bites (CRFB) is an immunologically mediated reaction, characterized by an intensely pruritic eruption occurring at the bite sites hours to days after the bites, manifested by grouped urticarial papules, papulovesicles, and/or bullae which persist for days to weeks; patients are unaware of being bitten.

EPIDEMIOLOGY AND ETIOLOGY

Age   Any age but more common in children

Season   Summer in temperate climates

Etiology   The cat flea *Ctenocephalides felis,* the dog flea *C. canis,* human fleas of the *Pulex* and *Xenopsylla* species, fowl fleas of the *Ceratophyllus* species

HISTORY

Incubation Period   CRFB appears hours to days after the bite

Duration of Lesions   Days, weeks

Skin Symptoms   Individuals are not aware of being bitten by fleas. Most patients who present with CRFB are incredulous when first given the diagnosis. Their association is with poor housekeeping practices or poor personal hygiene. Fleas commonly live in carpeting, emerging to hop onto and bite the lower legs. If dogs or cats are allowed onto furniture or bed, bites may occur on the trunk. Individuals holding the animal may have bites on the frontal chest. CRFB is associated with intermittent, mild to severe, intense pruritus. Several members of a household may have similar lesions.

PHYSICAL EXAMINATION

Skin Lesions
TYPES   *Erythematous macules*   Occur at bite sites and are usually transient.

Papular urticaria   Persistent urticarial papules, some surmounted by a vesicle (Figure 81), usually less than 1.0 cm (lesions persist more than 48 hours). Excoriations and excoriated urticarial papules, vesicles. Crusted painful lesions, usually purulent, may represent impetigo, ecthyma, or cutaneous diphtheria. Excoriated or secondarily infected lesions may heal with hyper- or hypopigmentation, and/or raised or depressed scars, especially in more darkly pigmented individuals.

Bullous lesions   Tense bullae with clear fluid on a slightly inflamed base (Figure 82). Excoriation results in large erosive lesions.

COLOR   Red. Bullae have clear amber fluid.

SHAPE   Round. Domed.

ARRANGEMENT   Usually in groups of three ("breakfast, lunch, and dinner") (see Figure 81). Lesions may be clustered around areas where clothing is restricted.

DISTRIBUTION

Extent   Generalized groups or clusters

Pattern   The most common sites are the legs from ankles to knees. Thighs, forearms and arms, lower part of trunk, and waist, but sparing anogenital area and axillae.

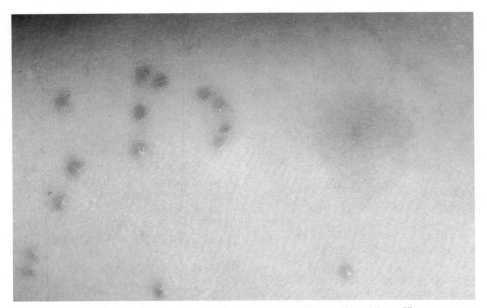

81   Papular urticaria   *Persistent urticaria-like papules, usually less than 1.0 cm. There are some excoriated papules also. Some lesions have a vesicle on the top, others an erosion or crust.*

DIAGNOSIS AND DIFFERENTIAL DIAGNOSIS

Diagnosis Clinical diagnosis at times confirmed by lesional biopsy

Differential Diagnosis Allergic contact dermatitis, especially to plants such as poison ivy or poison oak. Papular urticaria also follows bites of mites, bedbugs, mosquitoes.

LABORATORY AND SPECIAL EXAMINATIONS

Cultures Bacterial cultures are indicated if secondary infection is considered.

Dermatopathology *Epidermis:* intercellular and intracellular edema and occasional spongiotic vesicle. *Dermis:* chronic deep inflammatory infiltrate, perivascular, with eosinophils.

PATHOGENESIS

The cutaneous lesion following an arthropod bite is caused by an immunologic tissue response to an injected arthropodal antigen.

COURSE AND PROGNOSIS

Excoriation of CRFB commonly results in secondary infection of the eroded epidermis by group A β-hemolytic streptococcus, and/or *Staphylococcus aureus* causing impetigo or ecthyma. This is especially common in humid tropical climates. Less common is secondary infection with *Corynebacterium diphtheriae,* with resultant cutaneous diphtheria. Streptococcal skin infections are, at times, complicated by glomerulonephritis.

At times, fleas are vectors for infectious agents causing the following flea-borne diseases: bubonic plague, tularemia, murine typhus, boutonneuse fever, Q fever, lymphocytic choriomeningitis, tick-borne encephalitis.

TREATMENT AND PREVENTION

Avoidance of contact with cats and dogs

Treatment of cats and dogs for fleas

Spraying the household with insecticides (e.g., malathion 1 to 4% dust) with special attention to baseboards, rugs, floors, upholstered furniture, bed frames, mattresses, and cellar

Potent topical corticosteroids given for a short time are helpful for intensely pruritic lesions. Rarely, a short tapered course of oral corticosteroids can be given for extensive CRFB that is persistent.

Antibiotic treatment with topical agents such as mupirocin or antistaphylococcal/antistreptococcal agents if secondary infection is present.

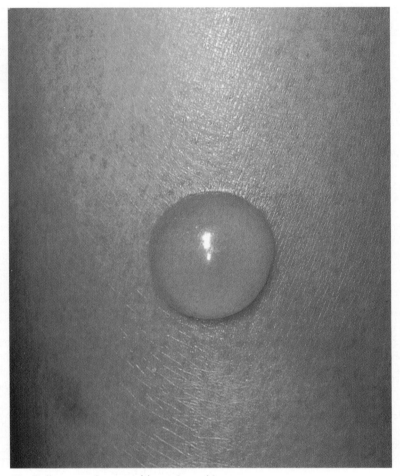

82   Bullous eruption caused by an insect bite

Cutaneous larva migrans is a cutaneous lesion produced by percutaneous penetration and migration of larvae of various nematode parasites, characterized by erythematous, serpiginous, papular or vesicular linear lesions corresponding to the movements of the larvae beneath the skin.
Synonym: creeping eruption.

ETIOLOGY AND EPIDEMIOLOGY

Etiology *Ancylostoma braziliense* in central and southeastern United States; *A. caninum, Uncinaria stenocephala* (hookworm of dogs), *Bunostomum phlebotomum* (hookworm of cattle); also *A. duodenale, Necator americanus.*

Epidemiology Ova of hookworms are deposited in sand and soil in warm, shady areas, hatching into larvae which penetrate human skin. Persons at risk include gardeners, farmers, sea bathers.

HISTORY

Skin Symptoms Local pruritus begins within hours after larval penetration.

PHYSICAL EXAMINATION

Skin Lesions
TYPE Serpiginous, thin, linear, raised, tunnel-like lesion 2 to 3 mm wide containing serous fluid (Figure 83). Several or many lesions may be present depending on the number of penetrating larvae. Larvae move a few to many millimeters daily, confined to an area several centimeters in diameter.
COLOR Erythematous
DISTRIBUTION Exposed sites, most commonly the feet and buttocks

Variant
LARVA CURRENS Caused by *Strongyloides stercoralis.* Papules, urticaria, papulovesicles at the site of larval penetration. Associated with intense pruritus. Occurs on skin around anus, buttocks, thighs, back, shoulders, abdomen. Pruritus and eruption disappear when larvae enter blood vessels and migrate to intestinal mucosa.

Systemic Findings Visceral larva migrans characterized by persistent hypereosinophilia, hepatomegaly, and frequently pneumonitis. Caused by *Toxocara canis, T. cati, A. lumbricoides*

DIAGNOSIS

Clinical findings

COURSE

Self-limited; humans are "dead-end" hosts. Most larvae die and the lesions resolve within 4 to 6 weeks.

TREATMENT

Thiabendazole topically and/or orally 50 mg per kg body weight per day in 2 doses (maximum, 3 g/day) for 2 to 5 days; liquid nitrogen applied to progressing end of larval burrow.

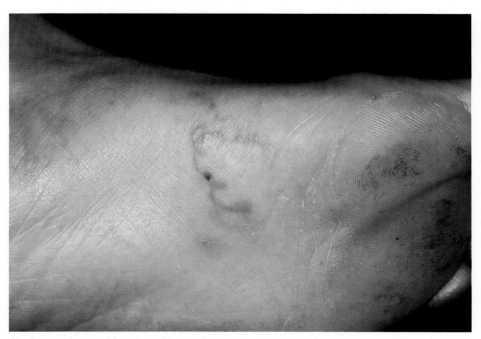

83   Larva migrans   *There is a thin, erythematous, serpiginous (snakelike), papular eruption.*

Benign Neoplasms and Hyperplasias

Seborrheic Keratosis

This very common, hereditary, benign tumor is usually pigmented; it occurs after age 30, especially on the trunk and face.

EPIDEMIOLOGY AND ETIOLOGY

Age   Rarely before 30 years of age

Sex   Slightly more common and more profuse in males

Other Features   Probably autosomal dominant inheritance

HISTORY

Duration of Lesions   Usually months to years

Skin Symptoms   Rarely pruritic; tender if secondarily infected

PHYSICAL EXAMINATION

Skin Lesions
TYPE *Early*   Small, 1.0- to 3.0-mm, barely elevated papule or plaque with or *without* pigment (Figure 84). The surface shows, with 7x to 10x magnification, fine stippling like the surface of a thimble.
Late   Plaque with warty surface and "stuck on" appearance (Figure 85), "greasy"; with a hand lens (7x to 10x) horn cysts can be seen often. Size from 1.0 to 6.0 cm (see Figure 85).
COLOR   Brown, gray, black, skin-colored
SHAPE   Round, oval
ARRANGEMENT   Scattered, discrete lesions
DISTRIBUTION   Isolated lesion or generalized
SITES OF PREDILECTION   Face, trunk (Figure 85), upper extremities

DIFFERENTIAL DIAGNOSIS

Early "flat" lesions confused with *solar lentigo* or *spreading pigmented actinic keratosis* (surface of seborrheic keratosis is more verrucous, also horn cysts are present); larger pigmented lesions are easily mistaken for *pigmented basal cell carcinoma* or *malignant melanoma* (only biopsy will settle this).

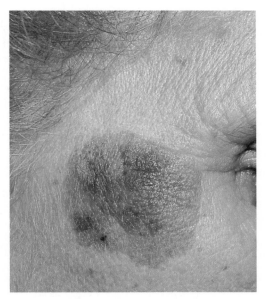

84   Seborrheic keratosis   *Large, slightly elevated, warty, keratotic, brown plaque. The lesion appears "stuck on" the skin.*

DERMATOPATHOLOGY

Site Epidermis

Process Proliferation of keratinocytes (with marked papillomatosis) and melanocytes, formation of horn cysts

TREATMENT

Light electrocautery will permit the whole lesion to appear to be easily rubbed off. Then the base can be lightly cauterized to prevent recurrence. Cryosurgery with liquid nitrogen spray.

BENIGN NEOPLASMS AND HYPERPLASIAS

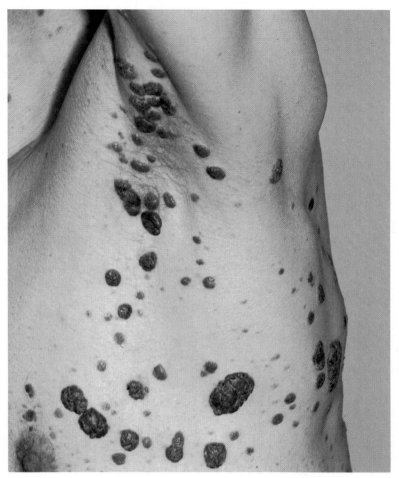

85 Seborrheic keratosis *A large number of pigmented lesions over the chest and back. These are dark brown, waxy, keratotic, and sharply demarcated, but some are light brown, yellowish, and flatter. All have a "stuck-on" appearance, giving the impression they can be picked off.*

Keratoacanthoma is a self-healing, rapidly developing, benign epithelial neoplasm that mimics squamous cell carcinoma.

EPIDEMIOLOGY

Age Over 50 years; rare below 20 years

Sex Males

Race Caucasians, rare in Orientals

HISTORY

Duration of Lesions Rapid growth, achieving a size of 2.5 cm within 6 weeks

Skin Symptoms None

PHYSICAL EXAMINATION

Skin Lesions
TYPE Nodule, dome-shaped often with a central keratotic plug (Figure 86)
COLOR Skin-colored or slightly red
PALPATION Firm but not hard
SIZE AND SHAPE 2.5 cm (range: 1.0 to 10.0 cm)
DISTRIBUTION Isolated single lesion. Uncommonly, may be multiple, eruptive.
SITES OF PREDILECTION Cheeks, nose, ears, and hands (dorsa)

DIFFERENTIAL DIAGNOSIS

Squamous cell carcinoma—a biopsy must be done as it is impossible to make a clinical distinction between keratoacanthoma and squamous cell carcinoma.

DERMATOPATHOLOGY

Site Epidermis

Process Proliferative. Central, large, irregularly shaped crater filled with keratin. The surrounding epidermis extends in a liplike manner over the sides of the crater. The keratinocytes are atypical, with many mitoses, and many are dyskeratotic.

PATHOPHYSIOLOGY

HPV has been identified in some keratoacanthomas. Other etiologic factors include ultraviolet radiation and chemical carcinogens (industrial: pitch and tar).

COURSE AND PROGNOSIS

Spontaneous regression in 2 to 6 months or sometimes more than 1 year

TREATMENT

The regressed lesion may result in a rather disfiguring scar; surgical excision or curettage followed by electrocautery is thus recommended. Histologic confirmation of the clinical diagnosis is important as this lesion can mimic squamous cell carcinoma.

BENIGN NEOPLASMS AND HYPERPLASIAS

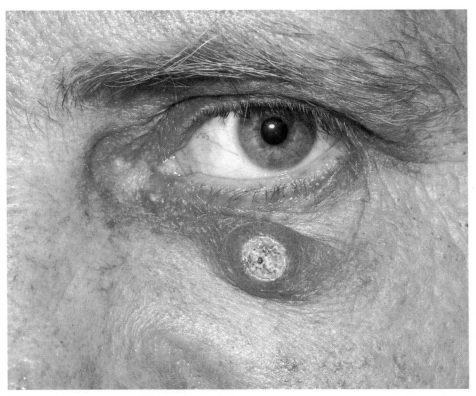

86 Keratoacanthoma *Oval, erythematous, violaceous tumor, 3.0 cm in diameter, with a horny plug in the center.*

Melanocytic nevocellular nevi are small (<1.0 cm), circumscribed, acquired pigmented macules or papules comprised of groups of melanocytic nevus cells located in the epidermis, dermis, and, rarely, subcutaneous tissue.

EPIDEMIOLOGY

Race
One of the most common acquired new growths in Caucasians (most adults have about 20 nevi), less common in blacks or pigmented peoples.

Dysplastic nevi, which are precursor lesions of malignant melanoma, occur in 30% of patients with primary melanoma and in 6% of their family members.

HISTORY

Duration of Lesions These lesions, which are commonly called *moles,* appear in early childhood and reach a maximum in young adulthood. There is a gradual involution of lesions and most disappear by age 60 (the dermal melanocytic nevocellular nevus does not disappear).

Skin Symptoms Nevocellular nevi are asymptomatic, and if a lesion begins to itch or is tender, it should be carefully followed, as pruritus, for example, may be an early indication of malignant change.

CLASSIFICATION

Nevocellular nevi (NCN) can be classified according to the site of the clusters of nevus cells.

Junctional Melanocytic NCN Cells at dermoepidermal junction above basement membrane (see Figure 87).

Dermal Melanocytic NCN Cells exclusively in the dermis (see page 153 and Figure 88)

Compound Melanocytic NCN A combination of the histologic features of the junctional and dermal (see Figure 89)

Junctional Melanocytic Nevocellular Nevi (Figure 87)

Skin Lesions
TYPE Macule, or only very slightly raised
SIZE If >1.0 cm, the mole is a congenital nevomelanocytic nevus or a dysplastic melanocytic nevus.
COLOR Uniform tan, brown, or dark brown
SHAPE Round or oval with smooth regular borders

ARRANGEMENT Scattered discrete lesions
DISTRIBUTION Random
SITES OF PREDILECTION Palms and soles, trunk, upper extremities, face, lower extremities

BENIGN NEOPLASMS AND HYPERPLASIAS

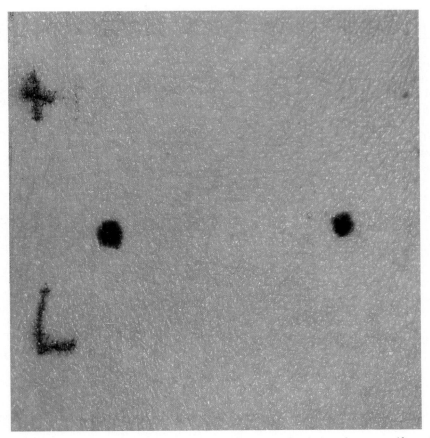

87　Junctional melanocytic nevomelanocytic nevus　*These macular lesions have a uniform tan, brown, or dark-brown color; there are round, smooth, regular borders.*

Skin Lesions

TYPE   Papule (Figure 88)

COLOR   Skin-colored, tan, brown, or flecks of brown, often with telangiectasia

SHAPE   Round, dome-shaped (Figure 88)

DISTRIBUTION   More common on the face and neck but can occur on the trunk or extremities

OTHER FEATURES   Usually appear in the second or third decade and do not spontaneously disappear

DIFFERENTIAL DIAGNOSIS

Dermal nevi are almost indistinguishable from basal cell carcinoma.

TREATMENT

Indications for removal of acquired melanocytic NCN are:

1. *Site*—lesions on the scalp, soles, all mucous membranes, anogenital area; any mole that is constantly exposed to trauma

2. *Color*—if color is or becomes variegated

3. *Border*—if irregularly irregular borders are present

4. *Symptoms*—if lesion begins to persistently itch, hurt, or bleed

These criteria are based on anatomic sites at risk for change of acquired nevi to malignant melanoma *or* changes in individual lesions (color, border) that indicate the development of a focus of cells with *dysplasia,* the precursor of malignant melanoma. Clark's dysplastic melanocytic nevi are *usually* >6.0 mm and darker, with distinctive variegation of color (tan, brown), and have irregularly irregular borders. These lesions occur over the trunk and upper extremities but also on the buttocks, groins, scalp, and female breasts.

Melanocytic NCN, if treated, should always be excised for histologic diagnosis and for definitive treatment. Electrocautery should never be used for removal.

See "Recommendations for the Management of Pigmented Lesions to Facilitate Early Diagnosis of Malignant Melanoma" in Appendix E.

Skin Lesions   Same color and shape as junctional melanocytic NCN except that they are not commonly seen on the palms and soles and are always distinctively elevated (papules).

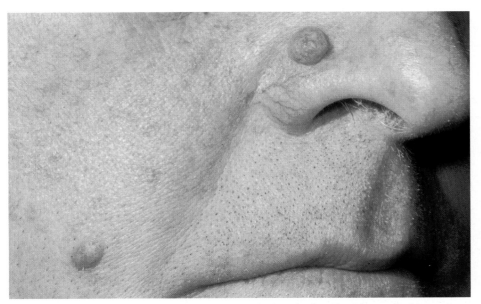

88 Dermal melanocytic nevus *There are two nevi; both are soft, pale red, pea-sized tumors.*

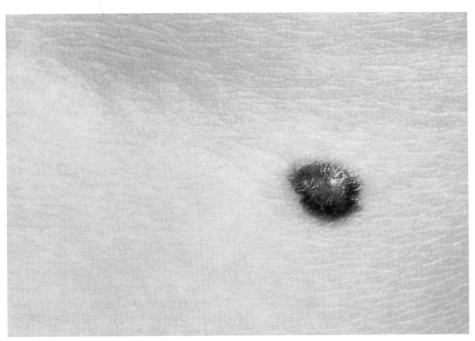

89 Compound melanocytic nevocellular nevus *This is a uniform, slightly elevated, dark-brown to black papule. The borders are only slightly irregular.*

COMMON MELANOCYTIC NEVOCELLULAR NEVI (MOLES) 153

This lesion is a nevomelanocytic nevus that is encircled by a halo of leukoderma. The leukoderma is based on a decrease of melanin in melanocytes at the dermoepidermal junction. Halo nevi often undergo spontaneous involution and often with regression of the centrally located pigmented nevus.

Synonym: Sutton's leukoderma acquisitum centrifugum.

EPIDEMIOLOGY AND ETIOLOGY

Age First three decades

Race and Sex All races, both sexes

Incidence In patients with vitiligo, 18 to 26%

Family History Halo nevi occur in siblings and with history of vitiligo in family

Associated Disorders Vitiligo, metastatic melanoma (around lesions and around nevus cell nevi)

"Halo" Depigmentation Around Other Lesions Blue nevus, congenital garment nevus cell nevus, Spitz's juvenile nevus, verruca plana, primary melanoma, dermatofibroma, and neurofibroma

HISTORY

Three Stages
1. Development (in months) of halo around preexisting nevus cell nevus
2. Disappearance (months to years) of nevus cell nevus
3. Repigmentation (months to years) of halo

PHYSICAL EXAMINATION

Skin Lesions
TYPE Papular brown nevus cell nevus (5.0 mm) with halo of sharply marginated hypomelanosis (Figure 90) The nevus is centrally located.
SHAPE Oval hypomelanosis (Figure 90).
ARRANGEMENT Scattered discrete lesions (1 to 90)
DISTRIBUTION Trunk (same as distribution of nevus cell nevus)

DERMATOPATHOLOGY AND ELECTRON MICROSCOPY

Nevus Cell Nevus Junctional dermal or compound nevus surrounded by lymphocytic infiltrate (lymphocytes and histiocytes) around and between nevus cells. Nevus cells develop evidence of cell damage and disappear.

Halo Epidermis Decrease or total absence of melanin and melanocytes (as shown by electron microscopy)

PATHOPHYSIOLOGY

Immunologic phenomena are responsible for the dynamic changes through the action of circulating cytotoxic antibodies and/or cytotoxic lymphocytes. This disease awaits a reevaluation using newer techniques.

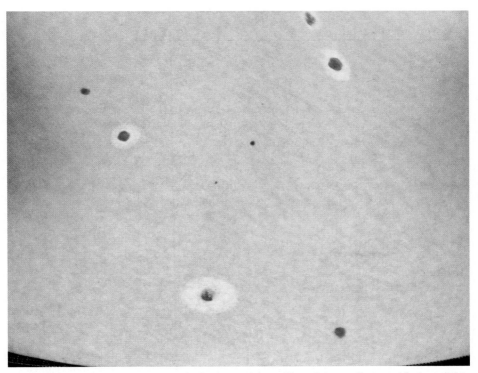

90   Halo nevus   *Disseminated over the back are eight uniform, brown, pigmented lesions, 2.0 to 5.0 mm in diameter. The lesions are slightly elevated and sharply demarcated; four are surrounded by a sharply marginated white zone 2.0 to 5.0 mm in diameter.*

TREATMENT

None. The lesions undergo spontaneous resolution. Nevus cell nevi must always be evaluated for clinical criteria of malignancy (variegation of pigment and irregular borders) as a "halo" can and does occasionally develop around primary malignant melanoma.

A blue nevus is an acquired, benign, firm, dark-blue to gray-to-black, sharply defined papule or nodule representing a localized proliferation of melanin-producing dermal melanocytes.

Synonyms: blue neuronevus, dermal melanocytoma.

EPIDEMIOLOGY AND ETIOLOGY

Age   Onset in late adolescence

Sex   Equal distribution

Variants   Cellular blue nevus, combined blue nevus-nevomelanocytic nevus

HISTORY

Nearly always asymptomatic, occasionally of cosmetic concern. Appearance gradual and often not observed by patient or parents.

PHYSICAL EXAMINATION

Skin Lesions
TYPE   Papules to nodules usually <10.0 mm in diameter (Figure 91)
COLOR   Blue, blue-gray, blue-black. Occasionally has targetlike pattern of pigmentation
SHAPE   Usually round to oval
PALPATION   Firm
SITES OF PREDILECTION   Most common on dorsa of hands or feet; may occur at any site.

DIAGNOSIS AND DIFFERENTIAL DIAGNOSIS

Diagnosis   Usually made on clinical findings, at times confirmed by excision and dermatopathologic examination.

Differential Diagnosis   Dermatofibroma, glomus tumor, primary or metastatic melanoma, pigmented spindle cell (Spitz's) nevus, traumatic tattoo

DERMATOPATHOLOGY

Melanin-containing fibroblast-like dermal melanocytes grouped in irregular bundles admixed with melanin-containing macrophages; excessive fibrous tissue production in upper reticular dermis. Epidermis normal.

PATHOGENESIS

Probably represents ectopic accumulations of melanin-producing melanocytes in the dermis during their migration from neural crest to sites in the skin.

COURSE AND PROGNOSIS

Most remain unchanged but may regress spontaneously.

TREATMENT

Blue nevi smaller than 10.0 mm in diameter and stable for many years usually do not need excision. Sudden appearance or change of an apparent blue nevus warrants surgical excision and dermatopathologic examination.

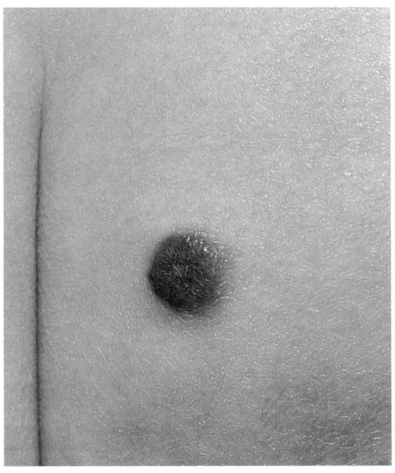

91 Common blue nevus *This is a solitary, asymptomatic, blue and blue-gray nodule.*

A port-wine stain (PWS) is an irregularly shaped, red or violaceous, macular, vascular malformation of dermal blood vessels which is present at birth and never disappears spontaneously; the malformation is usually confined to the skin but may be associated with vascular malformations in the eye and leptomeninges (Sturge-Weber syndrome).

Synonym: nevus flammeus.

EPIDEMIOLOGY

Age Congenital

Clinical Variants

Nevus flammeus nuchae (stork bite, erythema nuchae, salmon patch) occurs in approximately one-third of infants and tends to regress spontaneously. Similar lesions occur on eyelids and glabella.

Sturge-Weber syndrome (SWS) is the association of PWS with vascular malformations in the eye and leptomeninges and superficial calcifications of the brain.

Klippel-Trénaunay-Weber syndrome may have an associated PWS overlying the deeper vascular malformation of soft tissue and bone.

PWS on the midline back may be associated with an underlying arteriovenous malformation of the spinal cord.

HISTORY

Skin Symptoms None

Systemic Symptoms SWS may be associated with contralateral hemiparesis, muscular hemiatrophy, epilepsy, mental retardation; glaucoma and ocular palsy may occur.

PHYSICAL EXAMINATION

Skin Lesions
TYPE In infancy and childhood, PWS are macular. With increasing age of the patient, papules or nodules often develop, leading to significant disfigurement.

COLOR Varying hues of pink to purple (Figure 92).

SHAPE Irregular. Large lesions follow a dermatomal distribution and rarely cross the midline.

DISTRIBUTION Most commonly involve the face but may occur at any cutaneous site. In SWS, PWS occurs in the distribution of the trigeminal nerve, usually the superior and middle branches; mucosal involvement of conjunctiva and mouth may occur.

PATTERN Dermatomal in SWS

DIAGNOSIS

Made on clinical findings

LABORATORY AND SPECIAL EXAMINATIONS

Dermatopathology Developmental defect leading to ectasia of capillaries. No proliferation of endothelial cells.

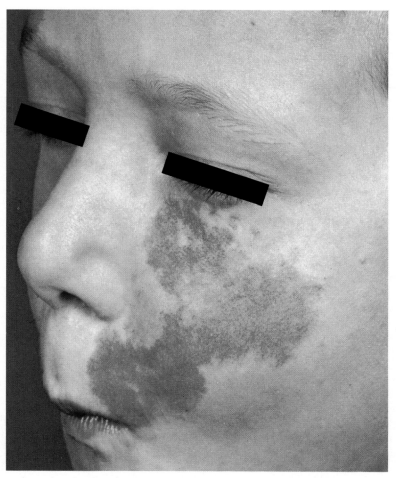

92 Port-wine stain   *On the left cheek is an extensive, macular, red to purplish-red lesion which is not indurated or elevated and which blanches under pressure. On close examination numerous telangiectases are seen.*

Radiography In SWS, skull x-rays show characteristic calcifications of angiomas or localized linear calcification along cerebral convolutions. CT scan should be done.

lar areas and are the cause of significant progressive cosmetic disfigurement.

TREATMENT

COURSE AND PROGNOSIS

PWSs do not regress spontaneously. The area of involvement tends to increase in proportion to the size of the child. In adulthood, PWSs usually become raised with papular and nodu-

- During the macular phase, PWS can be covered with makeup such as Covermark.

- Treatment with tunable dye or copper vapor lasers is very effective and increasingly available.

A capillary hemangioma of infancy (CHI) is a soft, bright-red to deep-purple, vascular nodule-to-plaque that develops at birth or soon after birth and disappears spontaneously by the fifth year.

Synonyms: strawberry nevus or mark, angiomatous nevus.

HISTORY

Duration of Lesion Lesion appears within the first month of life in the majority of patients and always by the ninth month. There is a rapid enlargement during the first year.

PHYSICAL EXAMINATION

Skin Lesions

TYPE Nodule, plaque, 1.0 to 8.0 cm. With the onset of spontaneous regression, a white-to-gray area appears on the surface of the central part of the lesion. Ulceration may occur with rapid regression. Ulcerated lesions may become secondarily infected. Multiple CHI may be associated with hemangiomas of CNS, GI tract, and/or liver.

COLOR The superficial CHI is bright red (Figure 93a); the deeper CHI is purple and lobulated.

PALPATION Soft or moderately firm, depending on the proportionate amount of vascular and fibrous elements. On diascopy, does not blanch completely.

DISTRIBUTION Localized or extending over an entire region (Figure 93a).

SITES OF PREDILECTION Face, trunk, legs, oral and vaginal mucous membrane

DIAGNOSIS AND DIFFERENTIAL DIAGNOSIS

Diagnosis Made on clinical findings

Differential Diagnosis The distinction between a *CHI* and a *cavernous angioma* is based on color and depth. Mixed angiomas (both superficial and deep) may occur.

DERMATOPATHOLOGY

Proliferation of endothelial cells in varying amounts in the dermis and/or subcutaneous tissue: there is more endothelial proliferation in the superficial type, and in the deep angiomas there is little or no endothelial proliferation.

PATHOPHYSIOLOGY

CHI is a localized proliferation of angioblastic mesenchyme.

COURSE AND PROGNOSIS

CHI spontaneously involutes by the fifth year, with some few percent disappearing only by age 10. There is virtually no residual skin change at the site in most lesions (80%) (see Figures 93a and 93b); in the rest there is a residual atrophy, depigmentation, and infiltration. Deeper lesions, especially those involving mucous membranes, may not involute completely. Synovial involvement may be associated with hemophilia-like arthropathy. Large CHI, usually associated with cavernous hemangiomas, may have platelet entrapment and thrombocytopenia (Kasabach-Merritt syndrome, see page 752). Rarely, morbidity associated with CHI occurs secondary to hemorrhage or high-output heart failure.

TREATMENT

Each lesion must be judged individually regarding the decision to treat or not to treat and the selection of a treatment mode. Surgical or

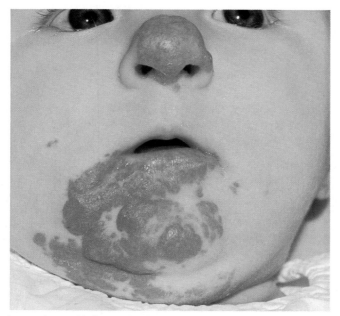

93*a* Capillary hemangioma of infancy *Bright red, nodular lesions with a smooth surface on the nose, chin, and neck of a child aged 4 months.*

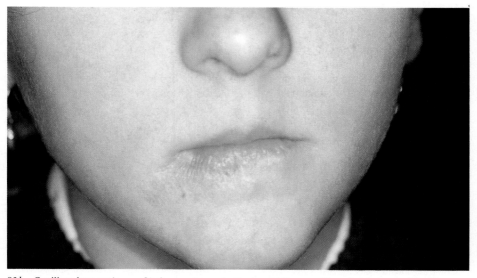

93*b* Capillary hemangioma of infancy *Same patient aged 5 years. There has been a virtually complete spontaneous remission with no scarring on the nose and very slight scarring on the right portion of the lip and chin.*

medical interventions include either continuous wave or pulsed dye laser, cryosurgery, or systemic corticosteroids. When possible, treatment should be avoided because spontaneous resolution gives the best cosmetic results.

CAPILLARY HEMANGIOMA OF INFANCY

A cavernous hemangioma (CH) is a deep vascular malformation, characterized by soft compressible deep-tissue swelling, which, at times, is associated with surface varicosities, arteriovenous shunts, or nevus flammeus-like changes.

ETIOLOGY AND EPIDEMIOLOGY

Age Lesions are not apparent at birth but become so during childhood.

HISTORY

Lesions usually asymptomatic except for cosmetic appearance. Limb hypertrophy may interfere with function.

PHYSICAL EXAMINATION

Skin Findings

TYPE Soft-tissue swelling, dome-shaped or multinodular (Figure 94). When vascular malformation extends to the epidermis, surface may be verrucous. Borders poorly defined. Considerable variation in size.

COLOR Often, normal skin color. Nodular portion blue to purple (Figure 94).

PALPATION Easily compressed, fills promptly when pressure released. Some types may be tender.

Variants

VASCULAR HAMARTOMAS CH with deep soft-tissue involvement and resultant swelling or diffuse enlargement of extremity. May involve skeletal muscle with muscle atrophy. Cutaneous changes include dilated tortuous veins and arteriovenous fistulas.

KLIPPEL-TRENAUNAY-WEBER SYNDROME Local overgrowth of soft tissue and bone with resultant enlargement of an extremity. Associated cutaneous changes include phlebectasia, arteriovenous aneurysms, and nevus flammeus-like cutaneous telangiectasia. Associated developmental abnormalities: nevus unius lateris, syndactylism, polydactylism.

BLUE RUBBER BLEB NEVUS Spontaneously painful and/or tender, compressible, soft, blue swelling in dermis and subcutaneous tissue. Size ranges from few millimeters to several centimeters. May exhibit localized hyperhidrosis over CH. Occur, often multiply, on trunk and upper arms. Similar vascular lesions occur in GI tract and may be a source of hemorrhage.

MAFFUCCI'S SYNDROME CH associated with dyschondroplasia, manifested as hard nodules on fingers or toes, bony deformities. Some CH may be blue rubber bleb variant.

DIAGNOSIS

Clinical diagnosis, at times, confirmed by arteriography

LABORATORY AND SPECIAL EXAMINATIONS

Dermatopathology Dilated, blood-filled vascular spaces lined with flattened endothelial cells. Vessels may be of cavernous, capillary, venous, and lymphatic types.

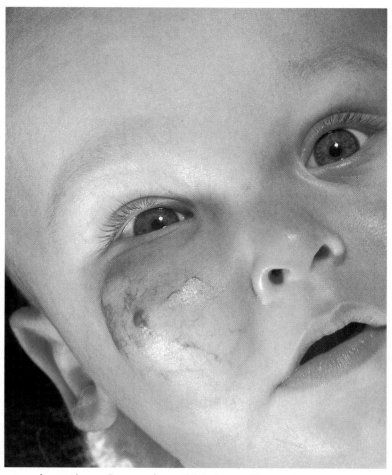

94 Cavernous hemangioma *Large, soft, semiglobular swelling with smooth surface. The color ranges from pale to purple; in the center is a small hemangioma in a 6-month-old child. At the age of 8 years this lesion entirely disappeared without scarring or discoloration.*

COURSE AND PROGNOSIS

CH may be complicated by ulceration and bleeding, scarring, secondary infection, and high-output heart failure in large lesions. Platelet sequestration and destruction may result in thrombocytopenia (Kasabach-Merritt syndrome, see page 752).

Cherry angiomas are exceedingly common, bright-red, domed vascular lesions, occurring on the trunk, becoming more numerous with advancing age, of no consequence other than their cosmetic appearance.

Synonyms: Campbell de Morgan spots, cherry (hem)-angioma.

EPIDEMIOLOGY AND ETIOLOGY

Age Middle aged to elderly

Sex Equal

Etiology Unknown. Very common with aging

HISTORY

Skin Symptoms Usually asymptomatic. May bleed and become crusted if traumatized.

PHYSICAL EXAMINATION

Skin Findings

TYPE Domed papule (Figure 95); surface dull to shiny; from barely perceptible to 8.0 mm in diameter.
COLOR Bright red to violaceous (Figure 95)
SHAPE Usually hemispherical, dome-shaped
PALPATION Soft, compressible. Often blanches completely with pressure.
SITES OF PREDILECTION Trunk, proximal extremities

DIAGNOSIS AND DIFFERENTIAL DIAGNOSIS

Diagnosis Clinical diagnosis

Differential Diagnosis Angiokeratoma (especially on genital skin), venous lake, pyogenic granuloma, nodular amelanotic melanoma, metastatic carcinoma (especially hypernephroma) to skin

DERMATOPATHOLOGY

Numerous moderately dilated capillaries lined by flattened endothelial cells; stroma edematous with homogenization of collagen. Epidermis thinned.

COURSE AND PROGNOSIS

Begin to appear in early adulthood, becoming more numerous with advancing age.

TREATMENT

Electro- or laser coagulation if indicated cosmetically.

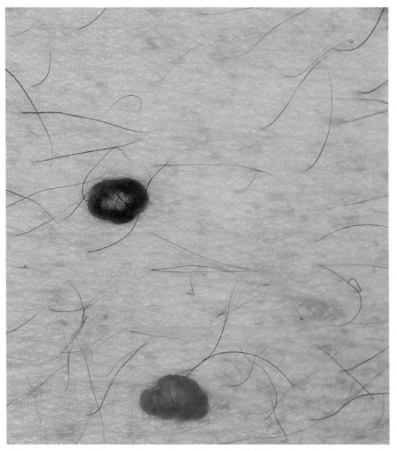

95   Senile hemangioma   *These are dome-shaped papules, bright-red to violaceous, soft and compressible.*

A venous lake is an angiomatous, dark-blue to violaceous dilatation occurring on the face, lips, and ears of elderly patients.

EPIDEMIOLOGY AND ETIOLOGY

Age Usually older than 50 years

Sex Equal incidence in males and females

Etiology Unknown

HISTORY

Skin Syndromes Asymptomatic. Bleeding if traumatized

PHYSICAL EXAMINATION

Skin Findings
TYPE Papule to nodule (Figure 96). Surface may be irregularly cobblestoned.
COLOR Dark blue to purple (Figure 96) with some variegation of color
SHAPE Round or oval
PALPATION Soft, completely compressible
SITES OF PREDILECTION Ears, face, lips

DIAGNOSIS AND DIFFERENTIAL DIAGNOSIS

Diagnosis Clinical diagnosis

Differential Diagnosis Pyogenic granuloma, nodular melanoma

DERMATOPATHOLOGY

Upper dermis shows either one greatly dilated space or several interconnected dilated spaces filled with red blood cells, lined by a single layer of flattened endothelial cells and a thin wall of fibrous tissue.

COURSE AND PROGNOSIS

Lesions stabilize in size after several years and usually do not regress spontaneously.

TREATMENT

If indicated cosmetically, electro- or laser coagulation, or surgical excision.

BENIGN NEOPLASMS AND HYPERPLASIAS

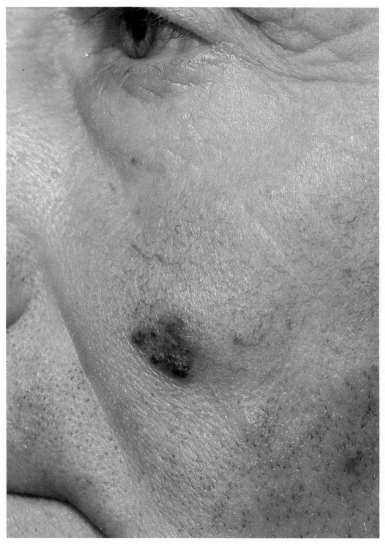

96 Venous lake *Irregular, cobblestone, purplish-red nodule on the cheek.*

A spider angioma is a focal telangiectatic network of dilated capillaries, radiating from a central arteriole (punctum), occurring in healthy individuals and, at times, associated with pregnancy or (rarely) hepatocellular disease.

Synonyms: nevus araneus, spider nevus, arterial spider, spider telangiectasia, vascular spider.

EPIDEMIOLOGY AND ETIOLOGY

Age Young children to old age, but most common in early adulthood

Sex Female > male

Incidence May occur in up to 15% of normal individuals. One or more spider angiomas are seen in two-thirds of pregnant women.

Etiology May be associated with hyperestrogenic states, such as pregnancy, or in hepatocellular disease, such as subacute and chronic viral hepatitis and alcoholic cirrhosis, or in estrogen therapy, i.e., oral contraceptive use.

PHYSICAL EXAMINATION

Skin Findings
TYPE Central papular punctum at the site of the feeding arteriole with macular radiating telangiectatic vessels (Figure 97); up to 1.5 cm in diameter. Usually solitary; when associated with pregnancy or liver disease may be multiple.
COLOR Red
SHAPE Round to oval

PALPATION On diascopy, radiating telangiectasia blanches and central arteriole may pulsate.
SITES OF PREDILECTION Above the nipple line, especially on face, forearms, and hands

DIAGNOSIS AND DIFFERENTIAL DIAGNOSIS

Diagnosis Made on clinical findings

Differential Diagnosis Hereditary hemorrhagic telangiectasia, ataxia-telangiectasia, progressive systemic sclerosis, CREST syndrome

COURSE AND PROGNOSIS

Spider angioma arising in childhood and pregnancy may regress spontaneously.

TREATMENT

Lesions may be treated with electro- or laser surgery.

BENIGN NEOPLASMS AND HYPERPLASIAS

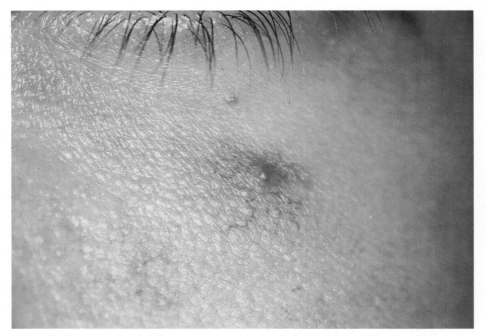

97   Spider hemangioma   *A red lesion with a central papular punctum at the site of the feeding arterial vessel, with macular, radiating, telangiectatic vesicles. On diascopy, the central arterial vessel can be seen to pulsate.*

Telangiectasia of the lateral nose appears as dilated parallel vascular ectasias appearing during middle age.

ETIOLOGY AND EPIDEMIOLOGY

Age Middle-age and older

Sex More common in men

Etiology Unknown. Tends to be familial

Predisposing Factors More common in fair-skinned individuals, chronic sun exposure, rosacea

HISTORY

Skin Symptoms None. However, lesions may become quite large and be cosmetically disfiguring.

PHYSICAL EXAMINATION

Skin Lesions
TYPE Numerous dilated blood vessels usually parallel on the lateral nose (see Figure 98) near the malar junction. May be raised and tortuous.
COLOR Red to purple
ARRANGEMENT Usually parallel at right angle to nasomalar junction

TREATMENT

Pulsed dye laser is quite effective and relatively painless.

BENIGN NEOPLASMS AND HYPERPLASIAS

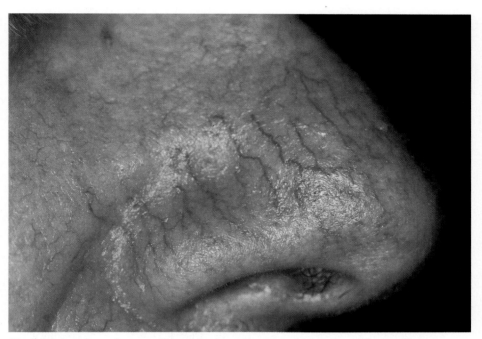

98   Telangiectasia on the nose   *Numerous streaming telangiectases in a 56-year-old man.*

Pyogenic granuloma is a rapidly developing, bright-red or violaceous or brown-black nodule that may be confused with malignant melanoma.

Synonym: granuloma telangiectaticum.

EPIDEMIOLOGY

Age Usually children or persons <30 years old

Sex Equal incidence in males and females

HISTORY

Duration of Lesions Weeks

Skin Symptoms None; recurrent bleeding from the lesion may occur

PHYSICAL EXAMINATION

Skin Lesions See Figure 99
TYPE Nodule with smooth or warty surface with or without crusts or erosions
COLOR Bright red, dusky red, violaceous, brown-black
SIZE AND SHAPE Less than 1.5 cm in diameter; usually lesion is pedunculated, base slightly constricted, or sessile
DISTRIBUTION Isolated single lesion
SITES OF PREDILECTION Fingers, lips, mouth, trunk, toes

DIFFERENTIAL DIAGNOSIS

Nodular malignant melanoma (especially amelanotic), *squamous cell carcinoma, glomus tumor, nodular basal cell carcinoma, metastatic carcinoma, bacillary angiomatosis*

DERMATOPATHOLOGY

Site Dermis with secondary epidermal involvement

Process Proliferation of capillaries with prominent endothelial cells embedded in edematous, gelatinous stromata

COURSE AND PROGNOSIS

Lesion does not spontaneously disappear and must be removed for a histologic diagnosis and treatment.

TREATMENT

Remove tissue for histology.

Electrocautery or laser treatment is also effective, especially with the tunable dye laser.

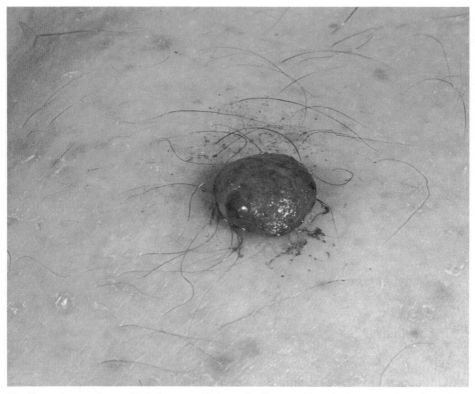

99 Pyogenic granuloma *Nodular tumor, 8.0 mm in diameter, sharply demarcated, erosive, with a partly hemorrhagic surface. The base is slightly constricted. Histologic examination of these lesions is essential to rule out amelanotic malignant melanoma.*

A dermatofibroma is a very common, buttonlike dermal fibroma, usually occurring on the extremities, important only because of its cosmetic appearance or its being mistaken for other lesions.

Synonyms: solitary histiocytoma, sclerosing hemangioma, nodulus cutaneus.

EPIDEMIOLOGY AND ETIOLOGY

Age Any age

Sex Females > males

Etiology Unknown, may be chronic histiocytic-fibrous reaction to insect bite.

PHYSICAL EXAMINATION

Skin Findings
TYPE   Papule or nodule (Figure 100), 3.0 to 10.0 mm in diameter. Surface variably domed but may be depressed below plane of surrounding skin. Texture of surface may be dull, shiny, or scaling. Top may be crusted or scarred secondary to excoriation or shaving. Borders ill-defined, fading to normal skin.

COLOR   Variable: skin color, pink, brown, tan, dark chocolate brown. Usually darker at center, fading to normal skin color at margin. Often center shows postinflammatory hypo- or hyperpigmentation secondary to repeated trauma.

PALPATION   Firm dermal button- or pealike papule or nodule. *Dimple sign:* lateral compression with thumb and index finger produces a depression or "dimple."

DISTRIBUTION   Legs > arms > trunk. Uncommonly occur on head, palms, soles. Usually solitary, may be multiple, and are randomly scattered.

DIAGNOSIS AND DIFFERENTIAL DIAGNOSIS

Diagnosis Clinical findings

Differential Diagnosis Primary malignant melanoma, scar, blue nevus, pilar cyst, metastatic carcinoma, Kaposi's sarcoma

DERMATOPATHOLOGY

Whorling fascicles of spindle cells with small amount of pale blue cytoplasm and elongate nucleus. Variable increase in vascular spaces. Overlying epidermis frequently hyperplastic.

COURSE AND PROGNOSIS

Lesions appear gradually over several months, may persist statically for years to decades, and may regress spontaneously.

TREATMENT

Surgical removal is not usually indicated in that resulting scar is often less cosmetically acceptable than the dermatofibroma. Indications for excision include repeated trauma, unacceptable cosmetic appearance, or uncertainty of clinical diagnosis. Lesion is removed by elliptical excision.

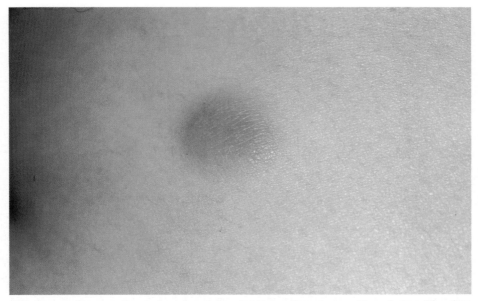

100   Dermatofibroma   *Dome-shaped nodule, slightly erythematous, with a button-like, firm consistency. Lateral compression with thumb and index finger produces a depression or "dimple."*

Hypertrophic scars and keloids are exuberant fibrous repair tissues following a cutaneous injury. A *hypertrophic scar* remains confined to the site of original injury; a *keloid,* however, extends beyond this site often with clawlike extensions.

EPIDEMIOLOGY AND ETIOLOGY

Age Third decade, but range from early first decade to senescence

Sex Equal incidence in males and females

Race Much more common in blacks than whites

Etiology Unknown. Usually follow injury to skin, i.e., surgical scar, laceration, abrasion, cryosurgery, electrocoagulation, as well as vaccination, acne, etc. May also arise spontaneously, without history of injury, usually in presternal site.

HISTORY

Skin Symptoms Usually asymptomatic. May be pruritic or painful if touched. May be cosmetically very unsightly.

PHYSICAL EXAMINATION

Skin Findings
TYPE   Papules to nodules (Figure 101) to tumors to large tuberous lesions.
COLOR   Usually color of the normal skin.
SHAPE   May be linear (Figure 101) following traumatic or surgical injury. Hypertrophic scars tend to be dome-shaped and are confined to approximately the site of the original injury. Keloids, however, may extend in a clawlike fashion far beyond any slight original injury.
PALPATION   Firm to hard; surface smooth
SITES OF PREDILECTION   Ear lobes, shoulders, upper back, chest

DIAGNOSIS AND DIFFERENTIAL DIAGNOSIS

Diagnosis Clinical diagnosis; biopsy not warranted unless there is clinical doubt, because it may induce new hypertrophic scarring.

Differential Diagnosis Scar, dermatofibroma, dermatofibrosarcoma protuberans, desmoid tumor, scar sarcoidosis, foreign body granuloma

DERMATOPATHOLOGY

Hypertrophic scar: whorls of young fibrous tissue and fibroblasts in haphazard arrangement. *Keloid:* added feature of thick, eosinophilic, acellular bands of collagen.

COURSE AND PROGNOSIS

Hypertrophic scars tend to regress, in time becoming flatter and softer. Keloids, however, may continue to expand in size for decades.

TREATMENT

Intralesional injection of triamcinolone (10 to 40 mg/mL) every month may reduce pruritus or sensitivity of lesion, as well as reduce its volume and flatten it. Response is often disappointing. Combined treatment of intralesional triamcinolone + cryotherapy may be a little more effective. Lesions that are excised surgically often recur larger than the original lesion.

BENIGN NEOPLASMS AND HYPERPLASIAS

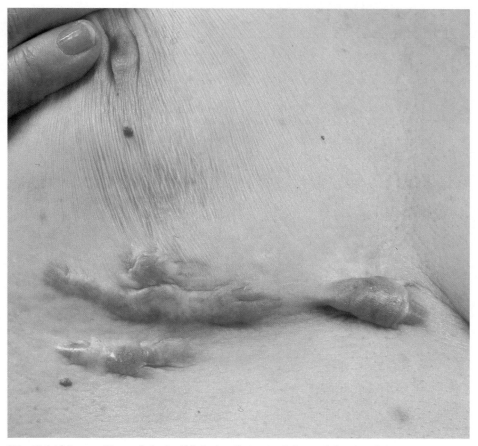

101   Keloidal scar   *Linear, hypertrophic lesion that extends beyond the site of the original lesion.*

A skin tag is a skin-colored pedunculated papilloma (polyp) occurring at intertriginous sites, important only because of any cosmetic disfigurement.

Synonyms: acrochordon, cutaneous papilloma, soft fibroma.

EPIDEMIOLOGY

Age Middle-aged and elderly

Sex Female > males

Incidence Very common

Etiology Unknown. Often familial. More common in obese individuals.

HISTORY

Skin Symptoms Usually asymptomatic but may be pesky nuisance, especially in the anogenital area. Occasionally may become tender following trauma or torsion.

PHYSICAL EXAMINATION

Skin Findings
TYPE Pedunculated papilloma, usually constricted at base, varying in size from <1.0 mm to, at times, >10.00 mm (Figure 102). At times, crusted or hemorrhagic following trauma. In obese individuals, frequently associated with acanthosis nigricans.
COLOR Skin color to tan to brown; varies with racial pigmentation of patient
SHAPE Usually round to oval
PALPATION Soft, pliable

SITES OF PREDILECTION Eyelids (upper > lower), neck, axillae, inframammary, groins

DIAGNOSIS AND DIFFERENTIAL DIAGNOSIS

Diagnosis Clinical findings

Differential Diagnosis Pedunculated seborrheic keratosis, dermal or compound melanocytic nevus, neurofibroma, molluscum contagiosum

DERMATOPATHOLOGY

Epidermis thinned, loose fibrous tissue stroma

COURSE AND PROGNOSIS

Lesions tend to become larger and more numerous over time, especially during pregnancy. Following spontaneous torsion, autoamputation can occur.

TREATMENT

Snipping off with scissor, or electrodesiccation, both of which are usually tolerated without local anesthetic.

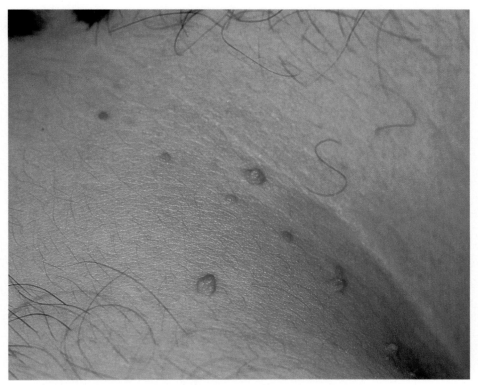

102 Skin tag *A cluster of tiny, papillomatous, skin-colored lesions.*

A true mucocutaneous cyst is a closed sac lined by epidermally or adnexally derived epithelium and filled with a liquid or semisolid material derived from that epithelium; various pseudocysts occur within the dermis and are not epithelial-lined.

Epidermoid Cyst

An epidermoid cyst is the most common cutaneous cyst, derived from epidermis or the epithelium of the hair follicle, and is formed by cystic enclosure of epithelium within the dermis that becomes filled with keratin and lipid-rich debris; because of their thin walls, rupture is common and accompanied by a painful inflammatory mass.

Synonyms: wen, sebaceous cyst, infundibular cyst, epidermal cyst.

EPIDEMIOLOGY AND ETIOLOGY

Age   Young to middle-aged adults

Sex   More common in men than in women

Histogenesis   Cyst with epidermal-like wall

PHYSICAL EXAMINATION

Clinical Appearance   Dermal-to-subcutaneous nodule, which often connects with the surface by keratin-filled pores. Cyst contents are cream-colored with a pasty consistency (Figure 103), and smell like rancid cheese. In blacks, cysts may be darkly pigmented. *Size:* 0.5 to 5.0 cm. *Number:* usually solitary, may be multiple. Scrotal lesions may calcify.

Distribution   Face, neck, upper trunk, scrotum

PATHOLOGY

Cyst Content   Keratinaceous material

Cyst Wall   Stratified squamous epithelium with well-formed granular layer

COURSE

Cyst wall is relatively thin. Following rupture of the wall, the irritating cyst contents initiate an inflammatory reaction, enlarging the lesion manyfold; the lesion is associated with a great deal of pain. Ruptured cysts are often misdiagnosed as being infected rather than ruptured. Bowen's disease, invasive squamous cell carcinoma, or basal cell carcinoma may rarely arise within the wall of the cyst.

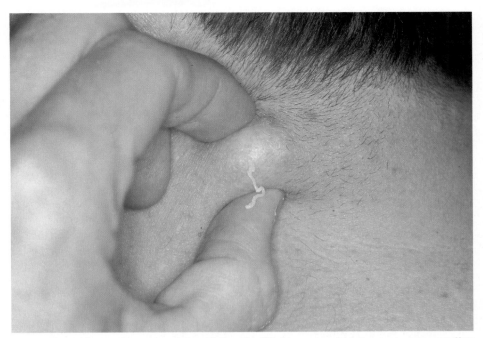

103   Epidermoid cyst   *Dermal nodule with keratin-filled pores in which pressure causes exuding of a cream-colored, pasty, rancid, cheeselike material.*

A trichilemmal cyst is the second most common type of cutaneous cyst (the most common being the epidermoid cyst), is seen most often on the scalp, is often familial, and occurs frequently as multiple lesions.

Synonyms: pilar cyst, isthmus catagen cyst. *Archaic terms:* wen, sebaceous cyst.

EPIDEMIOLOGY AND ETIOLOGY

Age   Middle-aged adults

Sex   More common in women than in men

Histogenesis   Derived from follicular isthmus of normal anagen hair. May be inherited as an autosomal dominant trait; usually multiple. Not connected to epidermis.

PHYSICAL EXAMINATION

Clinical Appearance   Smooth, firm, dome-shaped nodules to tumors (Figure 104). *Lacks the central punctum* seen in epidermoid cysts. Overlying scalp hair usually normal; may be thinned if cyst is large. *Size:* 0.5 to 5.0 cm. If cyst ruptures, may be inflamed and very painful.

Distribution   90% occur on scalp

PATHOLOGY

Cyst Content   Keratin, very dense, pink, homogeneous. Often calcified, cholesterol clefts

Cyst Wall   Usually thick; can be removed intact. Stratified squamous epithelium with a palisaded outer layer resembling that of outer root sheath of hair follicle. Inner layer is corrugated without a granular layer.

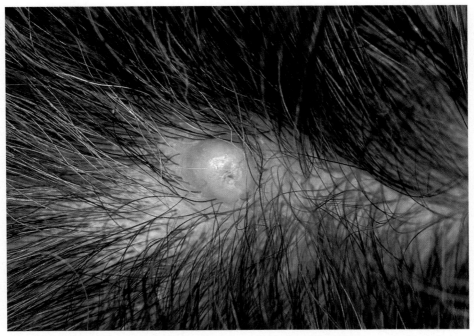

104　Trichilemmal (pilar) cyst　*A thick-walled, dome-shaped nodule without a central punctum as seen in epidermoid cysts.*

An epidermal inclusion cyst occurs secondary to traumatic implantation of epidermis within the dermis. Traumatically grafted epidermis grows in the dermis, with accumulation of keratin within cyst cavity.

Synonym: traumatic epidermoid cyst.

PHYSICAL EXAMINATION

Clinical Appearance Dermal nodule (Figure 105)

Distribution Palms and soles most commonly

PATHOLOGY

Cyst Content Thick, dense keratin

Cyst Wall Stratified squamous epithelium with a well-formed granular layer

---

| *Milium* |

A milium is a 1.0- to 2.0-mm, superficial, white-to-yellow, keratin-containing epidermal cyst, occurring multiply, located on the eyelids, cheeks, and forehead in pilosebaceous follicles and at sites of trauma.

EPIDEMIOLOGY AND ETIOLOGY

Age Infants to adults

Sex Equal incidence in men and women

Histogenesis Arises from pluripotential cells in epidermal or adnexal epithelium either *de novo* or in association with various dermatoses with subepidermal bullae or vesicles (pemphigoid, porphyria cutanea tarda, bullous lichen planus, epidermolysis bullosa, lichen sclerosus et atrophicus) and skin trauma (abrasion, burns, dermabrasion, radiation therapy)

PHYSICAL EXAMINATION

Clinical Appearance 1.0- to 2.0-mm, white-to-yellow papules (Figure 106)

Distribution Arising in normal skin: periorbital. At sites of trauma or dermatoses: i.e., porphyria cutanea tarda on dorsum of hand.

PATHOLOGY

Cyst Content Loose keratin

Cyst Wall Stratified squamous epithelium, only a few cells thick

TREATMENT

Incision and expression of contents

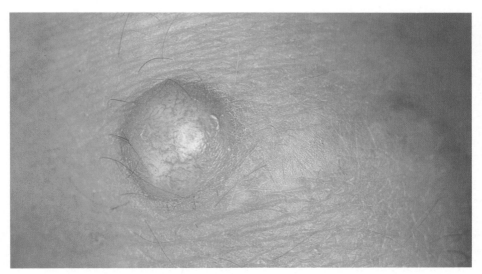

105 Epidermal inclusion cyst *A dermal nodule which contains thick, dense, keratin material, arising in a scar.*

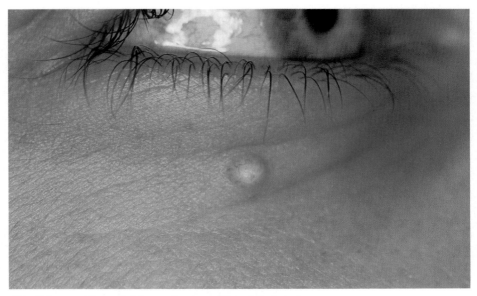

106 Primary milium *A 3.0-mm, hard, seedlike white papule.*

Digital Myxoid Cyst

A digital myxoid cyst is a pseudocyst occurring over the distal interphalangeal joint of the finger, formed by extrusion of mucin from an underlying joint space.

EPIDEMIOLOGY AND ETIOLOGY

Age   Middle-aged to elderly

Sex   More common in women than in men

Histogenesis   Escape of mucin from underlying joint space

PHYSICAL EXAMINATION

Clinical Appearance   Solitary. Firm rubbery, translucent cyst (Figure 107)

Distribution   Dorsal aspect of distal interphalangeal joint of finger, less commonly of toe

PATHOLOGY

Cyst Content   Clear gelatinous substance

Cyst Wall   No true cyst lining. Mucin may compress adjacent connective tissue.

COURSE

May cause nail dystrophy.

TREATMENT

Compression over several weeks can result in disappearance.

Mucocele

A mucocele is a pseudocyst occurring beneath the oral mucosa of the lower lip, formed by rupture of a minor salivary gland.

Synonyms: mucus retention phenomenon, retention cyst, ranula.

EPIDEMIOLOGY AND ETIOLOGY

Age   Young to middle-aged adults

Histogenesis   May arise following rupture of minor salivary duct

PHYSICAL EXAMINATION

Clinical Appearance   Solitary. Soft cyst with translucent bluish color (Figure 108)

Distribution   Mucosal surface of lower lip

PATHOLOGY

Cyst Content   Clear mucinous gel

Cyst Wall   Compressed connective tissue, variable amount of granulation tissue and granulomatous inflammation

BENIGN NEOPLASMS AND HYPERPLASIAS

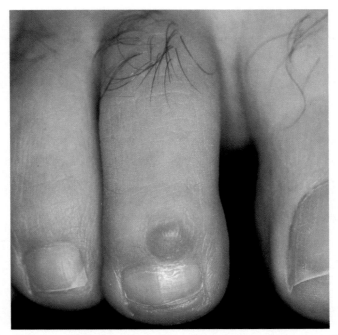

107 Digital myxoid cyst   *These are solitary, firm, rubbery, translucent cysts over the distal inter-phalangeal joint.*

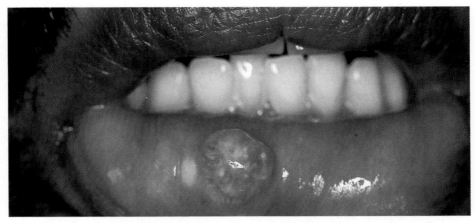

108 Mucocele   *A solitary, spherical, soft, translucent, slightly blueish cyst occurring on the mucosal surface of the lower lip.*

Section 10

Disorders of Hair

Hair growth on the scalp occurs in cycles of intermittent activity; periods of growth are followed by periods of quiescence. The period of active growth is referred to as *anagen*, which is followed normally by a brief transition phase, i.e., *catagen*, during which growth stops and follicles enter the resting or *telogen* phase.

Alopecia Areata

Alopecia areata is a localized loss of hair in round or oval areas without any visible inflammation on the scalp skin or any skin symptoms. All of the hair of the body may eventually be lost (alopecia universalis).

EPIDEMIOLOGY AND ETIOLOGY

Age Young adults (under 25 years); children are frequently affected.

Sex Equal in both sexes, although male:female ratio is 2:1 in Italy and Spain

Race In every race; 20% give a family history

Other Factors Not a sign of any multisystem disease, but may be associated with other autoimmune disorders such as vitiligo, familial multiendocrine syndrome, and thyroid disease (Hashimoto's disease). Emotional problems, especially life crises, can precipitate an attack.

HISTORY

Duration of Hair Loss Gradual over weeks

Skin Symptoms None, tenderness may occur early

PHYSICAL EXAMINATION

Skin Lesions None, possibly erythema in the area of hair loss

Hair Alopecia (Figure 109), occasionally with diagnostic broken-off stubby hairs called *exclamation point hairs*

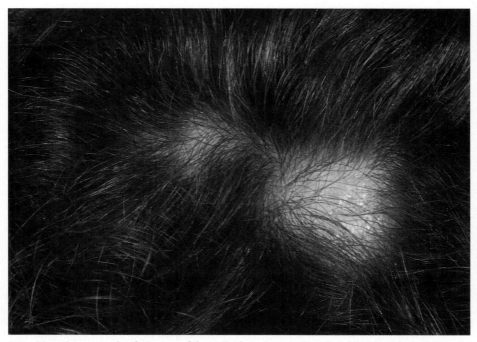

109   Alopecia areata   *On the crown of the scalp there are two sharply outlined patches of alopecia. There is no abnormal scaling or erythema, and there is no atrophy.*

ARRANGEMENT   Scattered discrete areas of alopecia, or confluent (total loss of hair)

DISTRIBUTION   Localized (to scalp or eyelids or cheek) (Figure 110) or generalized with total loss (alopecia universalis)

SITES OF PREDILECTION   Scalp, eyebrows, eyelashes, pubic hair, beard

Nails   Dystrophic changes (20%): fine stippling like "hammered brass" (Figure 110)

DIFFERENTIAL DIAGNOSIS

Secondary syphilis ("moth-eaten" appearance in beard or scalp); *tinea capitis* may be a problem in diagnosis but fluorescence and KOH examination are negative.

DERMATOPATHOLOGY

Follicles are reduced in size, arrested in anagen IV, and lie high in the dermis; perifollicular lymphocytic infiltrate with degenerative changes in the blood vessels that lead to the hair papillae. Increase of telogen hair from normal (less than 20%) to 25 to 40%

COURSE

If occurring after puberty, 80% of patients regrow hair. Alopecia universalis is rare. Following the first episode of hair loss about 33% completely regrow the hair within a year. Recurrences of alopecia, however, are frequent. Repeated attacks, nail changes, and total alopecia before puberty are poor prognostic signs.

TREATMENT

Topical clobetasol propionate ointment used for 6 weeks only, as skin atrophy can occur.

For small solitary spots intralesional triamcinolone acetonide is temporarily very effective (e.g., eyebrows, beard).

Wigs are very satisfactory, especially for women.

Avoid systemic corticosteroids.

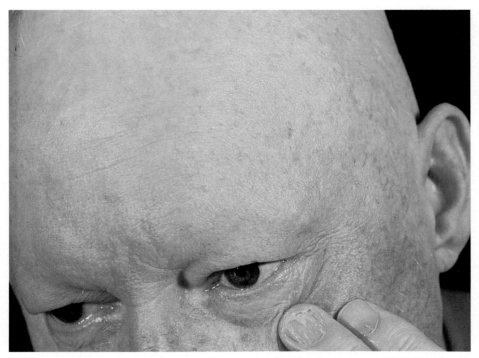

110   Alopecia areata   *There is loss of eyebrows and eyelashes and dystrophic nail changes.*

Androgenetic alopecia (AGA) is the common progressive balding which occurs through the combined effect of a genetic predisposition and the action of androgen on the hair follicles of the scalp.

Synonyms: male-pattern baldness, common baldness

EPIDEMIOLOGY AND ETIOLOGY

Age May begin anytime after puberty, as early as the second decade. Onset in females later—about 40% occur in the sixth decade.

Sex Males much more commonly than females

Race Occurs in all races

Heredity Polygenic or autosomal dominant in males, and autosomal recessive in females

Etiology Combined effects of androgen on predisposed hair follicles

HISTORY

Skin Symptoms Most patients present with complaints of gradually thinning hair or baldness. In males there is a receding anterior hair line, especially in the parietal regions, which results in an M-shaped recession. Following this a bald spot may appear on the posterior crown. If AGA progresses rapidly, some patients also complain of increased falling out of hair. In females, parietal and temporal recession is not a major feature and severe thinning is not common. The cosmetic appearance of AGA is very disturbing to many patients due to the high value which our society places on a "healthy head of hair."

Systems Review In young women, such manifestations of androgen excess should be sought as significant: acne, hirsutism, or virilization. However, most women with AGA are endocrinologically normal.

PHYSICAL EXAMINATION

Skin Lesions There are no skin lesions seen in AGA. In young women other signs of virilization should be sought, such as acne and excess facial or body hair or a male-pattern escutcheon. Findings of treatable causes of alopecia such as seborrheic dermatitis should be sought.

Hair Hair in areas of AGA becomes finer in texture, i.e., shorter in length and of reduced diameter. In time, hair becomes vellus and eventually atrophies completely. With complete alopecia, scalp is smooth and shiny, orifices of follicles barely perceptible with the unaided eye.

DISTRIBUTION

Males usually exhibit patterned loss in the frontotemporal and vertex areas (Figure 111). The end result may be only a rim of residual hair on the lateral and posterior scalp. Paradoxically, males with extensive AGA may have excess growth of secondary sexual hair, i.e., axillae, pubic area, chest, and beard. Hamilton (*Am J Anat* 71:451, 1941) classified male-pattern hair loss into stages: type I, loss of hair along the frontal margin; type II, increasing frontal as well as onset of loss on the occipital scalp (crown); types III, IV, V, increasing hair

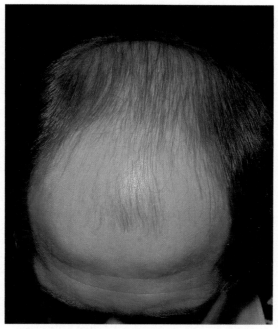

111　Androgenetic alopecia in a male　*There is loss of hair in the frontotemporal and vertex areas.*

loss in both regions with eventual confluent and complete balding of the top of the scalp with sparing of the sides.

Females, including those who are endocrinologically normal, also lose scalp hair according to the male pattern, but hair loss is far less pronounced (Figure 112).

Systemic Findings In young women with AGA, signs of virilization such as clitoral hypertrophy should be sought.

DIAGNOSIS AND DIFFERENTIAL DIAGNOSIS

Diagnosis Clinical diagnosis made on the history, especially family incidence of AGA, and the pattern of alopecia.

Differential Diagnosis Diffuse pattern of hair loss with alopecia areata, telogen effluvium, secondary syphilis, SLE, iron deficiency, hypothyroidism, hyperthyroidism, trichotillomania

LABORATORY AND SPECIAL EXAMINATIONS

Trichogram A trichogram determines the number of anagen and telogen hairs and is made by epilating (plucking) 50 hairs or more from the scalp with a needleholder, counting the number of anagen hairs (A) (growing hairs with a long encircling hair sheath) and the number of club or telogen hairs (T) (resting hairs with an inner root sheath and roots usually largest at base). Normally, 80 to 90% of hairs are in anagen phase. In AGA, the earliest changes are an increase in the percentage of telogen hairs.

Dermatopathology Abundance of telogen-stage follicles is noted, associated with hair follicles of decreasing size and eventually nearly complete atrophy.

PATHOPHYSIOLOGY

The mechanism of action of androgen on follicular cellular processes which results in AGA is unclear, but in most cases it is a local phenomenon (increased expression of androgen receptors, changes in androgen metabolism) of the scalp hair follicles. Consequently most patients (male and female) are endocrinologically normal. Terminal follicles are transformed into velluslike follicles, which in turn undergo atrophy. During successive follicular cycles, the hairs produced are of shorter length and of decreasing diameter. Conversely, androgens induce vellus-to-terminal follicle production of secondary sexual hair. Eunuchs and males castrated before or during puberty do not develop AGA in spite of a strong family history; administration of androgen produces baldness which does not progress if drug is withdrawn. Dihydrotestosterone, an intracellular hormone, causes growth of androgen-dependent hair (e.g., pubic, beard) and loss of non-androgen-dependent scalp hair. In males, testosterone produced by the testes is the major androgen. In females, androstenedione and dehydroepiandrostenone sulfate are the major peripheral androgens, and these two hormones are very slowly converted to dihydrotestosterone in the target cell (hair keratinocyte) by 5-alpha-testosterone reductase. The serum testosterone levels of men are much higher than in women and there are higher tissue levels and greater conversion to dihydrotestosterone.

COURSE

The progression of alopecia is usually very gradual, over years to decades.

TREATMENT

There is no highly effective therapy to prevent the progression of AGA. Topically applied minoxidil is helpful in reducing the rate of hair loss, or in partially restoring lost hair in some patients; in

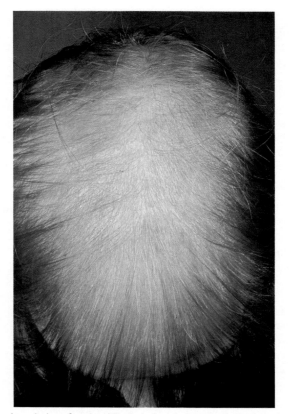

112 Androgenetic alopecia in a female *The hair loss is largely limited to the vertex.*

large clinical trials there has been noted moderate growth at 4 and 12 months in 40% of males; the efficacy of minoxidil in females is not yet known from large clinical trials. Combinations of higher concentrations of minoxidil with topical retinoic acid are promising improvements.

Antiandrogens such as spironolactone, cyproterone acetate, flutemide, and cimetidine which bind to androgen receptors and block the action of dihydrotestosterone have been reported to be effective in treating women with AGA who have elevated adrenal androgens; these are not used in men.

Hair transplantation using multiple punch grafts of follicles taken from androgen-insensitive hair sites (peripheral occipital and parietal hairy areas) to bald androgen-sensitive scalp areas are effective in some patients with AGA. These micrografts are a successful technique in many patients and help restore more normal appearance.

Telogen effluvium is the transient increased shedding of normal club hairs (telogen) from resting scalp follicles secondary to accelerated shift of anagen (growth phase) into catagen and telogen (resting phase), which results clinically in increased daily hair loss and, if severe, thinning of hair.

EPIDEMIOLOGY AND ETIOLOGY

Age Any age

Sex More common in women due to parturition, cessation of an oral contraceptive, and "crash" dieting

Etiology Factors which affect follicle growth resulting in telogen effluvium include: pregnancy followed either by abortion or parturition, discontinuing or changing type of oral contraceptive, major surgical procedure, major traumatic injury, "crash" diet with significant weight loss in a short period of time, significant medical illness (especially with high fever).

HISTORY

Skin Symptoms Patient presents with complaint of increased hair loss on the scalp which may be accompanied by varying degrees of hair thinning. Most patients are very anxious, fearing they will become bald. The physician is often presented with a plastic bag containing the shed hair. The precipitating event precedes the telogen effluvium by 6 to 16 weeks.

PHYSICAL EXAMINATION

Skin Lesions No abnormalities of the scalp are detected.

Hair Diffuse shedding of the scalp is seen. In running the fingers through the patient's hair, several to many hairs may be shed with each passage. These hairs are all telogen or club hairs.

DISTRIBUTION Hair loss occurs diffusely throughout the scalp (Figure 113). If hair loss is significant enough to result in thinning of hair, alopecia is noted diffusely throughout the scalp. Short regrowing new hairs are present close to the scalp; these hairs are finer than older hairs and have tapered ends. In patients with subclinical androgenetic alopecia, the thinning may be more pronounced on the vertex.

SITE OF PREDILECTION Scalp

Nails The precipitating stimulus for telogen effluvium may also affect the growth of nails, resulting in Beau's lines, which appear as transverse lines or grooves on the fingernail plates.

DIAGNOSIS AND DIFFERENTIAL DIAGNOSIS

Diagnosis Made on clinical findings and trichogram

Differential Diagnosis That of nonscarring, noninflammatory alopecia: androgenetic alopecia, diffuse-pattern alopecia areata, hyperthyroidism, hypothyroidism, SLE, secondary syphilis

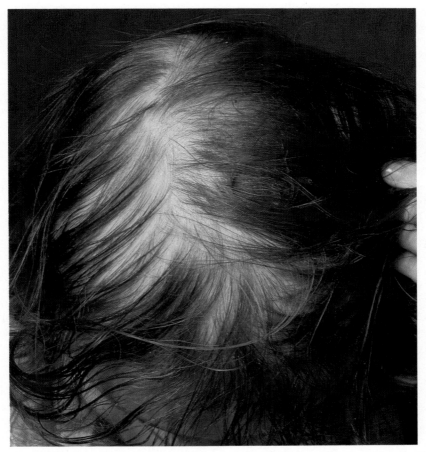

113   Telogen effluvium   *There is a decreased density of hair follicles without any abnormality in the scalp skin.*

LABORATORY AND SPECIAL EXAMINATIONS

Trichogram Compared with the normal trichogram, in which 80 to 90% of hair is in the anagen phase, telogen effluvium is characterized by a reduced percentage of anagen hairs, varying with the intensity of hair shedding. See page 194 for explanation of trichogram.

Histopathology No abnormality other than an increase in the proportion of follicles in telogen.

PATHOPHYSIOLOGY

The precipitating stimulus for telogen effluvium results in a premature shift of anagen follicles into the telogen phase, which is characterized by club, or resting, hairs. As a new anagen cycle begins, the old resting telogen hairs are "pushed out" by the new anagen hairs, resulting in a telogen effluvium. Normal hair loss from the scalp is up to 50 to 100 hairs per day; with telogen effluvium many more hairs than this are shed daily.

COURSE AND PROGNOSIS

Complete regrowth of hair is the rule. In postpartum telogen effluvium, if hair loss is severe and recurs after successive pregnancies, regrowth may never be complete. Telogen effluvium may continue for up to a year after the precipitating cause.

TREATMENT

No intervention is needed or required. The patient should be reassured that the process is part of a normal cycle of hair growth and shedding and that full regrowth of the hair is to be expected in most cases.

Section 11

Disorders of Keratinization

The ichthyosiform dermatoses are a group of hereditary disorders, characterized by an excess accumulation of cutaneous scale, whose severity varies from very mild and asymptomatic to life-threatening.

CLASSIFICATION

Dominant ichthyosis vulgaris (DIV)

X-linked ichthyosis (XLI)

Lamellar ichthyosis (LI)

HISTORY

All three types of ichthyosis tend to be worse during the dry, cold winter months and improve during the hot humid summer. Patients living in tropical climates may remain symptom free but may experience appearance or worsening of symptoms on moving to a temperate climate.

DIAGNOSIS

Usually made on clinical findings

PATHOPHYSIOLOGY

LI shows increased germinative cell hyperplasia and increased transit rate through the epidermis. In DIV and XLI, formation of thickened stratum corneum is caused by increased adhesiveness of the stratum corneum cells and/or failure of normal separation. Abnormal stratum corneum formation results in variable increase in transepidermal water loss.

TREATMENT

Hydration of stratum corneum Pliability of stratum corneum is a function of its water content. Hydration is best accomplished by immersion in a bath followed by the application of petrolatum. Urea-containing creams may help bind water in stratum corneum.

Keratolytic agents Propylene glycol, glycerin, lactic acid mixtures are effective without occlusion. Another effective preparation is 6% *salicylic acid in propylene glycol and alcohol;* this is used under plastic occlusion. Alpha-hydroxy acids such as lactic acid bind water or control scaling. *Urea*-containing preparations (2 to 20%) are effective; some preparations contain both urea and lactic acid.

Systemic retinoids such as isotretinoin and etretinate are effective for LI, but careful monitoring for toxicity is required. Severe cases may require intermittent therapy over long periods of time.

Ichthyosis vulgaris (IV) is characterized by mild generalized hyperkeratosis with xerosis most pronounced on the lower legs and by perifollicular hyperkeratosis (keratosis pilaris) and is frequently associated with atopy.

EPIDEMIOLOGY

Age of Onset   Childhood

Sex   Equal incidence in males and females

Mode of Inheritance   Autosomal dominant

Incidence   Very common

HISTORY

Very commonly associated with atopy, i.e., atopic dermatitis, allergic rhinitis, intrinsic asthma. Xerosis and pruritus worse in winter months. Keratosis pilaris and less commonly xerosis are of cosmetic concern to many patients.

PHYSICAL EXAMINATION

Skin Lesions

TYPE   Xeroderma (dry skin) with fine powdery scaling. Follicular keratosis, i.e., keratosis pilaris. Accentuated creases of palms and soles.

COLOR   Normal skin color (compare with X-linked ichthyosis)

SHAPE   Fish-scale pattern, especially on the shins (Figure 114)

DISTRIBUTION   Diffuse involvement, accentuated on the shins, arms, and back, but *sparing the axillae and the fossae (antecubital and popliteal);* face is spared (see Figure X). Follicular keratosis (keratosis pilaris): lateral upper arms (Figure 115), buttocks, lateral thighs; in childhood keratosis pilaris may be most prominent on the cheeks.

Eye Lesions   Keratopathy (rare)

DIFFERENTIAL DIAGNOSIS

Acquired ichthyosis occurring in later life may be a paraneoplastic syndrome and must be distinguished from dominant ichthyosis vulgaris.

LABORATORY AND SPECIAL EXAMINATIONS

Dermatopathology   Hyperkeratosis; reduced or absent granular layer; germinative layer flattened.

COURSE AND PROGNOSIS

May show improvement in the summer and in adulthood. Keratosis pilaris occurring on the cheeks during childhood usually improves during adulthood.

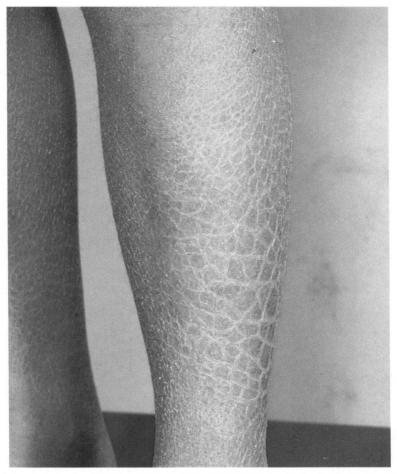

114 Ichthyosis vulgaris *Hyperkeratotic scaling, predominantly on the flanks, arms, and lower legs. The skin of the elbows, the axillae, and the knee folds is free of scaling.*

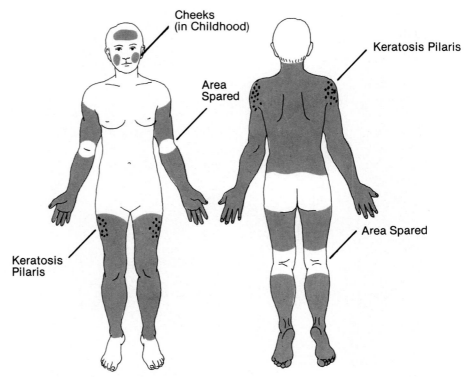

Cheeks
(in Childhood)

Keratosis Pilaris

Area
Spared

Keratosis Pilaris

Area Spared

Keratosis
Pilaris

Figure X   Ichthyosis vulgaris (dominant)

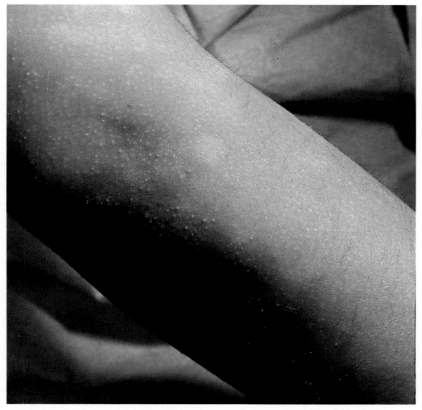

115 Keratosis pilaris *These lesions are discrete, keratotic, follicular papules.*

X-Linked Ichthyosis

X-linked ichthyosis (XLI) occurs only in males and is characterized by prominent dirty brown scales occurring on the neck, extremities, trunk, and buttocks, with onset soon after birth.

EPIDEMIOLOGY

Age of Onset Birth or infancy

Sex Males

Mode of Inheritance X-linked recessive. Gene has been cloned; prenatal diagnosis is possible.

Genetic Defect Steroid sulfatase deficiency

Incidence Uncommon

HISTORY

In addition to the discomfort due to xerosis, the dirty brown scales on the neck, ears, scalp, and arms are a major cosmetic disfigurement, causing the patient to appear dirty. Pituitary hypogonadism and delayed testicular descent are commonly present.

PHYSICAL EXAMINATION

Skin Lesions
TYPE Large scales which are not powdery as in ichthyosis vulgaris
COLOR Scales appear brown or dirty (Figures 116a and 116b).
SHAPE Fish-scale pattern, especially on the shins.

DISTRIBUTION (See Figure 116a.) Lateral neck (Figure 116b), upper lateral arms, chest, abdomen; *antecubital and popliteal fossae* are not spared. Prominent scalp scaling may occur. Palms and soles are normal. No follicular keratoses.

Eye Lesions Stromal corneal opacities (Descemet's membrane) develop during second and third decades which usually do not interfere with vision; may also be present in female carriers of XLI.

LABORATORY AND SPECIAL EXAMINATIONS

Dermatopathology Hyperkeratosis; granular layer present.

PATHOGENESIS

Steroid sulfatase deficiency is associated with failure to shed senescent keratinocytes normally, resulting clinically in hyperkeratosis.

COURSE AND PROGNOSIS

No improvement with age.

DISORDERS OF KERATINIZATION

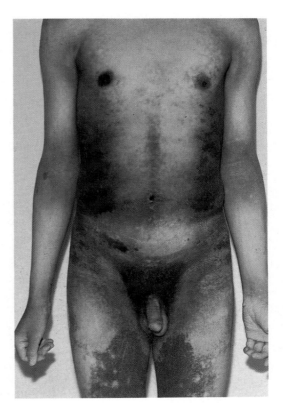

116a X-linked ichthyosis *The scales are large and dark and most evident on the flexural areas.*

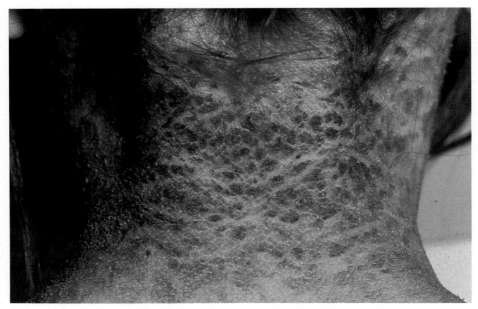

116b X-linked ichthyosis *The scales are large, dark, and dirty ("dirty neck").*

X-LINKED ICHTHYOSIS

Lamellar ichthyosis often presents at birth with the infant encased in a collodion-like membrane (collodion baby), which is soon shed. There is subsequent formation of large, coarse scales involving all flexural areas as well as palms and soles.

EPIDEMIOLOGY

Age of Onset Birth

Sex Equal incidence in males and females

Mode of Inheritance Autosomal recessive

Incidence Rare

HISTORY

During exercise and hot weather, hyperpyrexia may occur due to inability to sweat. Fissuring of stratum corneum may result in excess water loss and dehydration. Young children have increased nutritional requirements due to rapid growth and shedding of stratum corneum. Fissures on hands and feet are painful.

PHYSICAL EXAMINATION

Skin Lesions
TYPE At birth, infant presents as a collodion baby, encased in a collodion-like membrane, which is shed in 10 to 14 days. Subsequently, large parchment-like scales develop over the entire body (Figure 117), and frequent fracturing of the hyperkeratin plate results in a tessellated (tilelike) pattern (Figure 118). Scales are large and very thick. Fissuring of hands and feet common. Hyperkeratosis results in obstruction of eccrine sweat glands with resultant impairment of sweating. Secondary pyogenic infections.

DISTRIBUTION Generalized. Hyperkeratosis around joints may be verrucous. Involvement of eyelids results in ectropion.
HAIR AND NAILS Hair bound down by scales; frequent infections result in scarring alopecia. Nails show ridges and grooves.
MUCOUS MEMBRANES Usually spared. Ectropion may result in secondary infection.

Eye Lesions Ectropion

LABORATORY AND SPECIAL EXAMINATIONS

Dermatopathology Hyperkeratosis; granular layer present; acanthosis variable.

TREATMENT

Topical application of alpha-hydroxy acids, such as glycolic acid and lactic acid, is very effective.

COURSE AND PROGNOSIS

Collodion baby is a life-threatening condition in the first days of life; treatment in an incubator (moist climate) is usually necessary. Collodion membrane present at birth is shed; there is usually an interval with almost normal-appearing skin until lamellar ichthyosis develops. The disorder persists throughout life. No improvement with age.

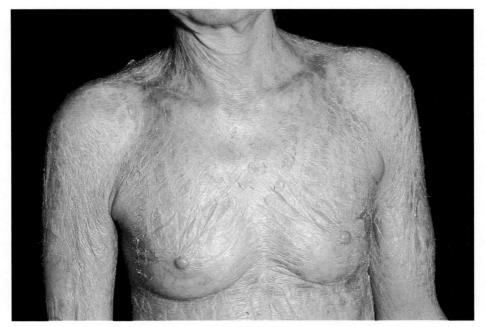

117 Lamellar ichthyosis *Large, parchment-like scales over the entire body. Mild ectropion is also present.*

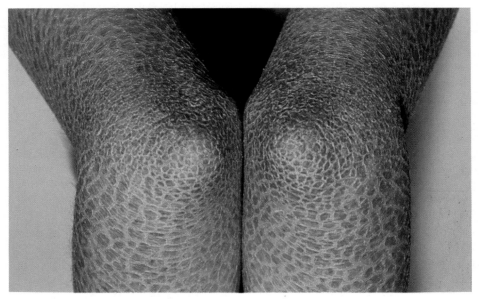

118 Lamellar ichthyosis *Tessellated (tilelike) scales*

LAMELLAR ICHTHYOSIS

Section 12

Skin Reaction to Sunlight Exposure

Photosensitivity: Important Abnormal Reactions to Light

Clinicians are always excited when, in a confusing eruption, they discover a clue to the etiology—this narrows the differential diagnostic list. Once the etiologic role of light is established, there is, moreover, a possibility of control of the disorder by discontinuing drugs or by topical or systemic treatment. The term ''photosensitivity'' describes an abnormal response to light, usually sunlight. Two broad types of acute photosensitivity are:

1. A ''*sunburn*-type'' response with the development of morphologic skin changes simulating a normal sunburn: erythema, edema, vesicles, and bullae. Examples are porphyria cutanea tarda, phytophotodermatitis.
2. A ''*rash*'' response to light exposure with development of varied morphologic expressions: macules, papules, plaques, eczematous dermatitis, urticaria. Examples are polymorphous light eruption, urticaria, eczematous drug reaction to sulfonamides.

Chronic repeated sun exposures over time result in polymorphic skin changes that have been termed *dermatoheliosis* (see page 214).

The skin response to light exposure is strictly limited to the areas that have been exposed, and sharp borders are usually noted. The light-exposed areas in males and females are presented in Figures XI and XII. It should be emphasized that *sparing* of certain skin areas may provide the clue to photosensitivity: the upper eyelids, the skin on the upper lip and under the chin (submental area), a triangle behind the ears, under the watch band, or in the area covered by a bra, in body creases on the back and sides of the neck, or on the abdomen in obese persons (see Figures XI and XII). While the distribution pattern of photoinduced abnormal reactions is presented in Figures XI and XII, it should be noted that UVR and visible light can penetrate clothing, regardless of the color or the type of fabric: the *tightness of the knit* is the most important feature of a cloth, not color or fabric, in filtering the passage of UVR and visible light.

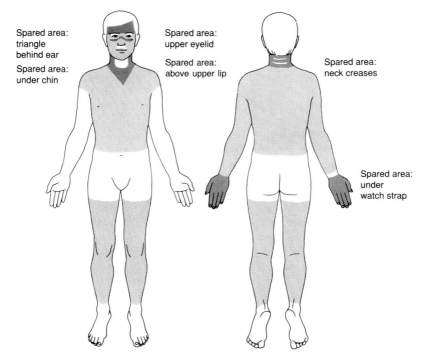

Figure XI *Variations in solar exposure on different body areas: Male.*

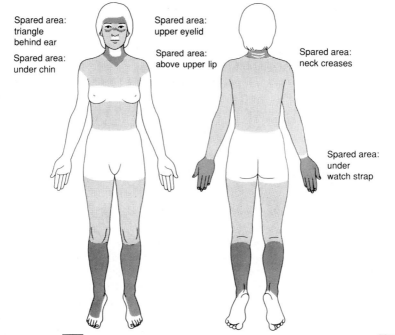

Figure XII *Female.*☐, *Rarely or never exposed (including doubly covered areas);* ☐, *often exposed;* ■, *habitually exposed.*

Sunburn is an acute, delayed, and transient inflammatory response of the skin following exposure to ultraviolet radiation (UVR) obtained from sunlight or artificial sources. Sunburn is characterized by erythema and, if severe, by vesicles and bullae, edema, tenderness, and pain; in normal sunburn there are never "rashes," i.e., scarlatiniform macules, papules, or plaques that occur in abnormal reactions to UVR. UVR in photomedicine is divided into two principal types: UVB (290 to 320 nm), the "sunburn" spectrum, and UVA (320 to 400 nm). The unit of measurement of sunburn is the *minimum erythema dose,* or MED, which is the minimum ultraviolet exposure that produces a clearly marginated erythema in the irradiated site following a single exposure. The MED is expressed in the amount of energy per unit area: mJ/cm^2 (UVB) or J/cm^2 (UVA). The MED for UVB in Caucasians is 20 to 40 mJ/cm^2 (about 20 minutes in northern latitudes at noon in June) and for UVA 15 to 20 J/cm^2 (about 120 minutes in northern latitudes at noon in June). UVB erythema develops in 12 to 24 hours and fades within 72 to 120 hours. UVA erythema peaks between 4 and 16 hours and fades within 48 to 120 hours.

EPIDEMIOLOGY

Incidence and Skin Phototypes Sunburn is most frequently seen in individuals who have white skin and a limited capacity to develop *facultative* melanin pigmentation (tanning) following exposure to UVR. Skin color (*constitutive* melanin pigmentation) is divided into white, brown, and black. Not all persons with white skin have the same capacity to develop tanning and this is the principal basis for the classification of individuals into four *skin phototypes* (SPT). The SPT is based on a *person's own estimate* of sunburning and tanning. Regardless of their phenotype (hair and eye color), SPT I persons sunburn easily with short exposures (30 minutes) and *never* tan. SPT IV persons tan with ease and do not sunburn with short exposures. SPT II persons are a subgroup of SPT I and sunburn easily but *tan with difficulty,* while SPT III persons have some sunburn with short exposures but can develop, over time, marked tanning. It is estimated that about 25% of white-skinned persons in the United States are SPT I and II. Persons with constitutive brown skin are termed SPT V, and with black skin SPT VI.

Race Persons with brown and black skin color can, in fact, sunburn following long exposures. The SPT of various races has not yet been determined, but it is known that some Asiatics and Hispanics have SPT I and II.

Age Very young children and elderly persons appear to have a reduced capacity to sunburn.

Geography Sunburn can occur at any latitude and may be less frequently observed in the indigenous populations near the equator who respect the sun; sunburn is seen more often in people who frequent beaches or who travel in winter to sunny vacation areas and obtain severe sunburns

HISTORY

Relationship of Sunburn to Medications An "exaggerated" sunburn response can occur in persons who are taking phototoxic drugs: sulfonamides, tetracyclines (particularly demethylchlortetracycline), chlorothiazides, doxycycline, phenothiazines, furosemide, nalidixic acid, amiodarone, naproxen, psoralens.

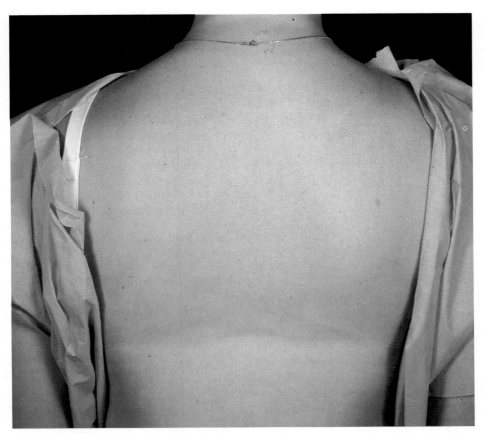

119   Acute sunburn   *Tender, pinkish-red, slightly edematous involvement of the back with sharp demarcation of the sun-protected areas.*

Skin Symptoms Pruritus may be severe even in mild sunburn; pain and tenderness with severe sunburn.

Constitutional Symptoms Headache, chills, feverishness, and weakness are not infrequent in severe sunburn; some SPT I and II persons develop headache and malaise even following short exposures.

Family History Skin phototypes are genetically determined.

PHYSICAL EXAMINATION

Appearance of Patient In severe sunburn the patient is "toxic"—with fever, weakness, and lassitude.

Vital Signs In severe sunburn pulse rate is rapid.

Skin
TYPE OF LESION Confluent erythema (Figure 119), edema, vesicles, and bullae confined to areas of exposure, no "rash"
COLOR Bright red
PALPATION Edematous areas are raised and tender.
DISTRIBUTION OF LESIONS Strictly confined to areas of exposure; sunburn can occur in areas covered with clothing, depending on the degree of exposure and the SPT of the person.

Mucous Membranes Sunburn of the tongue can occur rarely in mountain climbers who hold their mouth open "panting"; is frequent on the vermilion border of the lips.

LABORATORY AND SPECIAL EXAMINATIONS

Dermatopathology
LIGHT MICROSCOPY *Site* Epidermis, dermis, and subcutis

Process Inflammation
Cell Types
> Epidermis: "Sunburn" cells (damaged keratinocytes); also exocytosis of lymphocytes, vacuolization of melanocytes and Langerhans cells.
> Dermis: Endothelial cell swelling of superficial blood vessels and in the subcutaneous fat. Dermal changes are more prominent with UVA erythema with a denser mononuclear infiltrate and more severe vascular changes.

Special Techniques EM: wide gaps between endothelial cells, damaged pericytes, platelet aggregations, and perivascular fibrin deposition.

Laboratory Examination of Blood
SEROLOGIC ANA To rule out SLE
HEMATOLOGIC Leukopenia may be present in SLE.

Illumination (Allow for dark adaptation.)

> Partially darkened room—this permits the examiner to better see the eruption, as the contrast is accentuated.
> Completely darkened room—oblique lighting: place a flashlight at the side of the lesion to detect subtle surface changes (edema).

Wood's Lamp Examination Erythema is accentuated.

DIAGNOSIS AND DIFFERENTIAL DIAGNOSIS

Diagnosis History of UVR exposure and sites of reaction on exposed areas

Differential Diagnosis Obtain history of *medications* that can induce phototoxic erythema; *SLE* can cause a sunburn-type erythema. *Erythropoietic protoporphyria* causes erythema, vesicles, edema, and purpura.

PATHOGENESIS

The chromophores (molecules that absorb UVR) for UVB sunburn erythema are not known but damage to DNA possibly may be the initiating event. The mediators that cause the erythema include histamine for both UVA and UVB. Also in UVB erythema, other mediators include serotonin, prostaglandins, lysosomal enzymes, and kinins.

SIGNIFICANCE

History of "blistering" sunburns in youth is definitely a risk factor for development of malignant melanoma of the skin in later years.

Repeated sunburns result in dermatoheliosis, or "photoaging," over time.

COURSE

Sunburn, unlike thermal burns, cannot be classified on the basis of depth into "first-degree, second-degree, or third-degree," and scarring rarely, if ever, is seen following sunburn. At most, there can be a permanent hypomelanosis, probably related to destruction of melanocytes.

PREVENTION

There are many highly effective topical chemical filters (sunscreens) in lotion, gel, and cream formulations.

Persons with SPT I or II should avoid sunbathing, especially between 1100 and 1400 hours.

TREATMENT

Moderate
TOPICAL   Cool wet dressings, topical corticosteroids
SYSTEMIC   Acetylsalicylic acid, indomethacin

Severe   Bed rest. If very severe, a "toxic" patient is best managed in a specialized "burn unit" for fluid replacement, prophylaxis of infection, etc.
TOPICAL   Cool wet dressings, topical corticosteroids
SYSTEMIC   Oral corticosteroids are usually given but have not been established to be efficacious by controlled studies.

Dermatoheliosis ("Photoaging")

Repeated solar injuries over many years can ultimately result in the development of a skin syndrome, *dermatoheliosis*. Dermatoheliosis (DHe) results from excessive and/or prolonged exposure of the skin to ultraviolet radiation (UVR). The syndrome results from the cumulative effects of sun exposure following the first exposures in early life. DHe describes a polymorphic response of various components of the skin, especially cells in the epidermis, the vascular system, and the dermal connective tissue, to prolonged and/or excessive sun exposure. The severity of DHe depends principally on the duration and intensity of sun exposure and on the indigenous (constitutive) skin color and the capacity to tan (facultative melanin pigmentation). It is observed almost exclusively in persons with white skin, but especially in skin phototypes I and II (SPT, see page 210).

EPIDEMIOLOGY

Incidence In persons of SPT I–V who have had prolonged exposure to sunlight or UVR from artificial sources. The population susceptible to development of DHe are persons with SPT I and II, who comprise around 25% of the white population in the United States.

Age DHe is most often observed in persons over 40 years; young white children (age 10) living in southern Borneo (cool climate with high UVR) have been observed to have DHe.

Skin Phototype I and II are most susceptible, but III and IV and even V (brown skin color) can develop DHe.

Sex Higher incidence in males

Occupation Farmers ("farmer's skin"), telephone linemen, sea workers ("sailor's skin"), construction workers, lifeguards, swimming instructors, sportspersons, and "beach bums"

Geography DHe is more severe in the white population living in areas with high solar UVR (at high altitudes, in lower latitudes)

HISTORY

Personal History There is a history of intensive exposure to sun in youth (before 35 years); sun exposure may have been limited in later years.

Family History Skin phototypes are genetically determined, and therefore there is often a family history of DHe.

PHYSICAL EXAMINATION

Appearance of Patient Wrinkled, wizened, leathery, "prematurely aged" (Figures 120 and 121), or "looks old, but is young." Persons with brown and black skin color are deceptively young-looking because of the virtual absence of DHe. Persons with black skin who are albinos can develop DHe and sun-induced skin cancers.

Skin
EPIDERMIS *Keratinocytes*
   Atrophy: increased translucence

   Solar keratosis (see Figure 120)

   Xerosis (dryness)

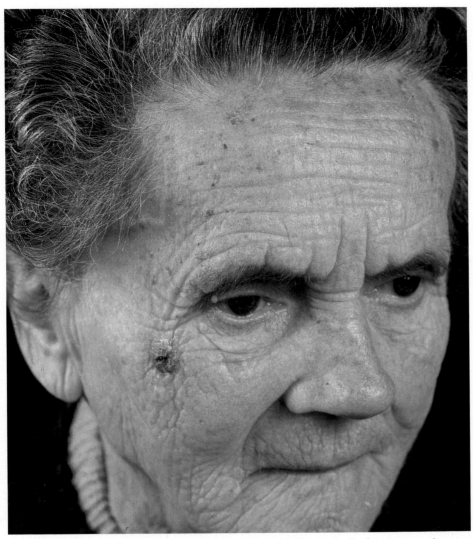

120 Dermatoheliosis   *Solar lentigines, telangiectases, wrinkling, and solar keratoses can be seen.*
There is also a basal cell carcinoma on the right malar area.

Melanocytes

Solar lentigo (see Figures 120 and 121)

Ephelides (freckles) of "old age" (less seasonal dependency than juvenile ephelides)

Guttate hypomelanosis

DERMIS   *Vascular System*

Permanent dilatation of vessels (telangiectasia)

Purpura, easy bruising

Connective Tissue   Wrinkling (fine surface, deep furrows), roughness, and elastosis (fine nodularity and inelasticity), yellowing of the skin

Pilosebaceous Unit   Comedones (especially periorbital) (Favre-Racouchot disease)

DISTRIBUTION

Exposed areas (see Figures 120 and 121)

Scalp (bald males)

Nuchal area: cutis rhomboidalis ("red neck" with rhomboidal furrows)

Periorbital areas: wrinkling

DERMATOPATHOLOGY

Epidermis

Acanthosis of epidermis, increased horny layer

Flattening of the dermoepidermal junction

Atypia of the keratinocytes

Dermis

Marked alteration in microcirculation with loss of small vessels in the papillary dermis

Elastosis: degraded elastic tissue with formation of coarse amorphous masses and increase in glycosaminoglycans

Increase in fibroblasts but a decrease in collagen and increase in elastin

DIFFERENTIAL DIAGNOSIS

Xeroderma pigmentosum exhibits severe DHe in addition to skin cancers (squamous cell and basal cell carcinoma, melanoma, fibrosarcoma, angiosarcoma); however, the disorder is present at a very young age. In *progeria* there is little or no wrinkling but atrophy of skin and subcutis with marked increase in translucency of the epidermis. There are no pigmentary changes and no xerosis of the skin or solar keratoses.

PATHOGENESIS

While UVB is the most obvious damaging UVR, it is now known that UVA can, in high doses, produce connective tissue changes in mice. In addition, visible (400 to 700 nm) radiation and infrared (1000 to 1,000,000 nm) have been implicated, e.g., infrared has been shown to augment the action of UVB on induction of elastosis in guinea pigs. The action spectrum for DHe is not known for certain; there is some experimental evidence in mice that infrared radiation is implicated, in addition to UVB and UVA.

SIGNIFICANCE

There is evidence based on case-control studies that severe sunburns in youth can lead to the development of malignant melanoma 2 or 3 decades later in life. This may result from sun-induced mutations in the gene regulating melanocytes present in common acquired nevomelanocytic and in dysplastic melanocytic nevi. The appearance of DHe marks a relatively young person as "old," a state that everyone tries to put off. There is a current wave to prevent skin cancers and to prevent the development of DHe by the use of protective sunblocks, by change of behavior in the sun, and by the use of topical chemotherapy that reverses some of the changes that occur in DHe (solar keratoses, solar lentigo, vascular and connective tissue changes).

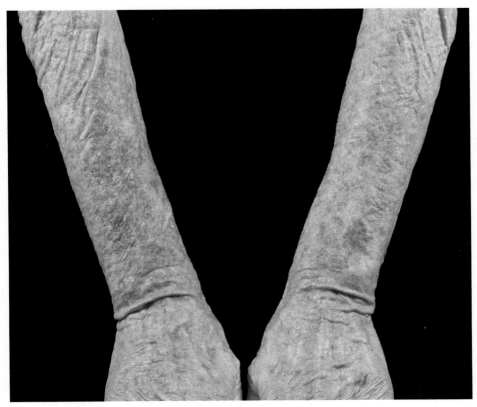

121 Dermatoheliosis *The same features as in Figure 120 are seen.*

COURSE AND PROGNOSIS

DHe is inexorably progressive and irreversible, but some repair of connective tissue effects can occur if the skin is protected. Some processes leading to DHe continue to progress, however, even when sun exposures are severely restricted in later life: solar keratoses and lentigo develop in the sun-damaged skin that is now being protected by avoidance and sunblocks. Yet there are documented examples of spontaneous reversal of solar keratoses and solar lentigo.

TREATMENT AND PREVENTION

Topical Treatment
1. Tretinoin in lotions, gels, and creams in varying concentrations has been demonstrated in controlled studies to effect a reversal (clinical and histologic) of some aspects of DHe, especially the connective tissue and vascular changes. There is a current notion that topical tretinoin can alter the progression of incipient epithelial skin cancers.
2. 5-Fluorouracil in lotions and creams is highly effective in causing a disappearance of solar keratoses.

Prevention Persons of SPT I and II should be identified early in life and advised that they are susceptible to the development of DHe and skin cancers, including melanoma. These persons should never sunbathe and should, from an early age, adopt a daily program of self-protection using substantive and effective topical sun-protective solutions, gels, or lotions that can filter DNA-damaging UVB; UVA filters are less effective. SPT I and II persons should avoid the peak hours of UVB intensity, which are the 2 hours before and after solar noon (1200 GMT).

Solar lentigo is a circumscribed 1.0- to 3.0-cm brown macule resulting from a localized proliferation of melanocytes due to chronic exposure to sunlight.

EPIDEMIOLOGY AND ETIOLOGY

Age Usually over 40 years, but may occur at 30 years in sunny climates

Sex No data available, probably equal incidence

Race Most common in Caucasians, but seen also in Orientals

Predisposing Factors Generally correlated with skin phototypes I to III and duration and intensity of solar exposure

PHYSICAL EXAMINATION

Skin Lesions
TYPE Strictly macular (Figure 122), 1.0 to 3.0 cm, as large as 5.0 cm
COLOR Light yellow, light brown (Figure 122) or dark brown (Figure 123); variegated mix of brown and not uniform color, as in café-au-lait macules.
SHAPE Round, oval, with slightly irregular border
ARRANGEMENT Often scattered, discrete lesions
DISTRIBUTION Exclusively exposed areas: forehead, cheeks, nose, dorsa of hands and forearms, upper back, and chest

DERMATOPATHOLOGY

Site Epidermis

Process Proliferative. Club-shaped elongated rete ridges which show hypermelanosis and increased number of melanocytes in the basal layer

DIFFERENTIAL DIAGNOSIS AND TREATMENT

"Flat," acquired, brown lesions of the exposed skin of the face, which may on cursory examination appear to be similar, have distinctive features:

Solar lentigo, the most frequently observed lesion, has a medium-brown color and is completely flat without evidence of epidermal change, even when carefully examined with a hand lens and oblique lighting. The lesions may gradually enlarge to 3.0 to 4.0 cm or more and completely disappear for 1 to 3 years following very short exposures (10 seconds) to liquid nitrogen applied with a cotton tip.

Seborrheic keratosis may be indistinguishable in its early stages from solar lentigo, but usually epidermal change is barely perceptible in seborrheic keratosis when examined with a hand lens and oblique lighting.

Pigmented solar keratosis, also called "spreading pigmented actinic keratosis," is indistinguishable from an early seborrheic keratosis (q.v.). This can be resolved with a small punch biopsy. This rather uncommon lesion is a mixture of atypical keratinocytic and atypical melanocytic proliferative processes. The lesion responds well to topical fluorouracil preparations. Ten days of 5% 5-fluorouracil in an ointment base will cause the lesion to disappear.

Lentigo maligna is completely flat, without any epidermal alteration, and simulates solar lentigo except for a distinct variegation of color: brown, dark brown, and flecks of black. These lesions should always be biopsied and, if proved histologically, excised; depending on size, a skin flap or split-thickness graft may be necessary.

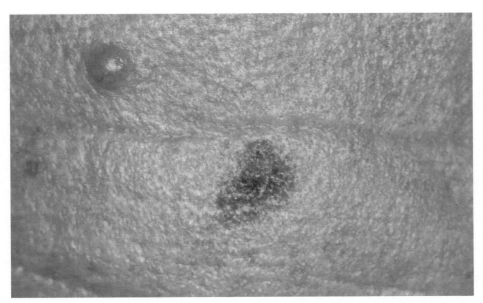

122 Solar lentigo *Dark-brown, slightly variegated, pigmented macule. A dermal nevus is also seen at the upper left.*

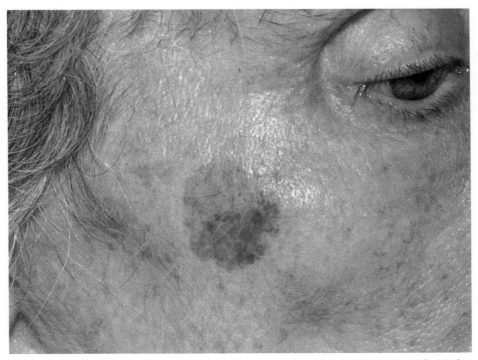

123 Solar lentigo *In the right zygomatous region, a round, sharply demarcated macule varying from light- to dark-brown. The surrounding skin shows patchy hyperpigmentation and telangiectases, as found after lifelong sun exposure.*

SOLAR LENTIGO   219

These single or multiple, discrete, dry, rough, adherent scaly lesions occur on the habitually sun-exposed skin of adults.
Synonym: actinic keratosis.

EPIDEMIOLOGY AND ETIOLOGY

Age Middle age, although in Australia and southwestern United States solar keratosis may occur in persons under 30

Sex More common in males

Race Skin phototypes (SPT) I, II, and III, rare in SPT IV, and almost never in blacks or East Indians

Occupation Outdoor workers (especially farmers, ranchers, sailors) and outdoor sportspersons (tennis, golf, mountain climbing, deep-sea fishing)

HISTORY

Duration of Lesions Months

Skin Symptoms Some lesions may be tender

PHYSICAL EXAMINATION

Skin Lesions
TYPE Adherent hyperkeratotic scale (Figure 124), which is removed with difficulty and pain. May be papular.
COLOR Skin-colored, yellow-brown (Figure 125), or brown; often there is a reddish tinge.
PALPATION Rough, like coarse sandpaper (see Figure 124)

SIZE AND SHAPE Most commonly <1.0 cm; oval or round
DISTRIBUTION Isolated single lesion or scattered discrete lesions
SITES OF PREDILECTION Face (forehead, nose, cheeks, temples, vermilion border lower lip), ears (in males), neck (sides), forearms and hands (dorsa)

DIFFERENTIAL DIAGNOSIS

Flat solar keratoses, especially red, may be confused with *discoid lupus erythematosus.* Biopsy is necessary.

DERMATOPATHOLOGY

Site Epidermis

Process Proliferative and neoplastic. Large bright-staining keratinocytes, with mild to moderate pleomorphism in the basal layer, parakeratosis, and atypical (dyskeratotic) keratinocytes.

PATHOPHYSIOLOGY

Prolonged and repeated solar exposure in susceptible persons (SPT I, II, and III) leads to cumulative damage to keratinocytes by the action of ultraviolet radiant energy, principally, if not exclusively, UVB (290 to 320 nm).

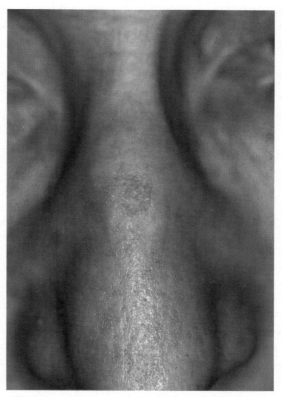

124 Solar keratosis *The lesion on the nose, a typical site, is ill-defined, with an adherent keratotic scale. Scratching the lesion often causes pain or sensitivity.*

COURSE AND PROGNOSIS

Solar keratoses may spontaneously disappear, but in general they remain for years. The actual incidence of squamous cell carcinoma in preexisting solar keratoses is unknown, but has been estimated at 1 squamous cell carcinoma developing annually in each 1000 solar keratoses.

TREATMENT AND PREVENTIVE MEASURES

Most solar keratoses react to local application to the lesion of 5% 5-fluorouracil cream over a period of several days to weeks and then erode and disappear. Short exposure to liquid nitrogen alone or followed in 3 days by topical application of 5% 5-fluorouracil cream is most effective; the latter avoids depigmented areas that occur when therapeutic exposures of liquid nitrogen are used alone.

Nodular lesions should be excised.

Prevention is afforded by use of highly effective UVB/UVA sunscreens, which should be applied daily to the face and ears during the summer in northern latitudes for SPT-I and -II persons and for those SPT-III persons who obtain prolonged sunlight exposures.

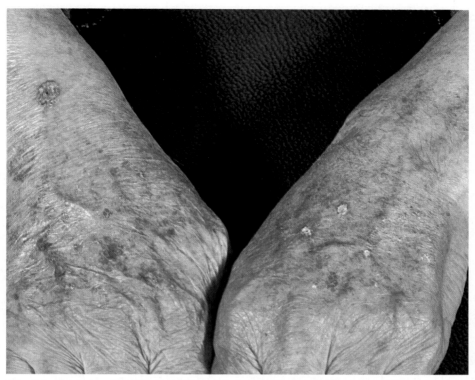

125 Solar keratoses *The skin is atrophic and shows delicate wrinkling, several brown macules, and small, white, keratotic patches which are rough on palpation.*

Phytophotodermatitis (Plant + Light = Dermatitis)

Phytophotodermatitis (PPD) is an inflammation of the skin caused by contact with certain plants during, and subsequent to, recreational or occupational exposure to sunlight. The inflammatory response is a phototoxic reaction to photosensitizing chemicals present in several plant families; a common type of PPD is due to exposure to limes.

EPIDEMIOLOGY

Age PPD can occur at any age; in children, exposure to plants in the grassy meadows near beaches may occur.

Race All skin colors; brown- and black-skinned peoples may develop only marked spotty dark pigmentation without erythema or bullous lesions.

Occupation Celery pickers, carrot processors, gardeners [exposed to carrot greens or to "gas plant" *(Dictamnus albus)*], and bartenders

HISTORY

History The patient gives a history of exposure to certain plants (lime, lemon, wild parsley, celery, giant hogweed, parsnips, carrot greens, figs). Lime juice is a frequent cause: making lime drinks, hair rinses with lime juice. Women who use perfumes containing oil of bergamot (which contains bergapten, 5-methoxypsoralen) may develop only streaks of pigmentation in areas where the perfume was applied, especially the sides of the neck, upper anterior chest, and wrists. This is called *berloque dermatitis* (*breloque,* French, "pendant"). Persons walking on beaches containing meadow grass will develop phytophotodermatitis on the legs; meadow grass contains agrimony.

Relationship of Skin Lesions to Season
Seen most often during the summer months in northern latitudes, or all year in tropical climates.

Skin Symptoms Marked pruritus

PHYSICAL EXAMINATION

Skin
TYPE OF LESION Acute: erythema, vesicles, and bullae (Figure 126), but not an eczematous dermatitis as seen in *Rhus* dermatitis. Residual dark hyperpigmentation in bizarre streaks (Figure 127)

SHAPE OF INDIVIDUAL LESIONS Bizarre streaks, artificial patterns which indicate an "outside job"

DISTRIBUTION AND ARRANGEMENT OF MULTIPLE LESIONS Scattered areas on the sites of contact, especially the arms and legs

SPECIAL EXAMINATIONS

Wood's Lamp Examination The sites of involvement can be detected by the enhancement of the erythema and pigmentation.

DIAGNOSIS

This is easily made if the pattern is recognized and a careful history is taken.

SKIN REACTION TO SUNLIGHT EXPOSURE

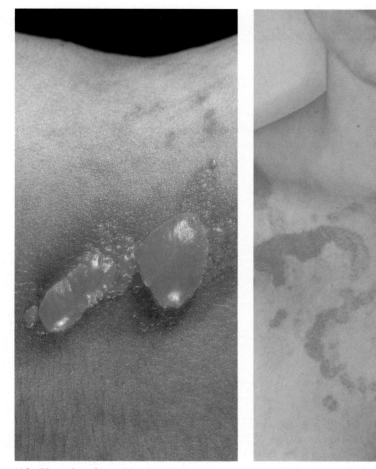

126 Phytophotodermatitis *Vesicles and bullae resulting from contact with wild celery, which contains furocoumarins.*

127 Phytophotodermatitis *Whorls of pigmentation occurring only in sites where a perfume-containing oil of bergamot had been applied. Oil of bergamot contains 5-methoxypsoralen.*

ETIOLOGY

The phototoxic reaction is caused by the presence of photoactive chemicals, mostly psoralens contained in the plants.

SIGNIFICANCE

May be an important occupational problem, as in celery pickers

COURSE

The acute eruption fades spontaneously, but the pigmentation may last for months.

TREATMENT

Wet dressings may be indicated in the acute vesicular stage.

PHYTOPHOTODERMATITIS (PLANT + LIGHT = DERMATITIS)

Drug-Induced Photosensitivity: Phototoxic

Drug-induced photosensitivity describes an adverse reaction of the skin which results from simultaneous exposure to certain drugs (via ingestion, injection, or topical application) and to ultraviolet radiation (UVR) or visible light. The chemicals may be therapeutic, cosmetic, industrial, or agricultural. There are two types of reaction: (1) "phototoxic," which *can* occur in all individuals and is essentially an exaggerated sunburn response (erythema, edema, vesicles, etc.) and (2) "photoallergic," which involves an immunologic response and in which the eruption is a "rash" (see page 228).

EPIDEMIOLOGY

Incidence Phototoxic drug reactions are more frequent than photoallergic drug sensitivity.

Age Can occur at any age

Race All types of skin color: black, white, and brown

HISTORY

History There are three patterns of phototoxic reaction: (1) immediate erythema and urticaria, (2) delayed sunburn-type pattern developing within 16 to 24 hours or later (48 to 72 hours in psoralen-related phototoxic reactions), or (3) delayed (72 to 96 hours) melanin hyperpigmentation.

Skin Symptoms Pruritus or burning or stinging

PHYSICAL EXAMINATION

Skin The skin lesions are those of an "exaggerated sunburn." In phototoxic drug reactions there is erythema, edema (Figure 128), and vesicle and bulla formation (e.g., pseudoporphyria). An eczematous reaction pattern is not seen in phototoxic reactions. Marked brown epidermal melanin pigmentation may occur in the course of the eruption, and, espe-

cially with certain drugs (chlorpromazine and amiodarone), a gray dermal melanin pigmentation develops. After repeated exposure some scaling and lichenification can develop.

DISTRIBUTION OF LESIONS Confined exclusively to areas exposed to light (see distribution pattern of light eruption, Figures XI and XII).

Nails Photo-onycholysis can occur with certain drugs (psoralens, demethylchlortetracycline, and benoxaprofen).

LABORATORY EXAMINATIONS

Dermatopathology Inflammation, "sunburn cells" in the epidermis, epidermal necrobiosis, intraepidermal and subepidermal vesiculation. Absence of eczematous changes.

DIAGNOSIS AND DIFFERENTIAL DIAGNOSIS

Diagnosis History of exposure to drug is most important as well as the type of morphologic changes in the skin characteristic of phototoxic drug eruptions: confluent erythema, edema, vesicles, and bullae.

Differential Diagnosis Phototoxic reactions due to excess of endogenous porphyrins (see Porphyrias, Section 22), photosensitivity due to other diseases, e.g., SLE

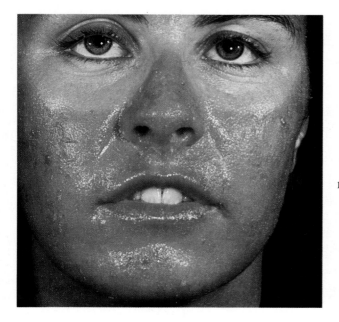

128 Photosensitivity to drugs: phototoxic *This patient was taking demethyl-chlortetracycline for acne and went skiing in the wintertime for 3 hours. There is an exaggerated sunburn reaction with exudation and edema.*

PHOTOTESTING

For verification of incriminated agent, template test sites are exposed to increasing doses of UVA (phototoxic reactions are almost always due to UVA) *while patient is on incriminated drug.* The UVA MED will be much lower than in normal individuals of the same SPT. After drug is excreted and then eliminated from the skin a repeat UVA phototest will reveal an *increase* of the UVA MED. This test may be important if patient was on multiple potentially phototoxic drugs.

ETIOLOGY

Amiodarone, thiazides, coal tar and derivatives, doxycycline, furosemide, nalidixic acid, demethylchlortetracycline, oxytetracycline, phenothiazines, piroxicam, psoralens (furo-coumarins), sulfonamides.

PATHOGENESIS

Formation of toxic photoproducts such as free radicals, or reactive oxygen species such as singlet oxygen. The principal sites of damage are nuclear DNA or cell membranes (plasma, lysosomal, mitochondrial, microsomal). The action spectrum is UVA.

SIGNIFICANCE

Phototoxic drug sensitivity is a major problem, as the abnormal reactions seriously limit or exclude the use of important drugs: diuretics, antihypertensive agents, drugs used in psychiatry. It is not known why some individuals show phototoxic reactions to a particular drug and others do not.

COURSE AND PROGNOSIS

Phototoxic drug reactions disappear following cessation of drug.

In photoallergic drug photosensitivity the chemical agent (drug) present in the skin absorbs photons and forms a photoproduct; this photoproduct then binds to a soluble or membrane-bound protein to form an antigen. As photoallergy depends on individual immunologic reactivity it develops in only a small percentage of persons exposed to drugs and light.

EPIDEMIOLOGY

Incidence Photoallergic drug reactions occur much less frequently than do phototoxic drug reactions.

Age Probably more common in adults

Race All types of skin color: black, white, and brown

HISTORY

History The history may be more difficult in that initial sensitization induces a delayed-hypersensitivity reaction, and the eruption occurs on subsequent sensitization. Topically applied photosensitizers are the most frequent cause of photoallergic eruptions, e.g., halogenated salicylanilides, benzocaine (in soaps and other household products used to inhibit bacterial overgrowth), or musk ambrette used in aftershave lotions.

Skin Symptoms Pruritus

PHYSICAL EXAMINATION

Skin The morphology of the skin reaction is much different than in phototoxic drug sensitivity. Acute photoallergic reaction patterns resemble: (1) allergic contact eczematous dermatitis (Figure 129) similar to poison ivy dermatitis, or (2) lichen planus-like eruptions. In chronic drug photoallergy there is scaling, li-chenification, and marked pruritus mimicking atopic eczematous dermatitis or chronic contact eczematous dermatitis.

Distribution of Lesions Confined primarily to areas exposed to light (see distribution pattern of photosensitivity, Figures XI and XII), but there may be spreading onto adjacent nonexposed skin. Therefore, not so well described as in phototoxic reactions.

LABORATORY EXAMINATIONS

Dermatopathology Acute and chronic delayed-hypersensitivity reaction: epidermal spongiosis with lymphocytic infiltration (see page 18).

DIAGNOSIS

History of exposure to drug is most important, as well as the types of morphologic change in the skin that are characteristic of photoallergic drug reactions; this is essentially a contact eczematous pattern, while phototoxic drug eruptions mimic an exaggerated sunburn.

ETIOLOGY

Halogenated salicylanilides, phenothiazines, sulfonamides; PABA esters, benzocaine, neomycin, benzophenones, and 6-methyl-coumarin in sunscreens; musk ambrette in aftershave lotions; and stilbenes in whiteners.

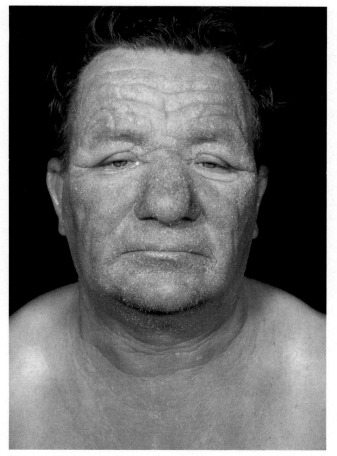

129   Photosensitivity to drugs: photoallergic   *Note chronic eczematous appearance.*

PATHOGENESIS

Formation of photoproduct which conjugates with protein producing an antigen. The action spectrum involved is UVA.

SIGNIFICANCE

Photoallergic drug reactions are difficult to diagnose and require the use of patch and photopatch tests. Photopatch tests are done in duplicate because photoallergens can also cause contact hypersensitivity. As in patch tests for contact hypersensitivity, photoallergens are applied to the skin and covered. After 24 hours one set of the duplicate test sites is exposed to UVA while the other remains covered, and test sites are read for reactions after 48 to 96 hours. An eczematous reaction in the irradiated site but not in the nonirradiated site confirms photoallergy to the particular agent tested.

COURSE AND PROGNOSIS

Contact photoallergic dermatitis can persist for months to years (Figures 130 and 131). This is known as "persistent light reaction" and was first observed in soldiers in World War II in whom topical sulfonamides were used and in persistent light reactors from chlorpromazine photoallergy. The classic generalized persistent light reactions were caused by exposure to salicylanilides. In the persistent light reactor the action spectrum usually broadens to involve UVB.

SKIN REACTION TO SUNLIGHT EXPOSURE

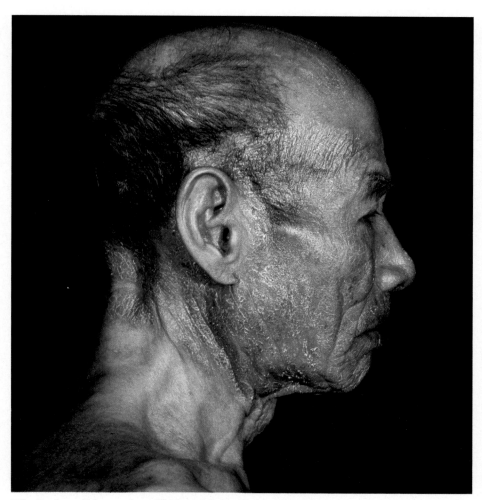

130   Persistent light eruption   *Thickened, lichenified, scaling dermatosis, sparing the creases of the neck and the covered areas.*

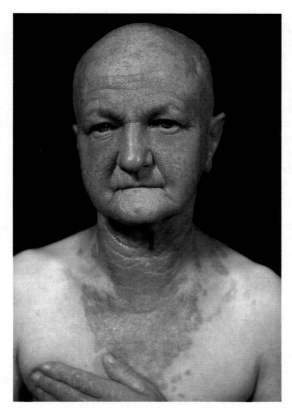

131 Persistent light eruption *Thickened, erythematous eruption confined to face and "V" neck area but sparing areas shaded by the nose.*

Polymorphous light eruption (PMLE) is a term that describes a group of heterogeneous, idiopathic, acquired, acute recurrent photodermatoses characterized by delayed abnormal reactions to ultraviolet radiation (UVR) and manifested by varied lesions. The various morphologic types include: erythematous macules, papules, plaques, and vesicles. However, in each patient the eruption is consistently monomorphous. By far the most frequent morphologic types are the papular and papulovesicular eruptions.

EPIDEMIOLOGY

Incidence Most common of the photodermatoses

Age Average age of onset is 23 years

Race All races, including brown and black peoples. In American Indians (North and South America) there is an hereditary type of PMLE which is also called *actinic prurigo*.

Skin Phototype (SPT) More often seen in SPT I, II, III, IV.

Sex Much more common in females

Geography PMLE is less frequently observed in areas that have high solar intensity throughout the year. PMLE often occurs for the first time in persons travelling for short vacations to tropical areas in winter from northern latitudes.

HISTORY

Onset and Duration of Lesions PMLE appears in spring or early summer, and not infrequently the eruption does not recur by the end of summer, suggesting a "hardening." The rash comes on suddenly, following minutes to days of sun exposure. PMLE most often appears within 18 to 24 hours of exposure and, once established, persists for 7 to 10 days, thereby limiting the vacationer's subsequent time in the sun.

Special Features The eruption is elicited most frequently by exposure to UVA but can also be caused by UVB or by both; as UVA is transmitted through window glass, PMLE can be precipitated while riding in a car. In patients who travel to sunny vacation areas such as the Caribbean the eruption will occur but is not noted even during the summer months in the northern latitudes; presumably the "threshold" for elicitation occurs with higher intensities. Also, areas of the skin habitually exposed (face and neck) are often spared, despite severe involvement of the arms, trunk, and legs.

Skin Symptoms Pruritus (may precede the onset of the rash) and paresthesia (tingling)

Systems Review Negative

Family History PMLE in American Indians is hereditary.

PHYSICAL EXAMINATION

Types of Lesions The papular and papulovesicular types (Figures 132 and 133) are the most frequent. Less common are plaques. The lesions are pink to red.

Distribution of Lesions The eruption

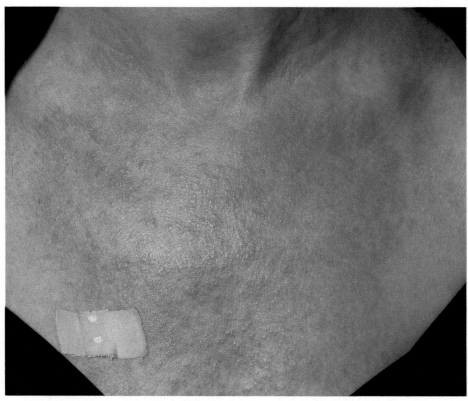

132   Polymorphous light eruption   *Clusters of papulovesicles involving the "V" area.*

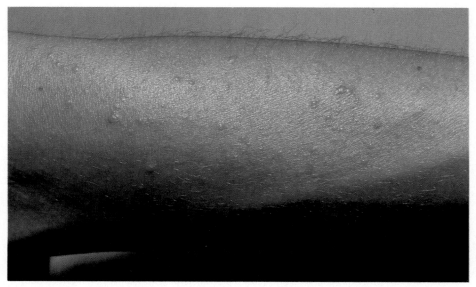

133   Polymorphous light eruption   *On the arm there is a rash composed of papulovesicular lesions.*

often spares the face and is most frequently seen on the forearms and "V" area of the neck. The lesions may also occur on the trunk, if there has not been previous exposure.

LABORATORY AND SPECIAL EXAMINATIONS

Dermatopathology (Characteristic but not diagnostic)

LIGHT MICROSCOPY In papular and eczematous lesions there is edema of the epidermis, spongiosis, vesicle formation, and mild liquefaction degeneration of the basal layer, but no atrophy or thickening of the basement membrane. A dense lymphocytic infiltrate is present in the dermis, with occasional neutrophils. There is edema of the papillary dermis and endothelial swelling.

IMMUNOFLUORESCENCE (DIRECT) Negative

SPECIAL TECHNIQUES Monoclonal antibody-immunopathology techniques reveal that the mononuclear cells are predominantly T cells.

Laboratory Examination of Blood

SEROLOGIC ANA is negative.

HEMATOLOGIC There is no leukopenia.

Illumination (Allow for dark adaptation)

Partially darkened room—this permits the examiner to better see the eruption, as the contrast is accentuated.

Completely darkened room—oblique lighting: place a flashlight at the side of the lesion to detect subtle surface changes (elevation or depression).

Wood's Lamp Examination The eruption is exaggerated because of the erythema.

DIAGNOSIS AND DIFFERENTIAL DIAGNOSIS

Diagnosis The diagnosis is not difficult: delayed onset of eruption, characteristic morphology, histopathologic changes which rule out lupus erythematosus, and the history of disappearance of the eruption in days. In plaque-type PMLE, a biopsy and immunofluorescence studies are mandatory to rule out lupus erythematosus. *Phototesting* is done with both UVB and UVA. Test sites are exposed daily, starting with 2 MEDs of UVB and UVA, respectively, for 1 week to 10 days, using increments of the UV dose. In 50% of patients a PMLE-like eruption will occur in the test sites confirming the diagnosis. This also helps to determine whether the action spectrum is UVB, UVA, or both.

Differential Diagnosis Lupus erythematosus (SLE) is the most important disease to exclude, as is discussed above. Serologic study of ANA and anticytoplasmic antibodies (anti-Ro, and anti-La) is necessary in plaque-type PMLE. Photosensitivity eruptions caused by systemic or topical drugs and cosmetics can be ruled out by history.

PATHOGENESIS

A delayed hypersensitivity reaction to an antigen induced by UVR is possible because of morphology of the lesions and the histologic pattern, which shows an infiltration of T cells. Immunologic studies thus far have not been rewarding.

SIGNIFICANCE

This is a pesky problem that severely limits recreational or occupational exposure to the sun.

COURSE AND PROGNOSIS

The course is chronic and recurrent and may, in fact, become worse each season. Although some patients may develop "tolerance" by the end of the summer, the eruption usually recurs again the following spring, and/or when they travel to tropical areas in the winter. However, spontaneous improvement or even cessation of eruptions occurs after years.

236

TREATMENT

Topical Sunblocks, even the potent UVA-UVB sunscreens are rarely effective but should be tried first in every patient. Even when systemic drugs or photochemotherapy is used, potent topical UVA-UVB sunblocks should be used in addition.

Systemic Beta-carotene has not been very effective but can be tried before antimalarials. Antimalarials (hydroxychloroquine and chloroquine) are the effective drugs for the treatment of PMLE in some patients and should be used in selected patients not helped by topical sunblocks or oral beta-carotene.

PUVA Photochemotherapy This treatment given in early spring induces "tolerance" for the following summer. PUVA treatments are given 3 times weekly for 4 weeks. It is not known whether their effectiveness is based on the production of an increase in the "filtering" capacity of the epidermis (increase in the stratum corneum and in melanin content of the epidermis) or to an effect of PUVA on T cells.

Solar urticaria is a distinctive reaction pattern of wheals that develops within minutes after exposure to sunlight or artificial UVR and disappears within 1 hour.

EPIDEMIOLOGY

Incidence   Uncommon

Sex   More common in females

Age   All ages from childhood to over 80 years. One series of 15 patients reported a median age of 25 years.

HISTORY

History   Itching and burning occur within a few minutes of exposure to sunlight. Soon after, erythema appears which develops into wheals, only in the sites of exposure. The wheals disappear within several hours.

Systems Review   Some patients experience giddiness, nausea, and headache. Bronchospasm has been rarely reported. Sudden exposure of large surface areas can result in a generalized urticaria and an anaphylactic-like reaction.

PHYSICAL EXAMINATION

Skin Findings
TYPE OF LESION   Urticarial wheals (Figure 134), usually with an axon flare in the periphery.
DISTRIBUTION OF LESIONS   The urticarial wheals occur less frequently on the habitually exposed areas (face and dorsa of the hands) than on the covered areas (arms, legs, and trunk).

LABORATORY EXAMINATIONS

Dermatopathology   Not diagnostic

Stool Examination   Determination of the levels of protoporphyrins should be done in all patients to rule out erythropoietic protoporphyria, although urticarial wheals are extremely rare in this disorder.

SPECIAL EXAMINATIONS

Phototesting is helpful in discovering the wavelengths involved and can aid in the management of the disorder (see Figure 135). Solar urticaria has been classified into several types depending on the action spectrum that elicits the eruption. Solar urticaria can be caused by UVB, UVA, and visible light, and by any combination of the above. The action spectra of solar urticaria most frequently seen is 320 to 400 nm (so-called type II) or 400 to 500 nm (so-called type III).

DIAGNOSIS

The history is typical; the disorder that can be confused with solar urticaria is that rare type of polymorphic light eruption (PMLE) in which the lesions appear within a few minutes. In PMLE, however, the lesions do not disappear in hours but last for days.

SKIN REACTION TO SUNLIGHT EXPOSURE

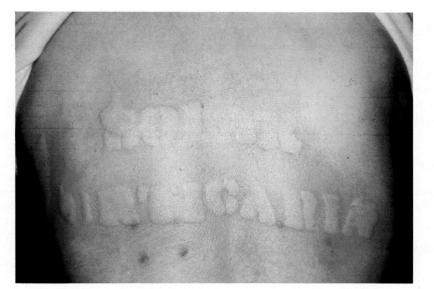

134   Solar urticaria   *These lesions were provoked in a patient with solar urticaria while sitting in the sun behind window glass for 10 minutes.*

PATHOGENESIS

Some few patients with solar urticaria have a serum factor which can be transferred and which has several features of an IgE-class immunoglobulin. Elevation of histamine levels has been detected in patients following exposure to UVR.

COURSE AND PROGNOSIS

Spontaneous remission can occur within 5 to 8 years.

TREATMENT

Topical Sunblocks are sometimes useful in patients with the rare type of solar urticaria elicited by UVB (290 to 320 nm). Oral beta-carotene is sometimes helpful.

Systemic Antihistamines are not effective. Some patients can be made unresponsive to solar radiation by plasmapheresis, presumably by the removal of serum factor(s) responsible for the eruption.

Phototherapy Desensitization is performed with the specific wavelengths that elicit the eruption. This has been successful in maintaining a symptom-free life using simple light sources taken at home. UVA home units are also commercially available for treatment of type II (320 to 400 nm). Nevertheless, desensitization is better done by the physician in control. PUVA photochemotherapy is effective and protects solar urticaria patients as it does patients with PMLE. Prophylactic PUVA treatment must be done under the supervision of a physician.

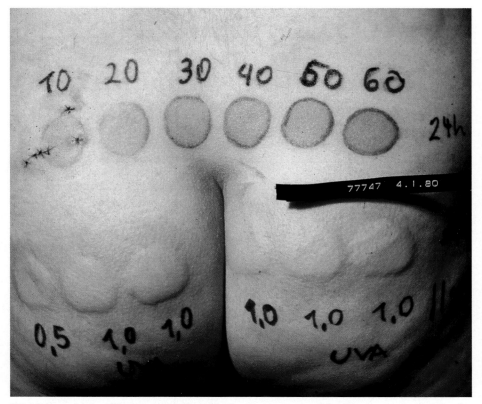

135 Solar urticaria *These test sites illustrate the dose response of the skin in a patient with solar urticaria. Note the urticarial lesions to the extremely low doses of UVA (whealing reaction to 0.5 J/cm², whereas the minimal erythema dose to UVA would be approximated at 40 to 60 J/cm² in this SPT). The upper row of test sites was exposed to UVB (10 to 60 mJ/cm²) 24 hours before. These tests were not urticarial in type and now show only erythema.*

Noninfectious Inflammatory Skin Disorders

Lichen Planus

This acute or chronic inflammation of the skin and mucous membranes has characteristic flat-topped (Latin *planus,* ''flat''), violaceous, shiny, pruritic papules on the skin, and milky-white papules in the mouth.

EPIDEMIOLOGY AND ETIOLOGY

Age 30 to 60 years

Sex Females more than males

Other Factors The etiology is unknown. Severe emotional stress can precipitate an attack. Drugs may induce a lichen planus-like eruption.

HISTORY

Duration of Lesions Acute (days) or insidious onset over weeks

Symptoms
SKIN Pruritus, which may be severe or may not be present at all
MUCOUS MEMBRANE Painful, especially when ulcers present

PHYSICAL EXAMINATION

Skin Lesions
TYPE Papules, 1.0 to 10.0 mm, shiny

COLOR Violaceous, with white lines (Wickham's striae, Figure 136) seen best with hand lens after application of mineral oil
SHAPE Polygonal or oval
ARRANGEMENT Grouped, linear (isomorphic phenomenon), annular, or disseminated scattered discrete lesions
DISTRIBUTION Wrists (flexor, see Figure 136), lumbar region, eyelids, shins (thicker, hyperkeratotic lesions), and scalp. Lichen planus actinicus occurs in sun-exposed sites.

Mucous Membranes 40% to 60% of patients. See Figure 137.
SITES OF PREDILECTION Buccal mucosa, tongue, lips
LESIONS Milky-white papules, with white lacework on the buccal mucosa. Carcinoma may very rarely develop in mouth lesions (see Figure 137).

Hair and Nails
SCALP Atrophic scalp skin with alopecia
NAILS 10% of patients. Destruction of the nail fold and nail bed, especially in the large toe.

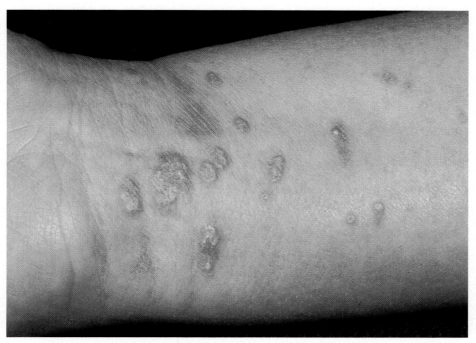

136   Lichen planus.   *Flat-topped papules on the wrist. Some are isolated and some have coalesced. The color is violaceous with lacy lines (Wickham's striae).*

DIFFERENTIAL DIAGNOSIS

Drug eruption caused by contact with chemicals used in color film developing. *Chloroquine* or *gold salts*. *Lichenoid graft-versushost reactions*.

DERMATOPATHOLOGY

Site Epidermis and dermis

Process Inflammation with hyperkeratosis, increased granular layer, irregular acanthosis, liquefaction degeneration of the basal cell layer, and bandlike mononuclear infiltrate that hugs the epidermis

COURSE

Spontaneous resolution in weeks is possible; lesions may also persist for years, especially on the shins and in the mouth.

TREATMENT

Topical corticosteroids with occlusion.

Oral prednisone is rarely used, and only in short courses.

PUVA photochemotherapy may be substituted for oral prednisone in generalized or resistant cases.

Oral retinoids are helpful for erosive lichen planus of the mouth. In very resistant oral lesions, cyclosporin A mouth washes.

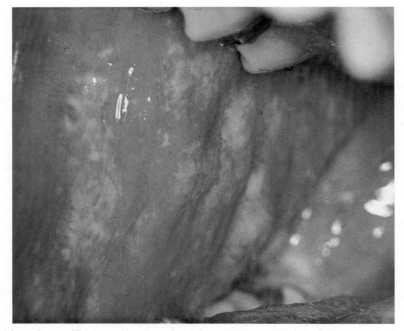

137 Lichen planus *The buccal mucosa shows irregularly marginated white areas which are not elevated or indurated. The surface is smooth and there is a lacelike pattern which is characteristic of oral lichen planus.*

This disease is a self-limited chronic inflammation of the dermis that exhibits papules in an annular arrangement.

EPIDEMIOLOGY AND ETIOLOGY

Age   Children and young adults

Sex   Female:male ratio 2:1

Other Factors   Etiology is unknown. The lesions are sometimes indistinguishable from necrobiosis lipoidica. Generalized granuloma annulare may very rarely be associated with diabetes mellitus.

HISTORY

Duration of Lesions   Weeks, months

Skin Symptoms   Usually asymptomatic, rarely pruritic

PHYSICAL EXAMINATION

Skin Lesions
TYPE
   Firm dermal papules 1.0 to 5.0 cm, rare epidermal change (so-called perforating granuloma annulare) (see Figure 138)
   Nodules, subcutaneous

COLOR   Skin-colored, erythematous, violaceous
SHAPE   Dome-shaped, annular
ARRANGEMENT   Complete circle (annular) or half-circle (arciform)
DISTRIBUTION   Isolated lesion (Figure 138), multiple lesions in certain regions, or generalized (older patients)
SITES OF PREDILECTION   *Dermal Papules* Dorsa of hands, fingers, feet, extensor aspects of arms and legs, trunk
Subcutaneous Nodules   Palms, legs, buttocks, scalp

DIFFERENTIAL DIAGNOSIS

Papular lesions (necrobiosis lipoidica, papular sarcoid, lichen planus, lymphocytic infiltrate of Jessner); subcutaneous nodules (rheumatoid nodules)

DERMATOPATHOLOGY

Site   Dermis or subcutaneous tissue

Process   Foci of chronic inflammatory and histiocytic infiltrations in superficial and mid-dermis with incomplete and reversible necrobiosis of connective tissue surrounded by a wall of palisading histiocytes and multinucleated giant cells.

COURSE

The disease disappears in 75% of patients in 2 years, but recurrences are common (40%).

TREATMENT

Either intralesional triamcinolone acetonide, 3.0 mg/mL, or topical corticosteroids with occlusion; corticosteroids incorporated in tape are somewhat useful. Superficial lesions respond to liquid nitrogen, but atrophy may occur. PUVA is effective in generalized granuloma annulare.

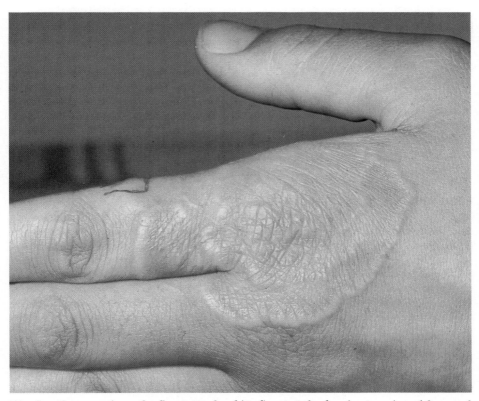

138 Granuloma annulare *Confluent, pearly white, firm papules forming two rings, 1.0 cm and 5.0 cm in diameter. There is no scale.*

Morphea is a localized cutaneous sclerosis characterized by early violaceous, later ivory-colored, plaques, which may be solitary, linear, generalized, and, rarely, accompanied by atrophy of underlying structures.

Synonyms: localized scleroderma, circumscribed scleroderma.

EPIDEMIOLOGY AND ETIOLOGY

Age Pansclerotic usually occurs in children before age 14 years.

Etiology Unknown. However, there is increasing evidence that at least some patients with classical morphea have sclerosis due to *Borrelia burgdorferi* infection.

HISTORY

Skin Symptoms Usually absent. No history of Raynaud's phenomenon.

PHYSICAL EXAMINATION

Skin, Hair, and Nail Lesions
CLASSIFICATION BY PATTERN OF INVOLVEMENT

Circumscribed or localized Plaques or bands

Linear Extremity

Frontoparietal (en coup de sabre) Linear morphea occurring on the head with or without hemiatrophy of face

Generalized plaques

Pansclerotic Involvement (trunk, extremities, face, scalp with sparing of fingertips and toes) of dermis, fat, fascia, muscle, bone. Pansclerotic morphea is usually generalized.

TYPE *Plaques*—initially, indurated but poorly defined areas; 2.0 to 15.0 cm in diameter (Figure 139). In time, surface becomes smooth and shiny; hair follicles and sweat duct orifices disappear. *Purpura, telangiectasia,* and, rarely, bullae may be seen later in course. Deep involvement of tissue may be associated with atrophy of muscle and bone, with resultant growth disturbance in children and flexion contracture; pseudo-ainhum-like lesion may occur circumferentially on limb with subsequent distal edema. Scalp involvement results in scarring alopecia.

COLOR Initially, purplish or mauve; after months to years may be hyperpigmented. Ivory with lilac-colored edge. In lesions of rapid onset, may be erythematous. With generalized morphea, may have hyperpigmentation in involved areas.

SHAPE Round or oval

PALPATION Indurated, hard. May be hypesthetic. Rarely, lesions become atrophic and hyperpigmented without going through a sclerotic stage *(atrophoderma of Pasini and Pierini).*

ARRANGEMENT Usually multiple, bilateral, asymmetric. May be linear on extremity or scalp.

HAIR AND NAILS Scarring alopecia with scalp involvement of plaque, generalized, or frontoparietal morphea. Nail dystrophy in linear lesions of extremity or in pansclerotic morphea.

DISTRIBUTION

Circumscribed Trunk, limbs, face, genitalia. Less commonly, axillae, perineum, areolae

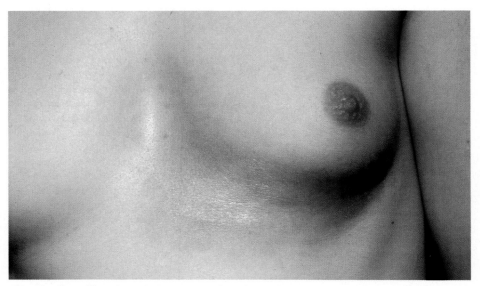

139   Morphea   *There is an indurated, poorly defined plaque under the left breast. The lesion is multicolored with a central, yellow, "carnauba-wax" area surrounded by a lilac border.*

Linear Usually on extremity

Frontoparietal Scalp and face

Generalized Initially on trunk (upper, breasts, abdomen) (Figure 140), thighs

MUCOUS MEMBRANES With linear morphea of head, may have associated hemiatrophy of tongue.

General Examination Involvement around joints may lead to flexion contractures, especially of hands and feet. Deeper involvement of tissue associated with atrophy and fibrosis of muscle. Extensive involvement may result in restricted respiration. With linear morphea of head, may have associated atrophy of ocular structures and atrophy of bone.

DIAGNOSIS AND DIFFERENTIAL DIAGNOSIS

Diagnosis Clinical diagnosis, at times confirmed by skin biopsy.

Differential Diagnosis Sclerotic plaque associated with *Borrelia burgdorferi* infection, progressive systemic sclerosis, lichen sclerosus et atrophicus, eosinophilic fasciitis, eosinophilia-myalgia syndrome associated with L-tryptophan ingestion, acrodermatitis chronica atrophicans, scleredema

LABORATORY AND SPECIAL EXAMINATIONS

Serology Appropriate serologic testing to rule out *B. burgdorferi* infection

Dermatopathology

EPIDERMIS Normal to atrophic with loss of rete ridges.

DERMIS Initially edematous with swelling and degeneration of collagen fibrils; later these become homogeneous and eosinophilic. Slight infiltrate, perivascular or diffuse; lymphocytes, plasma cells, macrophages. Later, dermis thickened with few fibroblasts and dense collagen; inflammatory infiltrate at dermal/subcutis junction; dermal appendages progressively disappear. Pansclerotic lesions show fibrosis and disappearance of subcutaneous tissue, fibrosis broadening as well as sclerosis of fascia. Silver stains should be performed to rule out *B. burgdorferi* infection.

COURSE

May be slowly progressive, but spontaneous remissions occur.

TREATMENT

There is no effective treatment for morphea, i.e., symptomatic interventions when indicated. In some patients with early morphea there is reversal of sclerosis with high-dose parenteral penicillin or ceftriaxone treatment given in several courses over a time span of several months (see Etiology).

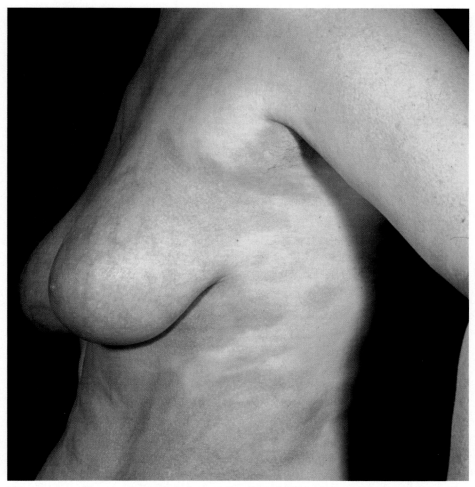

140   Morphea   *There are multiple lesions on the chest which are better felt as indurated plaques than seen. The lesions are light brown in color and are circumscribed.*

Lichen sclerosus et atrophicus (LSA) is a chronic atrophic mucocutaneous disorder, characterized by white, angular, well-defined, indurated papules and plaques and, at times, follicular keratotic plugs.

Synonyms: lichen sclerosus, guttate morphea, guttate scleroderma, white-spot disease.

EPIDEMIOLOGY AND ETIOLOGY

Age Occurs in children, 1 to 13 years. Mean age of onset: 50 years in females, 43 in males.

Sex Females > males (10:1)

Etiology Unknown

HISTORY

Duration of Lesions May be present for years prior to detection. May first be noted by gynecologist or internist doing pelvic examination.

Symptoms
NONGENITAL Usually asymptomatic
GENITAL Often asymptomatic even with striking clinical changes. In females, vulvar lesions may be sensitive especially while walking; pruritus; painful especially if erosions are present; dysuria; dyspareunia. In males, acquired phimosis, recurrent balanitis; in boys, may be discovered on pathologic examination of prepuce removed during circumcision.

PHYSICAL EXAMINATION

Skin Lesions
TYPE *Macules and papules:* whitish, sharply demarcated, individual lesions may become confluent, forming *plaques*. Surface of lesions may be elevated or in the same plane as normal skin; older lesions may be depressed. Dilated pilosebaceous or sweat duct orifices filled with keratin plugs (these are known as "dells"); if plugging is marked, surface appears verrucous. *Bullae and erosions;* may heal with milia formation. *Purpura* is a characteristic feature; *telangiectasia.* On vulva, hyperkeratotic plaques may become macerated; vulva may become atrophic, shrunken, especially clitoris and labia minora with vaginal introitus reduced in size. In uncircumcised males, prepuce becomes sclerotic and cannot be retracted; this was called in the past *balanitis xerotica obliterans.* Uncommonly, *squamous cell carcinoma* may develop in genital LSA, predominantly in females.
COLOR Ivory or porcelain-white (Figure 141); semitransparent, resembling mother-of-pearl
ARRANGEMENT Keyhole or figure-of-eight in anogenital area of females
DISTRIBUTION
Nongenital Trunk, especially upper back, periumbilical, neck, axillae; flexor surface of wrists; rarely palms and soles.

Genital Females: vulva and perianal regions as well as the perineum; inguinal line. Males: under surface of prepuce and glans (Figure 142).

ORAL MUCOSA Bluish-white plaques on buccal or palatal mucosa; tongue. Superficial erosions. Hyperkeratotic, macerated lesions may have reticulate pattern resembling lichen planus.

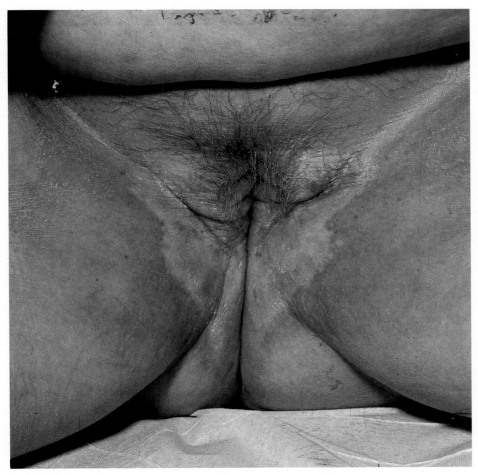

141 Lichen sclerosus et atrophicus *The process involves the inguinal area, the vulva, the perineum, and the perianal area. The color is ivory or porcelain-white, resembling mother-of-pearl. This disease has obliterated the clitoris and labia minora.*

DIAGNOSIS AND DIFFERENTIAL DIAGNOSIS

Diagnosis Clinical diagnosis at times confirmed by biopsy

Differential Diagnosis Morphea, lichen simplex chronicus, discoid lupus erythematosus, leukoplakia, lichen planus, intraepithelial neoplasia (bowenoid papulosis), extramammary Paget's disease, intertrigo, candidiasis

LABORATORY AND SPECIAL EXAMINATIONS

Dermatopathology *Epidermis:* early in course, variably thickened, hyperkeratotic, follicular plugging; later, epidermis atrophic. *Dermis:* band of homogenization of dermal collagen below epidermis; structureless, edematous; lymphocytic infiltrate, bandlike subepidermal in early lesions, later below the edematous, structureless, subepidermal zone. Dilated capillaries, hemorrhage.

COURSE AND PROGNOSIS

Waxes and wanes. In girls, may undergo spontaneous resolution. At times, coexisting lesions of morphea and vitiligo may be present. Patients should be followed every 12 months to check for occurrence of squamous cell carcinoma of the vulva.

TREATMENT

Symptomatic; no curative therapy. Topical anesthetics for sensitive or painful lesions give symptomatic relief. Corticosteroids, whether topical (triamcinalone acetate) or intralesional, may soften sclerotic lesions and are extremely effective in this condition. Testosterone propionate ointment 2.5% has been used to treat atrophic areas. Topical antiseptic preparations such as silver sulfadiazine or oral antibiotic for secondarily infected lesions. In males, circumcision relieves symptoms of phimosis.

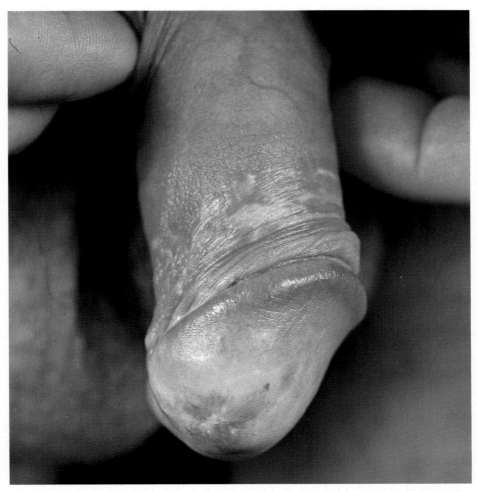

142 Lichen sclerosus et atrophicus in a male *The process involves the glans and the distal portion of the shaft. At the tip around the meatus there is a purpura that is characteristic. There is also a tiny ulcer.*

Pityriasis lichenoides (PL) is a self-limited eruption of unknown etiology, characterized clinically by successive crops of a wide range of morphologic lesions, i.e., macules, papules, vesicles, pustules, and crusts in the acute form, and by reddish-brown papules with adherent central scale in the chronic form.

Synonym: guttate parapsoriasis.

EPIDEMIOLOGY AND ETIOLOGY

Age Adolescents and young adults

Sex More common in males than females

Etiology Unknown

Classification PL has been classified into an acute form, pityriasis lichenoides et varioliformis acuta (PLEVA) (Mucha-Habermann disease), and a chronic form, pityriasis lichenoides chronica (PLC) (guttate parapsoriasis); however, a majority of patients have lesions of PLEVA and PLC simultaneously.

HISTORY

Duration of Lesions Lesions tend to appear in crops over a period of weeks or months.

Symptoms Uncommonly, patients with an acute onset of the disorder may have symptoms of an acute viral infection with fever, malaise, and headache. Cutaneous lesions are usually asymptomatic, but may be pruritic or sensitive to touch. In black patients, lesions may heal with significant scarring and postinflammatory hyperpigmentation.

PHYSICAL EXAMINATION

Skin Lesions

TYPE Initial edematous papules (i.e., lichen-

oides). Less commonly, vesicles-to-bullae which undergo necrosis with central vesiculation and hemorrhagic crusting (i.e., varioliformis) (Figures 143 and 144). In the chronic form, scaling papules are seen (Figure 145). Postinflammatory hypo- or hyperpigmentation often present after lesions resolve. May heal with depressed or elevated scars.

COLOR Acutely, pink to erythematous. Chronic lesion, reddish brown. Scars may be hypopigmented or depigmented.

ARRANGEMENT Random

DISTRIBUTION Most commonly, trunk, proximal extremities. Lesions may occur in a generalized distribution, including palms and soles.

ORAL AND GENITAL MUCOSA Inflammatory papules and necrotic lesions may occur.

DIAGNOSIS AND DIFFERENTIAL DIAGNOSIS

Diagnosis Clinical diagnosis, which may be confirmed by lesional skin biopsy

Differential Diagnosis Varicella, lichen planus, guttate psoriasis, prurigo nodularis, lymphomatoid papulosis

LABORATORY AND SPECIAL EXAMINATIONS

Dermatopathology *Epidermis:* spongiosis, keratinocyte necrosis, vesiculation, ul-

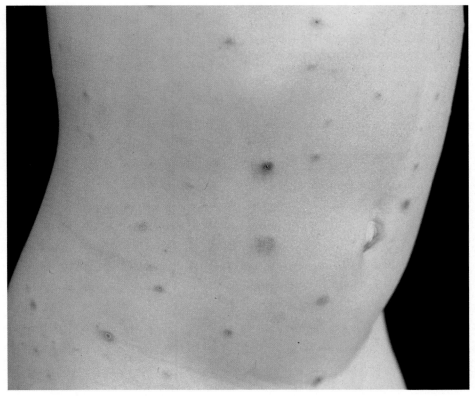

143　Pityriasis lichenoides, acute form (PLEVA)　*Erythematous papules, nodules, and crusted lesions are seen scattered on the trunk.*

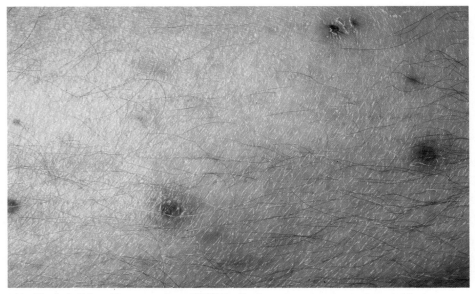

144　Pityriasis lichenoides, acute form (PLEVA)　*Erythematous papules and crusted lesions.*

ceration, exocytosis of erythrocytes within epidermis. *Dermis:* edema, chronic inflammatory cell infiltrate in wedge shape extending to deep reticular dermis; hemorrhage; vessels congested with blood; endothelial cells swollen.

COURSE AND PROGNOSIS

New lesions appear in successive crops. PL tends to resolve spontaneously after 6 to 12 months. In some cases, relapses after many months or years.

TREATMENT

Most patients do not require any therapeutic intervention. Both topical corticosteroid preparations and oral erythromycin and tetracycline are reported to be effective in some cases. On the other hand, ultraviolet radiation, whether natural sunlight, artificial UVB, or PUVA, is effective.

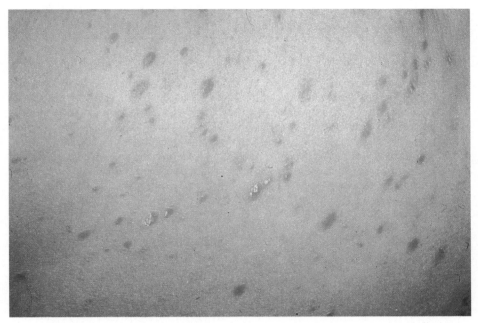

145 Pityriasis lichenoides chronica *A polymorphous eruption of round or oval, pink papules, some with scaling.*

PITYRIASIS LICHENOIDES

Two types are now generally recognized. (1) *"Small-plaque"* parapsoriasis (also known as *digitate dermatosis* or *chronic superficial dermatitis*). The lesions are round or oval, about 2.5 cm in diameter, and may be lightly yellow; they have a slight scale and a wrinkled cigarette-paper appearance. The lesions may have fingerlike (digitate) shapes. Small-plaque parapsoriasis is not regarded as a lesion in which mycosis fungoides (cutaneous T-cell lymphoma, CTCL) can occur. (2) *"Large-plaque"* parapsoriasis. The lesions are larger, more irregularly shaped, and less sharply defined than digitate dermatosis. Large-plaque parapsoriasis is an important disorder to follow carefully, obtaining repeated biopsies to rule out early mycosis fungoides. The précis below concerns large-plaque parapsoriasis.

EPIDEMIOLOGY

Age Middle age

HISTORY

Duration of Lesions Gradual development over months and years, starting with 1 or 2 plaques

Relationship of Skin Lesions to Season The lesions may disappear following exposure to sun.

Skin Symptoms Pruritus is rare.

PHYSICAL EXAMINATION

Skin Findings (Large-Plaque Parapsoriasis)
TYPE OF LESION Barely elevated plaque (Figure 146) with or without slight atrophy
COLOR Erythematous, dusky-red, sometimes yellowish hue
Palpation No "infiltration"
Surface Smooth or slight scaling
Size >10.0 cm
SHAPE OF INDIVIDUAL LESION Circular
ARRANGEMENT OF MULTIPLE LESIONS Randomly scattered (Figure 147)
DISTRIBUTION OF LESIONS Trunk, buttocks, breasts (females); anywhere

LABORATORY EXAMINATIONS

Dermatopathology
LIGHT MICROSCOPY *Site* Epidermis and dermis
Cell Types Nonspecific or, later, a bandlike mononuclear cell infiltrate with atrophy of the epidermis, vacuolization of the basal cell layer, capillary dilatation. There are no atypical lymphocytes.

DIAGNOSIS AND DIFFERENTIAL DIAGNOSIS

Large-plaque parapsoriasis is easily confused with "premycotic" stage of CTCL (mycosis fungoides) parapsoriasis-like lesions. The development of "infiltration" in the lesions, atrophy, and poikilodermatous changes are clues to early mycosis fungoides. Repeated biopsies may be necessary to establish the diagnosis of pre-lymphomatous disease.

COURSE AND PROGNOSIS

The lesions persist for life.

TREATMENT

Topical Temporary remission with topical corticosteroids

Phototherapy Good responses to PUVA photochemotherapy and sometimes to UVB

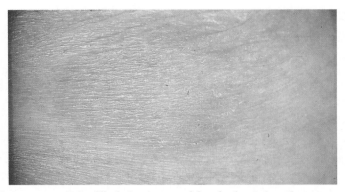

146   Large plaque parapsoriasis   *The lesion is an oval, barely elevated, erythematous plaque with a fine scale. This type of lesion must be repeatedly observed and biopsied to rule out cutaneous T-cell lymphoma.*

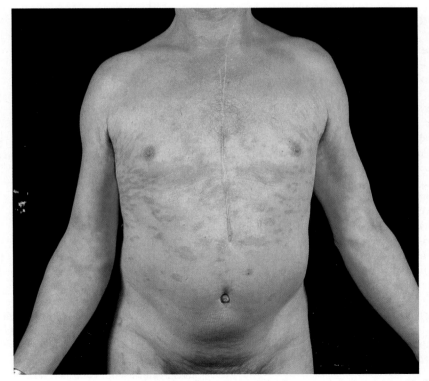

147   Large plaque parapsoriasis   *Multiple, barely elevated, erythematous plaques, some of which show slight atrophy, randomly scattered on the trunk.*

Rash and Fever

Consult Appendix D for differential diagnosis of rash and fever.

Infectious Exanthems

An infectious exanthem is a generalized cutaneous eruption associated with a primary systemic infection; it is often accompanied by oral mucosal lesions, i.e., an enanthem.

EPIDEMIOLOGY AND ETIOLOGY

Age Usually younger than 20 years

Etiology Adenoviruses, *Borrelia burgdorferi,* cytomegalovirus (CMV), enteroviruses (e.g., coxsackie viruses, echovirus), Epstein-Barr virus (EBV), flavivirus (dengue), hepatitis B virus, human herpesvirus-6 (exanthem subitum, roseola infantum), human immunodeficiency virus, *Legionella, Leptospira, Listeria,* meningococci, mycoplasma, orbivirus (Colorado tick fever), paramyxovirus (measles), parvovirus B19 (erythema infectiosum), reoviruses, respiratory syncytial virus, rhinovirus, *Rickettsia* (Rocky Mountain spotted fever, rickettsialpox, murine and epidemic typhus), rotaviruses, rubella virus, *Staphylococcus* (toxic shock syndrome), *Streptococcus* (scarlet fever). *Strongyloides, Toxoplasma, Treponema pallidum*

Transmission Respiratory, food, sexual, blood

Season Enterovirus infections: summer months

Geography Worldwide

HISTORY

Incubation Period Usually less than 3 weeks; hepatitis B virus several months

Prodrome Fever, malaise, coryza, sore throat, nausea, vomiting, diarrhea, abdominal pain, headache

PHYSICAL EXAMINATION

Skin Findings
TYPE OF LESION Erythematous macules and/ or papules (Figures 148*a* and 148*b*); less frequently, vesicles, petechiae
COLOR OF LESIONS Pink to red
DISTRIBUTION OF LESIONS Usually central, i.e., head, neck, trunk, proximal extremities (Figure 148*a*). Diffuse erythema of cheeks, i.e., "slapped cheek" with erythema infectiosum. Palms and soles usually spared, except in hand-foot-and-mouth dis-

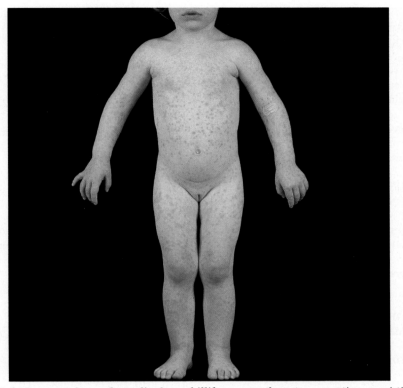

148*a*   Infectious exanthem   *Generalized, morbilliform, exanthematous eruption consisting of pink macules and papules suggesting infectious exanthem.*

ease (caused by coxsackie A16) and secondary syphilis

MUCOUS MEMBRANES Koplik's spots in measles; ulcerative lesions in herpangina due to coxsackie virus A; palatal petechiae in mononucleosis syndrome of EBV or CMV; conjunctivitis

General Examination Lymphadenopathy, hepatomegaly, splenomegaly

DIAGNOSIS AND DIFFERENTIAL DIAGNOSIS

Diagnosis Usually made on history and clinical findings

Differential Diagnosis Drug eruption

LABORATORY AND SPECIAL EXAMINATIONS

Cultures If practical

Serology Acute and convalescent titers most helpful in specific diagnosis

PATHOPHYSIOLOGY

Skin lesions may be produced by the direct effect of microbial replication in infected cells, the host response to the microbe, or the interaction of these two phenomena.

COURSE AND PROGNOSIS

Usually resolves in less than 10 days. Patient with primary EBV or CMV infection very often develops an exanthematous eruption if given ampicillin or amoxicillin.

TREATMENT

Symptomatic. Specific antimicrobial therapy when indicated.

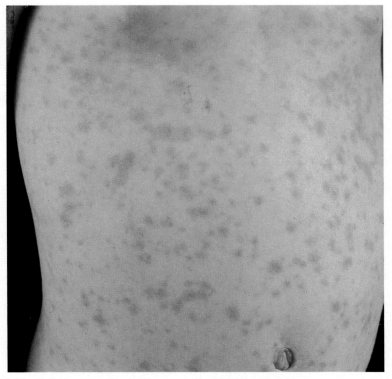

148*b* Infectious exanthem *Close-up of morbilliform lesions.*

Infective endocarditis (IE) is a microbial infection implanted on a heart valve or on the mural endocardium; it is characterized by fever, valve destruction, and peripheral embolization.

EPIDEMIOLOGY AND ETIOLOGY

Classification

ACUTE BACTERIAL ENDOCARDITIS (ABE) Caused by the more invasive organisms. Can attack normal valve or mural endocardium. *Agents: Staphylococcus aureus, Streptococcus pneumoniae* (alcoholics with pneumonia), group A *Streptococcus, Neisseria gonorrhoeae, Salmonella, Pseudomonas aeruginosa* (IVDUs)

SUBACUTE BACTERIAL ENDOCARDITIS (SBE) Defined as duration of more than 6 weeks. Caused by a variety of less virulent bacteria. Commonly, bacteria are members of the indigenous flora. Characteristically, infection is on deformed valves. *Agents:* streptococci of oral cavity, GI and GU tracts, *Haemophilus* organisms, *Staph. epidermidis*

Etiology Most usual is bacterial: (1) *Streptococcus viridans,* enterococci, and other streptococci account for about 50%, (2) *Staph. aureus, Staph. epidermidis:* 20%, (3) in 15 to 20% no causative agent can be isolated, (4) remainder uncommon bacterial and fungal organisms. Staphylococcal, fungal, gram-negative bacterial agents common in IVDUs, as well as polymicrobial IE. *Staph. aureus* most common cause with a normal valve. Also fungi, rickettsiae, chlamydiae.

Transmission Circumstances which result in transient bacteremia: dental procedures, IV drug use, various infections, induced abortions, intrauterine contraceptive devices, temporary transvenous pacemakers, prolonged IV infusions, endoscopic procedures.

Predisposing Factors

1. Underlying heart disease: (a) acquired heart disease—70% (rheumatic valvular disease, calcific stenosis, "floppy" mitral or aortic valves, prolapsing mitral valve leaflet (i.e., "click-murmur" syndrome), idiopathic hypertrophic subaortic stenosis, calcified mitral annulus, (b) congenital heart disease (intraventricular septal defect, patent ductus arteriosus, pulmonic valve in tetralogy of Fallot)
2. Prosthetic material (prosthetic heart valves, xenografts, intracardiac "patches," vascular prostheses)
3. IV drug use

HISTORY

History

ABE Onset abrupt with high fever and rigors, rapid downhill course

SBE Fever, sweats, weakness, myalgias, arthralgias, malaise, fatigability, anorexia, chilly sensations, cough. Recent history of dental extraction or scaling, cystoscopy, rectal surgery, tonsillectomy. Fever, weight loss, cerebrovascular accident, arthralgia, arthritis, diffuse myalgias.

IV Drug Use Occurs in 0.2 to 2% of users annually. Right-sided IE more common than left. *Staph. aureus* in 50%. 5% polymicrobial. Septic emboli common.

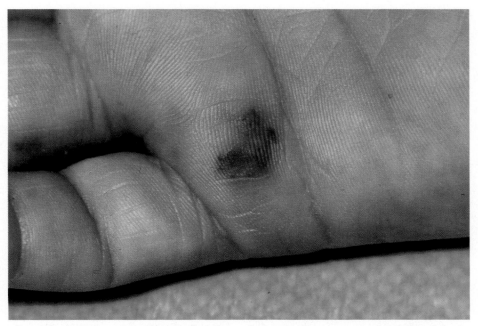

149*a* Infective endocarditis *Janeway lesions on the hands. These are nonpainful, hemorrhagic, infarcted macules on the palms and soles. This patient had an acute* Staphylococcus aureus *endocarditis. (Courtesy of David N. Silvers, M.D.)*

PHYSICAL EXAMINATION

Consider IE in any patient with fever and heart murmur.

Skin Findings
TYPE OF LESION

Janeway lesions (Figures 149*a* and 149*b*)—Small, erythematous or hemorrhagic, nonpainful macules or nodules of palms or soles. More common in ABE but occur in SBE.

Osler's nodes—Tender-to-painful, purplish, split-pea-sized, subcutaneous nodules in the pulp of the fingers and/or toes and thenar and hypothenar eminences. Transient, disappearing within several days (5% of patients). In ABE, associated with minute infective emboli; aspiration may reveal the causative organism, i.e., *Staph. aureus*. In SBE, associated with immune complexes and small-vessel arteritis of skin.

Subungual splinter hemorrhages—Linear in the *middle* of the nail bed (SBE). Distal hemorrhages are traumatic.

Petechial lesions—Small, non-blanching, reddish-brown macules. Occur on extremities, upper chest, mucous membranes (conjunctivae, palate). Occur in crops. Fade after a few days. 20 to 40% of patients.

Clubbing of fingers—Seen after prolonged course of untreated SBE (15%).

Gangrene of extremities—Secondary to embolism.

Pustular petechiae, purulent purpura—With *Staph. aureus*.

General Examination
HEART SBE, 90% have murmurs; ABE only 66% have murmurs, which may change, heart failure.

EYE Petechial and flame-shaped hemorrhages in retina, cotton-wool exudates in fundus, *Roth's spots* (oval or boat-shaped white areas in the retina that are surrounded by a zone of hemorrhage), endophthalmitis.

SPLEEN Splenomegaly (25 to 60%), splenic abscess

JOINTS Septic arthritis with ABE

THROMBOEMBOLIC PHENOMENA Significant embolic episodes occur in one-third of patients, resulting in stroke, seizures, monocular blindness, mesenteric artery occlusion with abdominal pain, ileus, melena, splenic infarction, pulmonary infarction, gangrene of extremities, mycotic aneurysms.

DIAGNOSIS AND DIFFERENTIAL DIAGNOSIS

Diagnosis Confirmed by isolating infecting organism with 4 to 6 blood cultures before antibiotic therapy

Differential Diagnosis
ABE Meningococcemia, disseminated intravascular coagulation

SBE Acute rheumatic fever, marantic endocarditis, collagen-vascular diseases (SLE with cardiac involvement, systemic vasculitis), dysproteinemia, atrial myxoma, organizing left atrial thrombus, atheromatous embolism, cytomegalovirus infection following cardiac surgery (postperfusion syndrome)

LABORATORY AND SPECIAL EXAMINATIONS

Dermatopathology Osler's nodes in SBE show aseptic necrotizing vasculitis.

Laboratory Examination of Blood Anemia, elevated ESR, leukocytosis in ABE but WBC often normal with SBE, depressed serum complement, immune complexes (90%), rheumatoid factor (50% with SBE)

Blood Cultures Establish the diagnosis; usually no more than 6 cultures are required.

Urinalysis Hematuria

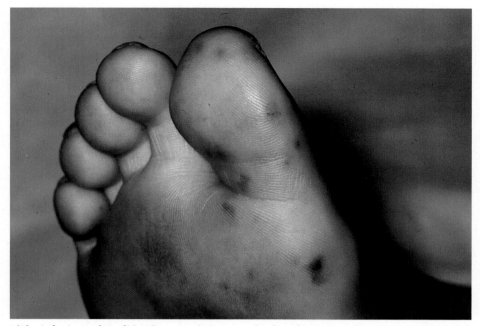

149*b*   Infective endocarditis *Janeway lesions on the feet. (Courtesy of David N. Silvers, M.D.)*

PATHOPHYSIOLOGY

During transient bacteremia, organisms adhere to the valve or mural endocardium or to overlying fibrin-platelet aggregate. Skin manifestations (Osler's nodes) in ABE result from septic embolism in most cases. In SBE, findings are caused by circulating immune complexes.

COURSE AND PROGNOSIS

Varies with the underlying cardiac disease and baseline health of the patient and with the complications that occur.

TREATMENT

Appropriate IV antibiotic therapy depending on the sensitivities of the infecting organism.

Disseminated Gonococcal Infection

Disseminated gonococcal infection (DGI) is a systemic gonococcal infection following the hematogenous dissemination of the organism from infected mucosal sites to skin, tenosynovium, and joints. It is characterized by fever, chills, scanty acral pustules, and septic polyarthritis.

Synonyms: gonococcemia, gonococcal arthritis-dermatitis syndrome.

EPIDEMIOLOGY AND ETIOLOGY

Age Young, sexually active

Sex Young females, homosexual males

Race Incidence higher in whites than blacks

Etiology Gonococcus, i.e., *Neisseria gonorrhoeae,* a gram-negative diplococcus

Geography Worldwide. Incidence varies with local incidence of DGI strains of gonococcus

Transmission Venereal. About 1% of patients with untreated mucosal gonococcal infection develop DGI.

HISTORY

Incubation Period 7 to 30 days of mucosal infection (range, from a few days to 1 year). Varies with host factors, such as menstruation, invasiveness of infecting organism.

Prodrome Fever, anorexia, malaise, ± shaking chills

History Recurring symptoms around menses, migratory polyarthralgias

PHYSICAL EXAMINATION

Skin Findings
TYPE OF LESION 1.0- to 5.0-mm erythematous macules evolving to hemorrhagic pustules (Figure 150) within 24 to 48 hours. Centers at times hemorrhagic/necrotic (Figure 150). Rarely, large hemorrhagic bullae. Lesions are few in number and usually countable, e.g., 3 to 20 lesions.

DISTRIBUTION OF LESIONS Acral, arms more often than legs, near small joints of hands (Figure 150) or feet. Difficult to detect in black patients; look in web spaces. Face spared.

MUCOUS MEMBRANES Usually asymptomatic colonization of oropharynx, urethra, anorectum, endometrium

General Examination
SPECTRUM OF DISEASE Fever 38° to 39°C usual. Severity varies: DGI with skin lesions alone, classic DGI with skin lesions and tenosynovitis, DGI with septic arthritis, DGI with metastatic infection at other sites.

TENOSYNOVITIS Common. Single or few sites, acrally. Extensor/flexor tendons and sheaths of hands/feet. Erythema, tenderness, swelling along tendon sheath aggravated by moving tendon.

SEPTIC ARTHRITIS Joint—red, hot, tender with effusion; asymmetric. Most commonly involved: knee, elbow, ankle, metacarpophalangeal/interphalangeal joints of hand, shoulder, hip. Usually only 1 or 2 joints involved.

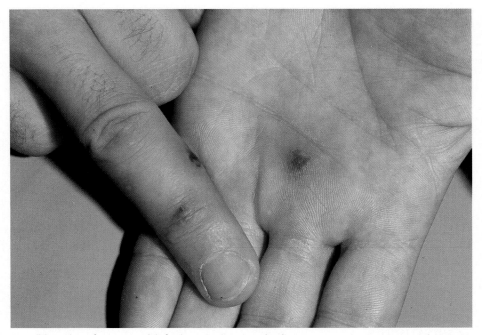

150   Disseminated gonococcal infection   *Lesions on the fingers and palm consisting of pustules and hemorrhagic, necrotic pustules, which are slightly tender.*

OTHER Hepatitis, perihepatitis (Fitz-Hugh–Curtis syndrome), myopericarditis, endocarditis, meningitis, perihepatitis. Rarely, pneumonitis, adult respiratory distress syndrome, osteomyelitis.

DIAGNOSIS AND DIFFERENTIAL DIAGNOSIS

Diagnosis Made on clinical criteria and confirmed by culture of gonococcus from mucosal sites.

Differential Diagnosis *Bacteremia:* meningococcemia, other bacteremias, endocarditis. *Tenosynovitis/arthritis:* infectious arthritis, infectious tenosynovitis, Reiter's syndrome, psoriatic arthritis, SLE.

LABORATORY AND SPECIAL EXAMINATIONS

Dermatopathology Immunofluorescence of skin lesion biopsy shows gonococcus in 60% of patients

Gram's Stain The male urethra or cervix, and occasionally the pharynx, may show gonococci.

Culture Mucosal sites yield 80 to 90% positive cultures. Skin biopsy, joint fluid, blood have only a 10 to 30% chance of positive culture.

PATHOPHYSIOLOGY

Most signs and symptoms of DGI are manifestations of immune-complex formation and deposition. Multiple episodes of DGI may be associated with abnormality of terminal complement-component factors.

COURSE AND PROGNOSIS

Untreated, skin and joint lesions often gradually resolve; endocarditis usually fatal.

TREATMENT

Hospitalization is recommended for initial therapy, especially for patients who cannot reliably comply with treatment, have uncertain diagnoses, or have purulent synovial effusions or other complications. Patients should be examined for clinical evidence of endocarditis or meningitis.

Recommended Regimens—DGI Inpatient

Ceftriaxone 1 g, IM or IV, every 24 hours
or

Ceftizoxime 1 g, IV, every 8 hours, *or*

Cefotaxime 1 g, IV, every 8 hours

Alternative Regimen for Patients Allergic to β-Lactam Drugs

Spectinomycin 2 g IM every 12 hours.

When the infecting organism is proven to be penicillin-sensitive, parenteral treatment may be switched to ampicillin 1 g every 6 hours.

Reliable patients with uncomplicated disease may be discharged 24 to 48 hours after all symptoms resolve and may complete the therapy (for a total of 1 week of antibiotic therapy) with an oral regimen of cefuroxime axetil 500 mg b.i.d. *or* amoxicillin 500 mg with clavulanic acid t.i.d. *or,* if not pregnant, ciprofloxacin 500 mg b.i.d.

Disseminated Herpes Simplex Infection

Disseminated herpes simplex infection is a potentially fatal systemic HSV infection, characterized by widespread mucocutaneous vesicles, pustules, erosions, and ulcerations, associated with signs of pneumonia, encephalitis, hepatitis, as well as involvement of other organ systems, usually occurring in an immunocompromised host.

EPIDEMIOLOGY AND ETIOLOGY

Age Any age

Etiology Herpes simplex virus (HSV) types 1 and 2

Incidence Uncommon, but incidence rising due to organ transplantation, AIDS, and chemotherapy.

Risk Factors Patients compromised by immunodeficiency, immunosuppression (organ transplantation, cancer chemotherapy, corticosteroid therapy), hematologic and lymphoreticular malignancies, malnutrition; rarely, pregnancy. Nasogastric tube in debilitated patient. Eczema herpeticum.

HISTORY

History Patients usually hospitalized with underlying condition or disease

Skin Symptoms Tender and painful mucocutaneous erosions

PHYSICAL EXAMINATION

Skin Findings
TYPE OF LESION *Recurrent herpetic lesion* (i.e., site from which systemic dissemination of HSV occurs) may be present: grouped crusts, erosions, ulcers; ulcers may be large (10.0 to 20.0 cm in diameter). With mucocutaneous dissemination, vesicles and pustules often hemorrhagic with inflammatory halo; quickly rupture and result in "punched-out" erosions (Figure 151). Lesions may be necrotic and then ulcerate. Ulcers may become confluent with polycyclic well-demarcated borders; edges may be slightly raised, rolled. Infarctive skin lesions if complicated by purpura fulminans.
DISTRIBUTION OF LESIONS Generalized, disseminated (Figure 151). Site of recurrent HSV infection, i.e., labial, oropharyngeal, esophageal, genital, perianal, may be apparent.
MUCOUS MEMBRANES Oropharyngeal erosions, HSV tracheobronchitis with erosions

General Examination HSV pneumonitis, HSV hepatitis

DIAGNOSIS AND DIFFERENTIAL DIAGNOSIS

Diagnosis Clinical suspicion confirmed by Tzanck preparation, negative stain electron microscopy, HSV cultures

Differential Diagnosis Eczema herpeticum, varicella, cutaneous dissemination of zoster, eczema vaccinatum, disseminated vaccinia in immunosuppressed patient (smallpox vaccination still given in U.S. military)

LABORATORY AND SPECIAL EXAMINATIONS

Tzanck Test Multinucleated giant cells present in scraping of mucocutaneous erosions, tracheobronchial washing

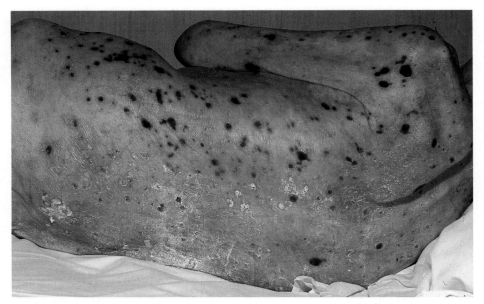

151 Disseminated herpes simplex infection *Generalized vesicles and pustules with hemorrhage and necrosis are seen; some have ruptured, resulting in erosions and ulcerations.*

Electron Microscopy Where available, negative stain of smear from lesions reveals HSV. Less than 30 minutes required.

Cultures Positive HSV cultures from involved site

Urinalysis Hematuria due to HSV cystitis

PATHOPHYSIOLOGY

60 to 80% of HSV seropositive transplant recipients and patients undergoing chemotherapy for hematologic malignancies will reactivate HSV. Following viremia, disseminated cutaneous or visceral HSV infection may follow. Factors determining whether severe localized disease, cutaneous dissemination, or visceral dissemination will occur are not well defined.

COURSE AND PROGNOSIS

When widespread, visceral dissemination of HSV may occur to liver, lungs, adrenals, GI tract, CNS. May be complicated by disseminated intravascular coagulation. Disseminated HSV infection with visceral involvement in neonates has a 50 to 80% mortality rate if untreated.

TREATMENT

Acyclovir prophylaxis for seropositive patients undergoing bone marrow transplantation, induction therapy for leukemia, and solid organ transplantation: acyclovir 5 mg per kg body weight IV every 8 hours *or* 200 mg orally every 6 hours, from the day of conditioning, induction, or transplantation for 4 to 6 weeks.

Disseminated HSV infection

Acyclovir 10 mg per kg body weight IV every 8 hours for 10 to 14 days *or*

Vidarabine 15 mg per kg body weight IV daily for 10 to 14 days

Eczema herpeticum is a cutaneous infection caused by herpes simplex virus types 1 and 2, occurring in abnormal skin most commonly in atopic dermatitis. It is characterized by widespread vesicles and erosions; it may occur as a primary or recurrent infection.

Synonym: Kaposi's varicelliform eruption.

EPIDEMIOLOGY AND ETIOLOGY

Age   Children > adults

Etiology   *Herpesvirus hominis* (HSV) type 1, less commonly type 2

Transmission   Commonly from parental herpes labialis

Risk Factors   Most commonly, atopic dermatitis; more serious infections occur in erythrodermic atopic dermatitis. Also, Darier's disease, thermal burns, pemphigus vulgaris, ichthyosis vulgaris, mycosis fungoides

HISTORY

Duration of Lesions   Lesions begin in abnormal skin and may extend peripherally for several weeks during the primary infection.

History   Primary eczema herpeticum often associated with fever, malaise, irritability. When recurrent, prior history of similar lesions; systemic symptoms less severe.

Skin Symptoms   Primary skin disease may be pruritic; onset of eczema herpeticum associated with pain and tenderness.

PHYSICAL EXAMINATION

Skin Findings
TYPE OF LESION   Umbilicated vesicles evolv-

ing into "punched-out" erosions (Figure 152). Vesicles are first confined to eczematous skin and are, in contrast to primary or recurrent HSV eruptions, not grouped but disseminated. Erosions may become confluent, producing large denuded areas. Larger crusted lesions and follicular pustules occur with staphylococcal superinfection. Successive crops of new vesiculation may occur.
SHAPE OF INDIVIDUAL LESION   Vesicle dome-shaped with umbilication
ARRANGEMENT OF MULTIPLE LESIONS   Disseminated
DISTRIBUTION OF LESIONS   Common sites: face, neck, trunk

General Examination   Primary infection often has fever and lymphadenopathy.

DIAGNOSIS AND DIFFERENTIAL DIAGNOSIS

Diagnosis   Clinical, confirmed by Tzanck test and HSV culture

Differential Diagnosis   Varicella zoster with dissemination, disseminated (systemic) HSV infection, widespread bullous impetigo, staphylococcal folliculitis, pseudomonal ("hot-tub") folliculitis, *Candida* folliculitis, Kaposi's varicelliform eruption caused by vaccinia virus

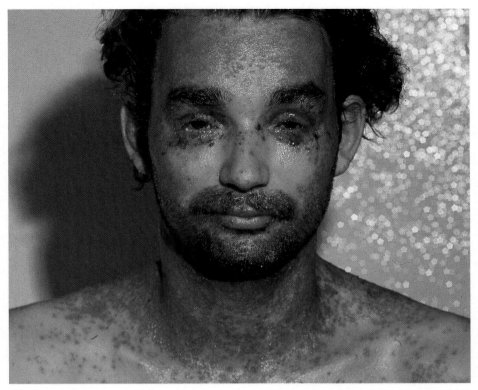

152 Eczema herpeticum *Vesicles, pustules, and erosions becoming confluent in areas of atopic dermatitis.*

LABORATORY AND SPECIAL EXAMINATIONS

Tzanck Test Wright's stain of vesicular fluid shows multinucleated giant epidermal cells

Electron Microscopy Negative stain of smears reveals herpesvirus-type particles.

Skin Culture Positive HSV. Frequently, superinfection with *Staph. aureus/S. pyogenes.*

Serology Much of humoral immune response to HSV is to common antigenic determinants, making it difficult to detect HSV-2 antibody in individuals with prior HSV-1 infection and HSV-1 infection in those with prior HSV-2.

PATHOPHYSIOLOGY

See "Nongenital HSV Infection" (Section 5)

COURSE AND PROGNOSIS

Primary episode of eczema herpeticum runs course with resolution in 2 to 6 weeks. Recurrent episodes tend to be milder and not associated with systemic symptoms. Systemic dissemination can occur, especially in immunocompromised patients. Rarely fatal.

TREATMENT

Most cases are mild and localized and may not require specific therapy. In more severe cases (usually primary infection), acyclovir should be given IV 1.5 g per m^2 per day. For milder cases, acyclovir can be given orally for 7 days. Impetiginization with *Staph. aureus* should be treated with erythromycin or dicloxacillin.

Meningococcemia is meningococcal bacteremia seeding from the nasopharynx, occurring as acute meningococcal septicemia, which may be fulminant (Waterhouse-Friderichsen syndrome), meningococcal meningitis, or chronic meningococcemia. It is characterized by fever, petechial or purpuric lesions, hypotension, signs of meningitis, and high morbidity and mortality.

EPIDEMIOLOGY

Age Highest incidence in children aged 6 months to 1 year; lowest in persons over 20 years.

Risk Groups Absence of spleen. Alcoholic. Complement deficiency, especially C5 to C8.

Etiology *Neisseria meningitidis,* meningococcus, a gram-negative coccus. Nasopharyngeal carrier rate in the general population: 5 to 15%.

Transmission Person-to-person through inhalation of droplets of infected nasopharyngeal secretions.

Season Highest incidence midwinter, early spring; lowest in midsummer.

Geography Worldwide. Occurs in epidemics or sporadically.

HISTORY

Prodrome Cough, headache, sore throat, nausea/vomiting. May be very short.

Systems Review
ACUTE MENINGOCOCCEMIA Spiking fever, chills, arthralgia, myalgia. Stupor, hemorrhagic lesions, hypotension may be evident within a few hours of onset of symptoms in fulminant meningococcemia.

CHRONIC MENINGOCOCCEMIA Intermittent fever, rash, myalgia, arthralgia, headache, anorexia

PHYSICAL EXAMINATION

Appearance Patient appears acutely ill with marked prostration.

Vital Signs High fever, tachypnea, tachycardia, mild hypotension

Skin Findings
TYPE OF LESION Characteristically petechial— small, irregular, "smudged," often raised with pale grayish vesicular centers. Transient urticarial, macular/papular lesions (Figure 153). Discrete pink macules/ papules/petechiae (1.0 to 3.0 mm) (Figure 154) in 75% of cases. Sparse. May have lighter halo. Transient, urticarial or maculopapular lesion. *Fulminant:* purpura, ecchymosis, and confluent, often bizarre-shaped grayish-to-black necrosis associated with disseminated intravascular coagulation (Figure 155).

DISTRIBUTION OF LESIONS Most commonly trunk, extremities, but can be anywhere, including palms and soles

MUCOUS MEMBRANES Petechiae

CHRONIC MENINGOCOCCEMIA Intermittent appearance of lesions. Macular and papular lesions, usually distributed about one or more painful joints or pressure points. Ery-

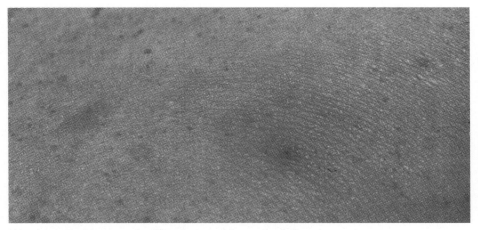

153 Acute meningococcemia *Transient maculopapular lesions.*

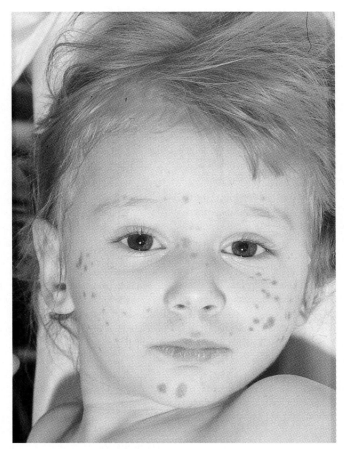

154 Acute meningococcemia *Discrete, pink-to-purple macules and papules, as well as purpura, are seen on the face of this young child. These lesions represent early disseminated intravascular coagulation.*

thema nodosum-like lesions on calves. Petechiae, which may evolve to vesicles or pustules. Minute hemorrhage with paler areola. Purpuric areas with pale blue-gray centers; hemorrhagic tender nodules.

GENERAL EXAMINATION

MENINGITIS 50 to 88% of patients with meningococcemia develop meningitis. Signs of meningeal irritation, altered consciousness. Agitated, maniacal behavior. Signs of increased intracranial pressure.

RARELY Septic arthritis, purulent pericarditis, bacterial endocarditis

VARIANTS Fulminant meningococcemia with adrenal hemorrhage (Waterhouse-Friderichsen syndrome)

CHRONIC MENINGOCOCCEMIA Intermittent fever, arthritis/arthralgia

DIAGNOSIS AND DIFFERENTIAL DIAGNOSIS

Diagnosis Clinical impression confirmed by cultures

Differential Diagnosis

ACUTE MENINGOCOCCEMIA AND MENINGITIS Acute bacteremias and endocarditis, acute "hypersensitivity" vasculitis, enteroviral infections, Rocky Mountain spotted fever, toxic shock syndrome

CHRONIC MENINGOCOCCEMIA Subacute bacterial endocarditis, acute rheumatic fever, Henoch-Schönlein purpura, rat-bite fever, erythema multiforme, gonococcemia

LABORATORY AND SPECIAL EXAMINATIONS

Dermatopathology In chronic meningococcemia, no bacteria demonstrable. Mononuclear perivascular infiltrate. Lesions probably immune-mediated.

Gram's Stain Scrapings from nodular lesions show gram-negative diplococci.

Laboratory Examination of Blood Polymorphous leukocytosis

Cultures *Blood:* acute meningococcemia, meningococcus in nearly 100%; meningitis 33% positive. *CSF:* usually positive. *Skin biopsy:* up to 85%.

PATHOPHYSIOLOGY

Primary focus is usually a subclinical nasopharynx infection. Hematogenous dissemination seeds the skin and meninges. Endotoxin felt to be involved in hypotension and vascular collapse. Disseminated intravascular coagulation seen in fulminant meningococcemia similar to Schwartzman reaction. Meningococci are found within endothelial and PMN cells. Local endothelial damage, thrombosis, and necrosis of the vessel walls occur. Edema, infarction of overlying skin, and extravasation of RBC are responsible for the characteristic macular, papular, petechial, hemorrhagic, and bullous lesions. Similar vascular lesions occur in the meninges and in other tissues. The frequency of hemorrhagic cutaneous manifestations in meningococcal infections, compared to infections with other gram-negative organisms, may be due to increased potency and/or unique properties of meningococcal endotoxins for the dermal reaction. On the other hand, lipopolysaccharide endotoxins from meningococci and *Escherichia coli* are equally potent producers of the generalized Schwartzman reaction and lethality in mice. In chronic meningococcemia, usually during periodic fevers, rash, and joint manifestations, meningococci can be isolated from the blood; unusual host-parasite relationship is central to this persistent infection.

COURSE AND PROGNOSIS

Acute Meningococcemia Untreated, ends fatally. Adequately treated, recovery rate for meningitis or meningococcemia is >90%. Mortality for severe disease or Waterhouse-Friderichsen syndrome remains very high.

RASH AND FEVER

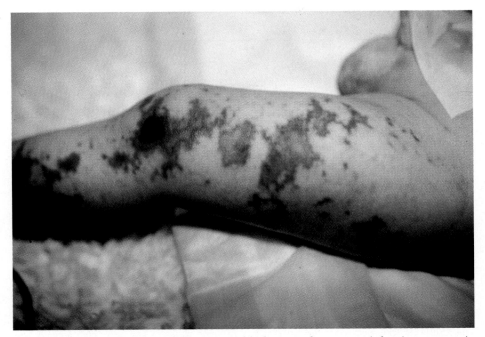

155　Acute meningococcemia　*Maplike, gray-to-black areas of cutaneous infarction are seen in this child with disseminated intravascular coagulation.*

Prognosis is poor when purpura and/or ecchymosis is present at time of diagnosis.

Chronic Meningococcemia　Untreated, may recur over few weeks to 8 months, average duration 6 to 8 weeks; may evolve into acute meningococcemia, meningitis, endocarditis. 100% cure with antibiotics.

TREATMENT

Penicillin G or ampicillin IV for 10 days.

Rocky Mountain spotted fever (RMSF), the most severe of the rickettsial spotted fevers, is characterized by sudden onset of fever, severe headache, myalgia, and a characteristic acral exanthem; it is associated with significant mortality.

EPIDEMIOLOGY AND ETIOLOGY

Age and Sex Majority of cases in young adult males

Etiology Caused by *Rickettsia rickettsii.*

Transmission Occurs through bite of an infected tick or inoculation through abrasions contaminated with tick feces or tissue juices. The reservoirs and vectors are the wood tick *Dermacentor andersoni* in the western United States and the dog tick *D. variabilis* in the east. Patient either lives in or has recently visited an endemic area; *however, only 62% have knowledge of a recent tick bite.*

Season 95% of patients become ill during the period April 1 to September 30

Geography Occurs only in the western hemisphere. In the United States, the highest endemic areas are centered around Virginia, the Carolinas–Georgia, and Kansas–Oklahoma–Texas. Also in New York City.

HISTORY

Incubation Period Range, 3 to 14 days (mean, 7 days)

Prodrome Anorexia, irritability, malaise, chilliness, and feverish feeling

History Onset of symptoms is usually abrupt with fever (94%), severe headache (94%), generalized myalgia (especially the back and leg muscles) (87%), a sudden shaking rigor, photophobia, prostration, and nausea with occasional vomiting, all within the first 2 days. However, onset is at times less striking. Symptoms are similar to those of many acute infectious diseases, making specific diagnosis difficult during the first few days. Characteristic rash (87%), which is the most helpful diagnostic sign, appears on the fourth day of the illness (range, 2 to 6 days). In some patients, however, rash appears late (10%) or not at all (13%).

PHYSICAL EXAMINATION

Skin Findings The temporal evolution of the rash is extremely helpful in the diagnosis.
TYPE OF LESION Early lesions 2.0 to 6.0 mm, pink blanching macules. In 1 to 3 days evolve to deep red papules. In 2 to 4 days become hemorrhagic, no longer blanching (Figures 156a and 156b). Rarely an eschar (round crusted ulcer associated with an acute rickettsial infection) is present at the site of the tick bite. With DIC, skin infarcts (gangrene) occur.
COLOR Pink, evolving to deep red, evolving to violaceous.
DISTRIBUTION OF LESIONS *Characteristically, rash begins on wrists, forearms, and ankles and somewhat later on palms and soles.* Within 6 to 18 hours rash spreads centripetally to the arms, thighs, trunk, and face. Gangrene occurs in acral areas.

General Findings Fever to 40°C. Hypotensive shock later in course. Hepatomegaly,

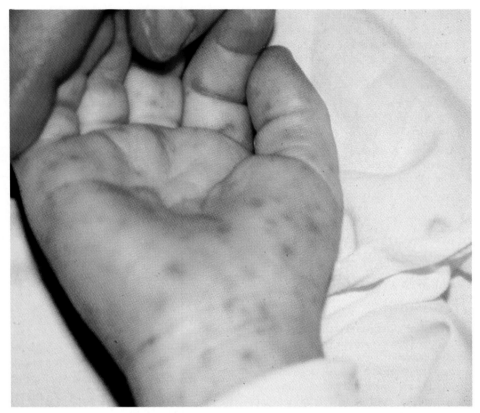

156*a*   Rocky Mountain spotted fever *Erythematous and hemorrhagic macules and papules appeared initially on the wrists and later on the palms, soles, and trunk. (Courtesy of Richard L. Dobson, M.D.)*

splenomegaly, GI hemorrhage, altered consciousness, transient deafness, incontinence, oliguria, and secondary bacterial infections of the lung, middle ear, and parotid gland may occur.

VARIANTS

"*Spotless fever*" 13% of cases. Associated with higher mortality because diagnosis is overlooked.

Abdominal syndrome Can mimic acute abdomen, acute cholecystitis, acute appendicitis.

Thrombotic thrombocytopenic purpura

DIAGNOSIS AND DIFFERENTIAL DIAGNOSIS

Diagnosis Must be made clinically and confirmed later

Differential Diagnosis Meningococcemia, *Staphylococcus aureus* septicemia, other rickettsioses (ehrlichiosis, murine typhus, epidemic typhus, rickettsialpox), leptospirosis, typhoid fever, viral exanthem (measles, varicella, rubella, enterovirus), drug reaction, immune complex vasculitis

LABORATORY AND SPECIAL EXAMINATIONS

Skin Biopsy

H&E Necrotizing vasculitis. Rickettsia can at times be demonstrated within the endothelial cells.

DIRECT IMMUNOFLUORESCENCE Specific *R. rickettsii* antigen within endothelial cells

Serodiagnosis Immunofluorescent antibody test (IFA) can be used to measure both IgG and IgM antibodies. Fourfold rise in titer between acute and convalescent stages is diagnostic.

PATHOPHYSIOLOGY

Following inoculation, initial local replication in endothelial cells is followed by hematogenous dissemination. Focal infection of vascular smooth muscle causes a generalized vasculitis. Hypotension, local necrosis, gangrene, and DIC may follow. Rash results from extravasation of blood after vascular necrosis.

COURSE AND PROGNOSIS

Untreated the fatality rate is 20%, treated 3% (6% if age >40 years). Fatality rate 1.5% with known tick bite but 6.6% if no known tick exposure.

TREATMENT

Tetracycline or chloramphenicol, 2 g per day for adults, is given as soon as the diagnosis is made clinically. Some patients require treatment for shock.

RASH AND FEVER

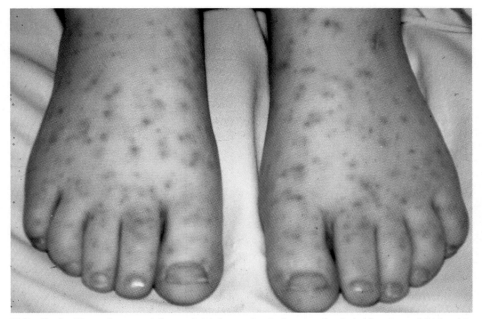

156*b*   Rocky Mountain spotted fever   *Initial macular lesions on the feet. (Courtesy of Richard L. Dobson, M.D.)*

Rubella is a common benign childhood infection manifested by a characteristic exanthem and lymphadenopathy; however, occurring in pregnancy, it may result in the congenital rubella syndrome with serious chronic fetal infection and malformation.

Synonyms: German measles, "3-day measles."

EPIDEMIOLOGY AND ETIOLOGY

Age Prior to widespread immunization, children <15 years. Currently young adults.

Etiology Rubella virus

Occupation Young adults in hospitals, colleges, prisons, prenatal clinics

Transmission Inhalation of aerosolized respiratory droplets; moderately contagious; 10 to 40% of cases asymptomatic; period of infectivity from end of incubation period to disappearance of rash.

Incidence Following immunization begun in 1969, incidence has decreased by 99%.

Risk Factors Lack of active immunization, lack of natural infection.

Season Prior to 1969, epidemics in United States every 6 to 9 years, occurring in spring

Geography Worldwide. Marked reduction in incidence in developed countries following immunization

HISTORY

Incubation Period 14 to 21 days

Prodrome Usually absent, especially in young children. In adolescents and young adults: anorexia, malaise, conjunctivitis, headache, low-grade fever, mild upper respiratory tract symptoms

History Arthralgia, especially in adult women following immunization

Immune Status *In women, rubella-like illness frequently follows administration of attenuated live rubella virus.*

PHYSICAL EXAMINATION

Skin Findings
TYPE OF LESION Pink macules, papules. Truncal lesions may become confluent, creating a scarlatiniform eruption.
DISTRIBUTION OF LESIONS *Initially on forehead, spreading inferiorly to face* (Figure 157a), *trunk* (Figure 157b), *and extremities during first day. By second day facial exanthem fades. By third day exanthem fades completely without residual pigmentary change or scaling.*
MUCOUS MEMBRANES Petechiae on soft palate (Forchheimer's sign) during prodrome (also seen in infectious mononucleosis)

General Examination
LYMPH NODES Enlargement noted during prodrome. Postauricular, suboccipital, and posterior cervical lymph nodes enlarged and possibly tender. Mild generalized lymphadenopathy may occur. Enlargement usually persists for one week but may last for months.
SPLEEN May be enlarged

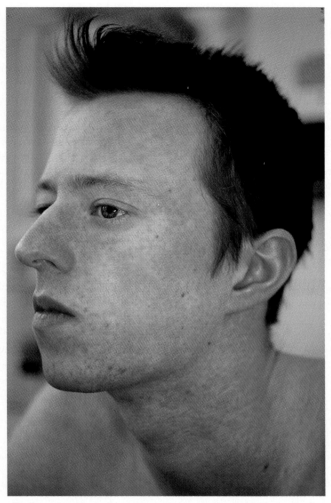

157a   Rubella   *Erythematous macules and papules appearing initially on the face and spreading inferiorly to the trunk and extremities, usuallly within the first 24 hours.*

JOINTS   Arthritis occurs in adults. Possible effusion.

DIAGNOSIS AND DIFFERENTIAL DIAGNOSIS

Diagnosis   Clinical diagnosis. Can be confirmed by serology.

Differential Diagnosis   *Of exanthem:* viral exanthems, drug eruption, scarlet fever. *With arthritis:* acute rheumatic fever, rheumatoid arthritis

LABORATORY AND SPECIAL EXAMINATIONS

Serology   Acute and convalescent rubella antibody titers show fourfold or greater rise.

Culture   Virus can be isolated from throat, joint fluid aspirate

COURSE AND PROGNOSIS

In most persons rubella is a mild, inconsequential infection. However, when rubella occurs in a pregnant woman during the first trimester, the infection can be passed transplacentally to the developing fetus. Approximately half of infants who acquire rubella during the first trimester of intrauterine life will show clinical signs of damage from the virus. Manifestations of the congenital rubella syndrome are congenital heart defects, cataracts, microphthalmia, deafness, microcephaly, hydrocephaly.

TREATMENT

Prophylaxis   Rubella is preventable by immunization. Prior rubella should be documented in young women; if antirubella antibody titers are negative, rubella immunization should be given.

Acute infection   Symptomatic

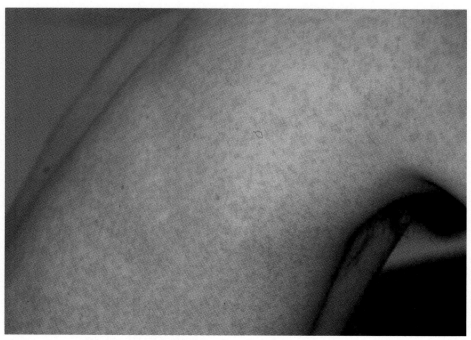

157*b*   Rubella   *Exanthem on the trunk.*

Measles is a highly contagious childhood viral infection characterized by fever, coryza, cough, conjunctivitis, pathognomonic enanthem (Koplik's spots), and an exanthem; it can be complicated, acutely and chronically, by significant morbidity and mortality.

Synonyms: rubeola, morbilli.

EPIDEMIOLOGY AND ETIOLOGY

Age Prior to measles immunization: 5 to 9 years in the United States. In underdeveloped countries, up to 45% of cases occur before the age of 9 months.

Etiology Measles virus, a paramyxovirus

Incidence *United States:* greater than fourfold increase, 1988 to 1989. *Worldwide:* hyperendemic in many underdeveloped countries, resulting in >1.5 million deaths annually.

Risk Factors Following immunization begun in 1963, incidence has decreased by 98%. Current outbreaks in the United States occur in inner city unimmunized preschool-age children, school-age persons immunized at early age, and imported cases. Most outbreaks are in primary or secondary schools, colleges or universities, daycare centers.

Transmission Spread by respiratory droplet aerosols produced by sneezing and coughing. Infected persons contagious from several days before onset of rash up to 5 days after lesions appear. Attack rate for susceptible contacts exceeds 90 to 100%. Asymptomatic infection rare.

Season Prior to widespread use of vaccine, epidemics occurred every 2 to 3 years, in late winter to early spring.

Geography Worldwide.

HISTORY

Incubation Period 10 to 15 days

History Symptoms of upper respiratory infection with coryza and *hacking, barklike cough,* photophobia, malaise, fever. As exanthem progresses, systemic symptoms subside.

PHYSICAL EXAMINATION

Skin Findings

TYPE OF LESION Exanthem: on the fourth febrile day, erythematous macules and papules. *Initial discrete lesions may become confluent, especially on face* (Figure 158), *neck, and shoulders. Lesions gradually fade in order of appearance with subsequent residual yellow-tan stain or faint desquamation. Exanthem resolves in 4 to 6 days.* Periorbital edema in prodrome.

COLOR Initially erythematous, fading to yellow-tan

DISTRIBUTION OF LESIONS Appear on forehead at hairline, behind ears; spread centrifugally and inferiorly to involve the face, trunk (Figure 159), and extremities, reaching the feet by third day.

MUCOUS MEMBRANES Koplik's spots: cluster of tiny bluish-white papules with an erythematous areola, appearing on or after second day of febrile illness, on buccal mucosa opposite premolar teeth. Bulbar conjunctivae: conjunctivitis

RASH AND FEVER

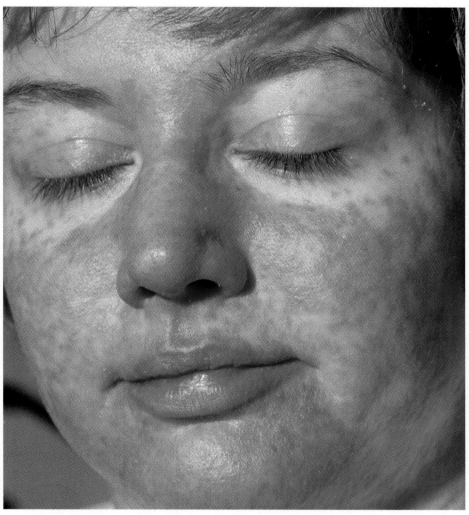

158   Measles   *Erythematous macules and papules becoming confluent, appearing initially on the face.*

General Examination Generalized lymphadenopathy common. Otherwise unremarkable.

DIAGNOSIS AND DIFFERENTIAL DIAGNOSIS

Diagnosis Clinical diagnosis

Differential Diagnosis The time course of rubella (3 days) versus measles (6 days) is distinctive as each moves from head to toe. Other viral exanthems, secondary syphilis, scarlet fever, drug eruption

LABORATORY AND SPECIAL EXAMINATIONS

Cultures Isolate virus from blood, urine, pharyngeal secretions.

Serology Demonstrate fourfold or greater rise in measles titer.

PATHOPHYSIOLOGY

Virus enters cells of respiratory tract, replicates locally, spreads to local lymph nodes, and disseminates hematogenously to skin and mucous membranes. Viral replication also occurs on skin and mucosa.

COURSE AND PROGNOSIS

Self-limited infection in most patients. Complications more common in malnourished third-world children, the unimmunized, and those with congenital immunodeficiency or leukemia. Acute complications (9.8% of cases): otitis media, pneumonia (bacterial or measles), diarrhea, measles encephalitis (1 in 800 to 1000 cases), thrombocytopenia. In unimmunized HIV-infected children, fatal measles pneumonia has occurred without rash. Chronic complication: subacute sclerosing panencephalitis.

TREATMENT

Prevention Prophylactic immunization

Acute infection Symptomatic

Secondary bacterial infections Administration of appropriate antibiotics

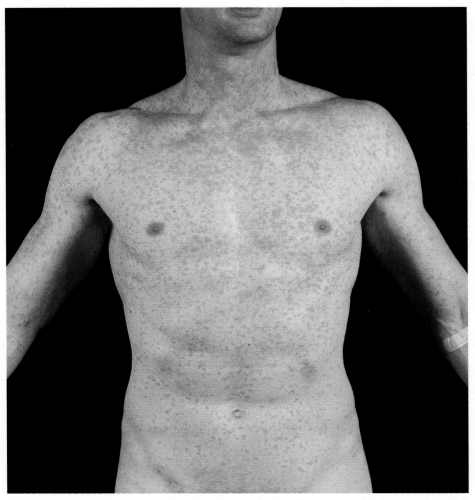

159 Measles *Exanthem spreads from head to toes in 2 to 3 days in contrast to rubella which spreads from head to toes in 1 day.*

Staphylococcal scalded-skin syndrome (SSSS) is a toxin-mediated epidermolytic disease characterized by erythema and widespread detachment of the superficial layers of the epidermis, resembling the effects of scalding. It occurs mainly in newborns and infants under 2 years of age. Severity ranges from a localized form, bullous impetigo, to a generalized form with extensive epidermolysis and desquamation. Clinical spectrum of SSSS includes: (1) bullous impetigo, (2) bullous impetigo with generalization, (3) scarlatiniform syndrome, (4) generalized scalded-skin syndrome.

Synonyms: pemphigus neonatorum, Ritter's disease.

EPIDEMIOLOGY AND ETIOLOGY

Age Infants and young children

Etiology *Staphylococcus aureus* of phage group II, mostly type 71

HISTORY

Immune Status Adults with immunosuppression or renal insufficiency are subject to SSSS.

Skin Symptoms Generalized SSSS: early erythematous areas are very tender.

PHYSICAL EXAMINATION

Skin Findings
TYPE OF LESION *Bullous impetigo:* intact flaccid purulent bullae, clustered. Rupture of the bullae results in moist red and/or crusted erosive lesions. *Generalized SSSS: tender, ill-defined erythema* (Figure 160*a*) occurs initially. With epidermolysis, epidermis appears wrinkled. Unroofed epidermis forms erosions with red, moist base (Figure 160*b*). *Scarlatiniform syndrome:* like scarlet fever (see page 298) but without pharyngitis, tonsilitis, and strawberry tongue.

PALPATION Gentle lateral pressure causes shearing off of superficial epidermis (Nikolsky's sign).
ARRANGEMENT OF MULTIPLE LESIONS In bullous impetigo, lesions often clustered in an intertriginous area.
DISTRIBUTION OF LESIONS *Bullous impetigo:* intertriginous areas. *Generalized SSSS:* Initially periorificially on face, neck, axillae, groins; becoming more widespread in 24 to 48 hours. Initial erythema and later sloughing of epidermis are most pronounced periorificially on face (Figure 160*a*) and in flexural areas on neck, axillae, groins, antecubital area, back (Figure 160*b*) (pressure points). *Scarlatiniform syndrome:* like scarlet fever.
MUCOUS MEMBRANES Usually uninvolved

General Examination Possible low-grade fever. Irritable child.

DIAGNOSIS AND DIFFERENTIAL DIAGNOSIS

Diagnosis By clinical findings

Differential Diagnosis Erythema multiforme, drug-induced toxic epidermal necrolysis

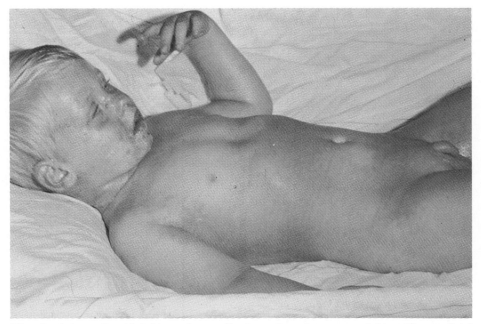

160*a* Staphylococcal scalded-skin syndrome *Tender erythematous areas of skin with superficial epidermis sloughing in sheets. Also seen in the axilla.*

LABORATORY AND SPECIAL EXAMINATIONS

Grams's Stain *Bullous impetigo:* pus in bullae, clumps of gram-positive cocci within PMN. *Generalized SSSS:* gram-positive cocci only at colonized site, not in areas of epidermolysis.

Bacterial Culture *Bullous impetigo: Staph. aureus. Generalized SSSS: Staph. aureus* only at colonized site of infection, i.e., umbilical stump, conjunctiva, external ear canal; culture of sloughing skin or bullae usually without pathogens.

PATHOPHYSIOLOGY

In newborns and infants, *Staph. aureus* colonizes in the nose, conjunctivae, or umbilical stump without causing clinically apparent infection, producing an exotoxin (exfoliatin, epidermolysin) which is transported hematogenously to the skin. At times purulent conjunctivitis, otitis media, or occult nasopharyngeal infection occurs at site of toxin production. The exfoliative toxin causes acantholysis and intraepidermal cleavage within the stratum granulosum. The few cases of SSSS reported in adults were associated with immunodeficiency or renal insufficiency. Local effects of the toxin result in bullous impetigo; however, with absorption of the toxin, a mild scarlatiniform rash accompanying the bullous lesions may be seen. Conversely, local effects of the toxin may be absent with systemic absorption resulting in a staphylococcal scarlet fever syndrome. More extensive epidermal damage is characterized by sloughing of superficial epidermis in generalized SSSS.

COURSE AND PROGNOSIS

Following adequate antibiotic treatment, the superficially denuded areas heal in 3 to 5 days with generalized desquamation in large sheets of skin.

TREATMENT

Newborn Hospitalization and treatment with IV oxacillin, 200 mg per kg body weight per day in divided doses every 4 hours, preferable. Hospitalize infants with extensive sloughing of skin or if parental compliance to treatment is questioned. With reliable home care and mild involvement, dicloxacillin, 30 to 50 mg per kg body weight per day, can be given orally.

Topical care Baths or compresses; mupirocin ointment, bacitracin, or silver sulfadiazine

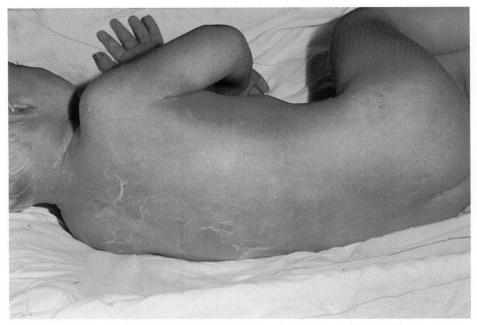

160*b*   Staphylococcal scalded-skin syndrome   *Back of patient shown in Figure 160a*

Scarlet fever is an acute infection of the tonsils *or* skin by an erythrogenic exotoxin-producing strain of group A streptococcus, associated with a characteristic exanthem, produced by the exotoxin.

EPIDEMIOLOGY AND ETIOLOGY

Age Children

Etiology Usually group A β-hemolytic *Streptococcus pyogenes* (GABHS). Uncommonly, exotoxin-producing *Staphylococcus aureus*.

HISTORY

Incubation Period Rash appears within 2 to 3 days after onset of infection.

Exposure Household member may be a streptococcal carrier.

PHYSICAL EXAMINATION

Skin Findings

TYPE OF LESION Finely punctate erythema is first noted on the upper part of the trunk. Face becomes flushed but with a perioral pallor (Figure 161). Initial punctate lesions become confluently erythematous, i.e., scarlatiniform. Linear petechiae (Pastia's sign) occur in body folds. Intensity of the exanthem varies from mild to moderate erythema confined to the trunk (Figure 162) to an extensive purpuric eruption. Exanthem fades within 4 to 5 days and is followed by brawny desquamation on the body and extremities and by sheetlike exfoliation on the palms and soles. In subclinical or mild infections exanthem and pharyngitis may pass unnoticed. In this case patient may seek medical advice only when exfoliation on the palms and soles is noted. Infected surgical or other wound. Impetiginous skin lesion.

COLOR Pink to scarlet

PALPATION Sandpaper "feel" as desquamation begins

DISTRIBUTION OF LESIONS Erythema first noted on chest. Spreads to extremities. Erythema accentuated at pressure points and in body folds. Pastia's sign noted in antecubital and axillary folds.

MUCOUS MEMBRANES Pharynx beefy red. Tongue initially is white with scattered red swollen papillae (white strawberry tongue). By the fourth or fifth day the hyperkeratotic membrane is sloughed, and the lingular mucosa appears bright red (red strawberry tongue). Punctate erythema and petechiae may occur in the palate. Acute follicular or membranous tonsillitis.

Variant Toxic strep syndrome: toxemia, organ failure, and a scarlatiniform rash associated with *GABHS* cellulitis.

General Examination Anterior cervical lymphadenitis

DIAGNOSIS AND DIFFERENTIAL DIAGNOSIS

Diagnosis Confirmed by detecting strep antigen in a rapid test, culturing GABHS from throat or wound, or documenting rise in the antistreptolysin O titer.

Differential Diagnosis Staphyloccal scar-

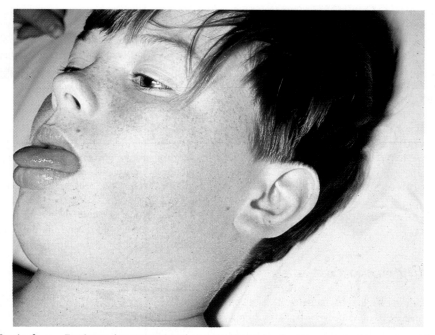

161 **Scarlet fever** *Erythema (scarlatiniform) sparing the perioral region and most pronounced in the body folds (not shown); a bright-red strawberry tongue. (Courtesy of Thomas C. Peebles, M.D.)*

let fever (pharyngitis, tonsillitis, strawberry tongue, and palatal enanthem not seen), viral exanthem, drug eruption

LABORATORY AND SPECIAL EXAMINATIONS

Microbiologic Examination of Skin Material   Gram's stain of infected wound or impetiginized skin lesion

Culture   For presence of GABHS

Serology   Fourfold rise in antistreptolysin O titer.

PATHOPHYSIOLOGY

Erythrogenic toxin production depends on the presence of a temperate bacteriophage. Patients with prior exposure to the erythrogenic toxin have antitoxin immunity and neutralize the toxin. The scarlet fever syndrome therefore does not develop in these patients. Since several erythrogenic strains of GABHS cause infection, it is theoretically possible to have a second episode of scarlet fever. Strains of *Staph. aureus* can synthesize an erythrogenic exotoxin producing a scarlatiniform exanthem.

COURSE AND PROGNOSIS

Nonsuppurative sequelae of streptococcal infections, i.e., acute rheumatic fever, acute glomerulonephritis, and erythema nodosum, may follow if the infection goes untreated. The incidence of acute rheumatic fever had markedly decreased during the past two decades but is currently on the rise.

TREATMENT

Penicillin V 250 mg 4 times a day for 10 days. Alternatively, erythromycin 250 mg 4 times a day for 10 days. Dose must be adjusted for pediatric patients.

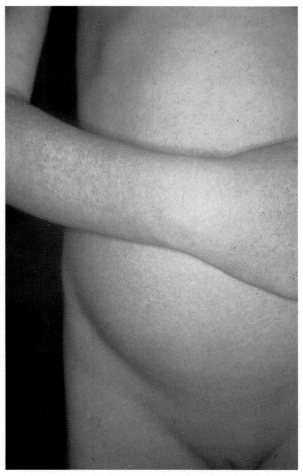

162　Scarlet fever　*Diffuse scarlatiniform rash on the trunk.*

Kawasaki's Disease

Kawasaki's disease (KD) is a rare acute febrile illness of infants and children, characterized by cutaneous and mucosal erythema and edema with subsequent desquamation, cervical lymphadenitis, and complicated by coronary artery aneurysms (20%).

Synonyms: mucocutaneous lymph node syndrome, juvenile periarteritis nodosa.

EPIDEMIOLOGY AND ETIOLOGY

Age Peak incidence at 1 year, mean 2.6 years, uncommon after 8 years

Sex Male predominance, 1.5:1

Race United States incidence: Japanese > African-American > Caucasian children

Etiology Idiopathic, probably infectious

Season Winter and spring

Geography First reported in Japan, 1961; United States, 1971. Epidemics in Japan and also several cities in the United States.

HISTORY

Constitutional symptoms of diarrhea, arthralgia, arthritis, meatitis, tympanitis, photophobia

PHYSICAL EXAMINATION

Skin Findings
TYPE OF LESION (See Figure 163). Scarlatiniform, morbilliform, erythema multiforme-like. Erythema, palms and soles. Edema, hands and feet. Subsequently, desquamation. Perineal: confluent macules to plaque-type erythema, followed by desquamation.
PALPATION Lesions may be tender.

DISTRIBUTION Hands and feet, striking erythema ± indurative edema; truncal erythema, perineal.
MUCOUS MEMBRANES Bulbar conjunctiva (Figure 164), hyperemic; lips, red, dry, fissured; pharynx, injected; strawberry tongue (Figure 164)

General Findings Meningeal irritation; pneumonia; lymphadenopathy, usually of cervical node, ≥1.5 cm, slightly tender, firm; arthritis and arthralgia, knees, hips, elbows; pericardial tamponade, arrhythmias, rubs, congestive heart failure, left ventricular dysfunction

DIAGNOSIS AND DIFFERENTIAL DIAGNOSIS

Diagnosis Diagnostic criteria: Fever spiking to >39.4°C lasting ≥ 5 days without other cause, associated with 4 of 5 criteria: (1) bilateral conjunctival injection; (2) at least one of following mucous membrane changes: injected/fissured lips, injected pharynx, strawberry tongue; (3) at least one of the following extremity changes: erythema of palms/soles, edema of hands/feet, desquamation (Figure 165), generalized/periungal desquamation; (4) diffuse scarlatiniform erythroderma, diffuse centrally/sharply demarcated borders on extremities; deeply erythematous maculopapular rash; iris lesions; (5) cervical lymphadenopathy (at least one lymph node ≥1.5 cm in diameter).

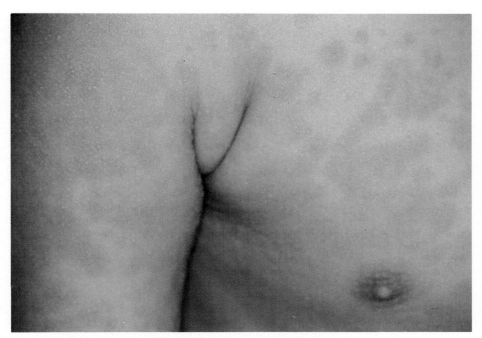

163   Kawasaki's disease   *Blotchy erythema on the trunk of a child.*

Differential Diagnosis Juvenile rheumatoid arthritis, infectious mononucleosis, viral exanthems, leptospirosis, Rocky Mountain spotted fever, toxic shock syndrome, staphylococcal scalded-skin syndrome, erythema multiforme, serum sickness, SLE, Reiter's syndrome

LABORATORY AND SPECIAL EXAMINATIONS

Echocardiography Coronary artery aneurysms

Cardiac Angiography Indications: symptoms of myocardial ischemia, coronary aneurysms on echocardiography

PATHOPHYSIOLOGY

Generalized vasculitis. Endarteritis of vasa vasorum involves adventitia/intima of proximal coronary arteries with ectasia, aneurysm formation, vessel obstruction, and distal embolization with subsequent myocardial infarction. Other vessels: brachiocephalic, celiac, renal, iliofemoral arteries.

COURSE AND PROGNOSIS

Clinical course triphasic. Uneventful recovery occurs in majority. CVS complications in 20%. Coronary artery aneurysms occur within 2 to 8 weeks; associated with myocarditis, myocardial ischemia/infarction, pericarditis, peripheral vascular occlusion, small bowel obstruction, stroke. Mortality 1%.

TREATMENT

Treatment is nonspecific, directed at prevention of the cardiovascular complications. Aspirin and/or high-dose IV γ-globulin may reduce risk of coronary aneurysms.

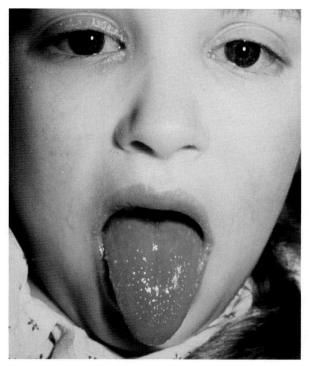

164　Kawasaki's disease　*Scarlet-red tongue and bulbar conjunctival erythema are seen on the face of this child. (Courtesy of Arthur R. Rhodes, M.D.)*

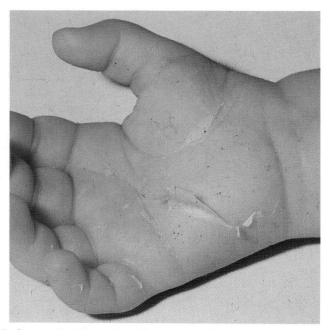

165　Kawasaki's disease　*Shedding of the skin is seen on the palm of this child, 10 days after the acute illness. (Courtesy of Arthur R. Rhodes, M.D.)*

KAWASAKI'S DISEASE

Varicella is the highly contagious primary infection caused by varicella-zoster virus, characterized by successive crops of pruritic vesicles which evolve to pustules, crusts, and, at times, scars. It is often accompanied by mild constitutional symptoms; primary infection occurring in adulthood may be complicated by pneumonia, encephalitis, or myocarditis.

Synonym: chickenpox.

EPIDEMIOLOGY AND ETIOLOGY

Age 90% of cases occur in children <10 years of age, less than 5% in persons >15 years.

Etiology Varicella-zoster virus (VZV), a herpesvirus

Incidence Nearly universal; 3,000,000 cases in the United States annually.

Transmission Airborne droplets as well as direct contact; indirect contact uncommon cause. Patients are contagious several days before exanthem appears and until last crop of vesicles. Crusts are not infectious.

Season In metropolitan areas in temperate climates, varicella epidemics occur in winter and spring.

Geography Worldwide.

HISTORY

Incubation Period 14 days (range, 10 to 23 days)

Prodrome Characteristically absent or mild. Uncommon in children, more common in adults: headache, general aches and pains, severe backache, malaise. Exanthem appears within 2 to 3 days.

History Exposure at daycare, school, by older sibling, relative with zoster.

Skin Symptoms Exanthem usually quite pruritic

PHYSICAL EXAMINATION

Skin Findings In most children, illness begins with appearance of exanthem, vesicular lesions appear in successive crops. Often single discrete lesions or scanty in number in children; much more dense in adults.

TYPE OF LESION Initial lesions are *papules* (often not observed) which may appear as wheals and quickly evolve to *vesicles* and initially appear as small "drops of water" or "dewdrops on a rose petal" (Figure 166), superficial and thin-walled with surrounding erythema. Vesicles become umbilicated and rapidly evolve to *pustules* and crusts over an 8- to 12-hour period. With subsequent crops, all stages of evolution may be noted simultaneously, i.e., papules, vesicles, pustules, *crusts* (Figure 167). Crusts fall off in 1 to 3 weeks, leaving a pink, somewhat depressed base. Characteristic punched-out permanent scars may persist. Uncommonly, hemorrhage into pustular lesions occurs in otherwise healthy children, i.e., hemorrhagic varicella. Complicated by superinfection by staphylococci or streptococci: impetigo, furuncles, cellulitis, and gangrene may occur.

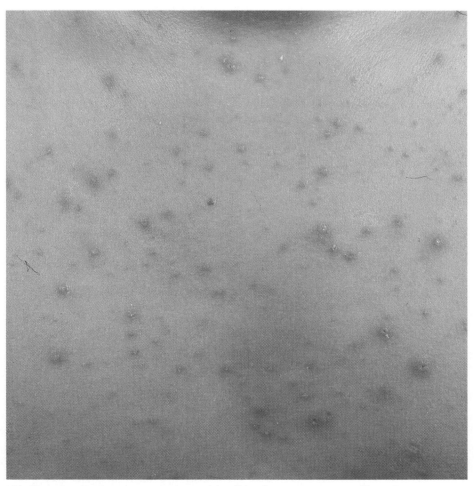

166 Varicella *Erythematous papules, vesicles ("dewdrops on a rose petal"), and crusts.*

COLOR Vesicles watery yellow. Pustules creamy white pus. Brownish-red crusts.

DISTRIBUTION OF LESIONS First lesions begin on face and scalp, spreading inferiorly to trunk and extremities. Most profuse in areas least exposed to pressure, i.e., back between shoulder blades, flanks, axillae, popliteal and antecubital fossae. Density highest on trunk and face, less on extremities. Palms and soles usually spared.

MUCOUS MEMBRANES Vesicles (not often observed) and subsequent shallow erosions (2.0 to 3.0 mm), most common on palate, but also occur on mucosa of nose, conjunctivae, pharynx, larynx, trachea, GI tract, urinary tract, vagina.

Variants Varicella gangrenosa occurs in children with leukemia or other severe underlying disease, characterized by gangrenous ulceration. Hemorrhagic varicella with disseminated intravascular coagulation (purpura fulminans).

General Examination Low-grade fever. Vesicopustules may occur in respiratory, GU, and GI tracts.

DIAGNOSIS AND DIFFERENTIAL DIAGNOSIS

Diagnosis Clinical diagnosis confirmed by Tzanck test

Differential Diagnosis Disseminated herpes simplex virus (HSV) infection, cutaneous dissemination of zoster, eczema herpeticum, eczema vaccinatum, disseminated vaccinia in immunosupressed patient (smallpox vaccination still given in the U.S. military), bullous form of impetigo

LABORATORY AND SPECIAL EXAMINATIONS

Tzanck Preparation Cytology of scraping from fluid or base of vesicle or pustule shows both giant and multinucleated giant epidermal cells (as does that of HSV infections).

Electron Microscopy VZV particles can be seen in negative stain preparations but cannot be distinguished from HSV.

Cultures Isolation of virus from skin lesions is possible, but more difficult than for HSV.

Serology Seroconversion, i.e., fourfold or greater rise in VZV titers.

PATHOPHYSIOLOGY

Virus enters through mucosa of upper respiratory tract and oropharnyx, followed by local replication and primary viremia; VZV then replicates in cells of reticuloendothelial system with subsequent secondary viremia and dissemination to skin and mucous membranes. Second episodes of varicella have been documented but are rare. As with all herpesviruses, VZV enters a latent phase, residing in sensory ganglion; reactivation of VZV results in zoster.

COURSE AND PROGNOSIS

In children, prodrome and rash may be very transient. In adults, prodromal symptoms are common and may be severe; exanthem may last for a week or more, with prolonged period of recovery. Primary varicella pneumonia is relatively common in adults, with 16% showing x-ray evidence of pneumonitis; however, only 4% have clinical signs of pneumonitis. VZV encephalitis may also complicate varicella in adults. Maternal varicella during first trimester of pregnancy may result in fetal varicella syndrome. Neonatal varicella has higher incidence of pneumonitis and encephalitis than in older children. Immunocompromised or corticosteroid-treated patients with varicella may manifest dissemination, hepatitis, encephalitis, and hemorrhagic complications. If varicella occurs at an early age when maternal antibody still present, a patient may have a second episode of varicella. In HIV-infected patients, reactivation of VZV may result in chronic painful ecthymatous varicella.

TREATMENT

Otherwise healthy patient: symptomatic treatment of pruritus; treatment of bacterial superinfection. Antipyretic administration is of concern because of a possible link between aspirin and Reye's syndrome in children with varicella.

In children, varicella is usually mild, and specific antiviral therapy is not indicated. In adults, orally administered acyclovir, 800 mg every 6 hours for 5 days, begun within the first 24 hours of illness may reduce the severity of the infection; however, its effect on the complications of pneumonitis and encephalitis are not yet determined.

Severe varicella, varicella pneumonitis, varicella encephalitis, or varicella occurring in immunocompromised host: IV acyclovir or vidarabine.

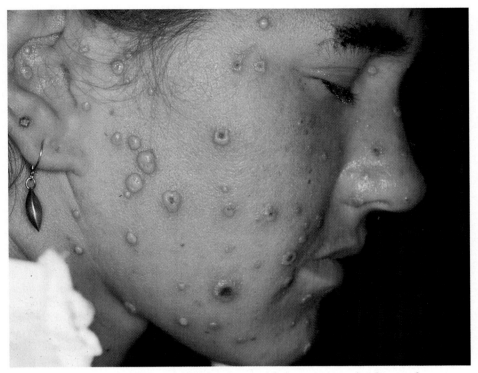

167   Varicella   *Discrete vesicles, pustules, and crusted lesions are seen simultaneously.*

Varicella-zoster immune globulin (VZIG) administration is indicated for individuals with the following illnesses or conditions following significant exposure to VZV: leukemia or lymphoma; cellular immune deficiency; immunosuppressive treatment; newborn of mother who had onset of varicella <6 days before or <2 days after delivery; premature infant (>28 weeks gestation) whose mother lacks previous history of varicella; premature infant (<28 weeks gestation or <1000 g) regardless of maternal history; pregnant women.

This can be a life-threatening medical problem with an abrupt onset. The skin involvement is distinctive and starts with a burning erythema which spreads in hours to result in large areas of fiery-red skin. Pinpoint pustules then appear in clusters, peppering the red areas of skin; these pustules become confluent and form "lakes" filled with purulent fluid. Fever, generalized weakness, severe malaise, and a leukocytosis are prominent features in almost every patient.

Synonym: syndrome of von Zumbusch.

EPIDEMIOLOGY

Age   Adults, rarely children

Precipitating Factors   There are no known precipitating factors, and the patient may or may not have had a stable plaque-type psoriasis in the past. Pustular, acral psoriasis of the Hallopeau type may, at times, progress to generalized acute pustular psoriasis.

HISTORY

Duration of Lesions   The constellation of fiery-red erythema followed by formation of pustules and "lakes" occurs over a period of less than 1 day. Waves of pustules may follow each other: as one set dries another will appear.

Skin Symptoms   Marked burning, tenderness

Constitutional Symptoms
ACUTE   Headache, chills, feverishness, marked fatigue, severe malaise

Systems Review   Arthralgia

PHYSICAL EXAMINATION

Appearance of Patient   Frightened, "toxic"

Vital Signs   Fast pulse, rapid breathing, fever which may be high

Skin Lesions
TYPE OF LESION   There is a sequence of burning erythema followed by the appearance of clusters of tiny nonfollicular and very superficial pustules that usually become confluent, forming lakes of pus (Figures 168a and 168b). Removal of top yields superficial, oozing erosions, and there will be crusting.
ARRANGEMENT OF MULTIPLE LESIONS   Closely set small pustules, circinate lesions, isolated pustules; pustules are interfollicular.
DISTRIBUTION OF LESIONS   Generalized, but especially involving the flexural areas and the anogenital regions

Mucous Membranes   Pustules, especially on the tongue

Hair and Nails   Nails become thickened, and there is onycholysis; subungual lakes of pus lead to shedding of nails; hair loss of the telogen effluvium type developing in 2 to 3 months may occur.

General Examination   Inflammatory polyarthritis

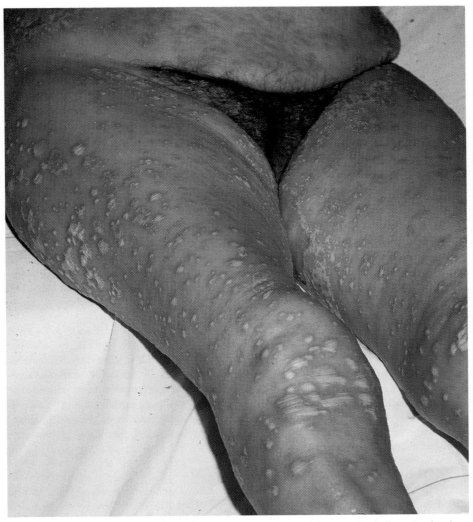

168*a* Generalized pustular psoriasis syndrome (von Zumbusch) *The pustular lesions develop in a fiery erythematous base. Pinpoint pustules appear and coalesce to form lakes, as are seen on the knees of this patient.*

GENERALIZED ACUTE PUSTULAR PSORIASIS

LABORATORY EXAMINATIONS

Dermatopathology
LIGHT MICROSCOPY Large spongiform pustules resulting from the migration of neutrophils from the capillaries in the dermal papilla to the upper stratum malpighii, where they aggregate within the interstices of the degenerated and thinned keratinocytes.

Microbiologic Examination of Skin Material
CULTURE OF TISSUE OR EXUDATE No pathogenic organisms can be cultured from the pustules.

Laboratory Examination of Blood
BACTERIOLOGIC Blood cultures are negative.

HEMATOLOGIC Polymorphonuclear leukocytosis as high as 20,000 WBC

CHEMISTRY Plasma albumin, zinc, and calcium may be low.

DIAGNOSIS

The abrupt onset, the typical evolution of erythema followed by pustulation is highly characteristic. Nevertheless, blood cultures should always be obtained because of possible superinfection, especially with staphylococcal bacteremia. Generalized herpes simplex has umbilicated pustules, and the Tzanck test and viral cultures establish the diagnosis.

PATHOGENESIS

The fever and leukocytosis probably result from the marked increase in the number of polymorphonuclear cells which invade the dermis and release their chemical mediators. This causes inflammation and necrosis of cells (leukocytes and keratinocytes).

SIGNIFICANCE

These patients are often brought to the emergency rooms of hospitals, and there is a serious question of overwhelming bacteremia until the blood cultures are shown to be negative.

COURSE AND PROGNOSIS

Relapses and remissions may occur over a period of years.

TREATMENT

The patient should be hospitalized and treated as a patient with extensive burns: bed rest, isolation, fluid replacement, repeated blood cultures.

Systemic Some patients undergo a rapid spontaneous remission without any therapy, and if they have had a previous spontaneous remission and are having a recurrence, specific systemic treatment is often omitted. For new patients, most are started on IV antibiotics pending the results of the blood culture. First-line therapy of generalized pustular psoriasis is oral etretinate or acitretin, 0.5 to 1.0 mg per kg body weight per day. It may result in rapid cessation of pustular eruptions but will have to be continued for a considerable time to prevent recurrence. PUVA photochemotherapy is also highly effective but is often difficult to perform in a toxic patient with fever. It is therefore added to etretinate once systemic symptoms have improved. *Parenteral* methotrexate, 15.0 to 25.0 mg once a week, is a second-line choice. Systemic corticosteroids should be avoided and may be indicated only in the initial toxic phases of an eruption.

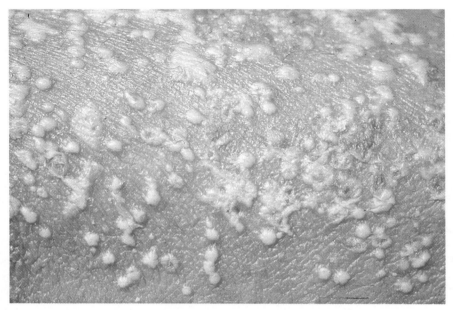

168*b* Generalized pustular psoriasis syndrome (von Zumbusch) *Superficial pustules becoming confluent and forming lakes of pus.*

Toxic epidermal necrolysis (TEN) is a cutaneous drug-induced or idiopathic reaction pattern characterized by tenderness and erythema of skin and mucosa, followed by extensive cutaneous and mucosal exfoliation. It is potentially life-threatening due to multisystem involvement.
Synonym: Lyell's syndrome.

EPIDEMIOLOGY AND ETIOLOGY

Age Adults >40 years

Sex Equal incidence

Etiology *Drugs* most commonly: antibiotics, barbiturates, hydantoins, pyrazolon derivatives (phenylbutazone), sulfonamides, sulfones. *Other:* infections (viral, fungal, bacterial septicemia), vaccinations, leukemia, lymphoma, graft-versus-host reaction. *Idiopathic.*

HISTORY

Prodrome Mild to moderate skin tenderness, fever, malaise, headache, conjunctival burning or itching, myalgias, arthralgias, nausea and vomiting, and/or diarrhea occur in the majority of patients.

Drug Ingestion Occurs within days of ingestion of the drug; newly added drug is most suspect.

Skin Symptoms Marked tenderness of rash, pain, pruritus, paresthesia

PHYSICAL EXAMINATION

Skin Findings
TYPE OF LESION Prodromal rash: morbilliform, erythema multiforme-like. Initial tender erythema. Small blisters then form,

becoming irregularly confluent. Entire thickness of epidermis becomes necrotic and shears off in large sheets, but large blisters only rarely form. Epidermal sloughing may be generalized, resulting in large denuded areas resembling a second degree thermal burn (Figure 169). The idiopathic form is usually not preceded by rash but starts with erythema which is rapidly followed by sloughing and denudation. Nails may be shed.
DISTRIBUTION OF LESIONS Initial erythema on face, extremities, becoming confluent over a few hours or days. Denudation most pronounced over pressure points. Scalp, palms, soles may be less severely involved or spared.
MUCOUS MEMBRANES Erythema and sloughing of lips, buccal mucosa, conjunctiva, genital and anal skin

General Findings Usually mentally alert. In distress due to severe pain. Acute renal failure; erosions in lower respiratory tract, gut.

DIAGNOSIS AND DIFFERENTIAL DIAGNOSIS

Diagnosis Clinical, confirmed by biopsy

Differential Diagnosis *Early:* exanthematous drug eruptions, scarlet fever, phototoxic eruptions, toxic shock syndrome, erythema multiforme, graft-versus-host disease (GVHD). *Full-blown:* staphylococcal scalded-

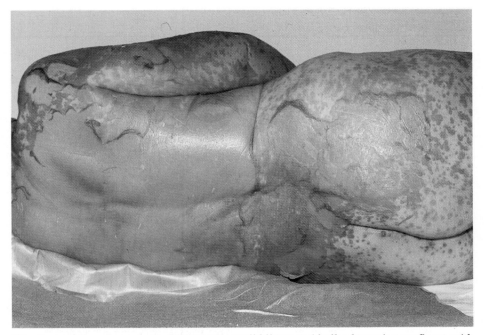

169 Toxic epidermal necrolysis *Widespread, small blisters and bullae becoming confluent, with epidermal sloughing, resulting in large denuded areas.*

skin syndrome, erythema multiforme, generalized bullous fixed drug eruption, GVHD.

LABORATORY AND SPECIAL EXAMINATIONS

Biopsy Confirms clinical diagnosis. *Early:* vacuolization/necrosis of basal keratinocytes and individual cell necrosis throughout the epidermis. *Late:* necrosis of entire epidermis with formation of subepidermal split above basement membrane. Little or no inflammatory infiltrate in dermis.

PATHOPHYSIOLOGY

Pathogenesis unknown. Behaves like second to third degree thermal burn.

COURSE AND PROGNOSIS

Currently, 25% mortality rate, mainly in elderly. Death due to sepsis, GI hemorrhage, fluid/electrolyte imbalance. If the patient survives the first episode of TEN, reexposure to the causative drug may be followed by recurrence within hours to days, more severe than the initial episode.

TREATMENT

Treat as a thermal burn patient in a burn unit of a hospital. Corticosteroid: role not determined. IV fluid replacement: water, electrolytes, albumin, plasma. Debridement: remove only frankly necrotic tissue. Watch for signs of sepsis (fever, hypotension, change in mental status). Conjunctival: erythromycin ointment. Frequent suctioning in oropharyngeal involvement to prevent aspiration pneumonitis.

Cat-scratch disease (CSD) is a benign, self-limited zoonotic infection characterized by a primary skin or conjunctival lesion following cat scratches or contact with a cat and subsequent tender regional lymphadenopathy.

Synonyms: cat-scratch fever, benign lymphoreticulosis, nonbacterial regional lymphadenitis.

EPIDEMIOLOGY AND ETIOLOGY

Age <21 years

Sex More common in males than females

Etiology CSD bacillus, a pleomorphic gram-negative rod

Transmission History of cat contact (scratch, bite, lick) in 95% of cases

Season Late fall, winter, or early spring in cooler climes; in July and August in warmer climes.

Geography Worldwide

HISTORY

Incubation Period 1 to 8 weeks

Duration of Lesions A local primary lesion occurs within 2 weeks at the site of scratch or injury in about half of patients.

Prodrome Mild fever and malaise occur in less than half the patients. Chills, general aching, and nausea are infrequently present.

PHYSICAL EXAMINATION

Skin Findings

TYPE OF LESION Innocuous-looking, small (1.5 cm) papule or nodule (Figure 170), vesicle, or pustule at the inoculation site; may ulcerate. Residual linear cat scratch.

COLOR Skin-color to pink to red

PALPATION Firm, at times tender

DISTRIBUTION OF LESIONS Primary lesion on exposed skin of head, neck, extremities

MUCOUS MEMBRANES If portal of entry is the conjunctiva, 3.0- to 5.0-mm whitish-yellow granulation on palpebral conjunctiva associated with tender preauricular and/or cervical lymphadenopathy; referred to as the *oculoglandular syndrome of Parinaud.*

OTHER SKIN FINDINGS Urticaria, transient maculopapular eruption, vesiculopapular lesions, erythema nodosum

HIV-INFECTED PATIENTS May develop bacillary angiomatosis, cutaneous hemangiomas which resemble Kaposi's sarcoma. Lesions vary in number from a few scattered to hundreds of generalized lesions.

General Examination Regional lymphadenopathy evident within a few days to a few weeks after the primary lesion. Nodes are usually solitary, moderately tender, freely movable, and *may be very large.* Nodes may suppurate. Generalized lymphadenopathy or involvement of the lymph nodes of more than one region is unusual. Less common: encephalitis, pneumonitis, thrombocytopenia, osteomyelitis, hepatitis, abscesses in liver or spleen.

DIAGNOSIS AND DIFFERENTIAL DIAGNOSIS

Diagnosis Demonstration of small, pleomorphic bacilli in Warthin-Starry-stained sections of primary skin lesion, conjunctiva, or lymph nodes

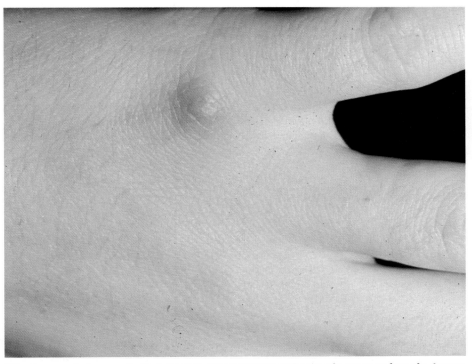

170 Cat-scratch disease *Erythematous nodule occurring at the site of a cat scratch on the dorsum of the hand.*

Differential Diagnosis Of regional lymphadenopathy: suppurative bacterial lymphadenitis, atypical mycobacteria, sporotrichosis, tularemia, toxoplasmosis, infectious mononucleosis, tumors, sarcoidosis, lymphogranuloma venereum, coccidioidomycosis. Large single nodes with only a small papular primary lesion may be confusing and Hodgkin's lymphoma can be ruled out only by a node biopsy.

LABORATORY AND SPECIAL EXAMINATIONS

Dermatopathology Primary lesion: mid-dermal, small areas of frank necrosis surrounded by necrobiosis and palisaded histiocytes; multinucleated giant cells and eosinophils may also be seen.

Culture CSD bacillus may be cultured by special techniques from primary lesion of lymph node.

Laboratory Examination of Blood WBC usually normal; ESR commonly elevated.

COURSE AND PROGNOSIS

Self-limited, usually within 1 to 2 months. Uncommonly, prolonged morbidity with persistent high fever, suppurative lymphadenitis, severe systemic symptoms.

TREATMENT

Symptomatic in most cases. Occasionally, surgical drainage of suppurative node is indicated. CSD bacillus is resistant to common orally administered antibiotics. Erythromycin is the drug of choice for treatment of bacillary angiomatosis, which is caused by a CSD-like organism.

Tularemia is an acute infection, transmitted by handling flesh of infected animals or by the bite of insect vectors, by inoculation of conjunctiva, by ingestion of infected food, or by inhalation; it manifests in four clinical patterns: ulceroglandular, oculoglandular, typhoidal, pulmonary.

Synonyms: rabbit fever, deerfly fever.

EPIDEMIOLOGY AND ETIOLOGY

Age, Sex Young males.

Occupation Rabbit hunters, butchers, cooks, agricultural workers, trappers, campers, sheepherders and -shearers, mink ranchers, muskrat farmers, *laboratory technicians.*

Etiology *Francisella tularensis,* a pleomorphic gram-negative coccobacillus

Transmission (1) Small abrasion or puncture wound, bites of infected deerflies/ticks; (2) conjunctival inoculation; (3) ingestion of infected meat; (4) inhalation. Animal reservoir—rabbits, foxes, squirrels, skunks, muskrats, voles, beavers. Insect vectors—ticks (*Ixodes, Dermacentor*), body lice, deerfly.

Season Greatest frequency in summer (tick season) and rabbit-hunting season.

Geography Throughout northern hemisphere. United States: midwest in summer; east of Mississippi in winter.

HISTORY

Incubation Period 2 to 10 days

Prodrome Headache, malaise, myalgia, high fever

History About 48 hours after inoculation, pruritic papule develops at the site of trauma or insect bite followed by enlargement of regional lymph nodes.

PHYSICAL EXAMINATION

Skin Findings
TYPE OF LESION *At inoculation site:* erythematous tender papule evolving to a vesicopustule, enlarging to crusted ulcer with raised, sharply demarcated margins (96 hours) (Figure 171). Depressed center which is often covered by a black eschar (chancriform). *Following bacteremia:* exanthem with macule, papule, petechiae; erythema multiforme; erythema nodosum.
DISTRIBUTION OF LESIONS Primary lesion on finger or hand at site of trauma or insect bite; in groin or axilla following tick bite. Exanthem on trunk and extremities.
MUCOUS MEMBRANES In oculoglandular tularemia, *F. tularensis* is inoculated into conjunctiva causing a purulent conjunctivitis with pain, edema, congestion. Small yellow nodules occur on conjunctivae and ulcerate.

General Findings Fever up to 40°C to 41°C.
REGIONAL LYMPH NODES As the ulcer develops, nodes enlarge and become tender (chancriform syndrome). If untreated, become suppurating buboes. Lung consolidation, splenomegaly, generalized lymphadenopathy, hepatomegaly may occur.
VARIANTS "Typhoidal" form occurs with ingestion of *F. tularensis* resulting in ulcer-

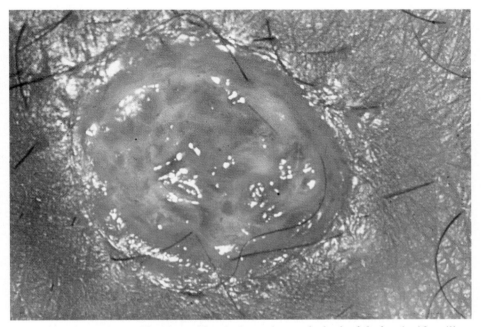

171   Tularemia   *A chancrelike ulcer with raised margins on the back of the hand with axillary adenopathy. The patient was a laboratory technician who handled rabbits.*

ative or exudative pharyngotonsillitis with cervical lymphadenopathy. Tularemic pneumonia occurs following bacteremia or inhalation of *F. tularensis*.

DIAGNOSIS AND DIFFERENTIAL DIAGNOSIS

Diagnosis   Clinical diagnosis in a patient with chancriform syndrome with appropriate animal exposure or insect exposure and systemic manifestations. Confirmed by serology.

Differential Diagnosis   *Inoculation site:* furuncle, paronychia, ecthyma, anthrax, *Pasteurella multocida* infection, sporotrichosis, *Mycobacterium marinum* infection. *Tender regional adenopathy (chancriform):* plague, cat-scratch disease, melioidosis or glanders, lymphogranuloma venereum.

LABORATORY AND SPECIAL EXAMINATIONS

Cultures   Routine culture media do not support the growth of *F. tularensis* from clinical specimens.

Serology   Diagnosis usually confirmed by demonstrating a fourfold rise in acute and convalescent *F. tularensis* antibody titers.

PATHOPHYSIOLOGY

Following inoculation, *F. tularensis* reproduces and spreads through lymphatic channels to lymph nodes and to blood stream.

COURSE AND PROGNOSIS

Untreated, mortality for ulceroglandular form 5%, typhoidal and pulmonary forms 30%.

TREATMENT

Drug of choice: streptomycin 1 to 2 g per day. Alternatives: gentamicin, tetracycline, chloramphenicol.

Section 15

Systemic Infections and Infestations

North American Blastomycosis

Blastomycosis is a chronic systemic mycosis characterized by primary pulmonary infection with hematogenous dissemination which uncommonly is followed by chronic infection of skin and other sites.

Synonyms: Gilchrist's disease, Chicago disease.

EPIDEMIOLOGY AND ETIOLOGY

Age Young, middle-aged

Sex 6 to 10 times more common in males than females

Etiology *Blastomyces dermatitidis,* a dimorphic fungus

Occupation Outdoor vocation or avocation, i.e., farm workers, manual laborers

Transmission Commonly, inhalation of spores with primary pneumonitis. Uncommonly, accidental cutaneous inoculation. Most cases isolated; epidemics rare.

Geography North America: endemic in basins of Great Lakes and great rivers; southeastern United States.

HISTORY

Incubation Period Estimated median 45 days

Symptoms Primary pulmonary infection: usually asymptomatic. Painless skin ulcers.

PHYSICAL EXAMINATION

Skin Findings
TYPE OF LESION Initial lesion, inflammatory nodule which enlarges and ulcerates (Figure 172); subcutaneous nodule, ± many small pustules on surface. Subsequently, verrucous/crusted plaque with sharply demarcated serpiginous borders. Peripheral border extends on one side, resembling a one-half to three-quarter moon. Pus exudes when crust lifted. Central healing with thin geographic atrophic scar.

SHAPE OF INDIVIDUAL LESION May be serpiginous

DISTRIBUTION OF LESIONS Usually symmetrically on trunk but also face, hands, arms. Multiple lesions in half of patients.

MUCOUS MEMBRANES 25% of patients have oral or nasal lesions, half of which have contiguous skin lesions. Laryngeal infection.

General Examination

LUNGS Infiltrates, miliary, cavitary lesions

BONES 50% involvement. Osteomyelitis in thoracolumbar vertebrae, pelvis, sacrum, skull, ribs, long bones. May extend to form large subcutaneous abscess. May occur in conjunction with cutaneous ulcer. Septic arthritis.

LYMPH NODES Regional, enlarged only with inoculation blastomycosis

GENITOURINARY TRACT Prostate, epididymis

DIAGNOSIS AND DIFFERENTIAL DIAGNOSIS

Diagnosis Clinical suspicion confirmed by culture of organism from skin biopsy, sputum, pus, urine

Differential Diagnosis Of verrucous skin lesion: squamous cell carcinoma, pyoderma gangrenosum tumor stage of mycosis fungoides, ecthyma, tuberculosis verrucosa cutis, actinomycosis, nocardiosis, mycetoma, syphilitic gumma, granuloma inguinale, leprosy, bromoderma

LABORATORY AND SPECIAL EXAMINATIONS

Dermatopathology Pseudoepitheliomatous hyperplasia. Seek budding yeast with thick walls and broad-based buds.

Direct Examination KOH preparation of pus shows large (8 to 15 μm), single, budding cells with a thick "double-contoured" wall and a wide pore of attachment.

Culture Of sputum, pus from skin lesion or biopsy, prostatic secretions.

PATHOPHYSIOLOGY

B. dermatitidis inhaled in dust; asymptomatic primary pulmonary infection most commonly resolves spontaneously. Hematogenous dissemination may occur to skin, skeletal system, genitalia, lungs. Reactivation may occur within lung or in sites of dissemination. Accidental inoculation into skin after trauma (laboratory workers).

COURSE AND PROGNOSIS

Greater majority of cases asymptomatic, self-limited. Skin most common site of hematogenous dissemination.

TREATMENT

Amphotericin. Alternative: ketoconazole in immunocompetent patients with mild to moderately severe nonmeningeal forms of the disease (800 mg per day).

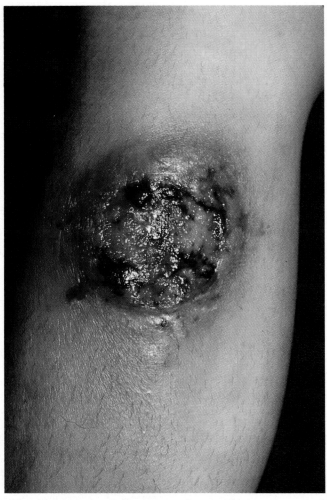

172　North American blastomycosis　*Inflammatory plaque with ulceration resembling pyoderma gangrenosum. (Courtesy of Elizabeth M. Spiers, M.D.)*

Coccidioidomycosis

Coccidioidomycosis is a systemic mycosis characterized by primary pulmonary infection which usually resolves spontaneously but which can disseminate hematogenously and result in chronic, progressive, granulomatous infection in skin, lungs, bone, meninges.

Synonyms: San Joaquin Valley fever, valley fever, desert fever.

EPIDEMIOLOGY AND ETIOLOGY

Race   Blacks, Filipinos

Sex   Risk of dissemination > in males, pregnant females

Incidence   Approximately 100,000 cases in the United States per year; most asymptomatic.

Geography   Southern California (San Joaquin Valley), southern Arizona, Utah, New Mexico, Nevada, southwestern Texas; adjacent areas of Mexico; Central and South America

Etiology   *Coccidioides immitis,* a dimorphic fungus

Season   Late spring through fall, i.e., dry season

Transmission   Inhalation of spores is followed by primary pulmonary infection. Rarely, percutaneous.

Risk Factors   Nonwhite, pregnancy, immunosuppression, HIV disease

HISTORY

Incubation Period   1 to 4 weeks

History   With primary pulmonary infection, influenza-like illness with fever, chills, malaise, anorexia, myalgia, pleuritic chest pain. With disseminated infection, headache, bone pain.

Travel History   Living in or visit to endemic area

PHYSICAL EXAMINATION

Skin Findings

TYPE OF LESION   *Primary Infection*   Toxic erythema (diffuse erythema, morbilliform, urticaria); erythema nodosum; erythema multiforme

Hematogenous Dissemination to Skin   Initially, papule evolving with formation of pustules, plaques, nodules; abscess formation, multiple draining sinus tracts, ulcers; subcutaneous cellulitis; verrucous plaques; granulomatous nodules; scars

Primary Cutaneous Inoculation Site (Rare)   Nodule eroding to ulcer (Figure 173). May have sporotrichoid lymphangitis, regional lymphadenitis.

DISTRIBUTION OF LESIONS   Central face, especially nasolabial fold; extremities.

MUCOUS MEMBRANES   Enanthem with primary infection

General Examination

BONE   Osteomyelitis. Draining abscess in psoas area.

CNS   Signs of meningitis

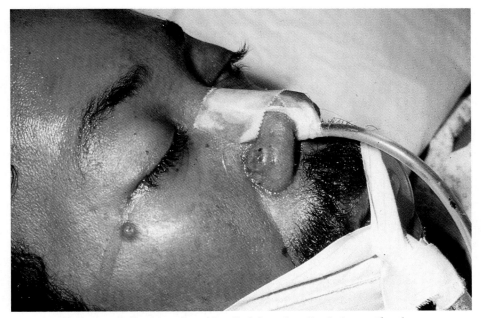

173　Coccidioidomycosis disseminated to skin　*Nodular, ulcerative lesion on the ala.*

DIAGNOSIS AND DIFFERENTIAL DIAGNOSIS

Diagnosis　Detection of *C. immitis* sporangia containing typical sporangiospores in sputum/pus; culture; skin biopsy.

Differential Diagnosis　*Of skin lesions:* warts, furuncles, ecthyma, bromoderma, rosacea, lichen simplex chronicus, prurigo nodularis, keratoacanthoma, blastomycosis, cryptococcosis, tuberculosis, tertiary syphilis, bacterial infection. *In HIV-infected patient:* may resemble folliculitis, molluscum contagiosum.

LABORATORY AND SPECIAL EXAMINATIONS

Dermatopathology　Granulomatous inflammation; arthroconidia in tissue

Culture　Pus. For best recovery the tissue specimen should be minced and cultured on Sabouraud's medium.

PATHOPHYSIOLOGY

Spores inhaled resulting in primary pulmonary infection, which is asymptomatic or accompanied by symptoms of coryza. Hematogenous may disseminate to various organs.

COURSE AND PROGNOSIS

Most infected residents of endemic areas heal spontaneously. Meningeal infection difficult to cure.

TREATMENT

Amphotericin B. Alternative: ketoconazole 400 mg daily

Cryptococcosis

Systemic cryptococcosis is a systemic mycosis acquired by the respiratory route, with the primary focus of infection in the lungs, and with occasional hematogenous dissemination, characteristically to the meninges, occasionally to the kidneys, and to the skin.

Synonyms: torulosis, European blastomycosis.

EPIDEMIOLOGY AND ETIOLOGY

Age   More common over the age of 40 years

Sex   Males > females, 2:1

Etiology   *Cryptococcus neoformans,* a yeast

Transmission   Inhalation of organism from dust. Associated with pigeon excreta.

Risk Factors   Defective host defenses: AIDS, diabetes mellitus, lymphoma, Hodgkin's disease, sarcoidosis

Geography   Worldwide

HISTORY

Headache most common symptom (80%), mental confusion, impaired vision for 2 to 3 months; pulmonary symptoms uncommon.

PHYSICAL EXAMINATION

Skin Findings   Occur in 10 to 20% of patients. *Papules or nodules* with surrounding erythema which occasionally break down and exude a liquid, mucinous material. *Acneform* lesions. *Cryptococcal cellulitis:* mimics bacterial cellulitis. Red, hot, tender, edematous plaque on extremity. Possibly multiple noncontiguous sites. Patient always immunocompromised. *Herpetiform* vesicular lesions. *Molluscum contagiosum-like* lesions commonly occur in HIV-infected patients with disseminated cryptococcosis on face (Figure 174). Note: All types of lesions may ulcerate.

General Findings   Meningitis

DIAGNOSIS AND DIFFERENTIAL DIAGNOSIS

Diagnosis   Confirmed by skin biopsy and fungal cultures.

Differential Diagnosis   Pyoderma, other bacterial or fungal skin lesions, blastomycosis, histoplasmosis

LABORATORY AND SPECIAL EXAMINATIONS

CSF   With meningitis see encapsulated budding yeast with India ink preparations in 40 to 60% of cases, lymphocytic pleocytosis, elevated protein, decreased glucose.

Culture   CSF, biopsy of skin lesion

Serology   Cryptococcal antigen latex agglutination system test is positive in 100% of patients with cryptococcal meningitis; the majority of patients also have antigenemia. Detection of anticryptococcal antibody is unreliable.

SYSTEMIC INFECTIONS AND INFESTATIONS

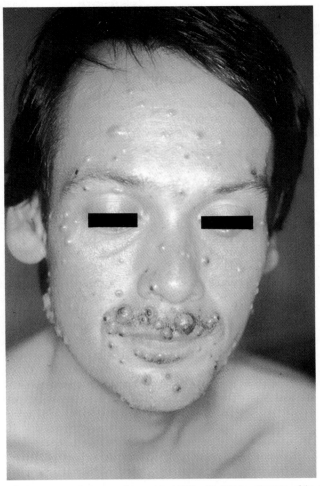

174 Disseminated cryptococcosis in a patient with AIDS *Multiple, discrete, skin-colored papules and nodules resembling molluscum contagiosum. (Courtesy of Loïc Vaillant, M.D.)*

PATHOPHYSIOLOGY

C. neoformans is inhaled in dust and causes a primary pulmonary focus of infection with subsequent hematogenous dissemination to meninges, kidneys, and skin. 10 to 20% of patients have skin lesions. Immune deficiency is an important factor in pathogenesis in many patients.

COURSE AND PROGNOSIS

Acute primary cryptococcosis usually mild.

Chronic cavitary forms lead to respiratory impairment. Progressive disseminated cryptococcosis in immunocompromised patients (AIDS) is fatal in >80%.

TREATMENT

Amphotericin B. Alternatives: flucytosine, ketoconazole, miconazole, fluconazole

CRYPTOCOCCOSIS

Histoplasmosis

Histoplasmosis is a relatively common systemic mycosis with a primary pulmonary infection but with rare hematogenous dissemination, characterized by chronic infection of mucous membranes, skin, and reticuloendothelial organs (liver, bone marrow, and spleen).

Synonyms: Darling's disease, cave disease, Ohio Valley disease.

EPIDEMIOLOGY AND ETIOLOGY

Age For disseminated infection, very old and very young

Etiology *Histoplasma capsulatum,* a dimorphic fungus. In Africa *H. capsulatum* var. *duboisii*

Occupation Farmers, construction workers, children, others involved in outdoor activities

Transmission Inhalation of spores in soil contaminated with bird (especially starlings) or bat droppings.

Risk Factors For dissemination: immunosuppressed host (HIV infection, post-organ transplant, lymphoma, leukemia, chemotherapy), very old patients

Geography North America: eastern and central United States especially Ohio/Mississippi River valleys; in some areas, 80% of residents are histoplasmin positive. Equatorial Africa

HISTORY

Incubation Period For acute infection, 7 to 14 days

History *Acute primary infection:* 90% of patients asymptomatic; if large number of spores inhaled, influenza-like syndrome may occur. *Dissemination:* chronic disease syndrome

PHYSICAL EXAMINATION

Skin Findings Occur in two different settings: *acute pulmonary infection* associated with hypersensitivity reactions; *disseminated disease* associated with tissue infection. Historically, lesions of mucous membranes much more common than those on skin. However, in HIV infection, 10% of patients with disseminated histoplasmosis have cutaneous lesions; in renal transplant patients, 4 to 6%. TYPE OF LESION *With acute pulmonary infection:* erythema nodosum, erythema multiforme. *With disseminated infection:* erythematous necrotic or hyperkeratotic papules and nodules (Figure 175); erythematous macules; folliculitis ± pustules ± acneform; ulcers; vegetative plaques; panniculitis; erythroderma. In HIV-infected patients, multiple scaling plaques resembling guttate psoriasis or nummular eczema. Diffuse hyperpigmentation with Addison's disease secondary to adrenal infection.
DISTRIBUTION OF LESIONS Face, extremities, trunk
MUCOUS MEMBRANES *Most common site of involvement;* nodules, vegetations, painful ulcerations of soft palate, oropharynx, epiglottis, nasal vestibule, esophagus.

General Examination Disseminated disease: hepatosplenomegaly, lymphadenopathy

SYSTEMIC INFECTIONS AND INFESTATIONS

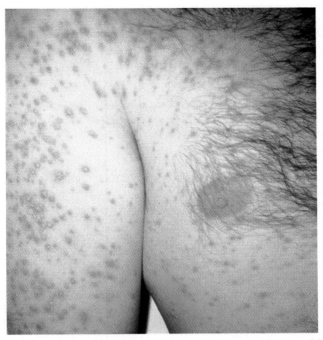

175 Disseminated histoplasmosis *Erythematous papules and small plaques with scale in a patient with AIDS. (Courtesy of J. D. Fallon, M.D.)*

DIAGNOSIS AND DIFFERENTIAL DIAGNOSIS

Diagnosis By clinical suspicion confirmed by culture of organism or by demonstration of *H. capsulatum* in a skin biopsy section

Differential Diagnosis Disseminated disease: miliary tuberculosis, coccidioidomycosis, cryptococcosis, leishmaniasis, lymphoma

LABORATORY AND SPECIAL EXAMINATIONS

Dermatopathology Identify *H. capsulatum* in tissue by size and staining. Differentiate from *Coccidioides immitis, Blastomyces dermatitidis, Leishmania donovani, Toxoplasma gondii.*

Culture Identify *H. capsulatum* from biopsy specimens of skin, oral lesions, bone marrow, sputum, blood, urine, lymph node, liver.

COURSE AND PROGNOSIS

Primary infection resolves spontaneously in most cases. Untreated progressive disseminated form has high mortality, 80% of patients dying within one year; prognosis linked to underlying condition; chronic maintenance often required.

TREATMENT

Amphotericin B. Alternative in normal host: ketoconazole.

Sporotrichosis is a cutaneous localized mycotic infection which follows accidental inoculation of the skin and is characterized by nodule and ulcer formation at the inoculation site, chronic nodular lymphangitis, and regional lymphadenitis.

EPIDEMIOLOGY AND ETIOLOGY

Sex Males > females, especially disseminated disease

Etiology *Sporotrix schenckii,* a dimorphic fungus commonly found in soil

Occupation Occupational exposure important: gardeners, farmers, florists, lawn laborers, agricultural workers, forestry workers, paper manufacturers, gold miners

Transmission Commonly, subcutaneous inoculation by a contaminated thorn, barb, splinter, or other sharp object (laboratory). Rarely, inhalation, aspiration, or ingestion causes systemic infection. Most cases isolated. Epidemics do occur.

Geography Ubiquitous, worldwide. More common in temperate and tropical zones. Present on rose and barberry thorns, wood splinters, sphagnum moss, straw, marsh hay, soils.

Predisposing Factors For disseminated disease: HIV infection, carcinoma, hematologic and lymphoproliferative disease, diabetes mellitus, alcoholism, immunosuppressive therapy

HISTORY

Incubation Period 3 weeks (range, 3 days to 12 weeks) after trauma or injury to site of lesion. Lesions are relatively asymptomatic, painful. Afebrile.

PHYSICAL EXAMINATION

Skin Findings
TYPE OF LESION *Local Cutaneous Type (Chancriform) (40%)* Subcutaneous papule, pustule, or nodule appears at inoculation site several weeks after puncture wound. Surrounding skin is pink to purplish. In time skin becomes fixed to deeper tissues. Painless indurated ulcer may occur, resulting in sporotrichoid chancre. Border ragged and undermined. Draining lymph nodes become swollen and suppurative.

Chronic Lymphangitic Type (Sporotrichoid) (60%) Follows lymphatic extension of local cutaneous type (Figure 176). Proximal-to-local cutaneous lesion, intervening lymphatics become indurated, nodular, thickened.

Fixed Cutaneous Sporotrichosis Crusted ulcers, ecthymatous, verrucous plaques (Figure 177), pyoderma gangrenosum-like, infiltrated papules and plaques

ARRANGEMENT OF MULTIPLE LESIONS Primary chancre, nodular linear lymphatic spread with enlarged regional lymph nodes described as "sporotrichoid"

DISTRIBUTION OF LESIONS Primary lesion most common on dorsum of hand or finger with chronic nodular lymphangitis up arm. Fixed cutaneous—face in children, upper extremities in adults. Dissemination of cutaneous lesions may follow hematogenous dissemination or autoinoculation.

General Examination Hematogenous dissemination results in bone, muscle, joint, visceral, CNS lesions.

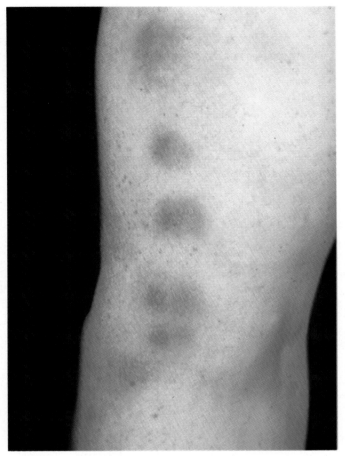

176 Sporotrichosis, chronic lymphangitic type   *The nodules follow the lymphatic extension of the local cutaneous type.*

DIAGNOSIS AND DIFFERENTIAL DIAGNOSIS

Diagnosis Clinical suspicion and isolation of organism on culture

Differential Diagnosis Tuberculosis, atypical mycobacterial infection, anthrax, tularemia, cat-scratch disease, primary syphilis, leishmaniasis, herpes simplex virus infection, staphylococcal lymphangitis, histoplasmosis, coccidioidomycosis, blastomycosis, cryptococcosis

LABORATORY AND SPECIAL EXAMINATIONS

Dermatopathology Granulomatous, Langhans'-type giant cells, pyogenic microabscesses. Organisms rare, difficult to visualize.

Culture Infected tissue should be minced and cultured for best recovery.

PATHOPHYSIOLOGY

Following subcutaneous inoculation, *S. schenckii* grows locally and slowly spreads along the draining lymphatics. Secondary skin lesions develop along the lymphatic chain.

COURSE AND PROGNOSIS

Shows little tendency to resolve spontaneously.

TREATMENT

Traditional treatment is with saturated solution of potassium iodide (SSKI) 3 to 4 g three times a day. Amphotericin B IV for those who cannot tolerate SSKI or those with pulmonary or disseminated infection. Alternative: ketoconazole.

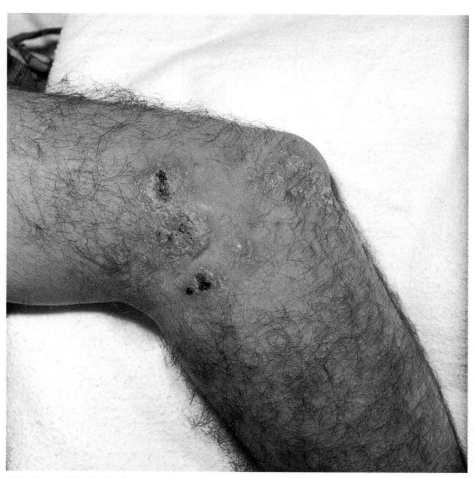

177　Sporotrichosis, fixed cutaneous type　*Crusted, ecthymatous, verrucous plaques.*

Leprosy is a chronic granulomatous disease caused by *Mycobacterium leprae* principally acquired during childhood or young adulthood. The skin, mucous membrane of the upper respiratory tract, and, in all forms of leprosy, the peripheral nerves are the major sites of involvement. The clinical manifestations, natural history, and prognosis of leprosy are related to the host response, and the various types of leprosy (tuberculoid, lepromatous, etc.) represent the spectra of the host's immunologic response (cell-mediated immunity).

Synonym: Hansen's disease.

CLINICOPATHOLOGIC CLASSIFICATION OF LEPROSY

Based on clinical, immunologic, and bacteriologic findings.

Tuberculoid Localized skin involvement and/or peripheral nerve involvement, few organisms present in the skin biopsies

Lepromatous Generalized involvement including skin, upper respiratory mucous membrane, the reticuloendothelial system, adrenal glands, and testes; many bacilli are present in tissue.

Borderline (or "Dimorphic") Has features of both tuberculoid and lepromatous leprosy. Usually many bacilli present, varied skin lesions: macules, plaques; progresses to tuberculoid or regresses to lepromatous.

Indeterminate and Transitional Forms (See Pathophysiology)

EPIDEMIOLOGY AND ETIOLOGY

Causative Organism and Transmission The organism, *M. leprae,* is a slender, straight or slightly curved, acid-fast rod, about 3.0 × 0.5 μm. The armadillo can be experimentally inoculated with *M. leprae* derived from human sources and one-half of those inoculated develop a progressive leprosy infection and die. Wild armadillos have been found in Louisiana with a leprosy-like skin infection caused by an organism thought to be *M. leprae*. The transmission of leprosy to humans is still not clearly understood—whether by droplet infection from nasal discharges, fomites, or arthropods.

World Health Problem Leprosy is a world health problem affecting over 12 million persons. At the present time it is more prevalent in hot and humid climates (Africa, Southeast Asia, and South and Central America). New lesions may first appear or suddenly flare during the hot rainy season. The disease is endemic in Texas, southern Louisiana, Hawaii, and California, and immigrants with leprosy are not uncommonly seen in Florida and New York City. There are approximately 2500 patients with leprosy in the continental United States and about 35 new cases of endemic leprosy are reported every year.

Sex Possibly more males than females

Race There appears to be an inverse relationship between the skin color and the severity of the disease: in the black African, susceptibility is high but there is a predominance of milder forms of the disease, i.e., the tuberculoid over lepromatous.

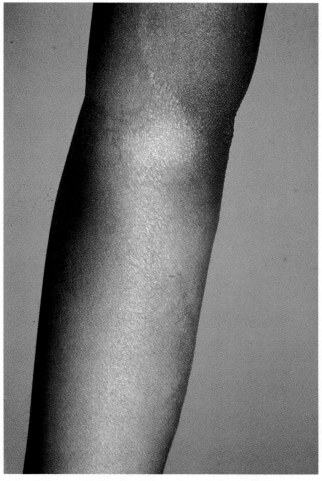

178 Leprosy, tuberculoid type *Well-defined, hypopigmented, anesthetic macule.*

Predisposing or Risk Factors (1) Residence in an endemic area, (2) having a blood relative with leprosy, (3) poverty (?malnutrition), and (4) contact with infected armadillos

HISTORY

Onset Insidious and painless, first affects the peripheral nervous system with persistent or recurrent paresthesias and numbness without any visible clinical signs. At this stage there may be transient macular skin eruptions.

Systems Review Neural involvement leads to muscle weakness, muscle atrophy, severe neuritic pain, and contractures of the hands and feet.

PHYSICAL EXAMINATION

Tuberculoid Leprosy
TYPE   A few well-defined hypopigmented *anesthetic* macules (Figure 178) with raised edges varying in size from a few millimeters to very large lesions covering the entire trunk.
COLOR   Erythematous or purple border and hypopigmented center
BORDER   May be a thickened nerve on the edge of the lesion; large peripheral nerve enlargement frequent (ulnar).
SHAPE   Often annular
DISTRIBUTION   Any site including the face

Lepromatous Leprosy
TYPE   Small erythematous or hypopigmented macules which are *anesthetic;* later, papules, plaques, nodules (Figure 179), and diffuse thickening of the skin, with loss of hair (eyebrows and eyelashes).
COLOR   Normal skin color or erythematous or slightly hypopigmented
DISTRIBUTION   Bilaterally symmetrical involving earlobes, face, arms, and buttocks, or, less frequently, the trunk and lower extremities.

Borderline Leprosy Lesions are intermediate between tuberculoid and lepromatous and consist of macules, papules, and plaques. Anesthesia and decreased sweating are prominent in the lesions.

DIAGNOSIS

A patient with macular hypopigmented lesions or erythematous papules and plaques and who has a history of living in an endemic area should be thoroughly examined for peripheral nerve enlargement (ulnar, posterior tibial). The lesions should be tested for anesthesia with a small wisp of cotton, and the discrimination of hot and cold should be checked in the lesions. A skin biopsy with a search for acid-fast bacilli is mandatory in every suspect patient, and their presence is proof of the diagnosis. Also, microbiologic examination of nasal mucosa and earlobes.

LABORATORY AND SPECIAL EXAMINATIONS

Microbiologic Examination of Skin and Nasal Mucosa Criteria have been established that permit the identification of *M. leprae* using dopa oxidase; pyridine extraction (abolition) of acid-fast staining (Figure 180) and growth in the mouse foot pad, but not on Loewenstein-Jensen media, appear to be restricted to *M. leprae*.

PATHOPHYSIOLOGY

Subclinical infection with leprosy is common among residents in endemic areas. Presumably the subclinical infection is handled readily by the host's cell-mediated immune response. Clinical expression of leprosy is the development of a granuloma, and the patient may develop a "reactional state," which may occur in some form in over 50% of certain groups of patients. The granulomatous spectrum of lep-

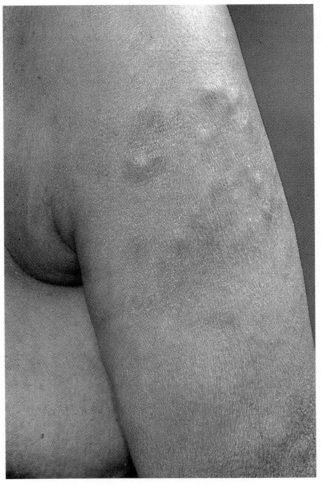

179 Leprosy, lepromatous type *Papules and nodules.*

rosy consists of: (1) a high-resistance tuberculoid response (TT); (2) a low- or absent-resistance lepromatous pole (LL); (3) a dimorphic or borderline region (BB); two intermediary regions: (4) borderline-lepromatous (BL) and (5) borderline-tuberculoid (BT). In order of decreasing resistance the spectrum is TT, BT, BB, BL, LL.

COURSE AND PROGNOSIS

After the first few years of drug therapy, the most difficult problem is the management of the changes secondary to neurologic deficits—contractures and trophic changes in the hands and feet. This requires a team of health care professionals: orthopedic surgeons, hand surgeons, podiatrists, ophthalmologists, neurologists, physical medicine and rehabilitation professionals, etc.

TREATMENT

The two most widely used drugs are dapsone and rifampin, which are generally available. Clofazimine is available through the National Hansen's Disease Center in Carville, Louisiana. Therapy of multibacillary leprosy requires three drugs: dapsone, rifampin, and clofazimine. For paucibacillary leprosy two drugs, dapsone and rifampin, are adequate. The duration of therapy is from 3 years to life. Thus, multibacillary disease (BB, BL, LL) should be treated for life because of high recurrence rates, however good the remission. Pure tuberculoid (TT) disease probably requires little if any treatment, but 3 years is recommended. BT disease is not an homogenous group. It contains some patients whose disease would remit spontaneously and others whose disease would progress to BL, if not treated.

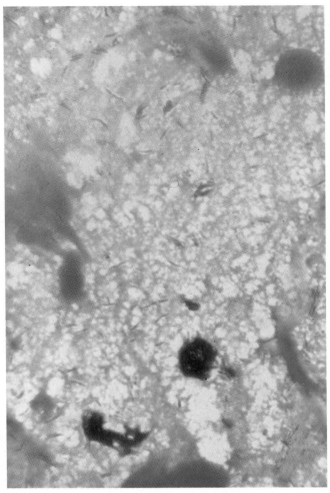

180   Leprosy, *Mycobacterium leprae*   *Acid-fast stain showing cigar-shaped, red-staining organisms.*

Cutaneous tuberculosis (CTb) is highly variable in its clinical presentation, dependent on the immunologic status of the patient and the route of inoculation of mycobacteria into the skin.

CLASSIFICATION OF CUTANEOUS TUBERCULOSIS

Exogenous Infection

Primary inoculation tuberculosis (PITb): Via percutaneous inoculation, CTb occurs at the inoculated site in a nonimmune host.

Tuberculosis verrucosa cutis (TbVC): Via percutaneous inoculation, CTb occurs at the inoculated site in an individual with prior tuberculosis infection.

Endogenous Spread

Lupus vulgaris (LV)

Scrofuloderma (SD)

Metastatic tuberculosis abscess (MTbA)

Acute miliary tuberculosis (AMTb)

Orificial tuberculosis (OTb)

Tuberculosis Due to BCG Immunization

ETIOLOGY AND EPIDEMIOLOGY

Age AMTb more common in infants and in adults with advanced immunodeficiency. PITb more common in infants. SD more common in adolescents, elderly. LV affects all ages.

Sex LV more common in females. TbVC more common in males.

Race Tuberculosis in blacks, in general, has a less favorable prognosis than in whites.

Occupation TbVC: previously in physicians, medical students, and pathologists as verruca necrogenica, anatomist's wart, post-mortem wart; in butchers and farmers from *Mycobacterium bovis*

Etiology The obligate human pathogenic mycobacteria: *M. tuberculosis, M. bovis,* and occasionally bacillus Calmette-Guérin (BCG)

Incidence CTb has steadily declined worldwide, paralleling the decline of pulmonary tuberculosis. Always rare in the United States compared to Europe. Incidence of various types of CTb varies geographically; LV, SD most common types in Europe; LV, verrucous lesions more common in tropics; TbVC a common type in Third World countries. Recently the incidence of CTb has been increasing, often associated with AIDS.

Epidemiology Predisposing factors for tuberculosis include poverty, crowding, HIV infection. The type of clinical lesion developing depends on the route of cutaneous inoculation and the immunologic status of the host. Cutaneous inoculation results in a tuberculous chancre in the nonimmune host, but TbVC in the immune host. Modes of endogenous spread to skin include: direct extension from underlying tuberculous infection, i.e., lymphadenitis or tuberculosis of bones and joints results in SD; lymphatic spread to skin results in LV; hematogenous dissemination results in either AMTb, LV, or MTbA.

Route of Cutaneous Infection May be exogenous, by autoinoculation, or endogenous.

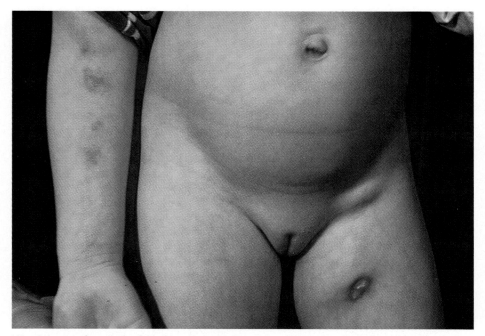

181 Primary tuberculosis of the skin   *An eroded nodule arising at the site of inoculation is seen on the thigh and is associated with regional lymphadenopathy. A positive tuberculin test is noted on the arm.*

CUTANEOUS TUBERCULOSIS   341

PHYSICAL EXAMINATION

Primary Inoculation Tuberculosis (PITb)

TYPE   Initially, papule occurs at the inoculation site 2 to 4 weeks after the wound. Lesion enlarges to a painless ulcer (Figure 181), i.e., a tuberculous chancre (up to 5.0 cm), with shallow granular base and multiple tiny abscesses, or alternatively may be covered by thick crust. Undermined margins; older ulcers become indurated with thick crusts. Deeper inoculation results in subcutaneous abscess. Intraoral inoculation results in ulcers on gingiva or palate. Regional lymphadenopathy occurs within 3 to 8 weeks.

COLOR   Ulcer margins reddish blue

DISTRIBUTION   Most common on exposed skin at sites of minor injuries. Oral lesions occur following ingestion of bovine bacilli in nonpasteurized milk; in the past, lesions in male babies have occurred on the penis after ritual circumcision.

Tuberculosis Verrucosa Cutis (TbVC)
(Figure 182)

TYPE   Initial papule with violaceous halo. Evolves to hyperkeratotic, warty, firm plaque. Clefts and fissures occur from which pus and keratinous material can be expressed. Border often irregular. Lesions are usually single but multiple lesions occur. No lymphadenopathy.

COLOR   Base brownish-red to purplish

DISTRIBUTION   Most commonly on dorsolateral hands and fingers. In children, lower extremities, knees.

Lupus Vulgaris (LV)   (Figure 183)

TYPE   Initial flat papule is ill-defined and soft and evolves into well-defined, irregular plaque. The consistency is characteristically soft; if the lesion is probed, the instrument breaks through the overlying epidermis. Surface is initially smooth or slightly scaly but may become hyperkeratotic. Hypertrophic forms result in soft tumorous nodules. Ulcerative forms present as punched-out, often serpiginous ulcers surrounded by soft, brownish infiltrate. Involvement of underlying cartilage but not bone results in its destruction (ears, nose). Scarring is prominent and, characteristically, new brownish infiltrates occur within the atrophic scars.

COLOR   Reddish brown. Diascopy (i.e., the use of a glass slide pressed against the skin) reveals an "apple-jelly" (i.e., yellowish-brown) color of the infiltrate.

DISTRIBUTION   Usually solitary but several sites may occur. Most lesions on the head and neck, most often on nose and ears or scalp. Lesions on trunk and extremities rare. Disseminated lesions after severe viral infection (measles).

Scrofuloderma (SD)   (Figure 184)

TYPE   Firm subcutaneous nodule which initially is freely moveable; the lesion then becomes doughy and evolves into an irregular, deep-seated plaque which liquefies and perforates. Ulcers and irregular sinuses, usually of linear or serpiginous shape, discharge pus or caseous material. Edges are undermined, inverted, and dissecting subcutaneous pockets alternate with soft, fluctuating infiltrates and bridging scars.

COLOR   Reddish blue, brownish

DISTRIBUTION   SD most often occurs in the parotidal, submandibular, supraclavicular, or axillary regions; lateral neck. SD most often results from continuous spread from affected lymph nodes or tuberculous bones (phalanges, sternum, ribs) or joints.

Metastatic Tuberculosis Abscess (MTbA)

TYPE   Also called tuberculous gumma. Subcutaneous abscess, nontender, "cold," fluctuant. Coalescing with overlying skin, breaking down and forming fistulas and ulcers.

COLOR   Initially normal skin color, later reddish blue.

DISTRIBUTION   Single or multiple lesions, often at sites of previous trauma.

Acute Miliary Tuberculosis (AMTb)

TYPE   Exanthem. Disseminated lesions are

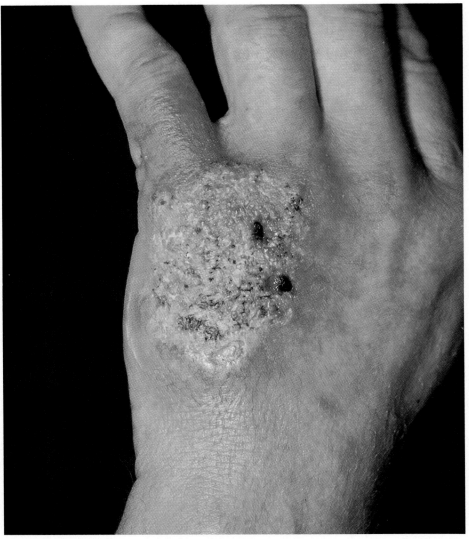

182   Tuberculosis verrucosa cutis   *Crusted and keratotic plaque arising at the site of inoculation. Not associated with axillary lymphadenitis.*

minute macules and papules or purpuric lesions. Sometimes vesicular and crusted. Removal of crust reveals umbilication.

COLOR   Red or purpuric

DISTRIBUTION   Disseminated on all parts of the body, particularly the trunk

Orificial Tuberculosis (OTb)

TYPE   Small yellowish nodule on mucosa breaks down to form painful circular or irregular ulcer with undermined borders and pseudomembranous material, yellowish tubercles and eroded vessels at its base. Surrounding mucosa swollen, edematous, and inflamed.

COLOR   Initially yellowish; ulcer red, hemorrhagic, and purulent

DISTRIBUTION   Since OTb results from autoinoculation of mycobacteria from progressive tuberculosis of internal organs, OTb is usually found on the oral, pharyngeal (pulmonary tuberculosis), vulvar (genitourinary tuberculosis), and anal (intestinal tuberculosis) mucous membranes. Lesions may be single or multiple, and in the mouth most often occur on the tongue, soft and hard palates, or lips. OTb may occur in a tooth socket following tooth extraction.

DIFFERENTIAL DIAGNOSIS

PITb, TbVC, SD, *M. marinum* infection, other chancriform syndromes (syphilis, tularemia, cat-scratch disease, sporotrichosis, discoid lupus erythematosus)

LABORATORY AND SPECIAL EXAMINATIONS

Dermatopathology   *PITb:* initially nonspecific inflammation; after 3 to 6 weeks, epithelioid cells, Langhans' giant cells, lymphocytes, caseation necrosis. *AMTb:* nonspecific inflammation and vasculitis. All *other forms* of CTb show more or less typical tuberculous histopathology; TbVC is characterized by massive pseudoepitheliomatous hyperplasia of epidermis and abscesses. Mycobacteria are found in PITb, SD, AMTb, MTbA, OTb, but only with difficulty or not at all in LV and TbVC.

Culture   Yields mycobacteria also from lesions of LV and TbVC.

Skin Testing   *PITb:* patient converts from intradermal skin test negative to positive during the first weeks of the infection. *AMTb:* usually negative. *SD, MTbA, and PTb:* may be negative or positive depending on state of immunity. *LV and TbVC:* positive.

PATHOPHYSIOLOGY

The clinical lesions occurring in the skin are dependent on whether the host has had prior infection with *M. tuberculosis,* and therefore delayed hypersensitivity to the organism, and the inoculation route and mode of spread.

COURSE AND PROGNOSIS

The course of CTb is quite variable, depending on the type of cutaneous infection, amount of inoculum, extent of extracutaneous infection, age of the patient, host immunity, immune status, and therapy. PITb: without treatment, usually resolves within 12 months, with some residual scarring. Rarely, LV develops at site of PITb. *Tuberculosis due to BCG immunization:* depends on general state of immunity. It may assume appearance and course of PITb, LV, or SD; in the immunocompromised it may lead to MTbA or AMTb.

TREATMENT

Prolonged antituberculous therapy with at least two drugs is indicated for all cases of CTb.

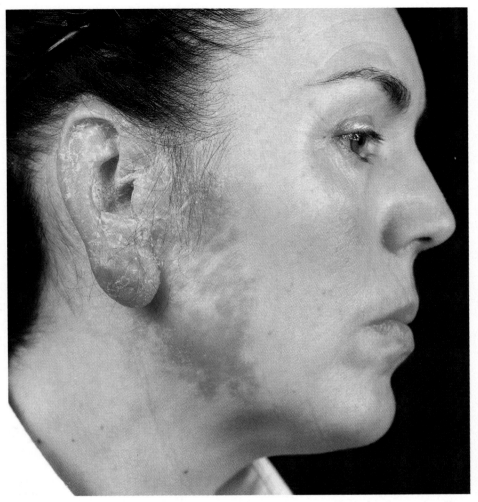

183 Lupus vulgaris *Reddish-brown plaque which, on diascopy, exhibits the diagnostic yellow-brown color.*

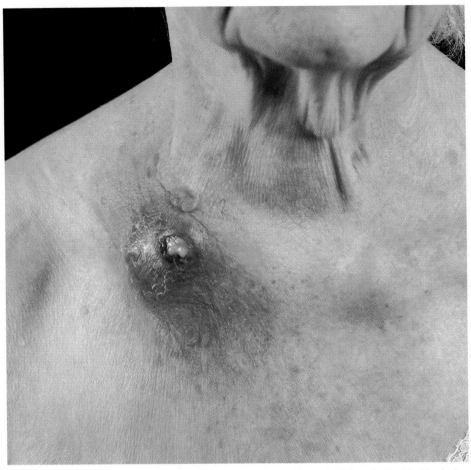

184 Scrofuloderma *Large, violaceous abscess associated with cervical lymphadenitis. The lesion represents an extension of the infection from the node into the skin, producing an ulcer.*

Cutaneous Atypical Mycobacterial Infection

Mycobacteria other than *Mycobacterium tuberculosis* (MOTT) are environmental mycobacteria, commonly found in water and soil, have low-grade pathogenicity, and are never transmitted person-to-person.

Synonyms: swimming pool granuloma, fish tank granuloma.

EPIDEMIOLOGY AND ETIOLOGY

Age Second to fourth decade

Sex Males > females

Etiology *Mycobacterium marinum,* most commonly

Occupation Occupation or avocation around water, maintenance of fish tank

Transmission Traumatic inoculation into skin during aquatic activity

Season Swimming pool granuloma usually begins in summertime. Fish tank granuloma, no seasonal variation.

HISTORY

Incubation Period Very variable. Most commonly few weeks to few months following inoculation.

Duration of Lesions Months to years

History Lesion at site of injury while in aqueous environment. Most commonly, asymptomatic. Afebrile. Cosmetic inconvenience. Possible local tenderness, limitation of movement if lesion over a joint, itching, painful when bumped.

PHYSICAL EXAMINATION

Skin Findings

TYPE OF LESION At site of inoculation, papule(s) enlarging to inflammatory nodule or plaque 1.0 to 4.0 cm with surface scale (Figure 185), crust, ulceration, ± serosanguinous or purulent discharge. In time, small satellite papules, draining sinuses, fistulae may develop. Atrophic scarring follows spontaneous regression.

Sporotrichoid Pattern Subcutaneous or intradermal cystlike swelling may occur, 1.5 to 2.0 cm in diameter some distance proximal to the original lesions. Deep-seated nodules in a linear configuration on hand and forearm exhibit sporotrichoid spread. Boggy inflammatory reaction may mimic bursitis, synovitis, or arthritis about the elbow, wrist, or interphalangeal joints.

Disseminated Cutaneous Infection Distinctly rare

DISTRIBUTION OF LESIONS Usually solitary, over bony prominence; may be multiple. Following trauma while swimming: most commonly on elbow, finger, knee; less commonly on ankle, toe or foot, leg, neck. Following aquarium exposure: most commonly on right hand.

General Examination

LYMPH NODES Regional lymphadenopathy and lymphangitis

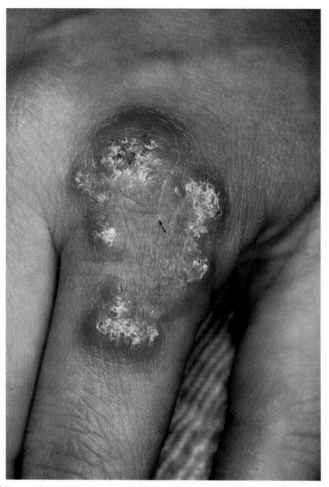

185   "Fish-tank" granuloma   *Verrucous, violaceous plaque with central spontaneous clearing occurring at the site of an abrasion sustained within a fish tank. Lesion was caused by* Mycobacterium marinum.

DIAGNOSIS AND DIFFERENTIAL DIAGNOSIS

Diagnosis Confirmed by isolating MOTT by culture of lesional tissue or exudate.

Differential Diagnosis Sporotrichosis, blastomycosis, histoplasmosis, coccidioidomycosis, erysipeloid, tularemia, *M. tuberculosis* (tuberculosis verrucosa cutis), nocardiosis, leishmaniasis, syphilis, yaws, iododerma, bromoderma, foreign body response to sea urchin or barnacle wound, benign or malignant skin tumors.

LABORATORY AND SPECIAL EXAMINATIONS

Skin Tests Intradermal testing with purified protein derivative-standard (PPD-S) often positive.

Skin Biopsy Suggestive but not pathognomonic. *Early:* dermal inflammatory reaction with lymphocytes, polymorphonuclear cells, histiocytes. Epidermal hyperkeratosis and acanthosis may be seen. *Older lesions:* more typical tuberculoid architecture is developed with epithelioid cells and Langhans' giant cells. No typical caseation necrosis.

AFB Stains Biopsy tissue: AFB infrequent. Smears of pus or exudates: AFB (few, scattered); however, may be seen in up to 50% of slides.

Culture Culture at 32°C. Biopsy specimen should be ground in saline solution with mortar and pestle or material secured by swab inoculated on Loewenstein-Jensen tubes and incubated at 32°C, 37°C, and at room temperature. *M. marinum will not grow at 37°C on primary isolation.* Grows out in 2 to 4 weeks; photochromogenic. Early lesions yield numerous colonies. Lesions 3 months or older generally yield few colonies.

COURSE AND PROGNOSIS

Most usually benign and self-limited but can remain active for a prolonged period. Single papulonodular lesions resolve spontaneously within 3 months to 3 years, whereas sporotrichoid form can persist up to 45 years.

TREATMENT

Initially, doxycycline or minocycline 100 mg twice a day or sulfamethoxazole-trimethoprim. Once *M. marinum* has been isolated, sensitivity studies should be performed. With sensitivities available, initial treatment can be continued if indicated. If sensitivities show drug resistance, then rifampin (600 mg q.i.d.)–ethambutol (800 mg q.i.d.) is an effective combination in 90% of patients and should be given in sporotrichoid form of infection.

Ecthyma gangrenosum (EG) is a skin infection characterized by hemorrhagic bullae evolving rapidly to gangrenous ulcers. EG occurs in immunocompromised and/or neutropenic patients and is usually associated with *Pseudomonas aeruginosa* bacteremia.

EPIDEMIOLOGY AND ETIOLOGY

Etiology Most commonly, the gram-negative bacillus *P. aeruginosa*. Also, *Staphylococcus aureus, Serratia marcescens, Escherichia coli, Neisseria meningitidis, Aeromonas hydrophila* and fungi of *Aspergillus* and *Rhizopus* genera.

Transmission Pseudomonal carriage increases with length of hospital stay and antibiotic administration. Entry sites for bacteremia at breaks in mucocutaneous barriers: sites of trauma, foreign bodies (IV or urinary catheter), aspiration/aerosolization into respiratory tract, decubitus or skin ulcers, thermal burns.

Risk Factors Hospitalization; immunocompromise; neutropenia; use of cancer chemotherapy, corticosteroids, antibiotics (recently); catheters (IV, urethral); cancer; debilitation. Pseudomonal carriage risk increases with length of hospital stay and antibiotic administration.

HISTORY

Symptoms High fever, chills

Immune Status Often immunocompromised

PHYSICAL FINDINGS

Skin Findings

TYPE OF LESION *Ecthyma Gangrenosum* (Figure 186) Begins as erythematous macule and quickly evolves into a large bulla or pustule. Epidermis eventually sloughs; dermal base becomes indurated, which results in a gunmetal-gray, indurated, relatively painless ulcer with surrounding erythema.

Other Lesions Associated with Pseudomonas *Septicemia* "Rose" spotlike lesions: erythematous macules and/or papules on trunk as in typhoid fever; occur with *Pseudomonas* infection of Gl tract, i.e., diarrhea, headache, high fever (Shanghai fever). Painful clustered vesicular-to-bullous lesions: multiple painful nodules representing small embolus-type lesions.

COLOR Initially erythematous progressing to hemorrhagic purple (i.e., bluish purple). Fully evolved EG: blackish central necrosis with erythematous halo.

PALPATION Frequently tender

DISTRIBUTION OF LESIONS Axillae, groin, perianal; may occur anywhere, including lip and tongue.

MUCOUS MEMBRANES May occur intraorally.

General Examination Septic shock

DIAGNOSIS AND DIFFERENTIAL DIAGNOSIS

Diagnosis Clinical suspicion confirmed by blood and skin exudate/biopsy specimen culture

Differential Diagnosis Hypersensitivity vasculitis, cryoglobulinemia, fixed drug eruption, polyarteritis nodosa.

LABORATORY AND SPECIAL EXAMINATIONS

Cultures In most cases *P. aeruginosa* can be cultured from both blood and ecthymatous skin lesions. However, EG can represent a localized cutaneous infection, not accompa-

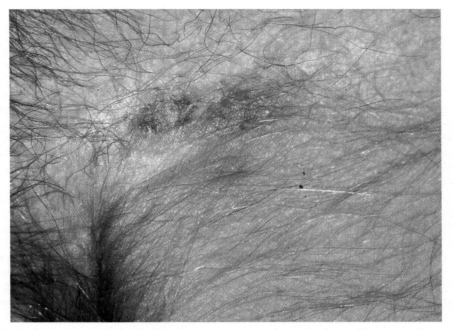

186 Ecthyma gangrenosum *Gunmetal gray, painless, infarcted lesions with surrounding erythema.*

nied by systemic infection; in this case only culture of exudate or biopsy specimen from the lesion is positive for *P. aeruginosa*.

Dermatopathology Vasculitis without thrombosis. Paucity of neutrophils at site of infection. Bacilli found in media and adventitia, but usually not in intima, of vessel.

PATHOPHYSIOLOGY

In general, EG is indicative of pseudomonal bacteremia/septicemia with seeding of cutaneous sites and subsequent development of vasculitic skin infection. Less commonly, EG may arise from local invasion of the skin. EG contraction depends primarily on altered susceptibility of the host rather than on spread from individual to individual or on increased pathogenicity.

COURSE AND PROGNOSIS

When arising as a result of pseudomonal bacteremia, prognosis for patient with EG poor; >50% mortality. When occurring as a local infection in the absence of bacteremia, prognosis much more favorable.

TREATMENT

Combination IV gentamicin-piperacillin. Antibiotic and dosage adjusted according to sensitivities and results of cultures.

Cutaneous and Mucocutaneous Leishmaniasis

Leishmaniasis is a parasitic infection caused by many species of the protozoa *Leishmania,* manifested clinically as four major syndromes—cutaneous leishmaniasis (CL) of Old and New World types, mucocutaneous leishmaniasis, diffuse cutaneous leishmaniasis, and visceral leishmaniasis. CL is characterized by development of single or multiple cutaneous papules at the site of a sandfly bite, often evolving into nodules and ulcers, which heal spontaneously with a depressed scar.

Synonyms: Old World leishmaniasis: Baghdad/Delhi boil or button; oriental/Allepo sore; bouton d'Orient. *Mucocutaneous:* espundia. *Visceral:* kala azar.

TAXONOMY

(1) Old World leishmaniasis: (*a*) urban, or dry, recidivans; (*b*) rural, or wet. (2) New World/ American leishmaniasis: (*a*) purely cutaneous (ACL); (*b*) mucocutaneous (MCL); (*c*) disseminated cutaneous (DCL)

EPIDEMIOLOGY AND ETIOLOGY

Incidence   Estimated 12 million people infected worldwide

Etiology

OLD WORLD CUTANEOUS LEISHMANIASIS (OWCL)   *L. tropica major* causes wet (rural). *L. t. minor* causes dry (urban)

AMERICAN CUTANEOUS LEISHMANIASIS (ACL) CL—*L. mexicana* complex (*L. m. mexicana, L. m. amazonensis*); *L. braziliensis guyanensis, L. b. peruviana.* Mucocutaneous leishmaniasis (MCL)—*L. b. braziliensis, L. b. panamensis, L. b. guyanensis*

DIFFUSE CUTANEOUS LEISHMANIASIS (DCL) *L. m. pifanoi* (Venezuela), *L. m. amazonensis* (Brazil), members of the *L. mexicana* complex (Dominican Republic), *L. aethiopica* (Africa)

Life Cycle   *Leishmania* dimorphic. In mammalian host: amastigote (leishmanial) form—2.0 to 3.0 μm in length, oval/round, aflagel-late; lives intracellularly in cells of reticuloendothelial system. In GI tract of sandfly/in culture: promastigote (leptomonad) form—10.0 to 15.0 μm in length, spindle-shaped, flagellated; extracellular. Speciation: isoenzyme patterns, kinetoplast DNA buoyant densities, specific phlebotomine vectors, monoclonal antibodies, DNA hybridization, DNA restriction endonuclease fragment analysis.

Reservoir   Varies with geography and leishmanial species. Zoonosis involves rodents/ canines. Mediterranean littoral—dogs. Southern Commonwealth of Independent States—gerbils.

Vector   Female sandflies of genus *Phlebotomus* (Old World) and *Lutzomyia* and *Psychodopygus* (New World). Breed in cracks in buildings, rubbish, rubble; rodent burrows, termite hills, rotting vegetation. Weak fliers; remain close to ground near breeding site. Ingest amastigotes while feeding on infected mammals, converting to promastigotes in the gut of the sandfly; replicate in gut.

Transmission   Promastigotes deposited on skin of host into a small pool of blood drawn by probing sandfly.

Season   *L. t. major*—summer through autumn epidemics. *L. t. minor*—year round. ACL—rainy season.

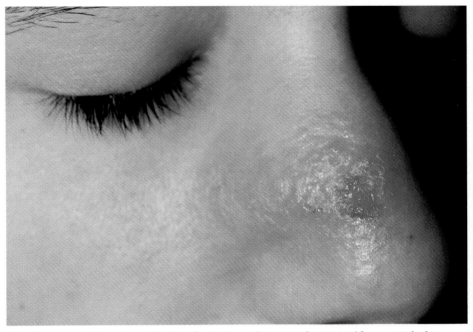

187   Cutaneous leishmaniasis, Old World   *Solitary plaque on the nose with a crusted ulcer.*

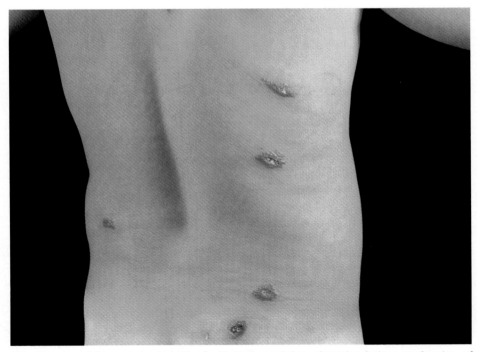

188   Cutaneous leishmaniasis, Old World   *Multiple, nodular, ulcerative lesions at the sites of sandfly bites.*

CUTANEOUS AND MUCOCUTANEOUS LEISHMANIASIS

Geography All inhabited continents except Australia.

OWCL Asia Minor, Middle East, southern Commonwealth of Independent States, China, the Mediterranean littoral, India, Africa (Sudan, Ethiopia, Congo basin)

ACL, MCL Forests of South and Central America. *L. mexicana* endemic in south-central Texas

DCL South America, Dominican Republic, Africa

HISTORY

Incubation Period Inversely proportional to size of inoculum; shorter in visitors to endemic area. *OWCL: L. t. major,* 1 to 4 weeks; *L. t. minor,* 2 to 8 months. *ACL:* 2 to 8 weeks or more.

Symptoms Noduloulcerative lesions usually asymptomatic. With secondary bacterial infection, may become painful.

PHYSICAL EXAMINATION

Skin Findings

TYPE OF LESION Primary lesions occur at site of sandfly bite.

OWCL

L. t. minor—single dry ulcer. Papule on face; evolves slowly (Figure 187), healing in >1 year with scar. After healing, peripheral papules may erupt and extend from scar (leishmaniasis recidivans)

L. t. major—multiple exudative ulcers (Figure 188). Erythematous papule. Numerous lesions may be present initially, some resolving, others evolving into CL. Persistent papule enlarges to nodule. Summit of nodule crusts, oozes; evolves to shallow ulcer with spongy base. Volcano sign: volcanic nodule with sloping sides, shallow apical crater covered with crust. Iceberg nodules: nodules with subcutaneous, endophytic component. Satellite papules: multiple

inflammatory papules surrounding (up to 2.0 cm distant) primary nodule, 2.0 to 5.0 mm, lack punctum or crust, appear late in evolution. Lesion fixed for months. Healing begins centrally, spreading centrifugally with resultant scar formation. Scar atrophic, hyperpigmented, irregular (cribriform). Recurrent CL (RCL) occurs several months to several years after the original lesion has healed; small firm papules to nodules appear on periphery or in scar; duration 60+ years.

ACL or New World CL L. m. mexicana: chiclero ulcer or bay sore. Small erythematous firm papule. Usually ulcerates, encrusted. Enlarges to 3.0 to 12.0 cm with raised border. Nonulcerating nodules may become verrucous. ±Lymphangitis, ±regional lymphadenopathy. Isolated lesions on hand or head usually do not ulcerate, heal spontaneously. Ear lesions may persist for years, destroying cartilage.

MCL L. b. braziliensis—one or several lesions on lower extremities, ulcerate, heal spontaneously. After months to years, metastatic lesions may appear in nasopharynx and/or perineum. Associated with nasal obstruction, epistaxis, painful mutilating erosions (espundia) (Figure 189).

DCL—resembles lepromatous leprosy (Figure 190).

SHAPE OF INDIVIDUAL LESION May be elongated with long axis along skin crease

DISTRIBUTION OF LESIONS *L. t. major*—exposed sites, especially ankles and legs; in children only, face

MUCOUS MEMBRANES MCL occurs 3 to 10 years after primary ACL in one-third of cases. Nasal mucosa—inflamed, edematous, ulcerative; associated with coryza, epistaxis. Perforation of septum. Ulceration with destruction of nasal fossa, mucosa, cartilage. Lips, pharynx, tonsils, floor of mouth, tongue may be affected; may extend to larynx, trachea, bronchi. Mucosa thick-

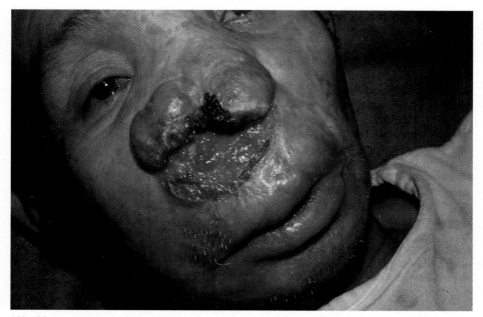

189　Mucocutaneous leishmaniasis, South American　*Painful, mutilating ulceration with destruction of portions of the nose. (Courtesy of Eric Kraus, M.D.)*

ened, granulomatous, bleeds easily. Complicated by difficulty in breathing, feeding, swallowing; malnutrition.

General Examination OWCL: regional lymphadenopathy common

DIAGNOSIS AND DIFFERENTIAL DIAGNOSIS

Diagnosis Clinical suspicion confirmed by demonstrating amastigotes on smear or in skin biopsy specimen or promastigotes on culture of aspirates or tissue.

Differential Diagnosis *Acute CL:* insect bite, furuncle, carbuncle, ecthyma, anthrax, orf, milker's nodule, tularemia, swimming pool granuloma, tuberculosis cutis, syphilitic gumma, yaws, sporotrichosis, blastomycosis, kerion, myiasis, dracunculosis, molluscum, pyogenic granuloma, tropical ulcer, foreign body granuloma, keratoacanthoma, squamous cell carcinoma, metastases, lymphoma, leukemia. *Chronic CL and relapsing CL:* lupus vulgaris, leprosy, sarcoidosis, granuloma faciale, Jessner's lymphocytic infiltrate, lymphocytoma cutis, discoid lupus erythematosus, cellulitis, Wegener's granulomatosis, syphilitic gumma

LABORATORY AND SPECIAL EXAMINATIONS

Leishmanin (Montenegro) Skin Test Of no use in endemic areas. Negative in DCL.

Serology Lacks specificity

Dermatopathology Large macrophages filled with 2.0- to 4.0-μm amastigotes (Leishman-Donovan bodies); mixed lymphocytic, plasmacytic infiltrate. In Wright- and Giemsa-stained preparations, the amastigote cytoplasm appears blue, nucleus relatively large and red, distinctive kinetoplast rod-shaped and stains intensely red.

Culture Novy-MacNeal-Nicolle medium at 22°C to 28°C for 21 days grows motile promastigotes.

Touch Prep Dark, slightly flattened nucleus and rod-shaped kinetoplast observed.

PATHOPHYSIOLOGY

Course determined by host's cellular immunity and species of *Leishmania*. MCL: destructiveness of metastatic lesions due to hypersensitivity to parasite antigens. *DCL:* leishmanin reaction negative, i.e., selective anergy.

COURSE AND PROGNOSIS

CL Whether caused by *L. tropica* or *L. mexicana,* CL is self-limited. Scarring is increased by secondary bacterial infection.

MCL May extend to secondary sites. Secondary infection common. Mortality from pneumonia.

DCL Progressive; refractory to treatment; cures rare.

TREATMENT

No chemoprophylaxis for travelers exists. *OWCL:* delay specific treatment until ulceration occurs, allowing protective immunity to develop, unless lesions are disfiguring, disabling, or persist >6 months.

Lesional Therapy Local injection of antimonials with or without steroids, cryosurgery, ultrasound-induced hyperthermia, excision, electrosurgery. Topical 15% paramomycin sulfate, 12% methylbenzethonium chloride in white paraffin twice daily for 10 days.

Systemic Therapy For selected CL, MCL, DCL. *Sodium antimony gluconate*—IV or IM

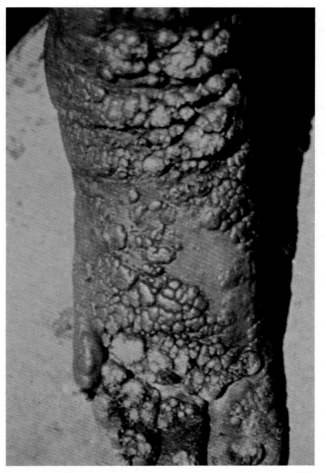

190 Disseminated (anergic) leishmaniasis *Confluent nodules on the foot resembling lepromatous leprosy; there was generalized cutaneous involvement as well. (Courtesy of David Wyler, M.D.)*

in single daily dose of 10 mg per kg body weight for adults and 20 mg per kg for patients <18 years of age for 10 days. *Meglumine antimoniate*—20 mg per kg daily for 10 days. Monitor ECG. *Amphotericin B* or *pentamidine* or *sodium antimony gluconate plus interferon gamma* for resistant cases. Ketoconazole.

Combined Immunotherapy Leishmanial antigen in BCG

Lyme Borreliosis

Lyme borreliosis (LB) is a spirochetal infectious disease transmitted to humans by the bite of an infected tick. Lyme disease (LD), the syndrome occurring early in the infection, is characterized by a pathognomonic rash, erythema migrans (EM), and lymphocytoma cutis, followed by late involvement that can include the joints, nervous system, and heart. Chronic LB is manifested by acrodermatitis chronica atrophicans and sclerotic plaques and nodules.

EPIDEMIOLOGY AND ETIOLOGY

Age Children (<15 years), adults (20 to 45 years and older)

Etiology *Borrelia burgdorferi*

Transmission Vector: in the United States, deer tick (*Ixodes dammini*) in Northeast and Midwest, *I. pacifica* in Northwest; in Europe, *I. ricinus*. Ticks cling to vegetation, are most numerous in brushy, wooded, or grassy habitats; not found on open sandy beaches. *B. burgdorferi* is transmitted to humans following biting and feeding of the tick or nymphs.

Incidence 4700 reported cases in the United States in 1988. Has been doubling annually.

Season Late May through early fall (80% of early LB begins in June and July) in the midwestern and eastern United States; January through May in the Pacific Northwest.

Geography Reported from at least 19 countries on three continents. In the *United States,* has been reported from all 50 states with indigenous cases occurring in all but 7 states. Indigenous cases concentrated along Northeast coast (Massachusetts, Rhode Island, Connecticut, New York, New Jersey, Pennsylvania, Delaware, Maryland), Midwest (Minnesota, Wisconsin) and Northwest (California, Oregon, Nevada, Utah); geographic area is widening. *Canada:* 30 reported cases in 1988 in 5 of 10 provinces. *Europe:* occurs widely throughout the continent and Great Britain. *Australia.*

Staging of LB
Stage I Acute
  Systemic symptoms (fever, chills, myalgia, headaches, weakness, photophobia)
  Erythema migrans
  Lymphocytoma

Stage II Intermediate
  Carditis
  Meningitis, cranial neuritis, radiculoneuropathy
  Arthralgia/myalgia

Stage III Chronic
  Arthritis
  Acrodermatitis chronica atrophicans
  Encephalomyelitis

HISTORY

Incubation Period Median 9 days (range, 1 to 36 days)

Prodrome Malaise, fatigue, lethargy, headache, fever, chills, stiff neck, arthralgia, myalgia, backache, anorexia, sore throat, nausea, dysesthesia, vomiting, abdominal pain, photophobia

SYSTEMIC INFECTIONS AND INFESTATIONS

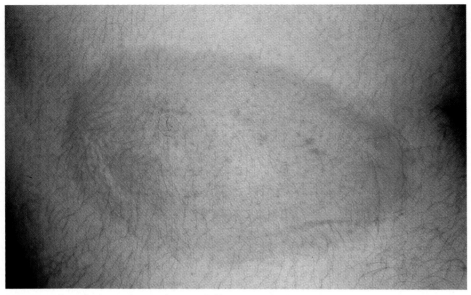

191   Lyme borreliosis, erythema migrans   *Solitary annular lesion on the lateral thigh occurring at the site of an asymptomatic tick bite.*

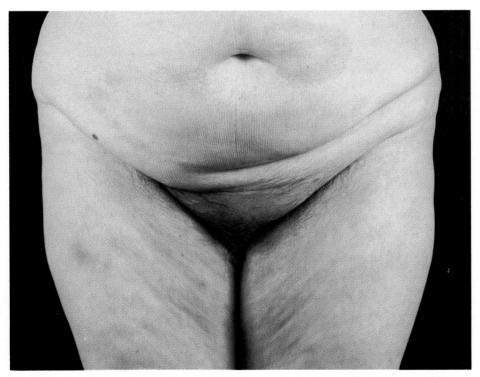

192   Lyme borreliosis, erythema migrans   *Multiple, annular lesions on the abdomen and leg, occurring at the sites of tick bites.*

History Ixodid tick bites are asymptomatic. Only 14% of LB patients are aware of a preceding tick bite. Transmission also occurs by nymphs that are very small (1 mm) and thus go unnoticed. Removal of the pinhead-sized tick within 18 hours of attachment may preclude transmission. EM may produce burning sensation, itching, or pain. Only 75% of patients with LB exhibit EM.

PHYSICAL EXAMINATION

Cutaneous Findings in Early LB

TYPE Initial macule or papule enlarges within days to form an expanding annular lesion with a distinct red border and partial central clearing (Figures 191 and 192), i.e., EM, at the bite site. Maximum median diameter is 15.0 cm (range, 3.0 to 68.0 cm). Center may become indurated, vesicular, or necrotic. At times concentric rings form. When occurring on the scalp, only a linear streak may be evident on the face or neck.

Secondary Lesions 17% develop multiple annular secondary lesions, ranging in number from 2 to >100. Secondary lesions resemble EM but are smaller, migrate less, and lack central induration. 17% of patients have multiple secondary EM lesions ranging in number from 2 to 36.

Other Cutaneous Findings Malar rash, diffuse urticaria, subcutaneous nodules (panniculitis)

COLOR Erythematous evolving to violaceous

DISTRIBUTION OF LESIONS EM: trunk and proximal extremities, especially the axillary and inguinal areas, most common sites. Secondary lesions: any site except the palms and soles; can become confluent.

MUCOUS MEMBRANES Red throat, conjunctivitis

Uncommonly, LB may occur without EM or secondary lesions and present only with the late manifestations. Also, late manifestations may occur in spite of treatment of early LB with tetracycline.

LYMPHOCYTOMA CUTIS Lymphocytoma cutis [*synonyms:* lymphadenosis benigna cutis (LABC), pseudolymphoma of Spiegler and Fendt] is an infiltrative cutaneous disorder, characterized most often by solitary (may be grouped) nodules or plaques; occasionally translucent; red-to-brown-to-purple in color; located on the head, especially earlobes (Figure 193), nipples, scrotum, and extremities; 3.0 to 5.0 cm in diameter; usually asymptomatic.

Cutaneous Findings in Long-Standing LB

ACRODERMATITIS CHRONICA ATROPHICANS (ACA)

Early Inflammatory Phase (Months to Years) Initially, diffuse or localized erythema (Figure 194) usually on one extremity, accompanied by mild to prominent edema, most commonly involving the extensor surfaces and periarticular areas. Asymptomatic dull-red and ill-defined plaques arise on the extremities, more commonly on lower legs than forearms, which slowly extend centrifugally over several months to years, leaving central areas of atrophy.

End Stage Skin becomes atrophic, veins and subcutaneous tissue become prominent, easily lifted and pushed into fine accordion-like folds, i.e., "cigarette paper" or "tissue paper" skin (Figure 195). Lesions may be single or multiple. Plaque(s) slowly extends centrifugally with an active inflammatory advancing border and a smooth, hairless, tissue paper-like atrophic central area with dull-red, poikilodermatous skin.

Sclerotic or Fibrotic Plaques and Bands Localized fibromas and plaques are seen as subcutaneous nodules around the knees and elbows (Figure 196); may involve the joint capsule with subsequent limitation of movement of joints in hand, feet, or shoulders; or extend like linear morphea from elbow down to wrist.

General Findings

ACUTE OR PRIMARY MANIFESTATIONS Fever: in adults, low-grade; in children, may be high and persistent. Regional lymphadenopathy, generalized lymphadenopathy, right upper quadrant tenderness,

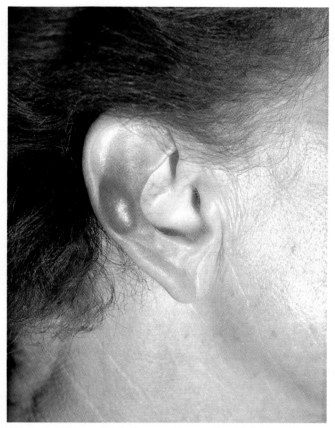

193   Lyme borreliosis, lymphocytoma   *Solitary, red-to-purple nodule occurring on the characteristic site of the earlobe.*

frank arthritis, splenomegaly, hepatomegaly, muscle tenderness, periorbital edema, and abdominal tenderness.

LATE OR TERTIARY MANIFESTATIONS *Arthritis* Occurs in 60% of untreated cases, 4 to 6 weeks after the tick bite (range, 1 week to 22 months), sudden in onset, involves one or a few joints. Knee (89%), shoulder (9%), hip (9%), ankle (7%), and elbow (2%) are commonly affected.

Neurologic Involvement Occurs in 10 to 20% of untreated LB cases, 1 to 6 weeks (or longer) following the tick bite. Manifested by meningitis (excruciating headache, neck pain), encephalitis (sleep disturbances, difficulty concentrating, poor memory, irritability, emotional lability, dementia); cranial neuropathies [unilateral or bilateral; optic neuropathy, sixth nerve palsy, facial (Bell's) palsy, eighth nerve deafness]; sensory and motor radiculopathies (severe radicular pain, dysesthesias, subtle sensory loss, focal weakness, loss of reflexes). Referred to as Bannwarth's syndrome or tick-borne meningopolyneuritis of Garin-Bujadoux-Bannwarth.

Cardiac Abnormalities Occur in 6 to 10% of untreated cases, usually within 4 weeks. Manifested by fluctuating degrees of atrioventricular block, myopericarditis, and left ventricular dysfunction. Usually transient and not associated with long-term sequelae.

Variants LB occurring in Europe usually milder than in United States, with more secondary EM-like skin lesions and fewer arthritic complications, probably due to strain differences in *B. burgdorferi*.

DIAGNOSIS AND DIFFERENTIAL DIAGNOSIS

Diagnosis

ACUTE Made on characteristic clinical findings in a person living in or having visited an endemic area.

LATE Confirmed by specific serologic tests. CDC case definition: physician-diagnosed EM in a person who acquired infection in a geographic area with endemic LB; or, for persons who acquired infection in a geographic area without endemic LB, laboratory evidence of infection in addition to the presence of EM.

ACA Made on clinical findings confirmed by lesional biopsy.

Differential Diagnosis

EM Tinea corporis, herald patch of pityriasis rosea, insect (e.g., brown recluse spider) bite, cellulitis, urticaria, erythema multiforme, fixed drug eruption. Secondary lesions: secondary syphilis, pityriasis rosea, erythema multiforme, urticaria.

ACA Arterial insufficiency of the lower leg, venous insufficiency with stasis dermatitis, and venous thrombosis/thrombophlebitis.

FIBROTIC NODULES Rheumatic nodules, gouty tophi, and erythema nodosum

LABORATORY AND SPECIAL EXAMINATIONS

Skin Biopsy

EM Deep and superficial perivascular and interstitial lymphohistiocytic infiltrate containing plasma cells. Spirochetes can be demonstrated in up to 40% of EM biopsy specimens.

ACA Early, perivascular inflammatory infiltrate and dermal edema. Subsequently, infiltrate broadens to a dense middermal bandlike infiltrate. Ultimately, epidermal and dermal atrophy, dilated dermal blood vessels, plasma cell infiltrate, elastin and collagen defects.

Serology The combination of an ELISA for detecting IgM and IgG anti-*B. burgdorferi* antibodies and a Western blot to confirm ELISA results (especially unexpected low-titer positive results) offer the greatest sensitivity and specificity. Initial antibody response is with IgM antibodies followed by IgG. Early in LB when only EM has occurred, as few as 50% of patients have positive serologies; adequate treatment may block seroconversion.

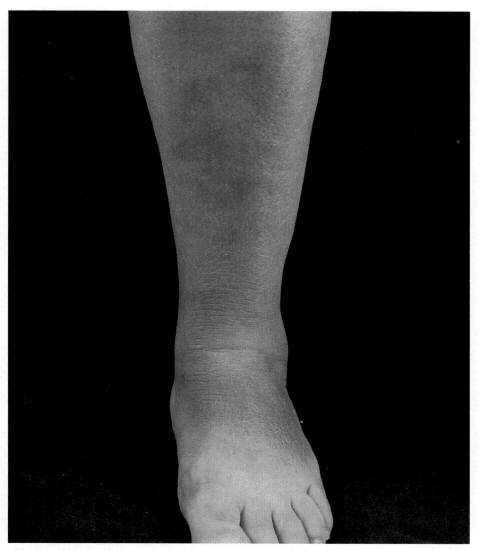

194 Lyme borreliosis, acrodermatitis chronica atrophicans *Early inflammatory phase exhibiting asymptomatic erythema.*

Virtually all cases with late manifestations are seropositive with a titer of 256 or greater.

PATHOPHYSIOLOGY

LB in many ways parallels the course of syphilis. EM, as with a syphilitic chancre, occurs at the site of entry of the spirochete soon after inoculation. Secondary lesions occur following hematogenous dissemination to the skin. The late joint manifestations appear to be mediated by immune-complex formation. Meningitis results from direct invasion of the cerebrospinal fluid. The pathogenesis of cranial and peripheral neuropathies in LB is unknown but might also result from immune mechanisms.

COURSE AND PROGNOSIS

Untreated EM and secondary lesions fade in a median time of 28 days, but this ranges from 1 day to 14 months. Both EM and secondary lesions can fade and recur during this time. However following adequate treatment, early lesions resolve within several days and late manifestations are prevented. Late manifestations identified early usually clear following adequate antibiotic therapy; however, delay in diagnosis may result in permanent joint or neurologic disabilities.

ACA shows little response to adequate antibiotic therapy once atrophy has supervened. Adequately treated patients show declining titers of anti-*B. burgdorferi* antibody within 6 to 12 months.

TREATMENT

Early LB

Doxycycline, 100 mg twice daily for 10 to 21 days

Amoxicillin, 500 mg 3 times daily for 10 to 21 days

Erythromycin, 250 mg 4 times daily for 10 to 21 days (less effective than doxycycline or amoxicillin)

Lyme Carditis

Ceftriaxone, 2 g daily IV for 14 days

Penicillin G, 20 million units IV for 14 days

Doxycycline, 100 mg p.o. twice daily for 14 to 21 days, may suffice

Amoxicillin, 500 mg p.o. 3 times daily for 14 to 21 days, may suffice

Neurologic Manifestations
FACIAL NERVE PARALYSIS

For an isolated finding, oral regimens for early disease, used for at least 21 days, may suffice

For a finding associated with other neurologic manifestations, IV therapy (see below)

LYME MENINGITIS

Ceftriaxone, 2 g daily by single dose for 14 to 21 days

Penicillin G, 20 million units daily in divided doses for 10 to 21 days

Possible alternatives for Lyme meningitis:

Doxycycline, 100 mg p.o. or IV for 14 to 21 days

Chloramphenicol, 1 g IV every 6 hours for 10 to 21 days

Lyme Arthritis

Doxycycline, 100 mg p.o. twice daily for 30 days

Amoxicillin and probenecid, 500 mg each p.o. 4 times daily for 30 days

Penicillin G, 20 million units IV in divided doses daily for 14 to 21 days

Ceftriaxone, 2 g IV daily for 14 to 21 days

In Pregnant Women

For localized early LB, amoxicillin 500 mg 3 times daily for 21 days

For disseminated early LB or any manifestation of late disease, penicillin G, 20 million units daily for 14 to 21 days

For asymptomatic seropositivity, no treatment necessary

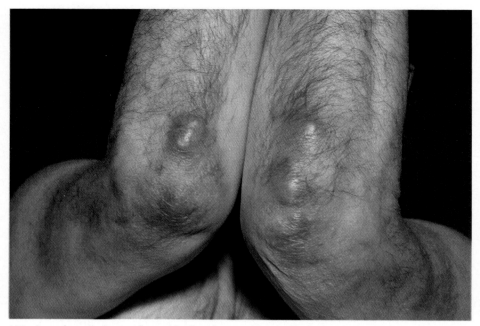

195 Lyme borreliosis, acrodermatitis chronica atrophicans *Typical endstage cutaneous atrophy is seen on both legs with prominence of the veins.*

LYME BORRELIOSIS

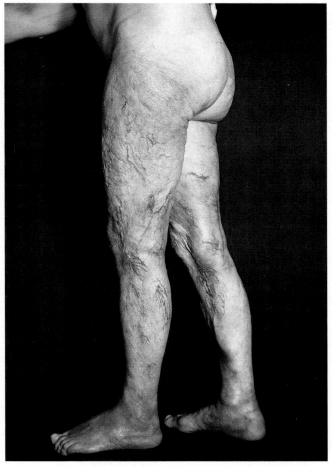

196 Lyme borreliosis, acrodermatitis chronica atrophicans *Asymptomatic, violaceous, fibromatous nodules and plaques occurring on the elbows.*

Cellulitis is an acute, spreading infection of dermal and subcutaneous tissues, characterized by a red, hot, tender area of skin, often at the site of bacterial entry, caused most frequently by group A β-hemolytic streptococci or *Staphylococcus aureus*.

EPIDEMIOLOGY AND ETIOLOGY

Age Children <3 years; older individuals

Etiology
MOST COMMON *Adults* Group A β-hemolytic *Streptococcus pyogenes, Staph. aureus.*
Children Haemophilus influenzae, group A streptococci, *Staph. aureus*
UNCOMMON *Adults H. influenzae*, group B streptococci, pneumococci. In diabetics or in patients with impaired immunity: *Escherichia coli, Proteus mirabilis, Acinetobacter, Enterobacter, Pseudomonas aeruginosa, Cryptococcus neoformans.* Other organisms: *Pasteurella multocida, Vibrio vulnificus; Mycobacterium fortuitum* complex
Children Pneumococci, *Neisseria meningitidis* group B (periorbital)

Transmission Entry via break in the skin (puncture, laceration, abrasion, surgical site), underlying dermatosis (tinea pedis, stasis dermatitis/ulcer), nasal fissures, injection by parenteral drug user. In children *H. influenzae* enters through middle ear or nasal mucosa.

Risk Factors Diabetes mellitus, hematologic malignancies, IV drug use, chronic lymphedema (postmastectomy, postcoronary artery grafting, previous episode of cellulitis), immunocompromise

HISTORY

Incubation Period Few days

Prodrome Occurs less often than commonly thought. Malaise, anorexia; fever, chills can develop rapidly, before cellulitis is apparent clinically. Higher fever (38.5°C) and chills usually associated with streptococci; lower fever (37.5°C) usually associated with staphylococci.

Previous Treatment Prior episode(s) of cellulitis in an area of lymphedema

Drug Ingestion IVDU

Immune Status Immunocompromised patients susceptible to infection with bacteria of low pathogenicity

PHYSICAL EXAMINATION

Skin Findings
TYPE OF LESION *Entry sites* Breaks in skin, ulcers, chronic dermatosis
Plaque Red, hot, edematous, and very tender area of skin of varying size; borders usually sharply defined, irregular, and slightly elevated; bluish-purple color with *H. influenzae*. Vesicles, bullae, erosions, abscesses, hemorrhage, and necrosis may form in plaque. Lymphangitis.
DISTRIBUTION OF LESIONS *Adults* Lower leg: most common site. Arm: in young male, consider IV drug use; in female, postmastectomy. Trunk: operative wound site.
Children Cheek, periorbital area, head, neck most common: usually *H. influenzae*. Extremities: *Staph. aureus,* group A streptococci.

SYSTEMIC INFECTIONS AND INFESTATIONS

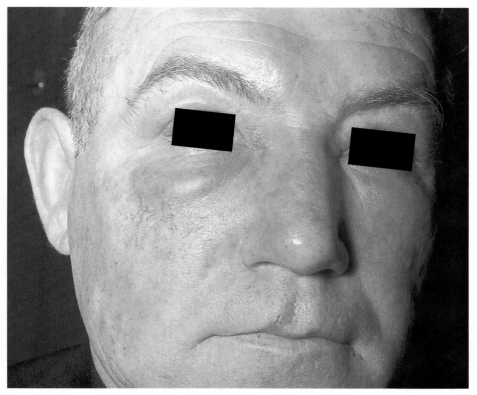

197   Cellulitis (erysipelas)   *Painful, erythematous, edematous involvement of the periorbital skin and left cheek.*

LYMPH NODES   Can be enlarged and tender, regionally

Variants

Erysipelas   Caused by group A streptococci. Superficial type of cellulitis involving lymphatics. Margin of lesion is raised, sharply demarcated from adjacent normal skin, often painful (Figure 197). Sites of predilection: face, lower legs (Figure 198), areas of preexisting lymphedema, umbilical stump

H. influenzae cellulitis   Cheek, periorbital area (Figure 199), head, neck most common sites. Occurs mainly in young children <3 years of age.

Erysipeloid   Erysipelothrix rhusiopathiae cellulitis on hand, especially finger after handling saltwater fish, shellfish, meat,

hides, poultry. Usually no systemic symptoms.

Ecthyma gangrenosum P. aeruginosa, usually extremity; rapidly becomes necrotic and leads to ulcer.

Vibrio vulnificus cellulitis   Follows exposure to seawater; usually on the extremities.

M. fortuitum complex cellulitis   Usually occurs on foot at site of nail puncture wound. Systemic findings lacking.

Cryptococcal cellulitis   Red, hot, tender, edematous plaque on extremity. Rarely multiple noncontiguous sites. Patient always immunocompromised.

Infectious gangrene (gangrenous cellulitis) Rapidly progressive, associated with extensive necrosis of subcutaneous tissue and overlying skin, guarded prognosis. Further subdivided into clinically different types depending on causative organisms, location, predisposing factors: *necrotizing fasciitis* (Figure 200) (streptococcal gangrene) (variant occurring about male genitalia referred to as Fournier's gangrene), *gas gangrene* (clostridial myonecrosis and anaerobic cellulitis), *progressive bacterial synergistic gangrene, synergistic necrotizing cellulitis* (perineal phlegmon), *gangrenous balanitis, gangrenous cellulitis in immunosuppressed patient,* and *localized areas of skin necrosis complicating conventional cellulitis.*

DIAGNOSIS AND DIFFERENTIAL DIAGNOSIS

Diagnosis Clinical diagnosis. Confirmed by culture in only 25% of cases in immunocompetent patients. Suspicion of necrotizing fasciitis requires immediate deep biopsy and frozen section histopathology.

Differential Diagnosis Deep vein thrombosis/thrombophlebitis, early contact dermatitis, giant urticaria, fixed drug eruption, erythema migrans, prevesicular herpes zoster. Necrotizing fasciitis and synergistic gangrene, which require early surgical debridement, must be ruled out.

LABORATORY AND SPECIAL EXAMINATIONS

Dermatopathology Diagnostic in necrotizing fasciitis and synergistic gangrene, helpful with cryptococcal cellulitis

Laboratory Examination of Blood WBC and ESR may be elevated

Cultures Primary lesion, aspirate or biopsy of leading edge of inflammation, blood; positive in only one-quarter of cases. Fungal and mycobacterial cultures indicated in atypical case.

PATHOPHYSIOLOGY

Bacterial multiplication follows entry into skin, although the number of organisms is scanty compared to the inflammatory response.

COURSE AND PROGNOSIS

Dissemination of infection (lymphatically, hematogenously) with metastatic sites of infection occurs if treatment is delayed. Abnormal or synthetic heart valve may be colonized and infected. In pre-antibiotic era, mortality was very high. Without surgical debridement necrotizing fasciitis is fatal.

TREATMENT

Supportive Rest, immobilization, elevation, moist heat, analgesia.

Antibiotics In that most cases are caused by group A β-hemolytic streptococci and/or *Staph. aureus,* initial therapy is best directed at both organisms.

For mild early cellulitis: If staphylococci suspected, or if agent not known, dicloxacillin 0.5 to 1.0 g p.o. every 6 hours. Alternative in penicillin-allergic patients, erythromycin 0.5 g p.o. every 6 hours.

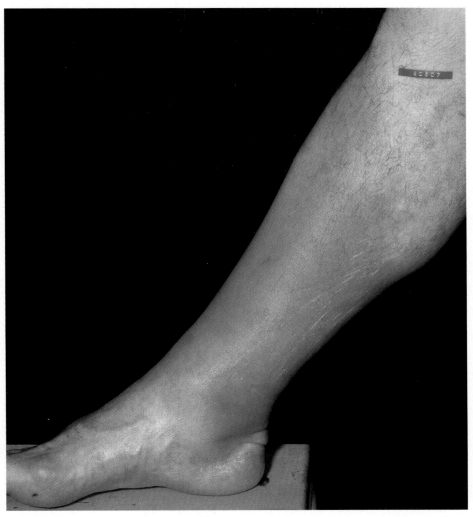

198 Cellulitis (erysipelas), streptococcal *There is extensive, brawny, erythematous edema and tenderness of the lower half of the leg.*

For more severe infection: Penicillin 10 million units + dicloxacillin 2 g t.i.d. IV. Nafcillin 1.0 to 1.5 g IV every 4 hours. Alternative in penicillin-allergic patients, vancomycin 1.0 to 1.5 g per day IV. Subsequent antibiotic therapy modified according to response and cultured bacteria.

For necrotizing fasciitis and synergistic gangrene: Wide surgical excision and debridement plus appropriate IV high-dose antibiotic treatment.

CELLULITIS

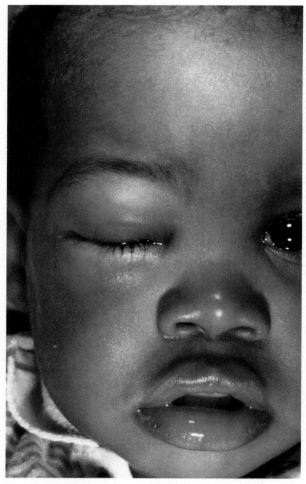

199 Cellulitis, *Haemophilus influenzae* There is inflammation in the right periorbital region and the right cheek of this 2-year-old child. (Courtesy of Arthur R. Rhodes, M.D.)

SYSTEMIC INFECTIONS AND INFESTATIONS

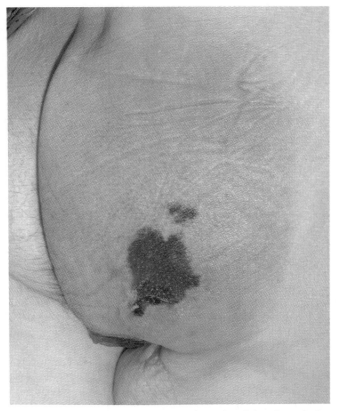

200　Necrotizing fasciitis　*Erythematous, edematous plaque involving the entire buttock, with rapidly progressing central area of necrosis. The patient was obtunded.*

Sexually Transmitted Diseases

Sexually Transmitted Diseases

The epidemiology of sexually transmitted diseases (STDs) in the 1990s has changed considerably from that of the past decade. The incidence of primary, secondary, and congenital syphilis, the STD most closely associated with dermatology, has nearly doubled during the past decade, a phenomenon associated with exchange of sex for illicit drugs. The incidence of genital herpes infection is probably unchanged, but this STD is no longer the subject of frequent media coverage, and, therefore, people's "herpesphobia" has lessened. The number of individuals infected with the genital human papillomavirus (HPV) infection is at an all time high, probably affecting 40 to 50 million persons in the United States. The HPV causes genital warts and is closely linked epidemiologically with both in situ and invasive squamous cell carcinoma of the anogenital region including the cervix and the bladder. Few patients are aware of this association. The guidelines for care of HPV-infected individuals are unclear in that current treatment options are not curative. The human immunodeficiency virus (HIV) epidemic, now a decade old, is associated with unprecedented morbidity and mortality. The focus of the HIV epidemic has shifted from the male homosexual population to the homeless, intravenous drug users and their sexual partners, and the inner city poor. In the United States and the rest of the world, successful management of STDs in the 1990s is closely linked to confronting and healing these epidemic social ills.

Gonorrhea

Gonorrhea is an acute sexually transmitted infection of the mucocutaneous surfaces of the lower genitourinary tract, characterized clinically in males by a purulent urethral discharge. In females, however, infection is often asymptomatic; if untreated, infection can spread to deeper structures with abscess formation and disseminated gonococcal infection (DCI).

Synonyms: blennorrhagia, blennorrhea.

EPIDEMIOLOGY AND ETIOLOGY

Age Young sexually active; infection of conjunctiva in newborns

Sex Symptomatic infection more common in males. Pharyngeal and anorectal infection in homosexual males.

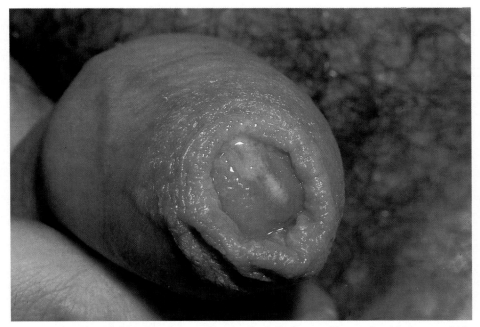

201   Gonococcal urethritis   *Purulent, copious urethral discharge with associated balanoposthitis.*

Etiology   *Neisseria gonorrhoeae,* the gono-coccus, a gram-negative diplococcus

Incidence   In United States in 1978, 1,000,000 cases reported with estimated 2,000,000 unreported. Associated with HIV epidemic and the practice of "safer sex," number of cases reported annually signifi-cantly decreased until 1988. Incidence is cur-rently rising, however.

Transmission   Sexually, from partner who is either asymptomatic or who has minimal symptoms. Neonate exposed to infected secre-tions in birth canal.

Geography   Worldwide

HISTORY

Incubation Period
MALES   90% of males develop urethritis within 5 days of exposure.
FEMALES   Usually >2 weeks when sympto-matic. However, up to 75% of women are asymptomatic.

Skin Symptoms   Urethral discharge, dys-uria. Vaginal discharge; deep pelvic or lumbar pain. Copious purulent anal discharge; burn-ing or stinging pain on defecation; tenesmus; blood in/on stool. Mild sore throat.

PHYSICAL EXAMINATION

Skin and Other Findings
TYPE OF LESION   *Males*   Urethral discharge ranging from scanty and clear to purulent and copious (Figure 201); meatal edema; preputial or penile edema. Balanoposthitis with subpreputial discharge in uncircum-cised men; balanitis in circumcised men. Folliculitis or cellulitis of thigh or abdomen. Rare complications of anterior urethritis include infection of: sebaceous glands of Tyson, paraurethral ducts, Littré's glands, lacunae of Morgagni, subepithelial and periurethral tissue of the urethra, median raphe, Cowper's ducts and glands.

Females Periurethral edema, urethritis. Purulent discharge from cervix but no vaginitis. In prepubescent females, vulvovaginitis. Bartholin's abscess.

DGI (see Section 14) Acral hemorrhagic pustules.

MUCOUS MEMBRANES Pharyngitis with erythema. In newborn or rarely in adult, copious purulent conjunctival discharge.

General Examination

MALES Prostatitis, epididymitis, vesiculitis, cystitis

FEMALES Pelvic inflammatory disease with signs of peritonitis, endocervicitis, endosalpingitis, endometritis

DIAGNOSIS AND DIFFERENTIAL DIAGNOSIS

Diagnosis Clinical suspicion confirmed by laboratory findings, i.e., presumptively by identifying gram-negative diplococci intracellularly in PMNs confirmed by culture

Differential Diagnosis Of urethritis: genital herpes with urethritis, *Chlamydia trachomatis* urethritis, *Ureaplasma urealyticum* urethritis, *Trichomonas vaginalis* urethritis, Reiter's syndrome

LABORATORY AND SPECIAL EXAMINATIONS

Gram's Strain Gram-negative diplococci intracellularly in PMNs in exudate

Culture Isolation on gonococcal selective media, i.e., so-called chocolatized blood agar, Martin-Lewis medium, Thayer-Martin medium. Antimicrobial susceptibility testing important due to resistant strains. Specimen collection sites: heterosexual men—urethra, oropharynx; homosexual men—urethra, anus, oropharynx; women—cervix, rectum, oropharynx.

Serologic Tests None available

PATHOPHYSIOLOGY

Gonococcus has affinity for columnar epithelium, while stratified and squamous epithelia are more resistant to attack; epithelium is penetrated between epithelial cells, causing a submucosal inflammation with PMN reaction and resultant purulent discharge.

COURSE AND PROGNOSIS

All patients with gonorrhea should have a serologic test for syphilis and should be offered HIV testing. Most patients with incubating syphilis may be cured by any of the regimens containing β-lactams or tetracyclines. There is a high frequency of chlamydial infections in persons with gonorrhea and treatment regimens cover this possibility. DGI more common in women with asymptomatic cervical, endometrial, or tubal infection and homosexual men with asymptomatic rectal or pharyngeal gonorrhea.

TREATMENT

Uncomplicated Urethral, Endocervical, or Rectal Infections

RECOMMENDED REGIMEN Ceftriaxone 250 mg IM once *plus* doxycycline 100 mg p.o. b.i.d. for 7 days

ALTERNATIVE REGIMEN

Spectinomycin 2 g IM *or* ciprofloxacin 500 mg p.o. once *or* norfloxacin 800 mg p.o. once *or* cefuroxime axetil 1 g p.o. once with probenecid 1 g *or* cefotaxime 1 g IM once *or* ceftizoxime 500 mg IM once

If gonococcus is known not to be penicillin-resistant, amoxicillin 3 g p.o. with 1 g probenecid

All of the above alternative regimens should be followed by doxycycline 100 mg p.o. b.i.d. for 7 days.

Pharyngeal Gonococcal Infection Ceftriaxone 250 mg IM once *or* ciprofloxacin 500 mg p.o. once

Syphilis is a sexually transmitted infection characterized by the appearance of a painless ulcer or chancre at the site of inoculation, often associated with regional lymphadenopathy; shortly after inoculation, syphilis becomes a systemic infection with characteristic secondary and tertiary stages. During the past few years, the incidence of syphilis has increased markedly and the clinical course and response to standard therapy may be altered in HIV-infected patients.

Synonyms: lues, the great imitator.

EPIDEMIOLOGY

Age In decreasing order: 20 to 39 years, 15 to 19 years, 40 to 49 years

Race All races; in the United States incidence increasing in African-Americans and Hispanics.

Sex Males outnumber females 2 to 4:1

Other Factors Until recently, nearly half of all males with syphilis in the United States were homosexual, but this percentage has decreased due to safer sexual practices. The incidence of syphilis, however, has markedly increased in minorities and is associated with exchange of sex for drugs. Associated with the increase in sexually transmitted syphilis is a marked increase in the number of cases of congenital syphilis.

Etiology *Treponema pallidum*

Primary Syphilis

HISTORY

Incubation Period 21 days (average); range, 10 to 90 days

PHYSICAL EXAMINATION

Skin Findings

TYPE OF LESION Chancre: buttonlike papule which develops into a painless erosion and then an ulcer with raised border with scanty serous exudate (Figure 202). Surface may be crusted. Size: few millimeters to 1.0 or 2.0 cm in diameter. Border of lesion may be raised.

COLOR Red, "meaty-colored"

PALPATION Most commonly, firm with *indurated* border. Painless. Extragenital chancres particularly on the fingers may be painful. Atypically, genital chancres painful, especially if secondarily infected with *Staphylococcus aureus*.

SHAPE OF INDIVIDUAL LESION Round or oval

ARRANGEMENT Single lesion. May be few or multiple; kissing lesions. Multiple chancres may occur in HIV-infected patients.

DISTRIBUTION OF LESIONS *Sites of Predilection* Male: inner prepuce, coronal sulcus of the glans, shaft, base. Female: cervix, vagina, vulva, clitoris, breast; chancres observed less frequently in women because of their location within vagina or on cervix.

Extragenital Chancres Anus or rectum, mouth (Figure 203), lips, tongue, tonsil, fingers (painful!), toes, breast, nipple

General Findings Syphilis is a systemic infection; all patients should have a thorough clinical examination. Regional lymphadenopathy appears within 1 week. Nodes are discrete, firm, rubbery, nontender, more commonly unilateral.

DIAGNOSIS AND DIFFERENTIAL DIAGNOSIS

Diagnosis Clinical suspicion confirmed by dark-field examination, or serologically.
SYPHILIS IN HIV-INFECTED PATIENTS HIV testing is advised for all sexually active patients with syphilis. Neurosyphilis should be considered in the differential diagnosis of neurologic disease in HIV-infected persons. When clinical findings suggest syphilis but serologic tests are negative or confusing, alternative procedures such as biopsy of lesions, dark-field examination, and direct fluorescent antibody staining of lesion material should be used.

Differential Diagnosis *In the differential diagnosis of any genital lesion, primary syphilis should be considered as suspect until ruled out clinically and by specific testing.* Chancroid, genital herpes, fixed drug eruption, lymphogranuloma venereum, donovanosis, traumatic ulcer, furuncle, aphthous ulcer.

SEXUALLY TRANSMITTED DISEASES

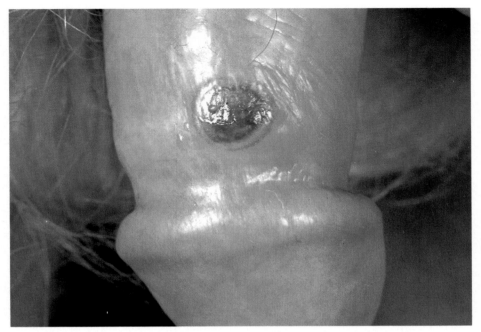

202　Primary syphilitic chancre　*Painless, firm, buttonlike, eroded nodule (chancre) occurring at the site of entry of treponeme.*

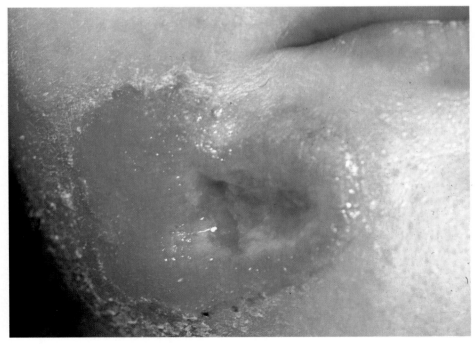

203　Primary syphilis　*Extragenital chancre.*

SYPHILIS

HISTORY

Secondary syphilis appears 2 to 6 months after primary infection, and 2 to 10 weeks after appearance of the primary chancre. Chancre may still be present when secondary lesions appear. Concomitant HIV infection may alter course of secondary syphilis. "Acute illness" syndrome: headache, chills, feverishness, arthralgia, myalgia, malaise, photophobia. Mucocutaneous lesions are asymptomatic.

Duration of Lesions Weeks

PHYSICAL EXAMINATION

Skin Findings

TYPE OF LESION Macules and papules 0.5 to 1.0 cm, round to oval (Figure 204). However, may be papulosquamous, pustular, or acneform. Vesiculobullous lesions occur only in neonatal congenital syphilis (palms and soles). Condylomata lata: soft flat-topped, moist, red-to-pale papules, nodules, or plaques, which may become confluent. Uncommonly, lesions of secondary syphilis and chancre of primary syphilis occur concomitantly.

COLOR Papules: brownish red, pink

PALPATION Papules—firm. Condylomata lata—soft

SHAPE Annular, polycyclic especially on face in dark-skinned individuals. In relapsing secondary syphilis, arciform lesions. Always sharply defined except for macular exanthem.

ARRANGEMENT Scattered discrete lesions (Figure 204). Symmetry usual. Asymmetric lesions in relapsing eruption.

DISTRIBUTION OF LESIONS Generalized eruption on the trunk (Figure 204); localized eruptions most commonly are scaling and papular localizing especially on the head (hairline, nasolabial, scalp), neck, *palms*

(Figure 205), and *soles*. Condylomata lata (Figure 206): broad-based, sharply defined plaques and flat nodules; erosive and oozing; most commonly in anogenital region and mouth; can be seen on any body surface where moisture can accumulate on intertriginous surfaces, i.e., axillae or toe webs.

HAIR Diffuse, or patchy, "motheaten" alopecia may occur on the scalp and beard area. Loss of eyelashes, lateral third of eyebrows.

MUCOUS MEMBRANES *Mucous patches,* i.e., small, asymptomatic, round or oval, slightly elevated, flat-topped macules and papules 0.5 to 1.0 cm in diameter, covered by hyperkeratotic white-to-gray membrane, occurring on the oral or genital mucosa; *split papules* at the angles of the mouth.

General Examination ±Fever. Generalized lymphadenopathy (cervical, suboccipital, inguinal, epitrochlear, axillary) and splenomegaly.

ASSOCIATED FINDINGS *Diffuse pharyngitis. Acute bacterial iritis. Periostitis* of long bones (nocturnal pain) and arthralgia or hydrarthrosis of knees or ankles without x-ray changes. *Meningovascular reaction* (CSF positive for inflammatory markers). Hepatosplenomegaly, cardiac arrhythmia, nephritis, cystitis, prostatitis, gastritis.

COURSE

In secondary syphilis there may be only one or several recurrent eruptions which appear after month-long asymptomatic intervals. Early secondary syphilis eruptions are macular or maculopapular; late eruptions are papular and tend to be more localized.

SEXUALLY TRANSMITTED DISEASES

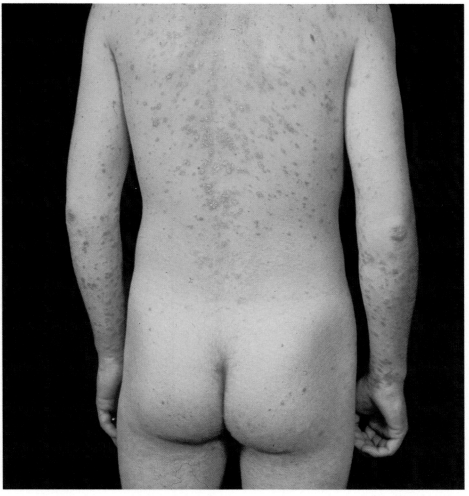

204 Secondary syphilis *Multiple, pinkish-brown to copper-colored macules and papules, occurring in a pityriasis rosea-like pattern on the trunk.*

DIAGNOSIS AND DIFFERENTIAL DIAGNOSIS

Diagnosis Clinical suspicion confirmed by dark-field examination and/or serology. Dark-field is positive in all secondary syphilis lesions except for macular exanthem.

Differential Diagnosis Drug eruption (e.g., captopril), pityriasis rosea, viral exanthem, infectious mononucleosis, tinea corporis, tinea versicolor, scabies, "id" reaction, condylomata acuminata, acute guttate psoriasis, lichen planus

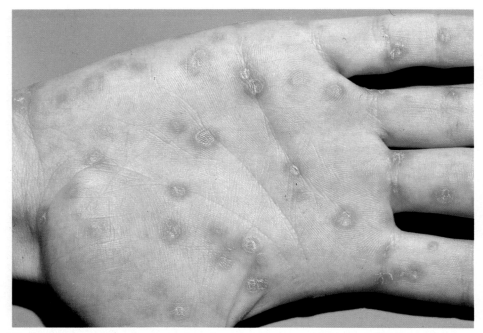

205   Secondary syphilis   *Characteristic palmar involvement with copper-colored, papulosquamous lesions.*

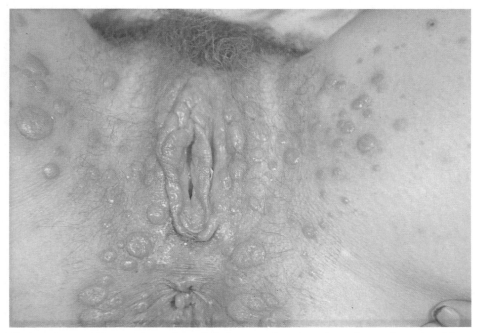

206   Secondary syphilis, condylomata lata   *Soft, flat-topped, moist, red-to-pale papules and nodules arising on the genital and perineal skin.*

COURSE

Latent syphilis is that stage in which there are no clinical signs or symptoms of the infection. The diagnosis is made only after a careful history and physical examination have ruled out symptoms and signs of active infection. The serologic tests for syphilis (STS) are positive; CSF is normal. All patients with syphilis have latent disease at some time during the course of the illness; some patients have only latent stage syphilis and are diagnosed by a positive STS. Latent disease does not preclude infectiousness nor development of gummatous skin lesions, cardiovascular lesions, or neurosyphilis. A pregnant woman with latent disease can infect her fetus.

HISTORY

Duration of Lesions   In *untreated* syphilis 15% of patients develop late benign syphilis, most commonly skin lesions; tertiary syphilis is now very rare. Previously, patients presenting with tertiary syphilis gave history of lesions of 3 to 7 years' duration (range, 2 to 60 years); gumma develop by fifteenth year.

Skin Symptoms   None

PHYSICAL EXAMINATION

Skin Findings

NODULOULCERATIVE SYPHILIDES   Simulates lupus vulgaris (cutaneous tuberculosis)

Type   Plaques and nodules (Figure 207) with scars healed in the center with or without psoriasiform scales and with or without ulceration. Typically, and in contrast to lupus vulgaris, syphilides do not occur in scars but rather on their periphery.

Palpation   Firm and superficial

Arrangement   Serpiginous (snakelike), annular, polycyclic, scalloped borders

Distribution   Solitary isolated lesions: arms (extensor aspects), back, or face

GUMMA   The term *gumma* (Latin, "gum") describes the rubbery lump or deep granulomatous lesion found in the subcutaneous tissue, having a tendency for necrosis and ulceration (Figure 208).

Type   Nodule, with ulceration, "punched out"

Palpation   Firm

Arrangement   Isolated

Distribution   Anywhere, but especially on the scalp, face, chest (sternoclavicular), and calf

General Examination   25% of patients have neurosyphilis or cardiovascular syphilis

DIAGNOSIS AND DIFFERENTIAL DIAGNOSIS

Diagnosis   Clinical findings confirmed by STS and lesional skin biopsy; dark-field examination always negative, silver impregnation of histologic sections for demonstration of spirochetes only very rarely positive.

Differential Diagnosis   Cutaneous tuberculosis, cutaneous atypical mycobacterial infection, malignancy such as lymphoma, deep fungal infections, furuncle

LABORATORY AND SPECIAL EXAMINATIONS

Serologic Tests

PRIMARY SYPHILIS Positive reactions develop in the third to fourth week after infection, or concomitantly and 1 week after appearance of the chancre. Untreated primary syphilis has a positive FTA-ABS and TPHA (*Treponema pallidum* hemagglutination) test (91%) at 6 weeks after infection, compared to VDRL (88%). Cardiolipin tests become nonreactive 1 year after adequate treatment. Specific *Treponema* antigen tests (FTA-ABS, TPHA) usually remain positive at low titers.

SECONDARY SYPHILIS Nontreponemal serologic tests (e.g., VDRL) are always positive (>1:32). FTA-ABS is 99.2% positive, as is TPHA. HIV-infected individual with secondary syphilis rarely may have negative STS. Beware of false-negative STS resulting from *prozone phenomenon* (presence of excess antibody results in failure of the flocculation reaction and thus a false nonreactive test). Nontreponemal serologic tests become nonreactive 24 months after adequate treatment, treponemal serologic tests usually remain reactive.

TERTIARY SYPHILIS STS is usually highly reactive, but false-negative nontreponemal tests are possible.

Note: Testing for HIV infection is advised for all patients with syphilis.

False-Positive Serologic Tests for Syphilis

FALSE-POSITIVE REACTIONS OCCUR WITH FTA-ABS FOR THE FOLLOWING REASONS Technical error, inefficient sorbents, healthy individuals without syphilis, genital herpes simplex, pregnancy, lupus erythematosus (systemic or skin only), alcoholic cirrhosis, scleroderma, mixed connective tissue disease

FALSE-POSITIVE REACTIONS OF NONTREP-ONEMAL TESTS ARE ASSOCIATED WITH THE FOLLOWING *Transient reactors:* technical error (low titer), *Mycoplasma* pneumonia, enterovirus infection, infectious mononucleosis, pregnancy, IVDU, and less common causes (advanced tuberculosis, scarlet fever, viral pneumonia, brucellosis, rat-bite fever, relapsing fever, leptospirosis, measles, mumps, lymphogranuloma venereum, malaria, trypanosomiasis, varicella

Chronic reactors: malaria, leprosy, SLE, IVDU, other connective tissue disorders, elder population, Hashimoto's thyroiditis, rheumatoid arthritis, reticuloendothelial malignancy, familial false-positives, idiopathic

Note: If no history of possible early lesions, or no evidence of congenital syphilis based on patient's history, or no sexual exposure except to individuals who are known to have a negative STS, then diagnosis of false-positive is probably correct.

Dark-Field Examination For spirochetes, obtain tissue fluid (without RBC) from chancre or do a needle aspiration of enlarged regional lymph nodes, or from papulosquamous lesions or condylomata lata of secondary syphilis.

Dermatopathology In primary and secondary syphilis, lesional skin biopsy shows central thinning or ulceration of epidermis. Lymphocytic and *plasmocytic* dermal infiltrate. Proliferation of capillaries and lymphatics with endarteritis; may have thrombosis and small areas of necrosis. Dieterle stain demonstrates spirochetes.

PATHOPHYSIOLOGY

Treponeme invades through mucous membrane or skin and divides locally, with resultant host inflammatory response and chancre

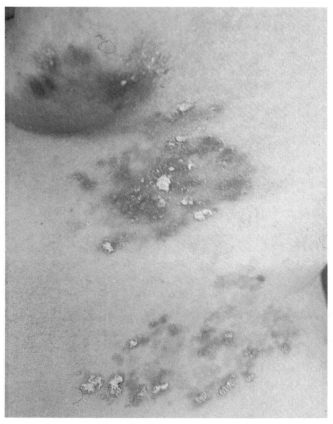

207 Tertiary syphilis *Granulomatous lesions characterized by reddish-brown, translucent papules and nodules becoming confluent.*

formation, either a single lesion or, at times, multiple lesions. Later syphilis is essentially a vascular disease, lesions occurring secondary to obliterative endarteritis of terminal arterioles and small arteries and by the resulting inflammatory and necrotic changes.

COURSE AND PROGNOSIS

Even without treatment, chancre will heal completely within a 4- to 6-week period; the infection either becomes latent or clinical manifestations of secondary syphilis appear. Secondary syphilis usually manifests as macular exanthem initially; after weeks lesions will resolve spontaneously and recur as maculopapular or papular eruptions. In 20% of untreated cases up to 3 to 4 such recurrences followed by periods of clinical remission may occur over a period of 1 year. The infection then enters a latent stage, in which there are no clinical signs or symptoms of the disease. After untreated syphilis has persisted for more than 4 years, it is rarely communicable, except in the case of the pregnant woman, who, if untreated, may transmit syphilis to the fetus, regardless of the duration of her disease. Gumma rarely heal spontaneously. Noduloulcerative syphilides undergo spontaneous partial healing but new lesions appear at the periphery.

TREATMENT

Primary and Secondary Syphilis and Early Latent Syphilis of Less Than 1 Year's Duration

RECOMMENDED REGIMEN Benzathine penicillin G, 2.4 million units IM, in one dose. Some authors advise that the dose should be repeated in 1 week.

ALTERNATIVE REGIMEN FOR PENICILLIN-ALLERGIC PATIENTS (NONPREGNANT)

Doxycycline, 100 mg p.o. b.i.d. for 2 weeks *or*

Tetracycline, 500 mg p.o. q.i.d. for 2 weeks *or*

Erythromycin, 500 mg p.o. q.i.d. for 2 weeks *or*

Ceftriaxone, 250 mg IM once a day for 10 days

JARISCH-HERXHEIMER REACTION An acute febrile reaction, often accompanied by chills, fever, malaise, nausea, headache, myalgia, arthralgia, that may occur after any therapy for syphilis. May occur within hours after treatment, subsiding within 24 hours. More common in patients with early syphilis; developing lesions of secondary syphilis may first appear at this time. Treatment: reassurance, bed rest, aspirin. Pregnant patients should be warned that early labor may occur.

Late Latent Syphilis of More Than 1 Year's Duration, Gummas, and Cardiovascular Syphilis

RECOMMENDED REGIMEN Benzathine penicillin G, 7.2 million units total, administered as 3 doses of 2.4 million units IM, given 1 week apart for 3 consecutive weeks

ALTERNATIVE REGIMEN FOR PENICILLIN-ALLERGIC PATIENTS (NONPREGNANT)

Doxycycline, 100 mg p.o. b.i.d. for 4 weeks *or*

Tetracycline, 500 mg p.o. q.i.d. for 4 weeks

Neurosyphilis

RECOMMENDED REGIMEN Aqueous crystalline penicillin G, 12 to 24 million units administered 2 to 4 million units every 4 hours IV, for 10 to 14 days

ALTERNATIVE REGIMEN (IF OUTPATIENT COMPLIANCE CAN BE ENSURED) Procaine penicillin, 2 to 4 million units IM daily *and* probenecid, 500 mg p.o. q.i.d., both for 10 to 14 days

Syphilis in HIV-Infected Patients
Penicillin regimens should be used whenever possible for all stages of syphilis in HIV-infected patients. Some authorities advise CSF examination and/or treatment with a regimen appro-

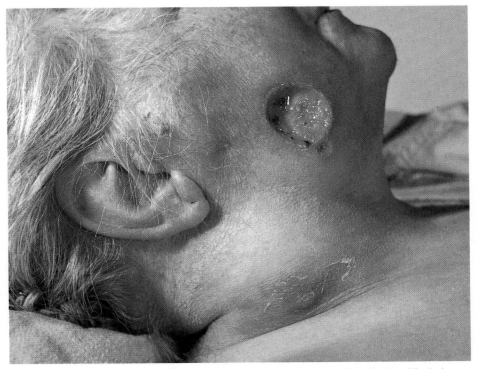

208 Tertiary syphilis (gumma) *Two deeply indurated, red, painless nodular lesions. The lesion on the right cheek has a sharply demarcated, punched-out ulcer with a necrotic base.*

priate for neurosyphilis for all patients coinfected with syphilis and HIV, regardless of the clinical stage of syphilis. Patients should be followed clinically and with quantitative nontreponemal serologic tests (VDRL, RPR) at 1, 2, 3, 6, 9, and 12 months after treatment.

Patients with early syphilis whose titers increase or fail to decrease fourfold within 6 months should undergo CSF examination and be re-treated. In such patients, CSF abnormalities could be due to HIV-related infection, neurosyphilis, or both.

SYPHILIS

Chancroid is an acute, sexually transmitted infection characterized by a painful ulcer at the site of inoculation, usually on the external genitalia, and the development of suppurative regional lymphadenopathy.

Synonyms: soft chancre, ulcus molle, sore sore, chancre mou.

EPIDEMIOLOGY AND ETIOLOGY

Sex Young males. Lymphadenitis more common in males.

Etiology *Hemophilus ducreyi,* a gram-negative streptobacillus

Transmission Most likely during sexual intercourse with partner who has *H. ducreyi* genital ulcer

Geography Uncommon in industrialized nations; microepidemics introduced sporadically from tropical countries. Endemic in tropical and subtropical Third World countries, especially in poor, urban and seaport populations.

HISTORY

Incubation Period 4 to 7 days

Prodrome None

Travel History Sexually active during visit to country where chancroid is endemic. Possible contact with prostitute.

PHYSICAL EXAMINATION

Skin Findings
TYPE OF LESION Primary lesion: tender papule with erythematous halo which evolves to pustule, erosion, and ulcer. Ulcer is usually quite *tender or painful*. Its borders are sharp, undermined, and *not* indurated (Figure 209). Its base is friable with granulation tissue and covered with gray-to-yellow exudate. Edema of prepuce common.
SHAPE OF INDIVIDUAL LESION Ulcer may be singular or multiple, merging to form large or giant ulcers (>2.0 cm) with a serpiginous shape.
DISTRIBUTION OF LESIONS Multiple ulcers (Figure 210) develop by autoinoculation. *Male:* prepuce, frenulum, coronal sulcus, glans, shaft. *Female:* fourchette, labia, vestibule, clitoris, vaginal wall by direct extension from introitus, cervix, or perianal. Extragenital lesions: breast, fingers, thighs, oral mucosa.

General Examination *Painful* inguinal lymphadenitis (usually unilateral) occurs in 50% of patients 1 to 2 weeks after primary lesion. Buboes occur with overlying erythema and may drain spontaneously.

DIAGNOSIS AND DIFFERENTIAL DIAGNOSIS

Diagnosis Made clinically by excluding other causes of genital ulcer or bubo.

Differential Diagnosis *Genital ulcer:* genital herpes, syphilis, donovanosis, lymphogranuloma venereum, secondarily infected human bites or traumatic lesions. *Tender inguinal mass:* incarcerated hernia, plaque, tularemia

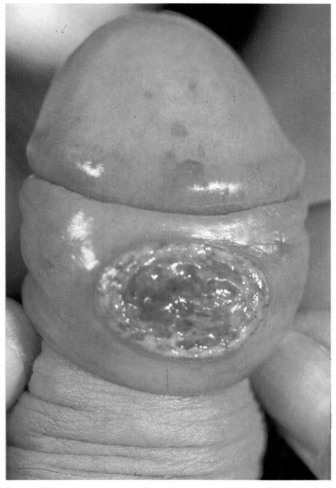

209 Chancroid *Tender, eroded nodule with marked surrounding erythema and edema. (Courtesy of Alfred Eichmann, M.D.)*

LABORATORY AND SPECIAL EXAMINATIONS

Gram's Stain Of scrapings from ulcer base or pus from bubo, attempt to see small clusters or parallel chains of gram-negative rods. Interpretation difficult due to presence of contaminating organisms in ulcers.

Culture Special growth requirements, isolation difficult.

Serologic Tests None available

Dermatopathology May be helpful. Organism rarely demonstrated.

PATHOPHYSIOLOGY

Poorly studied. *H. ducreyi* is inoculated through small breaks in the epidermis or mucosa. Primary infection develops at the site of inoculation followed by lymphadenitis. Bubo formation occurs with scant organisms and an exuberant acute inflammatory response. The role of the immune response is unknown.

COURSE AND PROGNOSIS

Chancroidal ulcers show symptomatic and objective improvement within 7 days after institution of therapy; clinical resolution of lymphadenopathy is slower. Because coexisting syphilis occurs in 10 to 15% of patients, STS is advisable within 3 months of therapy.

TREATMENT

Recommended Regimen
Erythromycin 500 mg p.o. q.i.d. for 10 days *or*

Ceftriaxone 250 mg IM in a single dose

Alternative Regimen
Trimethoprim/sulfamethoxazole 160/800 mg p.o. b.i.d. for 7 days *or*

Amoxicillin 500 mg plus clavulinic acid 125 mg p.o. t.i.d. for 7 days *or*

Ciprofloxacin 500 mg p.o. b.i.d. for 3 days

SEXUALLY TRANSMITTED DISEASES

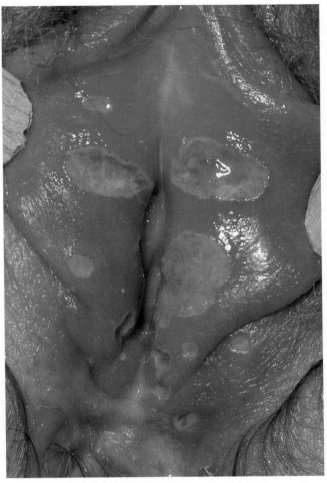

210   Chancroid   *Multiple, painful ulcers occurring by autoinoculation on the vulva.*

Donovanosis is a chronic progressively destructive bacterial infection of the genital region, characterized by ulceration and epitheliomatous hyperplasia.

Synonyms: granuloma inguinale, granuloma venereum.

EPIDEMIOLOGY AND ETIOLOGY

Sex Young males

Etiology *Calymmatobacterium granulomatis,* an encapsulated gram-negative rod

Transmission Mildly contagious. Repeated exposure necessary for clinical infection to occur. In most cases lesions cannot be detected in sexual contacts.

Geography Endemic foci in tropical and subtropical environments (India, Caribbean, Africa, aborigines in Australia). Rare in United States, Canada, Europe.

HISTORY

Incubation Period 8 to 80 days

Travel History Sexual exposure in endemic area

History Genital ulcers are relatively painless.

PHYSICAL EXAMINATION

Skin Findings
TYPE OF LESION Primary lesion: buttonlike papule (Figure 211) or subcutaneous nodule which ulcerates within a few days. Ulcers have beefy-red granulation tissue base with sharply defined edges. Fibrosis occurs concurrently with extension of ulcer. Lymph-

edema may follow with elephantiasis of penis, scrotum, vulva.
DISTRIBUTION OF LESIONS *Males* Prepuce or glans, penile shaft, scrotum
Females Labia minora, mons veneris, fourchette. Ulcerations then spread by direct extension or autoinoculation to inguinal and perineal skin. Extragenital lesions occur in mouth, lips, throat, face, GI tract, and bone.
VARIANTS *Ulcerovegetative* Develops from the nodular variant; large, spreading, exuberant ulcers (Figure 212)
Nodular Soft, red nodules which eventually ulcerate with bright-red granulating bases
Hypertrophic Proliferative reaction; formation of large vegetating masses
Cicatricial Spreading scar tissue formation associated with spread of infection
LATE SEQUELA Squamous cell carcinoma of genital skin

General Examination Regional lymph node enlargement is uncommon. Large subcutaneous nodule may mimic an inflamed lymph node, i.e., pseudobubo.

DIAGNOSIS AND DIFFERENTIAL DIAGNOSIS

Diagnosis Clinical diagnosis excluding other causes of genital ulcer(s) using touch preparation of biopsied tissue.

Differential Diagnosis *Genital ulcer(s):* chronic herpetic ulcer, syphilitic chancre, chancroid, lymphogranuloma venereum, cuta-

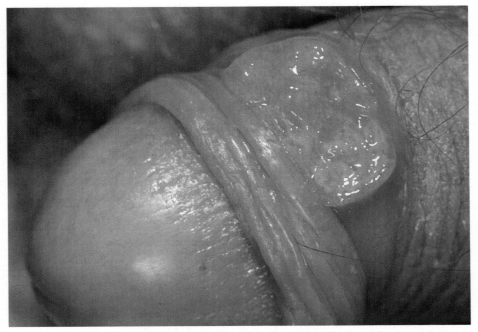

211 Donovanosis *A buttonlike papule with central ulceration, a beefy-red base, and a sharply demarcated margin. (Courtesy of Alfred Eichmann, M.D.)*

neous tuberculosis, cutaneous amebiasis, filariasis, squamous cell carcinoma. *Perianal hypertrophic donovanosis:* condylomata acuminata, condylomata lata

LABORATORY AND SPECIAL EXAMINATIONS

Touch or Crush Preparation Punch biopsy stained with Wright's or Giemsa's stain shows Donovan bodies in cytoplasm of macrophages. Clinical variants differ in quantity of organisms.

Dermatopathology Extensive acanthosis and dense dermal infiltrate, mainly plasma cells and histiocytes. Large mononuclear cells containing cytoplasmic inclusions (Donovan bodies), i.e., *C. granulomatis,* are pathognomonic.

Serology STS to rule out syphilis

COURSE AND PROGNOSIS

Little tendency toward spontaneous healing. Following antibiotic treatment, lesions often heal with depigmentation of reepithelialized skin.

TREATMENT

Most Effective Chloramphenicol 500 mg p.o. q8h *or* gentamicin 1 mg per kg body weight IV b.i.d. Tetracycline 500 mg p.o. q.i.d. for 3 to 4 weeks (until ulcers have healed).

Alternatives Streptomycin 1 g b.i.d. IM. Ampicillin 500 mg p.o. q.i.d. for up to 12 weeks. Erythromycin 500 mg p.o. q.i.d. Co-trimoxazole 2 tablets p.o. q12h for 10 days.

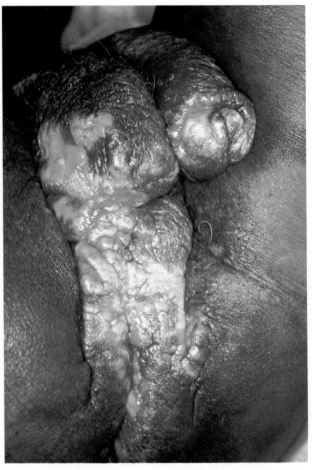

212   Donovanosis, ulcerovegetative type   *Extensive granulation tissue formation, ulceration, and scarring of the perineal and genital skin.*

Lymphogranuloma Venereum

Lymphogranuloma venereum (LGV) is a sexually transmitted infection manifested by an infrequent primary genital lesion, secondary lymphadenitis with bubo formation and/or proctitis, and late infrequent sequelae of fibrosis, edema, and fistula formation.

Synonym: lymphogranuloma inguinale.

EPIDEMIOLOGY AND ETIOLOGY

Age Third decade

Race Most cases in nonwhites; however, probably no true racial difference.

Sex Acute infection much more common in males. Anorectal syndrome more common in women and homosexual men.

Etiology *Chlamydia trachomatis,* immunotypes or serovars L_1, L_2, L_3

Transmission *Chlamydia* in purulent exudate is inoculated onto the skin or mucosa of a sexual partner and gains entry through minute lacerations and abrasions.

Geography Sporadic in North America, Europe, Australia, and most of Asia and South America. Endemic in east and west Africa, India, parts of southeastern Asia, South America, and the Caribbean.

HISTORY

Incubation Period 3 to 12 days or longer for primary stage; 10 to 30 days (but up to 6 months) for secondary stage.

Travel History In North America and Europe, most cases occur in patients who have traveled to endemic areas where they were sexually active.

History
PRIMARY STAGE Painless herpetiform abrasion or ulceration
SECONDARY STAGE *Inguinal Syndrome* Constitutional symptoms (fever, malaise) associated with inguinal buboes. Severe local pain in buboes. Lower abdominal and back pain.
Anogenitorectal Syndrome Anal pruritus, rectal discharge, fever, rectal pain, tenesmus, constipation, "pencil" stools, weight loss

PHYSICAL EXAMINATION

Skin Findings
PRIMARY STAGE *Type of Lesion* Papule, shallow erosion, or ulcer, grouped small erosions or ulcers (herpetiform), or nonspecific urethritis. In males, cordlike lymphangitis of dorsal penis may follow. Lymphangial nodule (bubonulus) may occur (Figure 213). Bubonuli may rupture, resulting in sinuses and fistulae of urethra and deforming scars of penis. In females cervicitis, perimetritis, salpingitis may occur.
Distribution of Lesions At the site of inoculation. *Males:* coronal sulcus, frenum, prepuce, penis, urethra, glans, scrotum. *Females:* posterior vaginal wall, fourchette, posterior lip of cervix, vulva. When primary lesion occurs intraurethrally, presentation is of a nonspecific urethritis with a thin, mucopurulent discharge.
Other Erythema nodosum in 10% of cases.

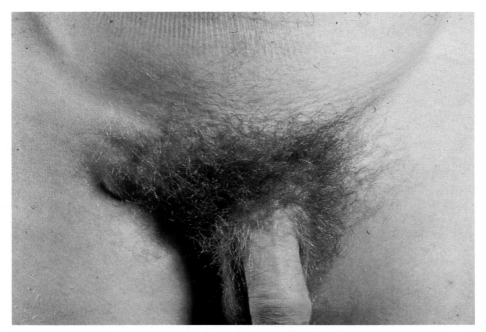

213 Lymphogranuloma venereum *Marked, tender, lymphadenopathy occurring in the femoral and inguinal lymph nodes separated by a groove made by Poupart's ligament ("groove" sign).*

Erythema multiforme, scarlatiniform eruptions, urticaria. Primary inoculation of mouth or pharynx results in lymphadenitis of submaxillary or cervical lymph nodes.

SECONDARY STAGE *Inguinal Syndrome* Unilateral bubo in two-thirds of cases. Marked edema and erythema of skin overlying node. One-third of inguinal buboes rupture; two-thirds slowly involute. "Groove" sign: inflammatory mass of femoral and inguinal nodes separated by depression or groove made by Poupart's ligament (Figure 213). 75% of cases have deep iliac node involvement with a pelvic mass which seldom suppurates.

Anogenitorectal Syndrome Proctocolitis, hyperplasia of intestinal and perirectal lymphatic tissue. Resultant perirectal abscesses, ischiorectal and rectovaginal fistulas, anal fistulas, rectal stricture. Overgrowth of lymphatic tissue results in lymphorrhoids (resembling hemorrhoids) or perianal condylomata.

Esthiomene Elephantiasis of vulva, which may ulcerate, occurring 1 to 20 years after primary infection.

General Examination

ANOGENITORECTAL SYNDROME Lower abdominal tenderness, pelvic colon thickened, enlarged perirectal nodes.

DIAGNOSIS AND DIFFERENTIAL DIAGNOSIS

Diagnosis By serologic tests or histologic identification of *Chlamydia* on biopsy

Differential Diagnosis

PRIMARY STAGE Genital herpes, primary syphilis, chancroid

INGUINAL SYNDROME Incarcerated inguinal hernia, plague, tularemia, tuberculosis, genital herpes, syphilis, chancroid, Hodgkin's disease

ANOGENITORECTAL SYNDROME Rectal stricture caused by rectal cancer, trauma, actinomycosis, tuberculosis, schistosomiasis

ESTHIOMENE Filariasis, mycosis

LABORATORY AND SPECIAL EXAMINATIONS

Frei Skin Test Of historical interest only. Positive delayed hypersensitivity to standardized antigen Lygranum indicates past or present infection. Positive 2 to 8 weeks after infection begins. Frei antigen is common to all *Chlamydia*. Positive test is not diagnostic of LGV.

Serologic Tests Complement-fixation (CF) test more sensitive and reactive earlier than Frei test. Active LGV usually has titer $\geq 1:64$. Microimmunofluorescence test most sensitive and specific test, identifying infecting serovar.

Culture *C. trachomatis* can be cultured on tissue-culture cell lines in up to 30% of cases.

Dermatopathology Not pathognomonic. *Primary stage:* small stellate abscesses surrounded by histiocytes, arranged in palisade pattern. *Late stage:* epidermal acanthosis/papillomatosis; dermis edematous, lymphatics dilated with fibrosis and lymphoplasmocytic infiltrate

PATHOPHYSIOLOGY

Primarily an infection of lymphatics and lymph nodes. Lymphangitis and lymphadenitis occur in drainage field of the inoculation site with subsequent perilymphangitis and periadenitis. Necrosis occurs and loculated abscesses, fistulas, and sinus tracts develop. As the infection subsides, fibrosis replaces acute inflammation with resultant obliteration of lymphatic drainage, chronic edema, and stricture. Inoculation site determines affected lymph nodes: penis, anterior urethra—superficial, deep inguinal; posterior urethra—deep iliac, perirectal; vulva—inguinal; vagina, cervix—deep iliac, perirectal, retrocrural, lumbosacral; anus—inguinal; rectum—perirectal, deep iliac

COURSE AND PROGNOSIS

Natural history is highly variable. Spontaneous remission is common.

TREATMENT

Drug of Choice

Doxycycline 100 mg p.o. b.i.d. for 21 days

Alternatives

Tetracycline 500 mg p.o. q.i.d. for 21 days *or*

Erythromycin 500 mg p.o. q.i.d. for 21 days *or*

Sulfisoxazole 500 mg p.o. q.i.d. for 21 days or equivalent sulfonamide course

Genital warts are soft, skin-colored, fleshy warts occurring on anogenital or oral mucosa or skin, resulting from infection by a human papillomavirus (HPV).

Synonyms: condyloma acuminatum, acuminate or venereal wart, verruca acuminata.

EPIDEMIOLOGY AND ETIOLOGY

Age Predominantly young sexually active adults

Etiology HPV, a DNA papovavirus which multiplies in nucleus of infected epithelial cells: types 6, 11 most common ''low-risk'' oncogenic types; also types 16, 18, 31, 33

Transmission Contagious, nonsexually and sexually transmitted. 90 to 100% of partners of infected females acquire HPV infection. In infants and children, HPV may be acquired during delivery.

Incidence Increased manyfold during the past two decades. Prevalence of HPV infection in women ranges from 3 to 28%, depending on the population studied.

HISTORY

Incubation Period Several weeks to months to years

Duration of Lesions Months to years

Skin Symptoms Usually asymptomatic. In infants and children, genital warts may be a marker for sexual abuse, although much less commonly so than initially thought.

PHYSICAL FINDINGS

Skin Lesions
TYPE Pinhead papules to cauliflower-like masses (Figure 214). May be subclinical on penis or vulva, visible only with aceto-whitening.
COLOR Skin colored, pink, or red
PALPATION Soft
SHAPE Filiform, sessile (especially on penis)
DISTRIBUTION Rarely solitary lesions, usually clusters
ARRANGEMENT May be solitary. Grouped into grapelike or cauliflower-like cluster. Perianal cauliflower lesions may be size of walnut to apple.
SITES OF PREDILECTION *Male* Frenulum, corona, glans, prepuce, shaft, scrotum
Female Labia (Figure 215), clitoris, periurethral area, perineum, vagina, cervix (flat lesions)
Both Sexes Perineal, perianal (Figure 216), anal canal, rectal; urethral meatus, urethra, bladder; oral

DIAGNOSIS AND DIFFERENTIAL DIAGNOSIS

Diagnosis Clinical diagnosis, occasionally confirmed by biopsy

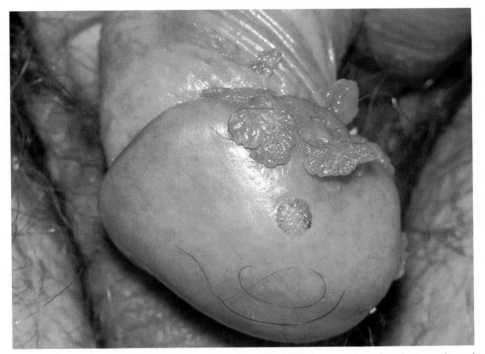

214 Condylomata acuminata *This is a soft, elongated, filiform mass on the glans penis and preputium.*

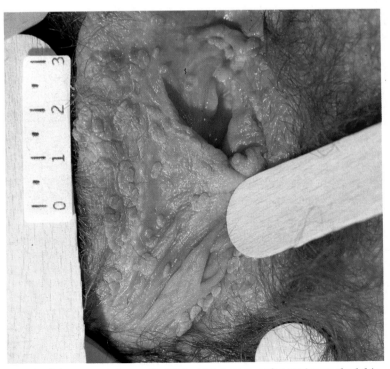

215 Condylomata acuminata *Multiple, pink-brown, soft papules on the labia.*

Differential Diagnosis Condylomata lata, intraepithelial neoplasia (bowenoid papulosis), invasive squamous cell carcinoma, molluscum contagiosum, lichen nitidus, lichen planus, normal sebaceous glands, angiokeratoma, pearly penile papules, folliculitis, moles, seborrheic keratoses, skin tags, pilar cyst, scabetic nodules

LABORATORY AND SPECIAL EXAMINATIONS

Acetowhitening Subclinical lesions can be visualized by wrapping the penis with gauze soaked with 5% acetic acid for 5 minutes. Using a 10x hand lens or colposcope, warts appear as tiny white papules.

STS Negative

COURSE AND PROGNOSIS

Condylomata recur even after appropriate therapy in a high percentage of patients due to persistence of latent HPV in normal-appearing perilesional skin. The major significance of HPV infection is the risk for malignancy. HPV types 16, 18, 31, and 33 are the major etiologic factors for cervical dysplasia and cervical squamous cell carcinoma, invasive carcinoma of both the vulva and penis, anal squamous cell carcinoma of homosexual/bisexual males. The importance of the annual Pap test must be stressed to women with genital warts.

Children delivered vaginally of mothers with genital HPV infection are at risk for developing anogenital condylomata and recurrent respiratory papillomatosis in later life.

TREATMENT

External Genital/Perianal Warts
RECOMMENDED REGIMEN Cryosurgery with liquid nitrogen.
ALTERNATIVE REGIMEN

Podophyllin (10 to 25%) in compound tincture of benzoin. Limit the total volume of podophyllin solution applied to <0.5 mL per treatment session. Thoroughly wash off in 1 to 4 hours. Treat <10 cm^2 per session. Repeat applications twice a week. Podofilox is less toxic and can be used for self-treatment. Mucosal warts are more likely to respond than highly keratinized warts on the penile shaft, buttocks, and pubic areas. *Contraindicated in pregnancy.*

Trichloracetic acid (80 to 90%). Apply only to warts; powder with talc or sodium bicarbonate (baking soda) to remove unreacted acid. Repeat application at weekly intervals.

Electrodesiccation/electrocautery; laser surgery. Highly effective in destruction of infected tissue and HPV. Should be attempted only by clinicians trained in the use of this modality. Electrodesiccation is contraindicated in patients with cardiac pacemakers.

Intralesional interferon is currently being used on an experimental basis.

URETHRAL MEATUS WARTS Cryosurgery, laser surgery. Alternative: podophyllin applied to dried mucosa; wash off in 1 to 2 hours; *or* 5-fluorouracil cream
ANAL WARTS Cryosurgery. Alternatives: trichloracetic acid (80 to 90%); surgical removal
ORAL WARTS Cryosurgery. Alternatives: electrodesiccation/electrocautery; surgical removal, laser surgery

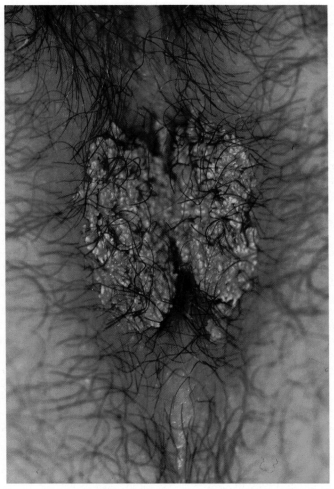

216 Condylomata acuminata *Cauliflower-like mass occurring on the perianal skin.*

Intraepithelial neoplasia (IN) of the anogenital skin is characterized by multifocal benign-appearing maculopapular lesions occurring on the mucosa and anogenital and crural skin, exhibiting histologic changes of squamous cell carcinoma in situ, but following a largely benign clinical course.

Synonyms: bowenoid papulosis, vulvar intraepithelial neoplasia, penile intraepithelial neoplasm, squamous intraepithelial neoplasia.

EPIDEMIOLOGY AND ETIOLOGY

Age Third and fourth decades

Etiology HPV 16, 18, 31, 33, i.e., "high-risk" oncogenic types

Transmission HPV transmitted sexually. Autoinoculation. Rarely, HPV 16 transmitted from mother to newborn, with subsequent development of bowenoid papulosis (BP) on penis.

Incidence Marked increase during past two decades associated with increased sexual promiscuity.

Risk Factors HIV-infected individuals are at increased risk of developing IN, as well as invasive squamous cell carcinoma.

HISTORY

Duration of Lesions Weeks to months to years to decades

Incubation Period Months to years

Systems Review Prior history of condylomata acuminata. Female partners of males may have cervical intraepithelial neoplasia (CIN)

Skin Findings

TYPE OF LESION Erythematous macules. Lichenoid (flat-topped) or pigmented papules (several millimeters); may show some confluence or form plaque(s). Leukoplakia-like plaque. Surface usually smooth, velvety.

COLOR Tan, brown, pink, red, violaceous, white

ARRANGEMENT Characteristically clusters (multifocal). May be solitary

DISTRIBUTION OF LESIONS *Males:* glans penis, prepuce (75%) (flat lichenoid papules or erythematous macules); penile shaft (25%) (pigmented papules) (Figure 217). *Females:* labia majora and minora (Figure 218), clitoris. *Both sexes:* inguinal folds, perineal/perianal skin (Figure 219).

ACETOWHITENING Application of 3 to 5% acetic acid to the area of involvement for 5 minutes may facilitate visualization of lesions.

OTHER May be associated with cervical dysplasia, cervical intraepithelial neoplasia, cervical squamous cell carcinoma. Rarely, IN of other sites, i.e., periungual, intraoral

DIAGNOSIS AND DIFFERENTIAL DIAGNOSIS

Diagnosis Clinical suspicion confirmed by lesional biopsy

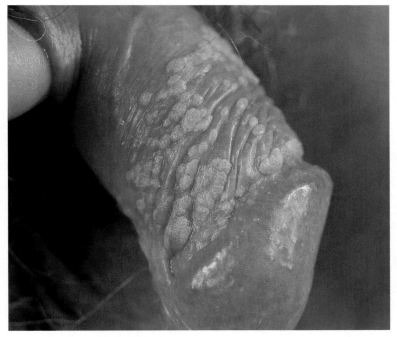

217 Penile intraepithelial neoplasia *Pink, flat-topped, confluent papules which may be clinically indistinguishable from condylomata acuminata, which at times may evolve into an invasive squamous cell carcinoma.*

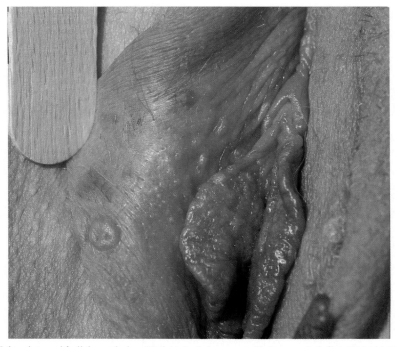

218 Vulvar intraepithelial neoplasia *Pink to dark-brown, well-demarcated, flat-topped papules on the vulva. These may progress to invasive squamous cell carcinoma.*

INTRAEPITHELIAL NEOPLASIA OF THE ANOGENITAL SKIN 407

Differential Diagnosis Psoriasis vulgaris; lichen planus; condylomata acuminata; angiokeratomas; extramammary Paget's disease; Bowen's disease, i.e., squamous cell carcinoma in situ (occurs as single lesion in older individual rather than as multiple lesions in younger person).

LABORATORY AND SPECIAL EXAMINATIONS

Dermatopathology Epidermal proliferation with numerous mitotic figures, abnormal mitoses, atypical pleomorphic cells with large hyperchromatic, often clumped, nuclei, dyskeratotic cells; basal membrane intact. ±Koilocytosis. Recent application of podophyllin to condyloma acuminatum may cause changes similar to IN.

Southern Blot Analysis Identifies HPV type

Pap Smear Koilocytotic atypia

COURSE AND PROGNOSIS

May resolve spontaneously. May persist for many years with the appearance of multiple new lesions. May rarely progress to invasive squamous cell carcinoma ± metastasis. Patients must be carefully followed, especially females.

TREATMENT

Current therapeutic options less than optimal: surgical excision, Mohs' surgery, electrosurgery, carbon dioxide laser vaporization, cryosurgery, topical 5-fluorouracil

SEXUALLY TRANSMITTED DISEASES

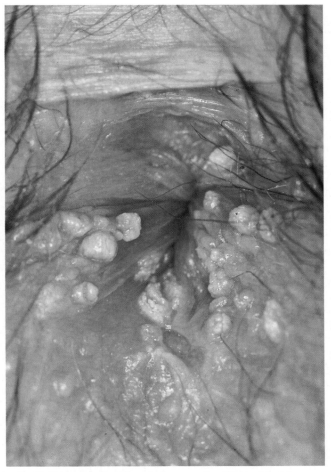

219   Perianal intraepithelial neoplasia   *These lesions can be distinguished from condylomata lata by biopsy and may also evolve to invasive anal carcinoma*

Genital Herpes Simplex

Genital herpes simplex is a sexually transmitted viral infection, characterized by primary infection with grouped vesicles at the site of inoculation and regional lymphadenopathy, and a course of recurring outbreaks of vesicles at the same site.

Synonyms: herpes progenitalis, herpes genitalis.

EPIDEMIOLOGY AND ETIOLOGY

Age   Young sexually active adults

Etiology   Herpes simplex virus (HSV) type 2 >> type 1. The presence of antibodies to HSV type 2 varies with the sexual history of the individual: nuns, 3%; middle class, 25%; heterosexuals at an STD clinic, 26%; homosexuals, 46%; lower classes 46 to 60%; prostitutes, 70 to 80%.

Transmission   Usually skin-to-skin contact

HISTORY

Incubation Period   2 to 20 days (average, 6 days)

Systems Review

PRIMARY GENITAL HERPES   May be accompanied by fever, headache, malaise, myalgia, peaking within the first 3 to 4 days after onset of lesions, resolving during the subsequent 3 to 4 days. Depending on location, pain, itching, dysuria, vaginal or urethral discharge are common symptoms. Tender inguinal lymphadenopathy occurs during second and third week. Deep pelvic pain associated with pelvic lymphadenopathy.

RECURRENT GENITAL HERPES   Prodrome of burning or itching sensation prior to eruption of vesicles

PHYSICAL EXAMINATION

Skin Findings

TYPE   *Primary Genital Herpes*   An erythematous papule is often noted initially, followed soon by grouped vesicles, which may evolve to pustules; these become eroded as the overlying epidermis sloughs. Erosions may enlarge to ulcerations, which may be crusted or moist. These epithelial defects heal in 2 to 4 weeks, often with resultant postinflammatory hypo- or hyperpigmentation, uncommonly with scarring. The area of involvement may be circumferential around the penis, or the entire vulva may be involved.

Recurrent Genital Herpes   Lesions similar to primary infection but on a reduced scale (Figure 220). Often a 1- to 2-cm plaque of erythema surmounted with vesicles. Heals in 1 to 2 weeks.

ARRANGEMENT   Herpetiform, i.e., grouped vesicles/erosions

DISTRIBUTION   *Males*   Primary infection: glans, prepuce, shaft, sulcus; scrotum, thigh, sacral region, buttocks. Recurrences: penile shaft.

Females   Primary infection: labia majora/minora (Figure 221), perineum, inner thighs. Recurrences: labia majora/minora

Anorectal infection   Occurs in male homosexuals (often HSV-1); characterized by tenesmus, anal pain, proctitis, discharge, and ulcerations as far as 10 cm into anal canal.

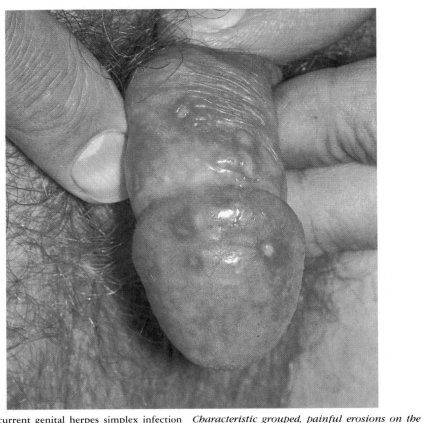

220 Recurrent genital herpes simplex infection *Characteristic grouped, painful erosions on the*
glans penis and foreskin. *glans penis and foreskin.*

General Findings Inguinal/femoral lymph nodes enlarged, firm, nonfluctuant, tender; usually unilateral. Signs of aseptic meningitis: headache, fever, nuchal rigidity, CSF pleocytosis with normal sugar content, and positive HSV CSF culture.

DIAGNOSIS AND DIFFERENTIAL DIAGNOSIS

Diagnosis Clinical suspicion confirmed by Tzanck test (acantholytic giant cells)

Differential Diagnosis Syphilitic chancre, fixed drug eruption, chancroid, gonococcal erosion, folliculitis, pemphigus, pemphigoid

LABORATORY AND SPECIAL EXAMINATIONS

Tzanck Test Optimally, fluid from intact vesicle is smeared thinly on a microscope slide, dried, and stained with either Wright's or Giemsa's stain. Positive if giant acanthocytes or multinucleated giant acanthocytes are detected. Positive in 75% of early cases, either primary or recurrent. (See Figure 37.)

Dermatopathology Ballooning and reticular epidermal degeneration, acanthosis and intraepidermal vesicles; intranuclear inclusion bodies, multinucleate giant acanthocytes; multilocular vesicles.

Viral Culture Documents the presence of HSV in 1 to 10 days.

Serology STS to rule out syphilis. Primary infection can be documented by obtaining acute and convalescent sera which show seroconversion for HSV antibodies. They also indicate whether HSV is type 1 or 2. In a patient with recurrent genital lesions, genital herpes can be ruled out if HSV antibodies are absent.

PATHOPHYSIOLOGY

Transmission of and infection with HSV occurs through close contact with a person shedding virus at a peripheral site or mucosal surface, or as a secretion. HSV is inactivated promptly at room temperature; spread by aerosol or fomites is unlikely. Infection occurs via inoculation onto susceptible mucosal surface or break in skin. Subsequent to primary infection at inoculation site, HSV ascends peripheral sensory nerves and enters sensory or autonomic nerve root ganglia, where latency is established. Latency can occur after both symptomatic and asymptomatic primary infection. Recrudescences may be clinically symptomatic or asymptomatic.

COURSE AND PROGNOSIS

As many as 50 to 70% of HSV-2 infections are asymptomatic. From 50 to 80% of patients with HSV-2 infections experience recurrence(s) in 1 year: 2% have monthly outbreaks, 13% every 2 to 11 months, 24% yearly or less often. Erythema multiforme may complicate genital herpes, occurring 1 to 2 weeks after an outbreak.

TREATMENT

First Clinical Episode of Genital Herpes
Acyclovir 400 mg p.o. 3 times a day for 7 to 10 days or until clinical resolution occurs.

First Clinical Episode of Herpes Proctitis Acyclovir 400 mg p.o. 5 times a day for 10 days or until clinical resolution occurs.

Inpatient Therapy For patients with severe disease or complications necessitating hospitalization: acyclovir 5 mg per kg body weight IV every 8 hours for 5 to 7 days or until clinical resolution occurs.

Recurrent Episodes In recurrent disease, some patients who start therapy at the beginning of the prodrome or within 2 days after onset of lesions may benefit from therapy, although this has not been proved.

> Acyclovir 400 mg p.o. 3 times a day for 5 days

Daily Suppressive Therapy for Recurrent Disease Daily treatment reduces frequency of recurrences by at least 75% among patients with frequent (more than 6 per year) recurrences. After 1 year of continuous daily suppressive therapy, acyclovir should be discontinued so that the patient's recurrence rate may be reassessed.

> Acyclovir 400 mg p.o. b.i.d.

Acyclovir for Treating Pregnant Patients As there is a high neonatal morbidity and mortality, women with a history of genital herpes who are asymptomatic at the onset of labor should be advised that the risk of exposure to excretion of HSV is low and that even if inadvertent exposure does occur, the risk that their neonate will acquire HSV infection is less than 8%. This risk can be weighed against the maternal and neonatal morbidity and the increased cost of childbirth associated with cesarean delivery. Viral cultures should be taken at weekly intervals in the final 2 months of pregnancy. If, however, a woman is experiencing her primary HSV genital infection around the time of delivery, the risk that her neonate will acquire an HSV infection is likely to be substantially higher. In this circumstance, a cesarean delivery is prob-

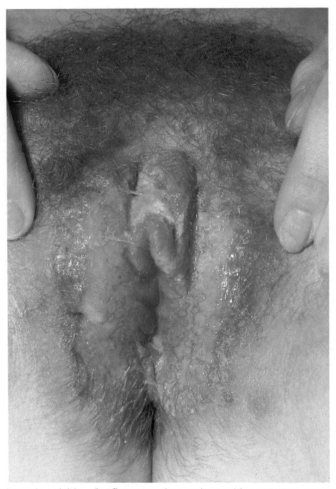

221　Primary herpetic vulvitis　*Confluent, tender erosions with exudation associated with very painful inguinal lymphadenopathy.*

ably prudent. The safety of systemic acyclovir therapy among pregnant women has not been established. Among pregnant women without life-threatening disease, systemic acyclovir treatment *should not* be used for recurrent genital herpes episodes or as suppressive therapy to prevent reactivation near term.

Genital Herpes Among HIV-Infected Patients　Neither the need for nor the proper increased dosage of acyclovir has been conclusively established. Patients with genital herpes who do not respond to the recommended dose of acyclovir may require a higher oral dose of acyclovir, IV acyclovir, or they may be infected with a resistant HSV strain, requiring IV foscarnet (side effects: genital ulcerations).

Mucocutaneous Manifestations of Human Immunodeficiency Virus (HIV) Disease

Mucocutaneous Findings in HIV Disease

The onset in 1981 of the human immunodeficiency virus (HIV) epidemic with its endstage, acquired immunodeficiency syndrome (AIDS), has profoundly changed the scope of dermatology, both for the patient and the practitioner. As of mid-1990, estimates are that about 1,500,000 individuals in the United States are HIV-infected, of which 140,000 have AIDS. More than 75,000 patients have already died of the disease. The majority of cases of HIV infection in the United States are yet to be diagnosed. The tally of the number of HIV-infected individuals and of those with AIDS in Western Europe is smaller than that in the United States but is rising steadily. Even more alarming are the statistics from West Africa where 20% of the population is HIV-infected in some countries. Worldwide, the number of cases of AIDS is currently over 600,000. It is estimated by the World Heath Organization that at least 3 million women and children will die of HIV disease during the 1990s. Nearly all HIV-infected individuals have some dermatologic problem attributable to the progressive immunodeficiency during the course of the disease.

Early diagnosis is critical in the management of HIV disease for several reasons, and cutaneous findings often raise the possibility of HIV infection. Findings such as epidemic Kaposi's sarcoma, oral hairy leukoplakia, multiple facial mollusca contagiosa, and bacillary angiomatosis are essentially pathognomonic of HIV disease. Other findings, such as herpetic infection, herpes zoster, dermatophytoses, and many others occur with increased severity in HIV disease, and their detection should raise the issue of HIV testing. In the 1990s, any patient presenting with a sexually transmitted disease should be tested serologically for syphilis as well as HIV infection.

Given the knowledge that they are HIV-infected and potentially contagious, most patients will reduce or eliminate behavior associated with transmission of HIV. Effective antiretroviral drugs such as zidovudine retard progression of HIV-induced immunodeficiency and can be prescribed to those identified as HIV-infected. Many of the opportunistic infections such as *Pneumocystis carinii* pneumonia (PCP) which plague HIV-infected patients are better treated by primary prophylactic regimens prior to development of clinical disease. Some dermatologic disorders such as psoriasis vulgaris in the HIV-infected patient are less responsive than would be anticipated to ordinary therapeutic regimens. The HIV-infected patient with psoriasis may improve if treated with zidovudine; however, Kaposi's sarcoma may occur if the patient is treated with methotrexate. (See page 419 for CDC Classification of HIV Infections.)

Primary Human Immunodeficiency Virus Infection

Primary human immunodeficiency virus (HIV) infection, when symptomatic, is characterized by an infectious mononucleosis-like syndrome or aseptic meningitis syndrome with fever, lymphadenopathy, meningitis, GI symptoms, and skin findings either of an infectious exanthem or urticaria.

EPIDEMIOLOGY AND ETIOLOGY

Age Commonly young, but any age from intrauterine to senescence

Sex Initially, in the United States and Europe, much more common in males due to male-male sexual intercourse; currently, incidence in females increasing due to heterosexual transmission. In Africa, nearly equal incidence in sexes due to pattern of male-female sexual transmission.

Etiology Nearly all cases in United States and Western Europe caused by HIV-1; some cases in West Africa caused by HIV-2.

Transmission and Risk Factors Sexual exposure, homosexual >> heterosexual in developed countries but may be equal in Africa; IVDUs; recipients of blood or blood products after 1978 but before 1985; child born to mother with HIV infection, i.e., intrauterine, during birthing, or by breast feeding

Geography Worldwide epidemic with many cases in United States, South America, Europe, Australia, and Africa

HISTORY

Incubation Period 3 to 6 weeks (from presumed exposure to development of acute febrile illness); varies according to route and size of virus inoculation. 10 to 20% of recently infected individuals experience symptomatic primary infection.

History Most patients are asymptomatic. Fever, rigors, malaise, lethargy, arthralgias, myalgias, lasting 2 to 3 weeks. Also, abdominal cramps, diarrhea, headache, stiff neck, photophobia.

PHYSICAL EXAMINATION

Skin Findings
TYPE OF LESION Urticaria. Maculopapular rash, i.e., infectious exanthem (Figure 222).
COLOR Pink to red
MUCOUS MEMBRANES Palatal ulcers. Esophageal ulcers. Uncommonly, oral candidiasis

General Examination Acute meningitis; acute reversible encephalopathy with loss of memory, alteration of consciousness, and personality change; lymphadenopathy

DIAGNOSIS AND DIFFERENTIAL DIAGNOSIS

Diagnosis Demonstrate seroconversion of HIV by ELISA or Western blot *or* isolation of HIV from blood or CSF *or* demonstration of p24 antigen.

Differential Diagnosis Febrile patient with risk factors for HIV infection who pre-

MUCOCUTANEOUS MANIFESTATIONS OF HIV DISEASE

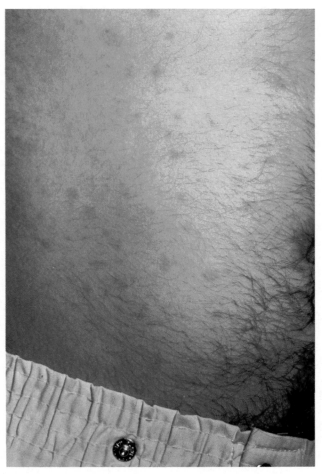

222   Infectious exanthem associated with HIV infection   *Multiple erythematous macules and papules (morbilliform) on the trunk. (Courtesy of Mark Drabkin, M.D.)*

sents with a maculopapular or urticarial rash. Lymphocytic meningitis.

LABORATORY AND SPECIAL EXAMINATIONS

Hematology Leukopenia, elevated ESR

Serology Demonstrate seroconversion of anti-HIV antibodies by ELISA confirmed by Western blot.

Viral Cultures HIV isolation from blood or CSF

CSF Lymphocytic pleocytosis, p24 antigenemia

PATHOPHYSIOLOGY

Following transmission and infection, 10 to 20% show symptoms of acute infection, including fever, rash, enlarged lymph nodes, aseptic meningitis.

COURSE AND PROGNOSIS

After an asymptomatic or symptomatic primary infection, HIV becomes latent. Some patients develop persistent generalized lymphadenopathy, which may be associated with constitutional symptoms. After 3 to 10 years some patients with this lymphadenopathy (5 to 10%) may revert to an asymptomatic state. In both asymptomatic patients and patients with persistent generalized lymphadenopathy, the condition may progress to acquired immunodeficiency syndrome (AIDS)-related complex (ARC), which is characterized by long-standing fever, weight loss, persistent diarrhea, oral candidiasis, multidermatomal herpes zoster, and hairy leukoplakia. Most patients with ARC, as well as an increasing number of asymptomatic carriers and patients with persistent lymphadenopathy, develop full-blown cases of AIDS that are characterized by opportunistic infections, Kaposi's sarcoma, and B-cell lymphomas. Persons with HIV infec-

tions may have thrombocytopenia as an isolated and early finding. Neurologic disease characterized by encephalopathy, myelopathy, or peripheral neuropathy can occur as a direct consequence of HIV infection regardless of the presence or absence of AIDS or ARC, although the disease occurs most commonly and most severely in those patients with profound immune defects.

In time most patients will experience progressive symptoms of persistent generalized lymphadenopathy, ARC, and/or AIDS. ARC is diagnosed with any 2 or more signs/symptoms which have been present for 3 months or longer and any 2 or more abnormal laboratory values:

> *Symptoms/signs:* Fever ≥38°C intermittent/continuous, weight loss ≥10%, persistent generalized lymphadenopathy, diarrhea intermittent/continuous, fatigue that reduces physical activity, night sweats
>
> *Laboratory abnormalities:* Lymphopenia, leukopenia, thrombocytopenia, anemia, reduced ratio of T4:T8 cells (>2SD), reduced T helper cells (>2SD), reduced blastogenesis, increased gamma globulins, cutaneous anergy

Approximately 50% of HIV-infected homosexual men in San Francisco developed AIDS 10 to 11 years after becoming infected. The percentage of persons infected with HIV who eventually go on to develop the tumors and opportunistic infections is uncertain. The incubation time for developing AIDS following infection by blood transfusion or antihemophiliac factor may be shorter than as a sexually transmitted disease in male homosexuals if a large inoculum was received. Positive antibody test to HIV indicates only exposure and not immunity to the virus.

TREATMENT

Symptomatic. The efficacy of specific antiretroviral therapy at this stage still controversial.

Centers for Disease Control Classification of HIV Infections (1986)

Group I   Acute infection: 3 to 6 weeks incubation period

Group II   Asymptomatic infection

Group III   Persistent generalized lymphadenopathy: after 3 to 10 years

Group IV   Other diseases: usually after 11 years
          A. Constitutional
             Fever   > 1 month
             Weight loss > 10% baseline
             Diarrhea   > 1 month
          B. Neurologic
          C. Secondary infections
             1. Opportunists diagnostic of AIDS
             2. Other specified secondary infections (e.g., buccal candidiasis, hairy leukoplakia, tuberculosis, multidermatome *Herpes zoster,* recurrent *Salmonella* bacteriaemia)
          D. Secondary cancers
             Kaposi's sarcoma
             Non-Hodgkin's lymphoma
             Primary cerebral lymphoma
          E. Other conditions

Oral hairy leukoplakia (OHL) is a benign, virally induced hyperplasia of the oral mucosa, most commonly of the inferolateral surface of the tongue, characterized by white, corrugated, verrucous plaques, occurring in patients with progressive HIV-induced immunodeficiency.

Synonym: oral viral leukoplakia.

EPIDEMIOLOGY AND ETIOLOGY

Sex By far most common in male homosexual risk group

Etiology Epstein-Barr virus

HISTORY

Risk Groups Occurs almost exclusively in HIV-infected individuals, especially homosexual men; has been detected in all groups at risk for HIV infection. Rarely noted in immunosuppressed organ transplantation patients.

Incubation Period Usually greater than 5 years after primary HIV infection

Symptoms Lesions are asymptomatic; uncommonly a cosmetic problem. Extent of lesions varies from day to day.

PHYSICAL EXAMINATION

Mucous Membranes
TYPE OF LESION Well-demarcated verrucous plaque (Figure 223). Surface appears irregular, with corrugated or hairy texture. Often present bilaterally, but size of plaques usually not equal.
COLOR White to grayish-white
DISTRIBUTION OF LESIONS Most commonly on the lateral and inferior surface of the tongue. Less commonly seen on the buccal and soft palatal mucosa.

PALPATION Lesion cannot be abraded off with a dry gauze pad.

DIAGNOSIS AND DIFFERENTIAL DIAGNOSIS

Diagnosis Clinical diagnosis. Does not rub off; does not clear with adequate anticandidal therapy.

Differential Diagnosis Hyperplastic oral candidiasis, condyloma acuminatum, geographic or migratory glossitis, lichen planus, tobacco-associated leukoplakia, mucous patch of secondary syphilis, squamous cell carcinoma either in situ or invasive, occlusal trauma

LABORATORY AND SPECIAL EXAMINATIONS

Dermatopathology Acanthotic epithelium with hyperkeratosis, hairlike projections of keratin, areas of koilocytes (ballooned cells with clear cytoplasm)

Cultures Not helpful. *Candida albicans* is commonly isolated.

Electron Microscopy Herpes viral structures within epithelial cells; positive for Epstein-Barr virus markers.

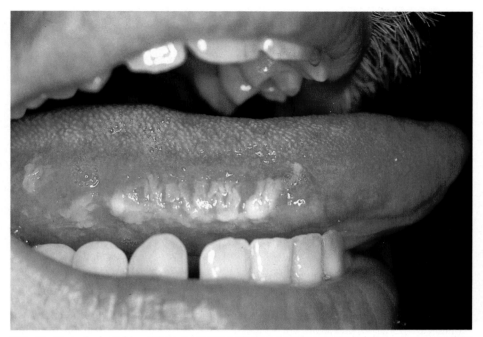

223   Oral hairy leukoplakia   *White, corrugated plaque occurring on the infralateral aspects of the tongue. Lesion cannot be removed by rubbing with a gauze.*

PATHOPHYSIOLOGY

Epstein-Barr viral infection of the oral mucosa appears to be responsible for the epidermal hyperplasia. Occurs by far most commonly in male homosexual risk group (>50% incidence); but also noted in HIV-infected IVDUs, hemophiliacs, and transfusion recipients. The presence of OHL correlates with advanced HIV-induced immunodeficiency. In those patients who do not carry the diagnosis of AIDS at the time of detection of OHL, the probability of developing AIDS has been reported to be 48% by 16 months after detection, and 83% by 31 months.

COURSE AND PROGNOSIS

The severity of OHL varies spontaneously from day to day. May clear completely during a course of treatment with zidovudine, acyclovir (oral or topical), p.o. desiclovir, IV ganciclovir, or foscarnet.

TREATMENT

None indicated. Lesion is usually asymptomatic.

Mucosal candidiasis is characterized, most often, by the presence of white, milklike, removable plaques on the oral or vaginal mucosa; its presence in HIV-infected individuals correlates with a moderate degree of immunodeficiency.

Synonyms: thrush, mycotic stomatitis, *Candida* leukoplakia, oropharyngeal candidiasis.

EPIDEMIOLOGY AND ETIOLOGY

Age All ages

Sex Equal

Etiology *Candida albicans*

Transmission Normal inhabitant of mucosal surfaces, overgrows with increasing immunodeficiency.

CDC Surveillance Case Definition for AIDS Candidiasis of the esophagus, trachea, bronchi, or lungs is an AIDS-defining condition if the patient has no other cause of immunodeficiency and is without knowledge of HIV antibody status.

HISTORY

Incubation Period *Candida* overgrowth occurs many years after primary HIV infection, with increasing immunodeficiency.

History Most patients are asymptomatic. At times, burning sensation, diminished taste sensation. Cosmetic concern about white curds on tongue. Odynophagia.

PHYSICAL EXAMINATION

Skin Findings
TYPE OF LESION *Pseudomembranous candidiasis (thrush):* removable white plaques on any mucosal surface; vary in size from 1.0 to 2.0 mm to extensive and widespread; removal with a dry gauze pad leaves an erythematous or bleeding mucosal surface (Figure 224). *Atrophic candidiasis:* smooth, red, atrophic patches (Figure 225). *Hypertrophic candidiasis (candidal leukoplakia):* white plaques which cannot be wiped off but regress with prolonged anticandidal therapy. *Angular cheilitis:* erythema, fissuring, i.e., intertrigo at the corner of mouth. *Intertrigo:* axillary, inguinal, perineal, balanoposthitis. *Vaginitis.*
COLOR *Thrush:* white to creamy.
PALPATION *Thrush:* removable with dry gauze
DISTRIBUTION OF LESIONS *Thrush:* dorsum of tongue, buccal mucosa, hard/soft palate, pharynx extending down into esophagus and tracheobronchial tree. *Atrophic candidiasis:* hard/soft palate, buccal mucosa, dorsal surface of tongue. *Leukoplakia:* buccal mucosa, tongue, hard palate.
NAILS *Candida* paronychia

DIAGNOSIS AND DIFFERENTIAL DIAGNOSIS

Diagnosis Clinical suspicion confirmed by KOH preparation of scraping from mucosal surface

Differential Diagnosis Oral hairy leukoplakia, condyloma acuminatum, geographic tongue, hairy tongue, lichen planus, bite irritation

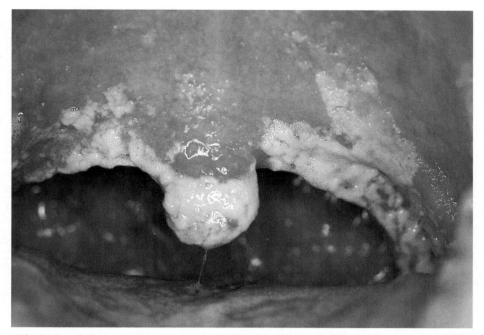

224   Oral candidiasis, pseudomembranous type (thrush)   *White, curdlike plaques with surrounding erythema on the posterior soft palate and uvula.*

LABORATORY AND SPECIAL EXAMINATIONS

KOH Preparation Scraping of an area suspected as candidiasis shows *Candida* pseudohyphae.

Cultures *C. albicans* is a commensural oral organism; isolation in culture, therefore, does not make a diagnosis of candidiasis.

Endoscopy Documents esophageal and/or tracheobronchial candidiasis.

PATHOPHYSIOLOGY

C. albicans is part of the normal oropharyngeal flora. Overgrowth with resultant mucosal candidiasis occurs when immunity is suppressed locally, as with use of corticosteroid inhalers, or with the profound immunodeficiency that occurs with advancing HIV disease. Onset of candidiasis correlates with moderate degree of immunodeficiency in HIV-infected patients and portends that AIDS is imminent. Cell-mediated immunity is felt to be responsible for protection against mucosal candidiasis, whereas humoral immunity protects against candidiasis of keratinized skin.

COURSE AND PROGNOSIS

Although rare, oral and esophageal candidiasis have been reported with primary HIV infection. Oral candidiasis responds to topical and/or systemic therapy; however, recurrence is the rule. May become refractory to intermittent therapy, requiring daily chemoprophylaxis, with either topical or systemic treatment.

TREATMENT

Topical Therapy
Nystatin: Vaginal tablets, 100,000 units t.i.d., dissolved slowly in the mouth; oral pastilles, 200,000 units, one pastille 5 times daily; oral suspension, 1 to 2 teaspoons, held in mouth for 5 minutes and then swallowed

Clotrimazole: oral tablets, 10 mg, one tablet 5 times daily

Systemic Therapy
Ketoconazole: 200 mg q.d. for 1 to 2 weeks. Adequate absorption dependent on acidic gastric pH.

Fluconazole: 200 mg p.o. or IV once, followed by 100 mg daily for at least 2 to 3 weeks

Recurrence is the rule; maintenance therapy is often required.

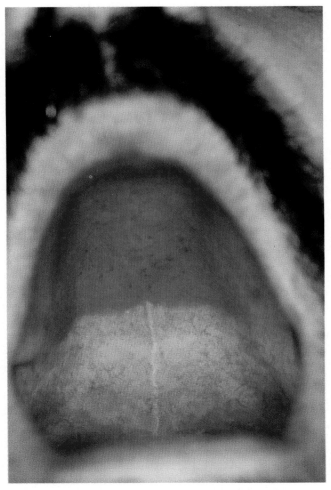

225   Oral candidiasis, atrophic type   *Erythema and atrophy of the palate under the area of the dentures in an HIV-infected patient.*

HIV-Associated Eosinophilic Folliculitis

HIV-associated eosinophilic folliculitis (HEF) is an extremely pruritic, papular and pustular follicular eruption of the upper trunk, face, neck, and proximal extremities.

EPIDEMIOLOGY AND ETIOLOGY

Sex Males

Etiology Unknown

HISTORY

History Moderate to intense itching unrelieved by usual means.

Systems Review Most patients have advanced immunodeficiency and meet the criteria for AIDS.

PHYSICAL EXAMINATION

Skin Findings
TYPE OF LESION 3.0- to 5.0-mm, edematous, follicular papules and pustules (Figure 226). Most patients have hundreds of lesions. Frequently, secondary changes of excoriations and crusting are apparent. Postinflammatory hyperpigmentation occurs in longstanding cases.
COLOR Erythematous
DISTRIBUTION OF LESIONS Trunk universally > head and neck > proximal extremities

DIAGNOSIS AND DIFFERENTIAL DIAGNOSIS

Diagnosis Clinical diagnosis confirmed by skin biopsy, with cultures ruling out infectious causes

Differential Diagnosis Allergic contact dermatitis, adverse cutaneous drug reaction, atopic dermatitis, scabies, papular urticaria, acne vulgaris, dermatophytosis, bacterial folliculitis (*Staphylococcus aureus, Pseudomonas aeruginosa*), fungal folliculitis (*Pityrosporum ovale, Candida albicans*), dermatitis herpetiformis

LABORATORY AND SPECIAL EXAMINATIONS

Serology HIV ELISA and Western blot positive. Elevated serum IgE levels.

Cultures Negative for pathogenic organisms

Dermatopathology Perifollicular and perivascular infiltrate with varying number of eosinophils. Epithelial spongiosis of follicular infundibulum and/or sebaceous glands associated with a mixed cellular infiltrate. Eosinophilic pustules occur uncommonly. Special stains for bacteria, fungi, and parasites are negative.

Hematology Most patients have either absolute or relative peripheral eosinophilia. CD4 usually <250 cells/mm^3.

PATHOPHYSIOLOGY

Unknown. Similar to the rare dermatosis, eosinophilic pustular folliculitis (Ofuji's disease), which is seen mainly in Japan.

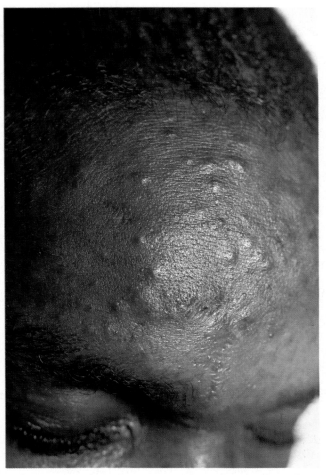

226 HIV-associated eosinophilic folliculitis *Edematous, erythematous papules and pustules, at times follicular. (Courtesy of Paul Bleicher, M.D.)*

COURSE AND PROGNOSIS

Course tends to be chronic, characterized by spontaneous exacerbations and remissions.

TREATMENT

Antihistamines: astemizole 10 to 20 mg/ day p.o.

Potent topical fluorinated corticosteroids, i.e., clobetasol propionate, applied twice daily, reported to be effective. Oral corticosteroids are effective but their use in patients with advanced immunodeficiency is risky.

Phototherapy with natural sunlight or UVB effective.

Chronic herpetic ulcers (CHU) are progressively enlarging ulcers occurring at the sites of recurrent herpes simplex virus (HSV) outbreaks, most commonly perianally, on the buttocks, or periorally, characterized by pain and hyperplastic edges; their occurrence correlates with an advanced degree of immunodeficiency. Also see "Nongenital Herpes Simplex Virus Infection" (page 70) and "Genital Herpes Simplex" (page 410)

EPIDEMIOLOGY AND ETIOLOGY

Age   Young adults

Sex   HSV infection is considerably more common in male homosexuals, and, thus, CHU occur most commonly in this group at risk for HIV infection. 95% of homosexual men with AIDS have latent HSV infection.

Etiology   HSV types 1 and 2 in the setting of immunodeficiency. CHU are thus most common in patients with AIDS but may also occur in other immunodeficiencies and lymphoma/leukemia.

CDC Surveillance Case Definition for AIDS
HSV infection causing a mucocutaneous ulcer that persists longer than 1 month; or HSV infection causing bronchitis, pneumonitis, or esophagitis for any duration in a patient older than 1 month, is an AIDS-defining condition if the patient has no other cause of immunodeficiency and is without knowledge of HIV antibody status.

HISTORY

Incubation Period   Most patients have previously been infected with HSV. Reactivated infection occurs commonly in HIV-infected patients. CHU occur late in the course of HIV disease.

Skin Symptoms   Ulcers are usually quite painful. Anorectal ulcers are associated with pain, constipation, pain on defecation, tenesmus, and, at times, sacral radiculopathy, impotence, neurogenic bladder. Herpetic whitlow is associated with severe pain.

PHYSICAL EXAMINATION

Skin Findings
TYPE OF LESION   Initial lesions are grouped vesicles on an erythematous base. Vesicles enlarge, merge, and become ulcerations, which continue to enlarge. Edges may be slightly rolled, hyperplastic. Coalescence of ulcerations may result in linear ulcers in intergluteal cleft, or inguinal fold. Base of ulcer may be crusted or moist. Ulcer may enlarge to 10.0 to 20.0 cm in diameter (Figure 227).
PALPATION   Very painful
SHAPE OF INDIVIDUAL LESION   Oval or round; polycyclic if individual ulcers merge
DISTRIBUTION OF LESIONS   Perianal and/or rectal > genital > orofacial > digital. Uncommonly, ulcer on face and perineum simultaneously. Esophageal.

General Examination
ESOPHAGOSCOPY, TRACHEOSCOPY   Mucosal erosions/ulceration
SIGMOIDOSCOPY   Friable mucosa, diffuse ulcerations, occasionally vesicular or pustular lesions

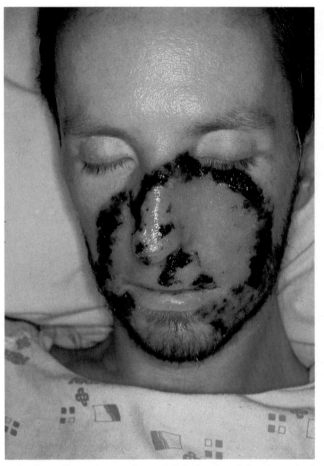

227　Chronic herpetic ulcer　*Extensive, erosive, painful ulcer involving the entire lower half of the face; it was unresponsive to IV acyclovir. (Courtesy of C. Lisa Kauffman, M.D.)*

DIAGNOSIS AND DIFFERENTIAL DIAGNOSIS

Diagnosis　Clinical suspicion confirmed by Tzanck test, HSV culture, and/or lesional biopsy.

Differential Diagnosis　Chronic cytomegalovirus ulcer, impetigo, ecthyma, decubitus ulcer, syphilitic chancre, ecthyma gangrenosum, deep mycotic (cryptococcal, histoplasmal, blastomycotic, coccidioidal) ulcer, fixed drug reaction

LABORATORY AND SPECIAL EXAMINATIONS

Tzanck Test Cytology of scraping of CHU border shows multinucleated giant cells. Negative stain for electron microscopy reveals herpes-type virus particles.

HSV Culture Culture exudate at floor of ulcer or biopsy specimen from ulcer

Dermatopathology Multinucleated giant epidermal cells with intranuclear viral inclusion bodies. Immunofluorescence staining demonstrates HSV.

PATHOPHYSIOLOGY

Majority of HIV-infected patients (especially homosexual male risk group) have latent HSV infection (documented by detection of type-specific IgG antibody). Primary HSV infection or infection with a different HSV type or strain can occur in the HIV-infected individual, but majority of herpetic infections occur by reactivation of the latent virus. With increasing immunodeficiency, HSV continues to infect contiguous epidermal cells, resulting in gradual enlargement and deepening of the CHU. Acyclovir resistance results from loss of synthesis of the viral enzyme thymidine kinase (TK). In the absence of TK, acyclovir is not activated to its monophosphate form and host cell enzymes cannot catalyze further phosphorylations that lead to acyclovir triphosphate.

COURSE AND PROGNOSIS

With increasing immunodeficiency, recurrences of HSV infection may not heal spontaneously, nor with low-dose oral acyclovir, but become persistent and progressive for a period of months. Erosions occurring at the usual sites (perianal, genital, orofacial) enlarge and deepen into painful ulcers with raised margins. Untreated, these ulcers may become confluent, involving half the face or becoming circumferential around the anus. Chronic perianal ulcers may be associated with herpetic colitis and are associated with painful defecation and diarrhea. Involvement of oropharynx with extension to esophagus, results in odynophagia.

CHU that fail to respond to acyclovir should be evaluated promptly for the presence of resistant virus. Infection with acyclovir-resistant strains result in chronic, progressive ulcerations which persist and/or continue to enlarge in spite of oral and IV acyclovir treatment. These ulcers can enlarge to 20.0 to 30.0 cm in diameter and are associated with major morbidity and pain.

HSV infection can disseminate hematogenously and result in hepatitis, pneumonitis, and encephalitis. Dissemination to the skin is characterized by varying numbers of grouped vesicles which quickly erode and form crusts, occurring on the trunk and extremities.

TREATMENT

Chronic herpetic ulcers are frequently superinfected with *Staphylococcus aureus* or *Streptococcus pyogenes* and should be treated with appropriate antibiotics if indicated.

Topical therapy Acyclovir cream applied every 3 hours

Systemic therapy Acyclovir: p.o. 200 mg every 4 hours for 5 to 7 days; recurrent infection, up to 800 mg 5 times daily; for severe mucocutaneous infection, IV 5 to 10 mg per kg body weight every 8 hours.

For acyclovir-resistant HSV infection: foscarnet (trisodium phosphonoformate) IV 50 mg/kg body weight every 8 hours or vidarabine IV 10 mg per kg per day

Epidemic or AIDS-associated Kaposi's sarcoma (KS) is a multicentric systemic vascular tumor characterized by violaceous nodules and by edema secondary to lymphatic obstruction, occurring mainly in homosexual males with AIDS.

Synonym: multiple idiopathic hemorrhagic sarcoma.

EPIDEMIOLOGY AND ETIOLOGY

Sex Homosexual males, uncommon in other risk groups for AIDS

Etiology Unknown. Evidence points to an infective agent, possibly a retrovirus, other than HIV.

Incidence Early in the HIV epidemic, 50% of homosexual men at time of initial diagnosis of AIDS had KS; currently, the incidence is 15% within this risk group.

Clinical Variants of KS Endemic (classic, European) KS occurs in elderly Mediterranean and Ashkenazi Jewish males, African (non-AIDS) KS, KS with iatrogenic immunosuppression, i.e., transplantation recipients.

CDC Surveillance Case Definition for AIDS KS in a patient <60 years is an AIDS-defining condition, if the patient has no other cause of immunodeficiency and is without knowledge of HIV antibody status.

HISTORY

Cutaneous KS lesions most often begin as an ecchymotic-like macule. Lesions are usually asymptomatic but are associated with significant cosmetic stigma. At times lesions may ulcerate and bleed easily. Large lesions on palms or soles may impede function. Progressive edema of extremity can be associated with progressive fibrosis and stricture, limiting movement. Urethral or anal canal lesions can be associated with obstruction. GI involvement rarely causes symptoms. Pulmonary KS can cause bronchospasm, intractable coughing, progressive respiratory failure, shortness of breath.

PHYSICAL EXAMINATION

Skin Findings
TYPE OF LESION Macules, papules, plaques, nodules (Figure 228), tumors located in dermis or hypodermis. Overlying epidermis is usually intact, but at times may become necrotic with formation of erosion or ulcer ± crusting. In time, individual lesions may enlarge and become confluent, forming tumorous masses. Lymphedema: confluent mass of lesions on an extremity may result in unilateral distal edema; deeper involvement of lymphatics and lymph nodes results in varying degrees of edema, usually symmetric, most pronounced on the lower legs, genitalia, and/or face; end stage may be atrophy and fibrosis of extremity.

COLOR Early dermal lesions violaceous, red, pink, or tan. Older lesions have purple-brownish hue with greenish hemosiderin halo.

PALPATION *Almost all KS lesions are palpable,* feeling firm to hard. Lesions that have the color of KS, but are not palpable, are probably ecchymoses except on the palate.

SHAPE OF INDIVIDUAL LESION Often oval initially

ARRANGEMENT OF MULTIPLE LESIONS Trun-

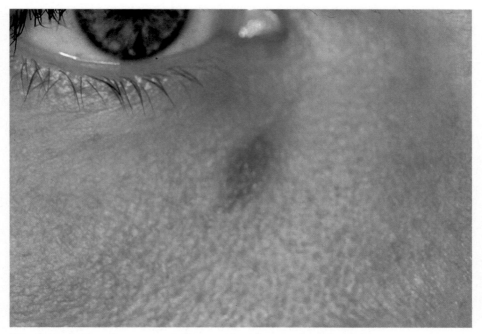

228 Epidemic Kaposi's sarcoma *Solitary, oval, violaceous, dermal nodule.*

cal lesions have pityriasis rosea-like pattern (Figure 229). Lesions may occur at sites of trauma, koebnerization, or isomorphic phenomenon.

DISTRIBUTION OF LESIONS   Widespread: trunk (Figure 230); head, especially tip of nose, periorbital, ears, scalp; penis; legs (Figure 231); palms and soles.

Mucous Membranes   Very common on the hard palate appearing as a violaceous stain. 15% of KS first appears intraorally. Gingiva, uvula.

General Examination

LUNG   Pulmonary infiltrates
GI TRACT   GI hemorrhage, rectal obstruction, protein-losing enteropathy can occur.

DIAGNOSIS AND DIFFERENTIAL DIAGNOSIS

Diagnosis   Confirmed on skin biopsy

Differential Diagnosis   Of single pigmented lesions: malignant melanoma, dermatofibroma; pyogenic granuloma, hemangioma, bacillary (epithelioid) angiomatosis, melanocytic nevus, ecchymosis, granuloma annulare, insect bite reactions, stasis dermatitis

LABORATORY AND SPECIAL EXAMINATIONS

Dermatopathology   Discrete intradermal nodule with vascular channels lined by atypical endothelial cells among a network of reticulin fibers and extravasated erythrocytes with hemosiderin deposition

Chest X-Ray   Difficult to distinguish pulmonary KS from *Pneumocystis carinii* pneumonia. In KS, pulmonary nodules and pleural effusions more common.

PATHOPHYSIOLOGY

Likely that KS cells are derived from the endothelium of the blood/lymphatic microvasculature. Probably not a true malignancy but rather a widespread cellular proliferation in response to angiogenic substances. KS lesions produce factors that promote their own growth as well as the growth of other cells.

COURSE AND PROGNOSIS

Cutaneous KS lesions slowly increase in size, may become tuberous and confluent. Patients with only a few lesions, present for several months, without history of opportunistic infections, and CD4 cell counts $>200/mm^3$ tend to respond better to therapy and probably have a better overall prognosis. Immunosuppression caused by prednisone or methotrexate may precipitate appearance of KS, which may regress when these agents are withheld. At the time of initial diagnosis, 40% of KS cases have GI involvement; 80% at autopsy. Reduced survival rate in patients with GI involvement. Pulmonary KS has high short-term mortality rate, i.e., median survival less than 6 months.

TREATMENT

Therapy is usually directed at individual lesions which are cosmetically disturbing, bulky, hemorrhagic, cause functional disturbance on the palms or soles, or lesions causing lymphatic obstruction and lymphedema.

Limited Intervention

LOCAL THERAPY   Radiotherapy (800 to 3000 rad), cryosurgery, laser surgery, excisional surgery
INTRALESIONAL THERAPY   Vinblastine (0.20 mg/mL) every 2 weeks. Interferon alpha 3 times a week

Aggressive Intervention

SINGLE-AGENT CHEMOTHERAPY   Adriamycin; vincristine, weekly IV bolus of 1.4 to 2.0 mg/kg body weight; vinblastine, weekly IV bolus 0.1 mg/kg
COMBINATION CHEMOTHERAPY   Vincristine (2.0 mg) + bleomycin (15 units/m^2) + adriamycin (20 mg/m^2) is given every other week in patients with relatively advanced KS. Interferon alpha (15 million units/day) + zidovudine (600 mg/day)

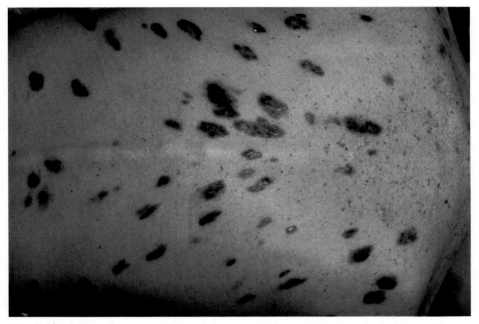

229   Epidemic Kaposi's sarcoma   *Large violaceous nodules occurring in a pityriasis rosea-like pattern on the trunk.*

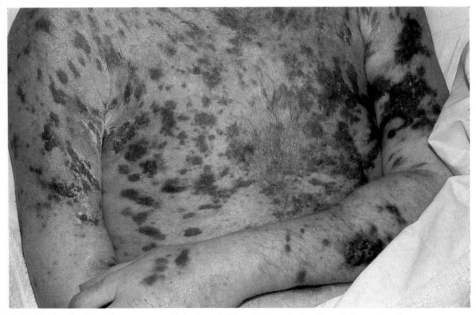

230   Epidemic Kaposi's sarcoma   *Fulminant KS, with myriads of nodules occurring over a one-month period; associated pulmonary KS was also present. (Courtesy of Jeffrey Dover, M.D.)*

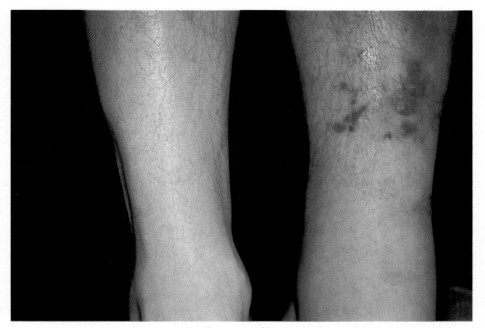

231 Epidemic Kaposi's sarcoma with edema *Confluent, violaceous nodules with associated marked edema of the lower leg.*

Mollusca contagiosa (MC) occur in approximately 10% of HIV-infected patients with advanced immunodeficiency, appearing as multiple facial umbilicated papules and nodules; lesions tend to become progressively more numerous, in spite of aggressive therapeutic attempts, and can create significant cosmetic disfigurement of the patient.

HISTORY

Duration of Lesions   Months

Symptoms of Skin Lesions   Usually asymptomatic unless secondarily infected with *Staphylococcus aureus*

PHYSICAL EXAMINATION

Skin Findings
TYPE OF LESION   Skin-colored, dome-shaped, 2.0- to 4.0-mm papules, which commonly have a central umbilication. Lesions may become superinfected with *Staph. aureus,* manifested as purulence or crusting. Treatment with cryo- or electrosurgery can be followed by postinflammatory hyper- or hypopigmentation. At times, MC are solitary or scanty, up to 1.0 cm in diameter, and confused with basal cell carcinoma or keratoacanthoma. In patients with moderate-to-advanced immunodeficiency, hundreds of facial lesions may occur (Figure 232).
COLOR   In fair-skinned patients, usually color of the skin, easily confused with dermal nevi. Usually more noticeable in darker-skinned patients, especially after treatment with resultant postinflammatory hyper- or hypopigmentation.
ARRANGEMENT   May occur in a linear arrangement, autoinoculated into a superficial scratch or abrasion. At times, the beard area becomes a confluent mass of MC, spread by shaving. Multiple MC are frequently clustered on the margins of the eyelids.
DISTRIBUTION   Most common on face; also clustered about the axillae, groins, or buttocks

DIAGNOSIS AND DIFFERENTIAL DIAGNOSIS

Diagnosis   Clinical; at times, confirmed by lesional skin biopsy

Differential Diagnosis   When solitary and large: keratoacanthoma, basal cell carcinoma. When multiple: multiple dermal nevi, verruca plana, hematogenous dissemination to skin of deep mycosis, i.e., cryptococcosis, histoplasmosis, coccidioidomycosis

COURSE AND PROGNOSIS

MC respond poorly to even aggressive treatment with liquid nitrogen, becoming more numerous and causing significant cosmetic disfigurement.

TREATMENT

MC may regress after beginning antiretroviral therapy with zidovudine. Regular treatment with cryosurgery often minimizes the size and number of MC. Bacterial superinfection should be treated with antibiotics.

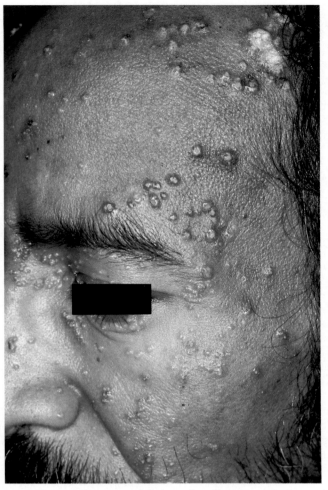

232 Molluscum contagiosum *The unusual feature of molluscum contagiosum in HIV-infected patients is the large number of lesions and their occurrence on the face.*

Bacillary angiomatosis (BA) is a newly described infection occurring in HIV-infected individuals, characterized by cutaneous vascular tumors which, at times, may disseminate systemically.
Synonym: bacillary epithelioid angiomatosis.

ETIOLOGY AND EPIDEMIOLOGY

Age Presumably an HIV-infected individual of any age

Etiology An agent similar or identical to the cat-scratch disease (CSD) bacillus, closely related to *Rochalimaea quintana* rickettsial organism

Transmission BA organism is probably harbored by cats. Presumably enters percutaneously through minor breaks in the epidermis. Latent infection or person-to-person infection is not known to occur in humans.

Risk Factors BA occurs almost exclusively in HIV-infected individuals with advanced immunodeficiency. BA occurring in an immunocompetent, non-HIV infected host has been reported.

Incubation Period Unknown, but probably days to weeks.

HISTORY

History of owning or having been scratched by a cat. Patients with localized infection may be free of systemic symptoms. Lesions are usually neither painful nor pruritic. Those with more widespread disseminated infection have fever, malaise, weight loss.

PHYSICAL EXAMINATION

Skin Lesions
TYPE Papules or nodules resembling angiomas. Up to 2.0 to 3.0 cm in diameter. Usually situated in dermis with thinning or erosion of overlying epidermis; may be located deeper in subcutaneous tissue. Number of lesions ranges from solitary lesions to more than a 100 and, rarely, greater than 1000 (Figure 233).
COLOR Red, bright red, violaceous, or skin colored
PALPATION Firm, nontender, nonblanching
SHAPE Dome-shaped
DISTRIBUTION Any site, but palms, soles, and the oral cavity are usually spared. Occasionally lesions occur at the site of a cat scratch. Solitary lesion presenting as a dactylitis has been reported.

Systemic Findings Infection may spread hematogenously or via lymphatics to become systemic, with involvement of bone marrow, bone, liver, and spleen.

DIAGNOSIS AND DIFFERENTIAL DIAGNOSIS

Diagnosis Demonstration of BA organism on a Warthin-Starry or similar silver stain of lesional biopsy.

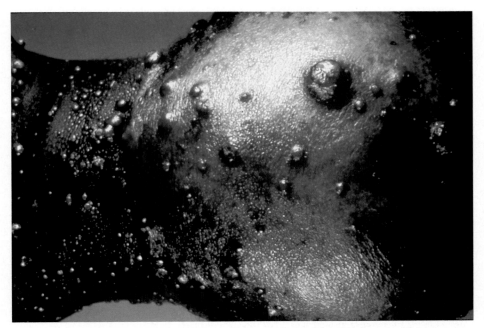

233 Bacillary angiomatosis *View of the posterior head of a patient with alopecia. Multiple vascular nodules occurring in a generalized distribution. (Courtesy of Clay Cockerell, M.D.)*

Differential Diagnosis Kaposi's sarcoma, pyogenic granuloma, epithelioid (histiocytoid) angioma, cherry angioma, sclerosing hemangioma, verruga peruana lesions of bartonellosis, disseminated cryptococcosis

PATHOPHYSIOLOGY

Cutaneous lesions of BA resemble the bacterial infection verruga peruana, i.e., bartonellosis, the chronic cutaneous infection by *Bartonella bacilliformis*. Vascular proliferation occurs in response to BA organism.

LABORATORY AND SPECIAL EXAMINATIONS

Dermatopathology Increased number of endothelial-lined vascular spaces in the dermis. The endothelial cells are typically large cuboidal cells with prominent nuclei. The amount of edema and infiltrate is variable. Clusters of bacteria with the structure of gram-negative rods are noted within the vascular proliferations.

Culture Culture of BA organism from lesional biopsy specimens of BA has been accomplished but is not possible in most microbiologic laboratories. Lacking the ability to culture the infecting organism, determination of antibiotic sensitivity is not possible.

COURSE AND PROGNOSIS

Course variable. In some patients, lesions regress spontaneously. Systemic involvement with the infection has occurred; death may occur secondary to pulmonary infection.

TREATMENT

Erythromycin 250 to 500 mg orally q.i.d. until the lesions resolve. Alternative: doxycycline 100 mg b.i.d. until resolved.

Erythroderma

Exfoliative Erythroderma Syndrome

The exfoliative erythroderma syndrome (EES) is a serious, often life-threatening, reaction pattern of the skin characterized by generalized and confluent redness and scaling and associated with systemic "toxicity," generalized lymphadenopathy, and fever. Two stages, acute and chronic, merge one to the other. In the acute and subacute phases there is rapid onset of generalized vivid red erythema and fine branny scales; the patient feels hot and cold, shivers and has fever. In the chronic EES there is a loss of scalp and body hair, the nails become thickened and separated from the nail bed (onycholysis), and there may be hyperpigmentation or patchy loss of pigment in patients whose normal skin color is brown or black. In about 50% of the patients with EES there is a history of a preexisting dermatosis, and this is recognizable only in the acute or subacute stages. The most frequent preexisting skin disorders are (in order of frequency): eczematous dermatitis (atopic, contact), psoriasis, lymphoma and leukemia, drug reaction, and pityriasis rubra pilaris. In 10 to 20% of patients it is not possible by the history or the histology to identify the cause. (See "Sézary's Syndrome," Section 26 for a special consideration of this form of EES.)

EPIDEMIOLOGY

Age >50 years; when in children EES results from pityriasis rubra pilaris or atopic dermatitis

Sex Males > females

HISTORY

Duration of Lesions Depending on the etiology, the acute phase may develop rapidly, as in a drug reaction, lymphoma, or eczema. At this early acute stage it is possible to identify the preexisting dermatosis (psoriasis, mycosis fungoides, lichen planus, etc.).

Skin Symptoms Pruritus

Constitutional Symptoms Fatigue, weakness, anorexia, weight loss, malaise, feeling cold

PHYSICAL EXAMINATION

Appearance of Patient Frightened, red, "toxic"

Skin

TYPE OF LESION Scaling dermatitis which is confluent and diffuse, without recognizable borders (Figures 234 and 235), except for pityriasis rubra pilaris, where EES spares sharply defined areas of normal skin (Figure 236). Edema of lower legs and ankles.

COLOR OF LESIONS Bright red

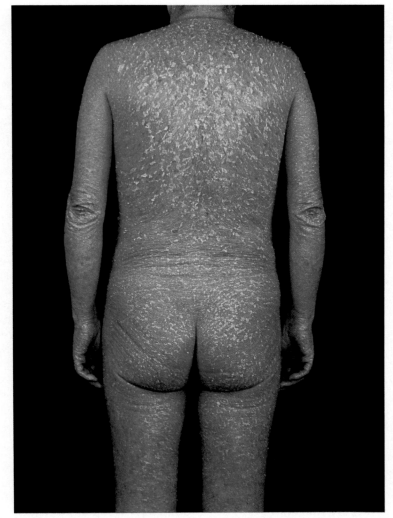

234 Erythroderma, psoriatic *This is a patient with universal psoriasis, showing extensive scaling.*

PALMS AND SOLES   Usually involved, with massive hyperkeratosis and deep fissures in pityriasis rubra pilaris, Sézary's syndrome, and psoriasis

Hair   Alopecia

Nails   Onycholysis, shedding of nails

General Examination   Lymph nodes generalized, rubbery, and usually small

LABORATORY EXAMINATIONS

Dermatopathology
LIGHT MICROSCOPY   Depends on type of underlying disease. Parakeratosis, inter- and intracellular edema, acanthosis with elongation of the rete ridges, and exocytosis of cells. There is edema of the dermis and a chronic inflammatory infiltrate.

Laboratory Examination of Blood
CHEMISTRY   Low serum albumin and increase of gamma globulins
BLOOD CULTURE   Should be performed.

IMAGING

CT scans should be used to find evidence of lymphoma.

DIAGNOSIS AND DIFFERENTIAL DIAGNOSIS

Diagnosis   This is not easy and the history of the preexisting dermatosis may be the only clue. Also, pathognomonic signs and symptoms of the preexisting dermatosis may help, e.g., typical nail changes of psoriasis; lichenification, erosions, and excoriations in atopic dermatitis and eczema; diffuse, relatively nonscaling hyperkeratoses with fissures in CTCL and pityriasis rubra pilaris; sharply demarcated patches of noninvolved skin within the erythroderma in pityriasis rubra pilaris; massive hyperkeratotic scale of scalp usually without hair loss in psoriasis; hair loss in CTCL and pityriasis rubra pilaris; in the latter, ectropion may occur.

Differential Diagnosis   In addition to those already discussed, EES can arise from: lichen planus, pemphigus foliaceus, ichthyosiform erythroderma, acute graft-versus-host disease.

PATHOGENESIS

The metabolic response to exfoliative dermatitis may be profound. Large amounts of warm blood are present in the skin due to the dilatation of the capillaries, and there is considerable heat dissipation through insensible fluid loss and by convection. Also the loss of scales through exfoliation can be considerable, up to 9.0 g per square meter of body surface per day; this may contribute to the reduction of serum albumin and the edema of the lower extremities, so often noted in these patients.

SIGNIFICANCE

This is an important medical problem that should be dealt with using a modern inpatient dermatology facility and personnel.

PROGNOSIS

Guarded. Despite the best attention to all details, patients may succumb to infections or, if they have cardiac problems, to cardiac failure ("high output" failure) or to the effects of the prolonged corticosteroid therapy that is required.

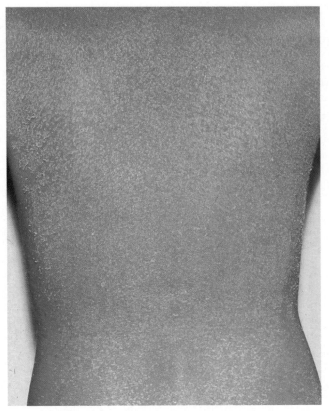

235　Erythroderma, drug-induced　*This patient has a drug reaction to gold, showing diffuse erythema and scaling involving the entire skin surface.*

TREATMENT

The patient should be hospitalized in a single room, at least for the beginning work-up and during the development of a therapeutic program. The hospital room conditions (heat and cold) should be adjusted to the patient's needs; most often these patients need a warm room with many blankets.

Topical Water baths with added bath oils, followed by application of bland emollients

Systemic

Oral corticosteroids for remission induction and for maintenance; systemic and topical therapy as required by underlying condition.

Supportive (cardiac, fluid, electrolyte, protein replacement) therapy as required.

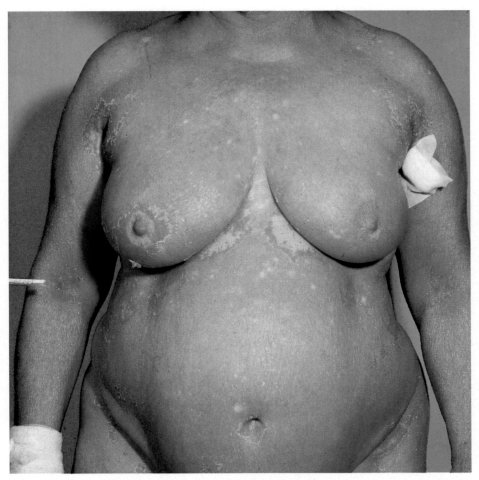

236   Erythroderma   *This patient has pityriasis rubra pilaris. There is an almost universal erythema and scaling. Note the areas of sparing in which normal skin can be seen; this is typical but is not pathognomonic for pityriasis rubra pilaris.*

Section 19

Skin Signs of Immune, Autoimmune, and Rheumatic Diseases

Systemic Amyloidosis

Amyloidosis is an extracellular deposition in various tissues of amyloid fibril proteins and of a protein, amyloid P component (AP); the identical component of AP is present in the serum and is called SAP. These amyloid deposits can affect normal body function, and *acquired systemic amyloidosis (amyloidosis AL)*, known previously as *primary amyloidosis,* occurs in patients with B-cell or plasma-cell dyscrasias in whom fragments of monoclonal immunoglobulin light chains form amyloid fibrils. AL amyloidosis also is associated with multiple myeloma. *AA or secondary amyloidosis* occurs in patients following chronic inflammatory disease in whom the fibril protein is derived from the circulating acute-phase lipoprotein known as *serum amyloid A.* Clinical features include a combination of macroglossia, cardiac, renal, hepatic, and GI involvement, as well as carpal-tunnel syndrome. Skin lesions occur in 30% of patients with amyloidosis AL (primary), and, as they occur early in the disease, they are an important clue to the diagnosis. There are few or no characteristic skin lesions in AA (secondary) amyloidosis.

Two not uncommon varieties of localized amyloidosis that are unrelated to the systemic amyloidoses are: *lichenoid amyloidosis* (discrete, very pruritic, brownish-red papules on the legs), and *macular amyloidosis* (pruritic, gray-brown reticulated macular lesions occurring principally on the upper back; the lesions often have a distinctive "ripple" pattern). The précis to follow discusses only amyloidosis AL (primary).

EPIDEMIOLOGY

Age Sixth decade

Sex Equal incidence

Precipitating Factors Multiple myeloma

in many but not all patients with AL amyloidosis

Systemic Involvement Chronic constitutional symptoms: fatigue, weakness, anorexia, weight loss, malaise. Dyspnea, paresthesia related to carpal-tunnel syndrome.

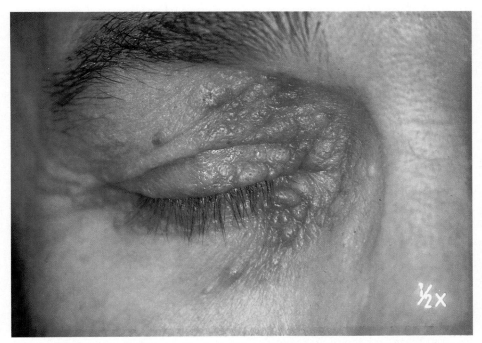

237 Primary systemic amyloidosis *The patient has multiple papules around the eye; these are flat-topped, nontender, nonpruritic. One portion exhibits purpura; this is sometimes called "pinch purpura" because it can be induced by pinching the lesions.*

PHYSICAL EXAMINATION

Skin

TYPES OF LESIONS

Purpura following trauma, "pinch" purpura (Figure 237), occurs on the face and especially around the eyes

Papules: smooth, waxy, with (Figure 237) or without purpura, sometimes involving large surface areas

Nodules

DISTRIBUTION OF LESIONS Purpuric lesions around the eyes, central face, body folds, axillae, umbilicus, anogenital area

Mucous Membranes Macroglossia: diffusely enlarged and firm, "woody" (Figure 238)

General Examination Kidney—nephrosis; nervous system—peripheral neuropathy, carpal-tunnel syndrome; CVS—partial heart block, congestive heart failure; hepatic—hepatomegaly

LABORATORY EXAMINATIONS

Dermatopathology

LIGHT MICROSCOPY *Site* Dermis and subcutis

Process Accumulation of faintly eosinophilic masses of amyloid near the epidermis, in sweat glands, around and within blood vessel walls. *Special stains:* use Congo red and examine the sections for an apple-green fluorescence, using a simple polarization microscope.

DIAGNOSIS

The combination of purpuric skin lesions, waxy papules, macroglossia, carpal-tunnel syndrome, and cardiac symptoms and signs. A tissue diagnosis can be made from the skin biopsy. Scintigraphy after injection of ^{123}I SAP is now available for estimating the extent of the involvement and can serve as a guide for treatment.

PATHOGENESIS

The various manifestations of the disease result from the impairment of normal function of the various organs because of the extracellular accumulation of large amounts of amyloid.

COURSE AND PROGNOSIS

Poor, especially if there is renal involvement. AL amyloidosis with multiple myeloma has an especially poor prognosis, with 18- to 24-month survival.

TREATMENT

Cytotoxic drugs can modify the course of amyloidosis AL associated with multiple myeloma.

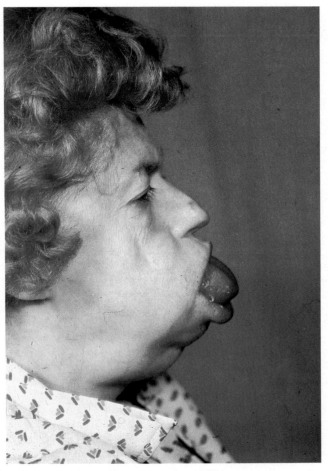

238 Primary systemic amyloidosis *This patient has striking macroglossia. (Courtesy of Evan Calkins, M.D.)*

Urticaria and angioedema are composed of transient wheals (edematous papules and plaques, usually pruritic) and of larger edematous areas that involve the dermis and subcutaneous tissue (angioedema). Urticaria and/or angioedema may be acute recurrent or chronic recurrent. There are some syndromes with angioedema in which urticarial wheals are rarely present (e.g., hereditary angioedema).

ETIOLOGY

Angioedema and urticaria can be classified as IgE-mediated, hypocomplementemic, or related to physical stimuli (cold, sunlight, pressure), or idiosyncratic. The syndrome, *angioedema-urticaria-eosinophilia syndrome,* is related to action of the eosinophil major basic protein.

Special Types

IMMUNOLOGIC *IgE-Mediated* Often with atopic background. Antigens: food (milk, eggs, wheat, shellfish, nuts), therapeutic agents, drugs (penicillin!), parasites

Complement-Mediated By way of immune complexes activating complement and releasing anaphylatoxins which induce mast cell degranulation. Serum sickness, administration of whole blood, immunoglobulins.

PHYSICAL URTICARIA *Dermographism* Although 4.2% of the normal population have it, symptomatic dermographism is a nuisance. Fades in 30 minutes.

Cold Urticaria Usually in children or young adults; "ice cube" test establishes diagnosis.

Solar Urticaria Action spectra 290 to 500 nm, histamine is one of the mediators.

Cholinergic Urticaria Exercise to the point of sweating provokes typical (small, papular) lesions and establishes diagnosis.

Vibratory (Pressure) Angioedema History of swelling induced by pressure (buttock swelling when seated, hand swelling after hammering, foot swelling after walking).

No laboratory abnormalities; no fever. Antihistamines are ineffective but corticosteroids are sometimes helpful. Biopsy reveals a prominent mononuclear infiltrate in the deep dermis. Urticaria may occur in addition to angioedema. Vibratory angioedema may be familial (autosomal dominant) or sporadic. It is believed to result from histamine release from mast cells caused by "vibrating" stimuli—rubbing a towel across the back will produce lesions but direct pressure (without movements) will not cause a response.

URTICARIA DUE TO MAST CELL RELEASING AGENTS Urticaria/angioedema and even anaphylaxis-like syndromes may occur with radiocontrast media and as a consequence of intolerance to salicylates, azo dyes, and benzoates.

HEREDITARY ANGIOEDEMA A serious autosomal dominant (positive family history) disorder; involves angioedema of face and extremities, episodes of laryngeal edema, and acute abdominal pain caused by angioedema of the bowel wall. Urticaria does not occur but there may be an erythema marginatum-like eruption. Laboratory abnormalities involve the complement system: decreased levels of C1 inactivator (85%) or dysfunctional inhibitor (15%), low C4 value in the presence of normal C1 and C3 levels. Angioedema results from bradykinin formation, as C1 inactivator is also the major inhibitor of the Hageman factor and kallikrein, the two enzymes required for kinin formation.

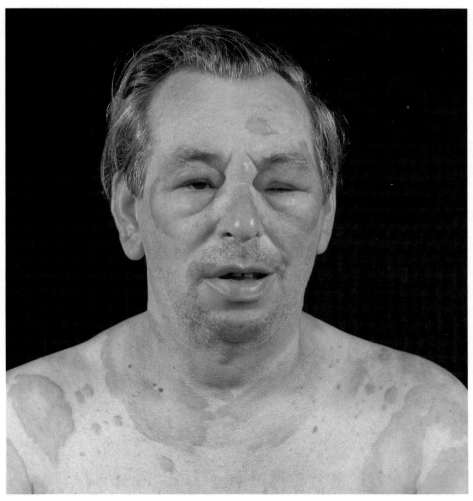

239   Urticaria   *This patient has obvious urticarial lesions occurring in the necklace pattern and around the eyes, with angioedema of the left eye particularly.*

ANGIOEDEMA-URTICARIA-EOSINOPHILIA SYNDROME Severe angioedema with pruritic urticaria involving the face, neck, extremities, and trunk that lasts for 7 to 10 days. There is fever and marked increase in normal weight (increased by 10 to 18%) owing to fluid retention. No other organs are involved. Laboratory abnormalities include striking leukocytosis (20,000 to 70,000 per μL) and eosinophilia (60 to 80% eosinophils) which are related to the severity of attack. There is no family history. Prognosis good.

General Types

ACUTE URTICARIA (<30 days) Often IgE-dependent with atopic background

CHRONIC URTICARIA (>30 days) Rarely IgE-dependent; etiology unknown in 80 to 90%; often emotional stress seems to be an exacerbating factor. Intolerance to salicylates.

HISTORY

Duration of Lesions Hours

Skin Symptoms Pruritus, pain on walking (in foot involvement), flushing, burning, and wheezing (in cholinergic urticaria)

Constitutional Symptoms Fever in serum sickness and in the angioedema-urticaria-eosinophilia syndrome; in angioedema, hoarseness, stridor, dyspnea

Systems Review Arthralgia (serum sickness, necrotizing vasculitis, hepatitis)

PHYSICAL EXAMINATION

Skin Lesions

TYPE

Transient papular wheals—many small (1.0 to 2.0 mm are typical in cholinergic urticaria), pruritic

Wheals—small (1.0 cm) to large (8.0 cm), edematous plaques (Figure 239)

Angioedema—skin-colored enlargement of portion of face (eyelids, lips, tongue) (Figures 240a and 240b) or extremity

COLOR Pink with larger lesions having white central area (Figure 239) surrounded by an erythematous halo

SHAPE Oval, arciform, annular, polycyclic (Figure 239), serpiginous, and bizarre patterns

ARRANGEMENT Annular, arciform, linear

DURATION Transient, hours

DISTRIBUTION Localized, regional, or generalized

SITES OF PREDILECTION Sites of pressure, exposed areas (solar urticaria), trunk, hands and feet, lips, tongue, ears

DIAGNOSIS AND DIFFERENTIAL DIAGNOSIS

Wheals in urticaria usually disappear in 24 hours or much less, while persistent urticaria (>96 hours) is suggestive of necrotizing vasculitis (urticarial vasculitis); a biopsy should be done. *Cholinergic urticaria* can best be diagnosed by exercise to sweating and intracutaneous injection of acetylcholine or mecholyl, which will produce whealing (micropapular). *Solar urticaria* is verified by testing with UV and visible light. The *angioedema-urticaria-eosinophilia syndrome* has the following unusual features: fever, high leukocytosis (mostly eosinophils), striking increase in body weight, and a cyclic pattern that may occur and recur over a period of years.

LABORATORY AND SPECIAL EXAMINATIONS

For general medical work-up, to rule out systemic disease in chronic urticaria (SLE, necrotizing vasculitis, lymphoma)

Dermatopathology *Site:* dermis. Edema of the dermis or subcutaneous tissue, dilatation of venules, mast cell degranulation. In necrotizing vasculitis, biopsy is diagnostic. In an-

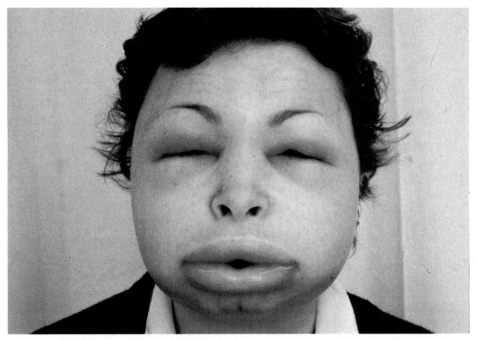

240*a* Hereditary angioedema *This grotesque-looking involvement is to be contrasted to this patient's normal facies shown in Figure 240*b.

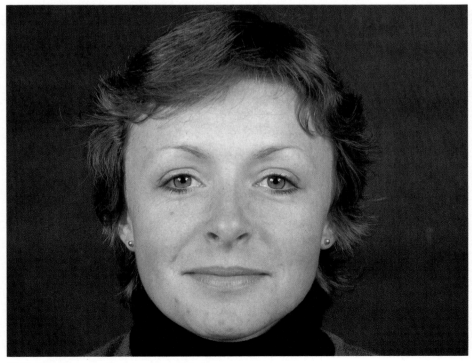

240*b* Hereditary angioedema, normal facies

gioedema-urticaria-eosinophilia syndrome, major basic protein is present outside the eosinophils around blood vessels and collagen bundles. There is dermal edema, a perivascular lymphocytic infiltration, and diffuse eosinophilic infiltration.

General Laboratory

SEROLOGIC Search for hepatitis-associated antigen, assessment of the complement system, assessment of specific IgE antibodies by RAST

HEMATOLOGIC The ESR is often elevated in persistent urticaria (necrotizing vasculitis) and there may be hypocomplementemia; transient eosinophilia in urticaria from reactions to foods and drugs; high levels of eosinophilia in the angioedema-urticaria-eosinophilia syndrome.

Special Examinations

Screening for functional Cl esterase inhibitor

Ultrasonography for early diagnosis of bowel involvement; if abdominal pain is present, this may indicate edema of the bowel.

PATHOPHYSIOLOGY

Lesions in acute IgE-mediated urticaria result from antigen-induced release of biologically active materials from mast cells or basophilic leukocytes sensitized with specific IgE antibodies (type I anaphylactic hypersensitivity). Mediators released increase venular permeability and modulate the release of biologically active materials from other cell types. In complement-mediated urticaria complement is activated by immune complexes, which results in the release of anaphylatoxins which, in turn, induce mast cell degranulation. The

pathogenesis of physical urticaria is unknown; intolerance to salicylates is presumably mediated by abnormalities of the arachidonic acid pathway; in hereditary angioedema decreased or dysfunctional esterase inhibitor leads to increased kinin formation. The angioedema-urticaria-eosinophilia syndrome may possibly result from the eosinophilia which is markedly elevated in the skin. In this syndrome the eosinophilia increases and decreases with the angioedema and urticaria; there are morphologic changes in the eosinophils, including destruction and release of their contents in the dermis; major basic protein is distributed following release from the eosinophil into the collagen bundles, and mast cells in the dermis show degranulation.

COURSE AND PROGNOSIS

Half of the patients with urticaria alone are free of lesions in 1 year, but 20% have lesions for more than 20 years. Prognosis is good in most syndromes except hereditary angioedema, which may be fatal if untreated.

TREATMENT

Try to prevent attacks by elimination of etiologic chemicals or drugs: aspirin and food additives, especially in chronic recurrent urticaria—rarely successful

Antihistamines: H_1 blockers, e.g., hydroxyzine, terfenadine; and if they fail, H_1 and H_2 blockers (e.g., doxepin)

Prednisone is indicated for angioedema-urticaria-eosinophilia syndrome

Danazol as long-term therapy for hereditary angioedema; whole plasma or Cl esterase inhibitor in the acute attack

This is a perplexing multisystem inflammation which, in the most recent definition of diagnostic criteria, has one basic major feature—recurrent *oral* ulceration of the aphthous type—and two of the following features: recurrent genital ulceration, eye lesions (uveitis or retinal vasculitis), skin lesions (erythema nodosum or papulopustular lesions or acneform nodules). Other manifestations include arthritis, neurologic disorders, and thrombophlebitis.

EPIDEMIOLOGY

Frequency In Japan 1:10,000

Age Third decade

Sex Males < females

Geography Most patients in the Middle East, Japan, and Korea

HISTORY

Duration of Lesions Days to weeks, with multiple oral aphthous type ulcerations

Skin Symptoms Pain in mouth lesions

Systems Review Recurrent painful oral and genital ulcers (100%), skin lesions (80%), eye inflammation (60%), blindness from infarction of retina, arthritis or arthralgia, thrombophlebitis (25%), inflammatory bowel disease with discrete ulcerations; CNS involvement (25%): meningoencephalitis, cerebral infarction, cranial nerve palsies, psychosis, hemiparesis and quadriparesis

PHYSICAL EXAMINATION

Skin and Mucous Membranes
TYPE OF LESION *Painful Ulcers* Punched-out (3.0 to >10.0 mm) with rolled or overhanging borders and necrotic base; red rim (Figure 241); occur in crops (2 to 10)

Erythema Nodosum Painful nodules on the arms and legs (40%)
Other Papulopustules
DISTRIBUTION Mouth (Figure 241), vulva (Figure 242), penis, and scrotum

LABORATORY AND SPECIAL EXAMINATIONS

Dermatopathology
LIGHT MICROSCOPY Lymphocytic (T cell) infiltrate, B cells and plasma cells in upper dermis, invading the epidermis; epidermal and subepidermal necrosis and neutrophils; small- and medium-sized vessel leukocytoclastic vasculitis.

Blood Circulating immune complexes can be demonstrated.

Pathergy Test At the site of a needle puncture a pustule surrounded by erythema may appear in some, but not all, patients.

DIAGNOSIS

Recurrent oral aphthosis is the cardinal and major feature. The other criterion is that two of the following be present: recurrent genital ulceration, eye lesions, skin lesions, or positive pathergy test. These then are the criteria for diagnosis.

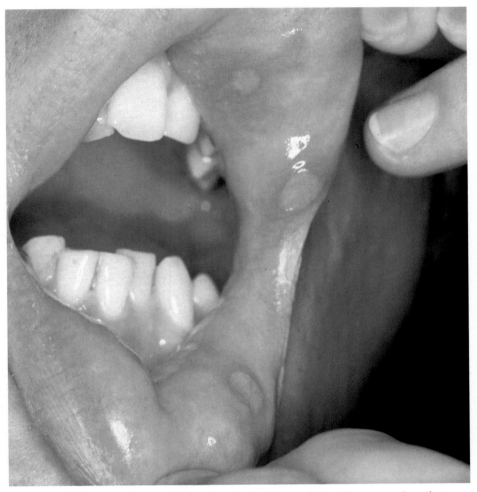

241 Behçet's syndrome *On the labial mucosa there are painful aphthous-type ulcerations.*

ETIOLOGY AND PATHOGENESIS

In the eastern Mediterranean and East Asia, HLA-B5 and HLA-B51; in the United States and Europe, no HLA association. Etiology unknown. The lesions could be the result of an accumulation of neutrophils in the sites of immune complex-mediated vasculitis.

COURSE AND PROGNOSIS

Highly variable course, with recurrences and remissions; the mouth lesions are always present; remissions may last for weeks, months, or years. With CNS involvement there is a higher mortality. In the eastern Mediterranean and East Asia, severe course, one of leading causes of blindness.

TREATMENT

Topical Mouth "retention enemas": tetracycline, 250 mg suspended in a small amount of water (15 mL) and held in the mouth for 15 minutes t.i.d. Intralesional triamcinolone 3 mg per mL injected into ulcer base.

Systemic Various treatments have been proposed: oral colchicine, dapsone, corticosteroids with or without azathioprine, chlorambucil, cyclosporine, and thalidomide. Most effective single agent is chlorambucil, 0.1 mg per kg body weight.

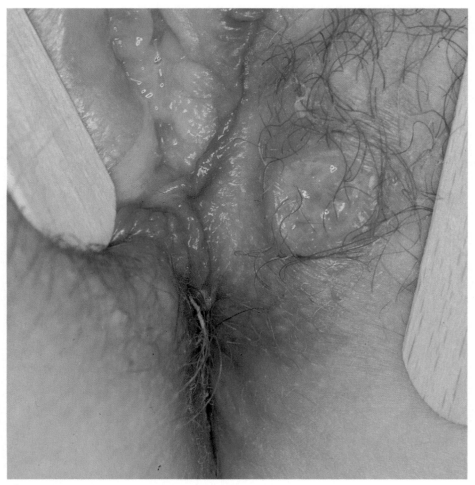

242 Behçet's syndrome *Large, painful aphthous-type ulcer on the vulva.*

This disease is a chronic, recurrent, intensely pruritic eruption occurring often in *symmetrical* groups and comprising three types of lesions: tiny vesicles, papules, and urticarial wheals.

EPIDEMIOLOGY

Age   20 to 60 years, but most common at 30 to 40 years; may occur in children.

Sex   Male:female ratio 2:1

HISTORY

Duration of Lesions   Days, weeks

Skin Symptoms   Pruritus, intense, episodic; burning or stinging of the skin; rarely, pruritus may not occur.

Systems Review   Laboratory evidence of small-bowel malabsorption is detected in 10 to 20%. Gluten-sensitive enteropathy occurs in nearly all patients and is demonstrated by small-bowel biopsy. There are usually no systemic symptoms.

PHYSICAL EXAMINATION

Skin Lesions   (Figures 243 and 244)
TYPES OF LESIONS   Erythematous papule, tiny firm-topped vesicle sometimes hemorrhagic, or urticarial wheal. Occasionally bullae. Excoriations, crusts. Postinflammation spotty pigmentation.
COLOR   Red
ARRANGEMENT   In groups (hence the name *herpetiformis*)
DISTRIBUTION   See Figure XIII. Regional (e.g., scalp) and strikingly symmetrical
SITES OF PREDILECTION   Extensor areas— elbows, knees. Buttocks, scapular, sacral area. Scalp, face, and hairline.

DIFFERENTIAL DIAGNOSIS

Often difficult. Biopsy of early lesions is usually pathognomonic, but immunofluorescence detecting IgA deposits in normal-appearing skin is the best confirming evidence.

LABORATORY AND SPECIAL EXAMINATIONS

Dermatopathology   Biopsy is best from early erythematous papule. (1) Microabscesses (polymorphonuclear cells and eosinophils) at the tips of the dermal papillae. Fibrin accumulation and necrosis occur also. (2) Dermal infiltration (severe) of neutrophils and eosinophils. (3) Subepidermal vesicle.

Immunofluorescence (of Normal-Appearing Skin, Usually the Buttocks)
IgA deposits: (1) *Granular* in tips of papillae— this correlates well with small-bowel disease. Granular IgA is found in the large majority of patients. In addition, complement is also deposited. (2) *Linear,* bandlike along the dermoepidermal junction (other bullous diseases have, in addition, IgG in bandlike pattern at the basement membrane zone). This pattern is not associated with small-bowel disease. Patients with linear IgA constitute only a minority of patients.

Malabsorption Studies   Steatorrhea (20 to 30%) and abnormal D-xylose absorption (10 to 73%)

Hematologic   Anemia secondary to iron or folate deficiency

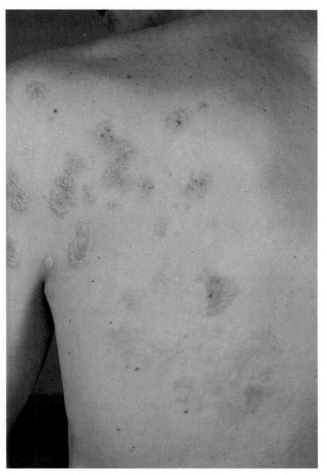

243 Dermatitis herpetiformis *This patient exhibits clusters of grouped vesicles and some residual pigmentation.*

Immunogenetic Findings 77 to 90% of patients with granular IgA have HLA-B8 and HLA-DR3.

RADIOGRAPHIC STUDIES

Small bowel: In the proximal areas of the small intestine there is blunting and flattening of the villi (80 to 90%), as in celiac disease. Lesions are focal and best seen by endoscopy. Verification by small-bowel biopsy.

PATHOPHYSIOLOGY

The relationship of the gluten-sensitive enteropathy to the skin lesions has been controversial. It is now known that circulating immune complexes are always found in patients with dermatitis herpetiformis. It is not known whether IgA binds to antigens in the bowel and complexes then circulate to bind in the skin or whether IgA has specificity for skin proteins. In skin, IgA is associated with microfibrils. IgA and complement mediate a cascade of events (possibly through the alternative complement pathway) leading to tissue injury by chemotaxis of neutrophils and release of enzymes. The absence of gluten sensitivity and gluten-sensitive enteropathy in patients with linear IgA deposits who also have normal prevalence of HLA-B8 and HLA-DR3 suggests that these patients have a different disease (linear IgA disease).

COURSE

Prolonged, for years, with a third of the patients eventually having a spontaneous remission

TREATMENT

Dapsone, 100 to 200 mg daily with gradual reduction to 25 to 50 mg. Obtain G-6-PD before starting treatment. Follow blood counts carefully.

Follow with weekly CBC for 1 month, then every 6 to 8 weeks.

If dapsone contraindicated or not tolerated, sulfapyridine 1.0 to 1.5 g daily, with plenty of fluids.

A gluten-free diet may completely suppress the disease or allow reduction of the dosage of dapsone or sulfapyridine.

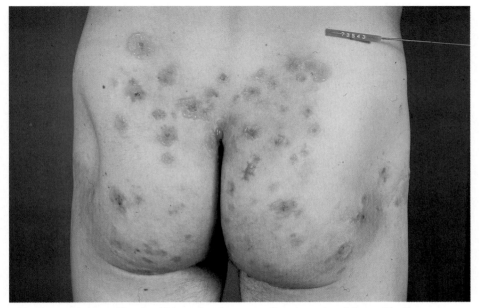

244 Dermatitis herpetiformis *This patient has many firm-topped vesicles and bullae, some erosions, and residual hyperpigmentation. Some of the vesicles are arranged in an annular pattern.*

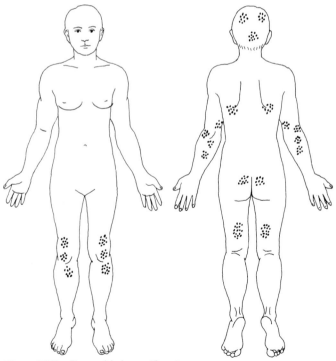

Figure XIII   Dermatitis herpetiformis

DERMATITIS HERPETIFORMIS

Dermatomyositis (DM) is a systemic disease characterized by violaceous (heliotrope) inflammatory changes of the eyelids and periorbital area, erythema of the face, neck, and upper trunk, and by flat-topped violaceous papules over the knuckles, associated with a polymyositis, interstitial pneumonitis, myocardial involvement, vasculitis.

EPIDEMIOLOGY AND ETIOLOGY

Age   Juvenile; >40 years

Etiology   Unknown, cases >55 years often associated with malignancy. Associated malignant tumors: breast, lung, ovary, stomach, colon, uterus.

Clinical Spectrum   Ranges from DM with only cutaneous inflammation to polymyositis with only muscle inflammation.

HISTORY

History   ±Photosensitivity, difficulty combing hair, muscle weakness

Systems Review   Difficulty in rising from supine position, climbing stairs, raising arms over head, turning in bed. Dysphagia.

PHYSICAL EXAMINATION

Skin Findings

TYPES OF LESIONS   Periorbital heliotrope (reddish-purple) flush usually associated with some degree of edema (Figure 245). Dermatitis with varying degrees of erythema (Figure 245) and scaling; may evolve to erosions and ulcers which heal with stellate, bizarre scarring. Flat-topped, violaceous papules (Gottron's papule/sign) (Figure 246) with varying degrees of atrophy. Periungual erythema, telangiectasia, throm-

bosis of capillary loops, infarctions. Calcification in subcutaneous/fascial tissues common later in course of juvenile DM; may evolve to calcinosis universalis.
COLOR   Facial lesions have a heliotrope hue.
PALPATION   ±Muscle atrophy, ±muscle tenderness
DISTRIBUTION OF LESIONS   Pressure points— elbows, knuckles. Dermatitis—forehead, malar area, neck, upper chest. Gottron's papules—dorsa of knuckles (sparing interarticular areas) and nape of neck. ±Sparing of dermatitis under chin and adjacent neck, i.e., photoprotection; accentuation in "V area" of neck; subcutaneous calcifications about elbows, trochanteric region.

General Examination   Progressive muscle weakness affecting proximal/limb girdle muscles. Difficulty or inability to rise from sitting or supine position without using arms. Occasional involvement of facial/bulbar, pharyngeal, and esophageal muscles. Deep tendon reflexes—within normal limits.

DIAGNOSIS AND DIFFERENTIAL DIAGNOSIS

Diagnosis   Proximal muscle weakness with 2 of 3 laboratory criteria, i.e., elevated serum "muscle enzyme" levels, characteristic electromyographic changes, diagnostic muscle biopsy.

Differential Diagnosis   Lupus erythematosus, mixed connective tissue disease, steroid myopathy, trichinosis, toxoplasmosis

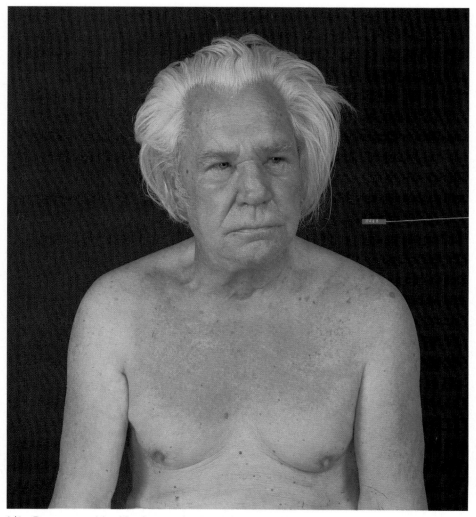

245 Dermatomyositis *The fiery erythema on the upper chest and neck is composed of numerous telangiectases. There is also considerable edema of the eyelids and a heliotrope color of the upper eyelids.*

LABORATORY AND SPECIAL EXAMINATIONS

Chemistry   During acute active phase: elevation of creatine phosphokinase (65%) most specific for muscle disease; also aldolase (40%), glutamic oxaloacetic transaminase, lactic dehydrogenase.

Urine   Elevated 24-hour creatine excretion (>200 mg per 24 hours)

Electromyography   Increased irritability on insertion of electrodes, spontaneous fibrillations, pseudomyotonic discharges, positive sharp waves: excludes neuromyopathy. With evidence of denervation, suspect coexisting tumor.

EKG   Evidence of myocarditis; atrial, ventricular irritability, atrioventricular block.

X-Ray of Chest   ±Interstitial fibrosis

Pathology

SKIN   Flattening of epidermis, hydropic degeneration of basal cell layer, edema of upper dermis, scattered inflammatory infiltrate, PAS+ fibrinoid deposits at dermoepidermal junction and around upper dermal capillaries, accumulation of acid mucopolysaccharides in dermis

MUSCLE   Biopsy shoulder/pelvic girdle; one that is weak or tender, i.e., deltoid, supraspinatus, gluteus, quadriceps. Histology— segmental necrosis within muscle fibers with loss of cross-striations; waxy/coagulative type of eosinophilic staining; ±regenerating fibers; inflammatory cells, histiocytes, macrophages, lymphocytes, plasma cells. Vasculitis may be seen in juvenile DM.

PATHOPHYSIOLOGY

Acute and chronic inflammation of striated muscle accompanied by segmental necrosis of myofibers resulting in progressive muscle weakness.

COURSE AND PROGNOSIS

Dermatitis and polymyositis usually are detected at the same time; however, skin or muscle involvement can occur alone initially, followed at some time by the other. Prognosis is good except in patients with malignancy and those with pulmonary involvement. Current recommendation is that patients >50 years be investigated for associated malignancy: carcinoma of the breast, ovary, bronchopulmonary, GI tract. Successful treatment of the neoplasm often followed by improvement/resolution of DM. Otherwise, course unpredictable. Two-thirds respond to steroid therapy. Subcutaneous calcification is a complication, especially in children.

TREATMENT

Prednisone 0.5 to 1.0 mg per kg body weight per day increasing to 1.5 mg per kg if lower dose ineffective. Taper when muscle enzyme levels approach normal.

Note: Onset of steroid myopathy may occur after 4 to 6 weeks of therapy. Alternative: methotrexate, cyclophosphamide.

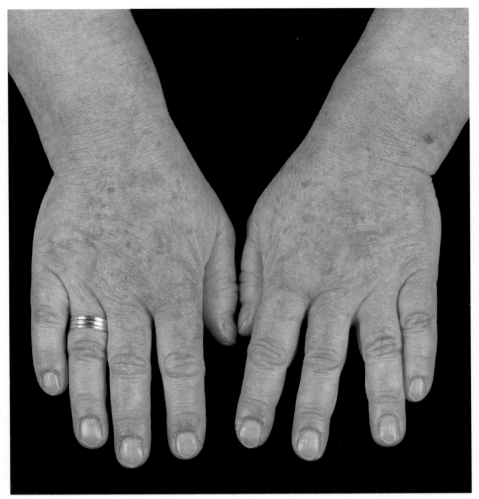

246 Dermatomyositis *In this patient can be seen a vivid red color of the nail fold which is produced by multiple telangiectases. Also on the knuckles there are plaques and papules, which tend to be over bony prominences; these are called* Gottron's papules *but are not specific for dermatomyositis.*

Eosinophilic fasciitis (EF) is an inflammatory disorder characterized by pain, swelling, and tenderness over the extremities, with subsequent induration of the skin and subcutaneous tissues, associated with peripheral eosinophilia.

Synonym: Shulman's syndrome.

EPIDEMIOLOGY AND ETIOLOGY

Age 30 to 60 years

Sex Equal incidence in males and females

Etiology Unknown

HISTORY

Onset may follow strenuous exercise or other physical stress. ±Tenderness, ±swelling, ±thickening of involved skin. History of carpal- and/or tarsal-tunnel syndrome, characterized by distal extremity paresthesias and pain. ±Arthralgia. No history of Raynaud's phenomenon or dysphagia.

PHYSICAL EXAMINATION

Skin Findings

TYPES OF LESIONS Initially, erythema and swelling of (upper > lower) extremities, that evolve to diffuse cutaneous and subcutaneous induration. Epidermis appears normal during early course; later has an indented, shiny, and leathery "orange-peel" appearance (Figure 247) with diffuse or patchy hyperpigmentation. *Presence of the groove sign* (Figure 247): reflects absence of dermal fibrosis around superficial veins, when affected limb raised, collapsed veins resemble a system of merging brooks. Pertinent negative findings: no mat telangiectases, no cutaneous signs of *acral* scleroderma.

COLOR May or may not be erythematous initially. Postinflammatory hyperpigmentation may occur.

PALPATION Skin feels sclerotic, firm, indurated; cannot be moved over fascia. Plaques, on palpation, are corrugated like an old-fashioned washboard. Skin may be tender.

DISTRIBUTION OF LESIONS Proximal limbs, chest, neck. Face, fingers tend to be spared.

Neurologic Findings Percussion over posterior tibial nerve or over carpal tunnel reproduces pain or paresthesia experienced in tunnel syndromes.

DIAGNOSIS AND DIFFERENTIAL DIAGNOSIS

Diagnosis Clinical findings must be confirmed by deep incisional biopsy extending to muscle.

Differential Diagnosis Progressive systemic sclerosis, generalized morphea, generalized lichen sclerosus et atrophicus, Lyme borreliosis with sclerotic plaques, L-tryptophan–induced eosinophilia-myalgia syndrome (criteria: eosinophil count ≥1000 cells/mm^3; myalgias of severity sufficient to interfere with patient's ability to pursue usual activities; exclusion of other infectious or neoplastic findings), scleromyxedema, scleredema of Buschke, chemically induced scleroderma-like sclerosis (polymerizing vinyl chloride, trichloroethylene, toxic oil), post silicone aug-

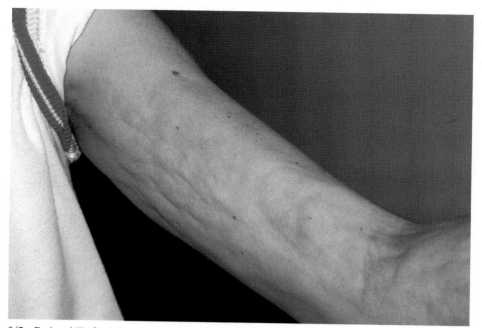

247   Eosinophilic fasciitis   *Illustrated is the diffuse cutaneous induration in which the epidermis is normal and the abnormality of the dermis is represented by the "groove" sign, in which the dermal fibrosis is absent around the superficial veins so that, when the affected limb is raised, the collapsed veins resemble a system of merging brooks.*

mentation mammoplasty, bleomycin chemotherapy, porphyria cutanea tarda, chronic graft-versus-host disease, carcinoid

LABORATORY AND SPECIAL EXAMINATIONS

CBC Eosinophilia may be found at some stage; 10% of patients have associated blood dyscrasias: bone marrow aplasia, autoimmune thrombocytopenia, leukemias, Hodgkin's disease.

ESR Elevated

Immunochemistry Hyperglobulinemia; ANA, rheumatoid factor negative.

Dermatopathology *Adequate biopsy specimen imperative for diagnosis, optimally including subcutaneous tissue, fascia, muscle. Epidermis:* within normal limits. *Dermis:* occasional mild inflammatory infiltrate of lymphocytes, plasma cells, histiocytes, occasional eosinophils, with subsequent fibrosis. *Subcutaneous tissue and fascia:* mixed inflammatory infiltrate of lymphocytes, plasma cells, histiocytes, occasional eosinophils, with subsequent sclerosis of fibrous septa of subcutaneous fat; collagen bundles appear homogeneous or hyalinized; fibrous septa between fat lobules of hypodermis are thickened, with expanded collagen bundles and a perivascular infiltrate. *Eccrine glands:* entrapped by collagen bundles. *Muscle:* mild to moderate perivascular infiltration of lymphocytes, plasma cells, histiocytes, eosinophils.

PATHOPHYSIOLOGY

Uncertain. Both cell-mediated and humoral forms of autoimmunity likely have a role. Primary vascular alterations, enhanced collagen synthesis, and immunologic abnormalities probably have major roles. The groove sign is probably caused by absence of fibrosis above superficial veins. Eosinophilic fasciitis originates in deep fascia and extends outward following connective tissue septa; superficial veins somehow cause sparing of overlying skin so veins collapse normally when limb is elevated.

COURSE AND PROGNOSIS

Most patients respond to systemic corticosteroids. After 1 to 3 years, eosinophilic fasciitis often regresses spontaneously. Prognosis for recovery is excellent in most patients. Residual flexion contractures are common.

TREATMENT

Prednisone, 40 mg daily, may produce marked improvement with decreased swelling and induration of skin, increased joint mobility, and improvement of joint contractures. Therapeutic response to corticosteroids is, however, variable; in 25 to 50% of patients there is little or no response. Moreover, corticosteroid therapy may not have a prolonged benefit. Carpal-/tarsal-tunnel syndrome: local steroid injection; decompressive surgical procedure.

Erythema Multiforme Syndrome

This reaction pattern of blood vessels in the dermis with secondary epidermal changes is exhibited clinically as characteristic erythematous iris-shaped papules and vesicobullous lesions typically involving the extremities (especially the palms and soles) and the mucous membranes.

EPIDEMIOLOGY AND ETIOLOGY

Age 20 to 30 years, with 50% under 20 years

Sex More frequent in males than females

Etiologies
DRUGS Sulfonamides, phenytoin, barbiturates, phenylbutazone, penicillin
INFECTION Especially following herpes simplex, *Mycoplasma*
IDIOPATHIC >50%

HISTORY

Duration of Lesions Several days. May have history of prior episode of erythema multiforme.

Skin Symptoms May be pruritic or painful

Mucous Membrane Symptoms Mouth lesions are painful, tender

Constitutional Symptoms Fever, weakness, malaise

PHYSICAL EXAMINATION

Skin Lesions Lesions may develop over 10 days or more
TYPE
    Macule (48 hours) → papule, 1.0 to 2.0 cm; lesions may appear for 2 weeks
    Vesicles and bullae (in the center of the papule)

COLOR Dull red
SHAPE Iris or target lesions are typical (Figures 248 and 249)
ARRANGEMENT Localized to hands or generalized
DISTRIBUTION Bilateral and often symmetrical
SITES OF PREDILECTION Dorsa of hands, palms, and soles; forearms; feet; elbows and knees; penis (50%) and vulva (see Figure XIV)

Mucous Membranes Mouth and lips (99%) (Figure 248)

Other Organs Pulmonary, eyes with corneal ulcers, anterior uveitis

COURSE

Mild Forms [Erythema Multiforme (EM) Minor] Little or no mucous membrane involvement, no bullae or systemic symptoms. Eruption usually confined to extensor aspects of extremities. Recurrent EM minor is usually associated with an outbreak of herpes simplex preceding it by several days. Chronic suppressive acyclovir therapy prevents recurrence of herpes as well as EM.

Severe Forms (EM Major) Most often occurs as a drug reaction, always with mucous membrane involvement, severe, extensive, tendency to become bullous, systemic symptoms, fever, prostration. Cheilitis and stomatitis interfere with eating, vulvitis and balanitis with micturition. Conjunctivitis can lead to

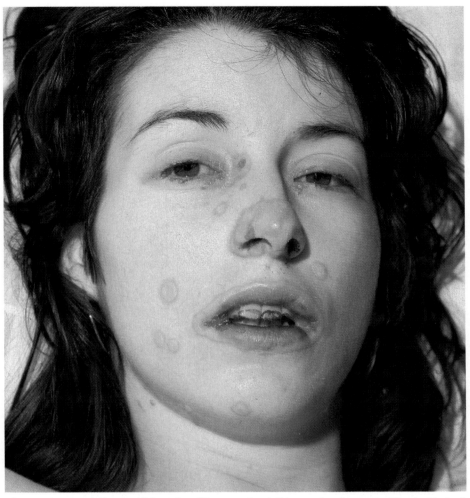

248 Erythema multiforme *This patient illustrates the striking eye involvement with scleritis, peri-orbital erythema, and frank bullae on the inner canthus. There are many targetoid lesions on the face and severe involvement of the oral mucous membrane.*

ERYTHEMA MULTIFORME SYNDROME

keratitis and ulceration; lesions also in pharynx, larynx, and trachea.

Maximal Variant Life-threatening. In addition to the above, necrotizing tracheobronchitis, meningitis, renal tubular necrosis.

DIFFERENTIAL DIAGNOSIS

The target lesion and the symmetry are quite typical, and the diagnosis is not difficult. In the absence of skin lesions, the mucous membrane lesions may present a difficult differential diagnosis: bullous diseases and primary herpetic gingivostomatitis. Urticaria.

DERMATOPATHOLOGY

Site Epidermis and dermis

Process Inflammation characterized by perivascular mononuclear infiltrate, edema of the upper dermis; if bulla formation, there is eosinophilic necrosis of keratinocytes with subepidermal bulla formation.

TREATMENT

Symptomatic. In severely ill patients, systemic corticosteroids are usually given (prednisone 50 to 80 mg daily in divided doses, quickly tapered), but their effectiveness has not been established by controlled studies.

Control of herpes simplex using oral acyclovir may prevent development of recurrent erythema multiforme.

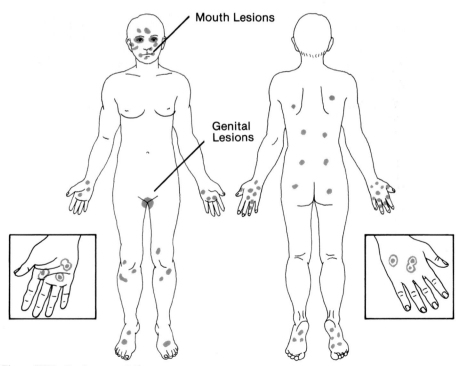

Figure XIV   Erythema multiforme

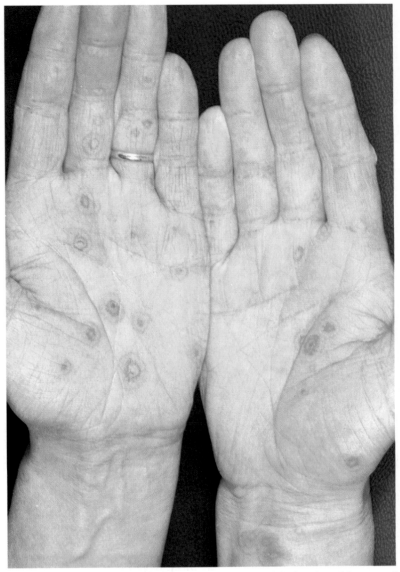

249   Erythema multiforme   *Symmetrically on the flexor sides of the hands and forearms there are edematous-looking, pale, erythematous macules with a vesicle or an erosion in the center surrounded by a few concentric rings. The whole lesion resembles a "target."*

ERYTHEMA MULTIFORME SYNDROME

Erythema nodosum is an important acute inflammatory/immunologic reaction pattern of the panniculus, characterized by the appearance of painful tender nodules on the lower legs and caused by multiple and diverse etiologies.

EPIDEMIOLOGY AND ETIOLOGY

Age 15 to 30 years, but age distribution related to etiology

Sex Three times more common in females than males

Etiologic Associations
INFECTIOUS AGENTS Rarely primary tuberculosis (children), coccidioidomycosis, histoplasmosis, β-hemolytic streptococcus, *Yersinia* organisms, lymphogranuloma venereum
DRUGS Sulfonamides, oral contraceptives
MISCELLANEOUS Sarcoidosis (quite often), ulcerative colitis, Behçet's syndrome, idiopathic ±40%

HISTORY

Duration of Lesions Days

Skin Symptoms Painful, tender lesions

Constitutional Symptoms Fever, malaise

Systems Review Arthralgia (50%), other symptoms depending on etiology

PHYSICAL EXAMINATION

Skin Lesions
TYPE Nodules (3.0 to 20.0 cm) not sharply marginated (Figure 250)

COLOR Bright to deep red, later violaceous
PALPATION Indurated, tender
SHAPE Oval, round, arciform
ARRANGEMENT Scattered discrete lesions (2 to 50)
DISTRIBUTION Bilateral but not symmetrical
SITES OF PREDILECTION Lower legs (most frequent) (Figure 250), knees, arms, rarely face and neck

LABORATORY AND SPECIAL EXAMINATIONS

Culture throat for GABHS (group A β-hemolytic streptococcus)

Radiologic examination of the chest is important to rule out sarcoidosis

DERMATOPATHOLOGY

Site Panniculus

Process Acute (polymorphonuclear) and chronic (granulomatous) inflammation in the panniculus and around blood vessels in the septum and adjacent fat

COURSE

Spontaneous resolution occurs in 6 weeks, but the course depends on the etiology.

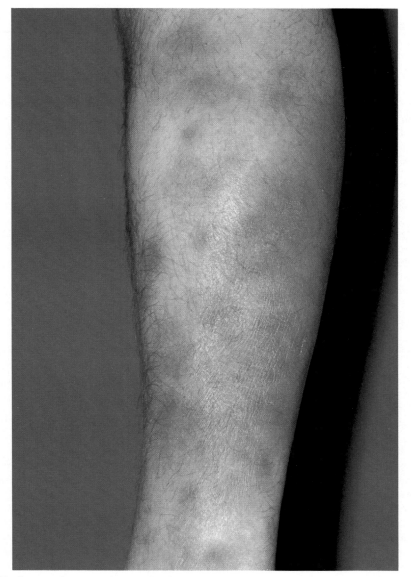

250 Erythema nodosum syndrome *On the sides and front of the lower leg there are tender, red, warm, nodular and indurated lesions. The borders are not well defined.*

TREATMENT

Bed rest or compressive bandages (lower legs). Symptomatic anti-inflammatory treatment: salicylates, iodides. The use of systemic corticosteroids is indicated only when the etiology is known (and infectious agents are excluded).

Graft-versus-host disease (GVHD) is an immune disorder caused by the response of histoincompatible, immunocompetent donor cells against the tissues of an immunoincompetent host (graft-versus-host reaction, GVHR), characterized by acute cutaneous changes ranging from maculopapular eruption to toxic epidermal necrolysis, diarrhea, and liver dysfunction, as well as a chronic sclerodermatous stage.

EPIDEMIOLOGY AND ETIOLOGY

Incidence Varies between 60 and 80% of successful engraftment with allogeneic marrow. Low incidence following blood transfusion in immunosuppressed patient, maternal-fetal transfer in immunodeficiency disease.

Etiology

HOST Recipients of marrow transplants: aplastic anemia, acute leukemia, some immunodeficiency disorders. Immunosuppressed patients receiving blood transfusions containing immunocompetent leukocytes. Immunodeficient fetus with maternal-fetal transfer of leukocytes.

TYPES OF GVHD *Acute* During first 3 months after bone marrow transplantation (usually between 14 and 21 days)

Chronic >100 days after bone marrow transplantation. Either evolving from acute GVHD or arising de novo. Acute GVHD is not always followed by chronic GVHD. Clinical classification thus distinguishes between "quiescent onset," "progressive onset," and "de novo" chronic cutaneous GVHD.

HISTORY

History Mild pruritus, localized/generalized; pain on pressure, palms/soles.

Systems Review Nausea/vomiting, right upper quadrant pain/tenderness; cramping abdominal pain, watery diarrhea. Cough.

PHYSICAL EXAMINATION

Skin Findings

CLINICAL GRADING OF ACUTE CUTANEOUS GVHD

1. Erythematous maculopapular eruption involving <25% of body surface
2. Erythematous maculopapular eruption involving 25 to 50% of body surface
3. Erythroderma
4. Bulla formation

TYPES OF LESIONS *Acute GVHD* Initially: subtle, discrete macules and/or papules (Figure 251); mild edema/violaceous hue, periungual and pinna. If controlled/resolves, erythema diminishes with subsequent desquamation and postinflammatory hyperpigmentation. If progresses, macules/papules become confluent and then generalized, i.e., erythrodermic. Subepidermal bullae, especially over pressure/trauma sites (Figure 252). If bullae widespread with rupture/erosion, toxic epidermal necrolysis-like (TEN-like) form of acute cutaneous GVHR.

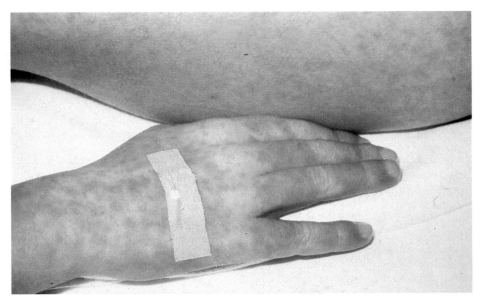

251 Acute graft-versus-host disease *There are discrete and confluent, erythematous, blanchable macules and papules involving the hands and the trunk.*

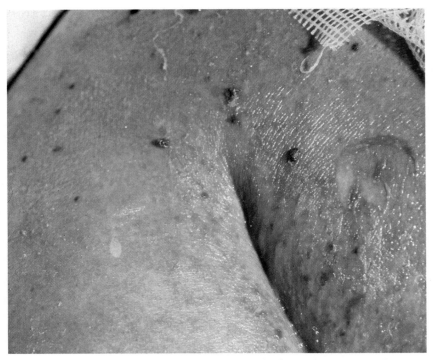

252 Acute graft-versus-host-disease *This is a later stage in the development, and there is epidermal necrolysis with erosions and hemorrhagic vesicles.*

Chronic GVHD Flat-topped papules, lichen planus-like (Figure 253). Confluent areas of dermal sclerosis (Figure 253) with overlying scale. Hair loss; anhidrosis, vitiligo-like hypopigmentation; lichen planus-like lesions in oral mucosa; erosive stomatitis, oral and ocular sicca-like syndrome; esophagitis, serositis. More common are severe sclerodermoid changes with necrosis and ulceration on acral and pressure sites.

COLOR *Acute GVHD* Erythematous

Chronic GVHD Violaceous

PALPATION *Acute GVHD* Pain at pressure points

Chronic GVHD Sclerotic

DISTRIBUTION OF LESIONS *Acute GVHD* Earliest findings—upper trunk, hands/feet especially palms/soles

Chronic GVHD Distal extremities. Sclerosis—trunk, buttocks, hips, thighs

General Examination ±Fever

DIAGNOSIS AND DIFFERENTIAL DIAGNOSIS

Diagnosis Clinical setting confirmed by skin biopsy

Differential Diagnosis

ACUTE GVHD Exanthematous drug reaction, viral exanthem, TEN, erythroderma

CHRONIC GVHD Lichen planus, lichenoid drug reaction, scleroderma, poikiloderma

LABORATORY AND SPECIAL EXAMINATIONS

Chemistry Elevated SGOT, bilirubin

Dermatopathology

ACUTE GVHD Basal vacuolization several days before clinically detectable lesions → focal vacuolization of basal cell layer, *necrosis of individual keratinocytes;* mild perivenular mononuclear cell infiltrate → increasing vacuolization/cellular necrosis; apposition of lymphocytes to necrotic kerat-inocytes; vacuoles coalesce forming subepidermal clefts; endothelial cell swelling → subepidermal blister formation. Immunocytochemistry: HLA-DR expression by keratinocytes precedes morphologic changes and thus represents important, early diagnostic sign.

CHRONIC GVHD Hyperkeratosis, mild hypergranulosis, mild irregular acanthosis, moderate basal vacuolization; mild perivascular mononuclear cell infiltrate; melanin incontinence → hyperkeratosis, epidermal atrophy or acanthosis, rare individual cell necrosis, mild perivascular mononuclear cell infiltrate, melanin incontinence; loss of hair follicles, entrapment of sweat glands; dense dermal sclerosis.

PATHOPHYSIOLOGY

GVHR associated with inflammatory reaction mounted by the donor cells against specific host organs—skin, liver, or GI tract. Severity of GVHD related to histocompatibility match between donor and recipient and preparatory regimen used. With successful engraftment there is replacement of host marrow by immunocompetent donor cells capable of reacting against the ''foreign'' tissue antigens of the host.

COURSE AND PROGNOSIS

Acute GVHD Mild to moderate GVHD responds well to treatment. Prognosis of TEN-like GVHR grave. Severe GVHD susceptible to infections—bacterial, fungal, viral (CMV, HSV, VZV). Acute GVHD is primary or associated cause of death in 15 to 70% of bone marrow transplant patients.

Chronic GVHD Sclerodermoid with tight skin/joint contracture may result in impaired mobility, ulcerations. Permanent hair loss; xerostomia, xerophthalmia → corneal ulcers → blindness. Malabsorption. Mild chronic cutaneous GVHD may resolve spontaneously.

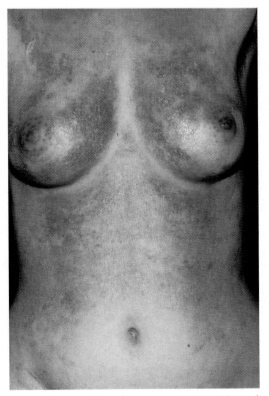

253 Chronic graft-versus-host disease *Sclerodermoid and lichenoid reaction. There is a striking pigmentation and induration over the upper chest, breasts, and upper abdomen.*

TREATMENT

Acute GVHD High-dose corticosteroids ± azathioprine or methotrexate. Hyperalimentation, protective isolation, antibiotics, physical therapy.

Chronic GVHD Corticosteroids, thalidomide (not easily available), supportive and symptomatic measures. Lichen planus-like skin lesions respond to PUVA.

Livedo reticularis (LR) is a mottled bluish (livid) discoloration of the skin that occurs in a netlike pattern. It is not a diagnosis in itself but a reaction pattern.

Synonyms: livedo racemosa, livedo annularis.

EPIDEMIOLOGY AND ETIOLOGY

Classification

Idiopathic livedo reticularis (ILR) Permanent bluish mottling for which no underlying disease is found.

Secondary or symptomatic livedo reticularis (SLR) Associated with underlying disorder such as *intravascular obstruction* [viscosity changes, stasis (paralysis, cardiac failure), organic (atheroemboli, thrombocythemia, cryoglobulinemia, cold agglutininemia, air)]; *vessel wall disease* [arteriosclerosis, hyperparathyroidism, vasculitis syndromes (polyarteritis nodosa, cutaneous polyarteritis nodosa, rheumatoid vasculitis, lupus erythematosus, dermatomyositis, lymphoma, syphilis, tuberculosis, pancreatitis)]; *drugs* (amantadine, quinine, quinidine)

Sneddon's syndrome Extensive livedo reticularis, hypertension, cerebrovascular accidents, and transient ischemic attacks

Age ILR: 20s to 50s

Sex ILR: more common in females

Etiology ILR: unknown. SLR: that of associated disorder.

Season Worse during winter months

HISTORY

Appearance or worsening with cold exposure. ±Numbness, tingling associated.

PHYSICAL EXAMINATION

Skin Findings

TYPE OF LESION Netlike, blotchy, or mottled pattern of cyanosis. Skin within webs of net (Figure 254) is normal to pallid. ILR: ulceration may occur in winter or spring/summer about ankles.

COLOR Reddish blue

PALPATION Skin feels cool

DISTRIBUTION OF LESIONS *ILR:* Symmetrical, arms/legs; less commonly, body; ulceration on lower legs. *SLR:* patchy, asymmetrical on extremities.

General Examination *ILR:* noncontributory. *SLR:* symptoms of underlying disease, thromboembolitic disease. Sneddon's syndrome: neurologic lesions (palsy, aphasia).

DIAGNOSIS AND DIFFERENTIAL DIAGNOSIS

Diagnosis Clinical diagnosis confirmed by laboratory data supporting diagnosis of associated disorder

Differential Diagnosis Cutis marmorata (transient physiologic mottling of skin which resolves on warming), livedoid vasculitis (segmental hyalinizing vasculitis causing atrophie blanche), erythema ab igne

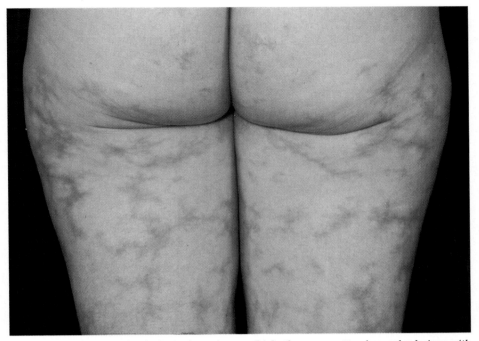

254 Livedo reticularis *On the buttocks and upper thighs there are scattered macular lesions with a netlike configuration. The skin within the webs of the net is normal and pale. The patient had labile hypertension and cerebrovascular ischemic attacks.*

LABORATORY AND SPECIAL EXAMINATIONS

Laboratory SLR: Varies with associated disorders

Dermatopathology ILR with ulceration: arteriolar intimal proliferation with dilated numerous capillaries, thickening of walls of venules; lymphocytic perivascular infiltration. In Sneddon's syndrome: vascular changes as in endarteritis obliterans.

PATHOPHYSIOLOGY

LR pattern due to vasospasm of perpendicular arterioles, perforating dermis from below. Cyanotic periphery of each web of net caused by deoxygenated blood in surrounding horizontally arranged venous plexuses. When factors such as cold cause increased viscosity/low flow rates in superficial venous plexus, further deoxygenation occurs and cyanotic reticular pattern becomes more pronounced. Elevation of limb decreases intensity of color due to increased venous drainage. LR may result from arteriolar disease causing obstruction to inflow and blood hyperviscosity, or from obstruction to outflow of blood in venules.

COURSE AND PROGNOSIS

ILR occurs on exposure to cold, but in time may become permanent. Course/prognosis of SLR depends on that of associated disorder.

TREATMENT

ILR: Keep from chilling extremity. Pentoxifylline 400 mg p.o. t.i.d. and low-dose aspirin may be helpful.

SLR: Treat associated disorder.

This serious multisystem disease involves connective tissue and blood vessels; the clinical manifestations include fever (90%); skin lesions (85%); arthritis; and renal, cardiac, and pulmonary disease. Systemic lupus erythematosus (SLE) may uncommonly develop in patients with chronic discoid lupus erythematosus (DLE), but lesions of DLE are common in SLE.

EPIDEMIOLOGY AND ETIOLOGY

Age 30 (females), 40 (males)

Sex Male:female ratio 1:8

Race More common in blacks

Other Features Family history (<5%); SLE syndrome can be induced by drugs (hydralazine, certain anticonvulsants, and procainamide), although rash is an uncommon feature of drug-induced SLE. Sunlight may cause an exacerbation of SLE (36%).

HISTORY

Duration of Lesions Weeks (acute), months

Skin Symptoms Pruritus (especially papular lesions), smarting

Constitutional Symptoms Fatigue (100%), fever (100%), weight loss, and malaise

Systems Review Arthralgia or arthritis, abdominal pain

PHYSICAL EXAMINATION

Skin Lesions
TYPE
  Erythematous, confluent, macular butterfly eruption (face) (Figure 255) with fine scaling; erosions and crusts

  Erythematous, discrete, papular or urticarial lesions (face and arms)

  Bullae, often hemorrhagic (acute flares)

  Discoid papules as in chronic DLE (face and arms)

  ''Palpable'' purpura (vasculitis)

  Urticarial lesions with purpura (''urticarial vasculitis'')

COLOR   Bright red (Figure 255)
SHAPE   Round or oval
ARRANGEMENT   Diffuse involvement of the face in light-exposed areas. Scattered discrete lesions (Figure 256) (face, forearms, and dorsa of hands)
DISTRIBUTION   Localized or generalized
SITES OF PREDILECTION   Face (80%); scalp (discoid lesions); presternal, shoulders; dorsa of the forearms, hands, fingers, fingertips (vasculitis); palms; periungual telangiectases and palmar erythema are also seen.

Hair Discoid lesions associated with patchy alopecia. Diffuse alopecia.

Mucous Membranes Ulcers arising in purpuric necrotic lesions on palate (80%), buccal mucosa, or gums

Extracutaneous Multisystem Involvement Arthralgia or arthritis (15%), renal disease (50%), pericarditis (20%), pneumonitis (20%), gastrointestinal (due to arteritis and

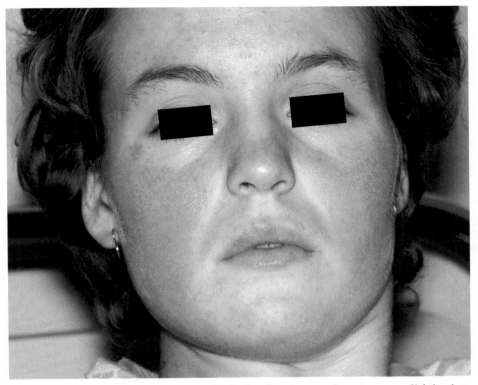

255   Systemic lupus erythematosus, acute   *On the face there is an erythematous, very slightly edematous, sharply outlined erythema in the "butterfly" area.*

sterile peritonitis), hepatomegaly (30%), splenomegaly (20%), lymphadenopathy (50%), peripheral neuropathy (14%), CNS disease (10%), seizures or organic brain disease (14%)

DERMATOPATHOLOGY

Skin Atrophy of epidermis, liquefaction degeneration of the dermoepidermal junction, edema of the dermis, dermal inflammatory infiltrate (lymphocytes), and fibrinoid degeneration of the connective tissue and walls of the blood vessels

Other Organs The fundamental lesion is fibrinoid degeneration of connective tissue and walls of the blood vessels, which is associated with an inflammatory infiltrate of plasma cells and lymphocytes.

Immunofluorescence of Skin The lupus band test (direct immunofluorescence demonstrating IgG, IgM, C1q) shows granular or globular deposits of immune reactants in a bandlike pattern along the dermoepidermal junction. This is positive in lesional skin in 90% and in clinically normal skin (sun-exposed, 70 to 80%; non-sun-exposed, 50%); in the latter case indicative of renal disease and hypocomplementemia.

LABORATORY AND SPECIAL EXAMINATIONS

Serologic ANA positive (>95%); peripheral pattern of nuclear fluorescence and anti-double-stranded DNA antibodies are specific for SLE; low levels of complement (especially with renal involvement). SS-A(Ro) autoantibodies are present in a subset of subacute cutaneous lupus erythematosus (SCLE) in which there is extensive skin involvement and photo-sensitivity. SS-B(La) antibodies also coexist in 50% of the cases.

Hematologic Anemia [normocytic, normochromic, or, rarely, hemolytic Coombs-positive, leukopenia (<4000/mm^3)], elevated ESR (a good guide to activity of the disease)

PATHOPHYSIOLOGY

The tissue injury in the epidermis results from the deposition of immune complexes at the dermoepidermal junction. Immune complexes selectively generate the assembly of the membrane-attack complex, which mediates membrane injury.

TREATMENT

General measures: rest, avoidance of sun exposure.

Indications for prednisone (60 mg daily in divided doses): (1) CNS involvement, (2) renal involvement, (3) severely ill patients without CNS involvement, (4) hemolytic crisis.

Concomitant immunosuppressive drugs (azathioprine or cyclophosphamide) depending on organ involvement and activity of disease.

Chloroquine sulfate or other antimalarials are useful for treatment of the skin lesions in subacute and chronic SLE, but do not reduce the need for prednisone. See precautions in the use of chloroquine on page 494.

PROGNOSIS

Five-year survival is 93%.

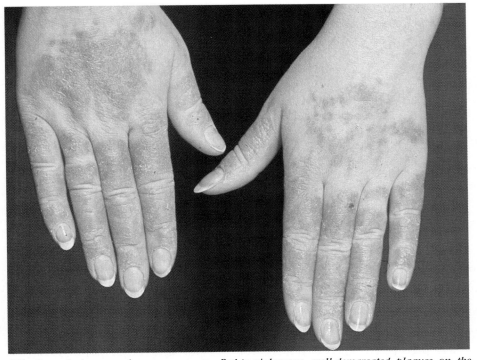

256 Systemic lupus erythematosus, acute *Red-to-violaceous, well-demarcated plaques on the dorsa of the fingers and hands with periungual erythema sparing the knuckles.*

Subacute cutaneous lupus erythematosus (SCLE) is regarded by many as a variant of chronic discoid lupus erythematosus (CDLE). There is, however, no follicular plugging and no scarring or atrophy as is frequently noted in CDLE. Patients with SCLE may have a few of the criteria of SLE as defined by the American Rheumatism Association, including photosensitivity, arthralgias, serositis, renal disease, and serologic abnormalities, especially anti-Ro (SS-A) and anti-La (SS-B) antibodies. The serious criteria of SLE are uncommon: severe vasculitis, severe CNS disease, or progressive renal disease. The clinical skin lesions are the distinctive feature of SCLE.

Synonyms: subacute LE, subacute disseminated LE.

EPIDEMIOLOGY

Incidence About 10% of the LE population

Age Young and middle aged

Race Uncommon in blacks or Hispanics

Sex Females > males

Precipitating Factors Sunlight exposure

HISTORY

Duration Rather sudden onset with diffuse, erythematous eruption appearing on the upper trunk, dorsa of the hands

Constitutional Symptoms Chronic: mild fatigue, malaise

Systems Review Some arthralgia, fever of unknown origin

PHYSICAL EXAMINATION

Skin Findings
TYPE OF LESION Psoriasiform. Papulosquamous, with slight delicate scaling (Figure 257), and occasionally vesicular lesions.

Telangiectasia. No scarring, atrophy, or follicular plugging; not sharply demarcated as in CDLE. Hypopigmentation.

SHAPE OF INDIVIDUAL LESION Annular, arciform, iris-shaped (erythema multiforme-like)

ARRANGEMENT OF MULTIPLE LESIONS Scattered diffuse (Figure 257), livedo pattern

DISTRIBUTION OF LESIONS In light-exposed areas (Figure 257): shoulders, extensor surface of the arms, dorsal surface of the hands, upper back, V-neck area of the upper chest. Only rarely on the face.

Hair Diffuse nonscarring alopecia

Nails Periungual telangiectasia

LABORATORY EXAMINATIONS

Dermatopathology
LIGHT MICROSCOPY Liquefaction degeneration of the basal layer and edema of the upper dermis which can sometimes lead to vesicle formation. Colloid bodies in the epidermis.

IMMUNOFLUORESCENCE Only 40% have immune deposits in dermoepidermal junction.

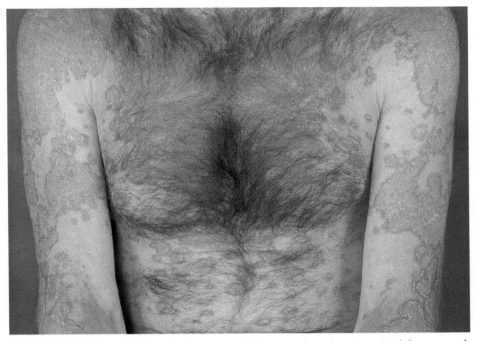

257　Subacute cutaneous lupus erythematosus　*Widely scattered, erythematous-to-violaceous, scaling, very well-demarcated plaques on the trunk, neck, and arms.*

UV TESTING　Most patients have a lower than normal UVB MED. Typical SCLE lesions may develop in UVB test sites.

Laboratory Examination of Blood

SEROLOGIC　Low titers of ANA. Antibodies to Ro/SS-A antigen present in more than 60%, as well as high levels of circulating immune complexes.

DIFFERENTIAL DIAGNOSIS

The extensive involvement is far more than is ever seen in CDLE, and the distinctive eruption is a marker for SCLE. The skin lesions could, however, be confused with atypical psoriasis or dermatomyositis.

COURSE AND PROGNOSIS

A better prognosis than for SLE. Some patients may have renal (and CNS) involvement and thus have guarded prognosis. The skin lesions can completely disappear, but occasionally a vitiligo-like leukoderma remains for some months.

TREATMENT

Topical　Anti-inflammatory corticosteroids are somewhat helpful.

Systemic　This is usually required. Hydroxychloroquine 400 mg per day; if this does not control the skin lesions, quinacrine hydrochloride, 100 mg per day, can be added. The bizarre yellow skin color caused by quinacrine can be somewhat modified by beta carotene, 60 mg t.i.d. Thalidomide (200 to 300 mg per day) very effective for skin lesions but not for systemic involvement.

This chronic, indolent skin disease is characterized by sharply marginated, scaly, atrophic, red plaques, usually occurring on habitually exposed areas.

EPIDEMIOLOGY

Age   20 to 45 years

Sex   Females > males

Race   Possibly more severe in blacks

CLASSIFICATION

Discoid lupus erythematosus (localized and generalized)

Lupus erythematosus panniculitis (lupus profundus)

HISTORY

Duration of Lesions   Months to years

Skin Symptoms   Usually none, sometimes slightly pruritic or smarting

Systems Review   Negative

PHYSICAL EXAMINATION

Skin Lesions

TYPE   *Early*   Papules and plaques, sharply marginated, with slight adherent scaling
Late   Atrophy and depression of lesions, with slightly raised border (Figure 258). Erythema contains fine telangiectases. Follicular plugging (closely set and often in clusters), dilated follicles, and scarring. Chronic untreated cutaneous lupus erythematosus results in marked scarring, with depressed and contracted lesions on the face, creating a wolflike, or lupus, facies.
COLOR   Active lesions bright red. "Burned out" lesions may be pink or white (hypomelanosis) macules and scars. Lesions may show hyperpigmentation, especially in persons with brown or black skin.
SHAPE   Round, oval, annular, polycyclic with irregular borders
DISTRIBUTION   Scattered discrete lesions
SITES OF PREDILECTION   Face and scalp; otherwise: nose, dorsa of forearms, hands, fingers, toes, and less frequently the trunk

Hair   Scarring alopecia associated with lesions in the scalp skin

Mucous Membranes   Less than 5% of patients have lip involvement (hyperkeratosis, hypermelanotic scarring, erythema) and atrophic erythematous areas with (Figure 259) or without ulceration on the buccal mucosa, tongue, and palate.

DIFFERENTIAL DIAGNOSIS

The lesions of chronic discoid lupus erythematosus (CDLE) may closely mimic *actinic keratosis*. *Plaque psoriasis* and scaling discoid lupus erythematosus without atrophy and scarring may be difficult to distinguish, especially on the dorsa of the hands; histopathology permits distinction. Polymorphous light eruption (PMLE) may pose a problem. PMLE disappears in the winter in northern latitudes, does not develop atrophy or follicular plugging, and does not occur in unexposed areas—mouth, hairy scalp. *Lichen planus* can be confusing

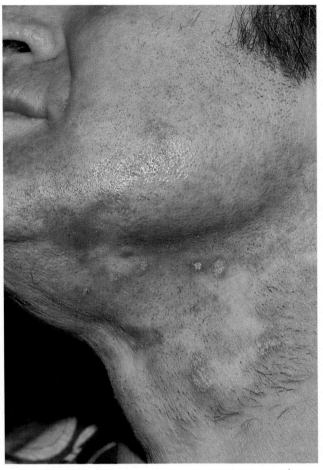

258   Chronic cutaneous lupus erythematosus   *Round-to-ovoid, slightly indurated, red-violaceous patches, fairly sharply demarcated, disseminated on the neck and face. Most patches show a slight follicular keratotic scaling, and some show central atrophy. Hypopigmentation and scarring mark the sites of lesions that have resolved.*

but the biopsy is distinctive. *Lupus vulgaris* and *tinea faciale*.

LABORATORY AND SPECIAL EXAMINATIONS

Dermatopathology Hyperkeratosis, atrophy of the epidermis, follicular plugging, liquefaction degeneration of the basal cell layer. In the dermis there is edema, dilatation of small blood vessels, and perifollicular and periappendageal inflammatory infiltrate (lymphocytes and histiocytes). Strong PAS reaction of the subepidermal, thickened basement zone.

Immunofluorescence Positive in active lesions at least 6 weeks old. Granular deposits of IgG (>IgM) at the dermoepidermal junction. This is known as the *lupus band test* (LBT) and is positive in 90% of active lesions not recently treated with topical corticosteroids but *negative in burnt-out (scarred) lesions and in the normal skin,* both sun-exposed and non-exposed. SLE, in contrast, has a positive LBT in lesional as well as both normal sun-exposed (70 to 80%) and nonexposed (50%) skin.

General Laboratory Examination
SEROLOGIC   Low incidence of ANA in a titer more than 1:16
HEMATOLOGIC   Occasionally leukopenia (<4500/mm^3)

COURSE AND PROGNOSIS

Only 1 to 5% may develop SLE; with localized lesions, complete remission occurs in 50%; with generalized lesions, remissions are less frequent (<10%). *Note:* CDLE lesions may be presenting cutaneous sign of SLE.

PRETREATMENT SCREENING WHEN USING ANTIMALARIALS

G-6-PD screening

Liver function tests

Slit-lamp and funduscopic examination

Assessment of visual acuity

Visual field testing by both static and kinetic techniques with a 3-mm red test object

Have patients test themselves with the Amsler grid every 2 weeks

TREATMENT

Topical suncreens (SPF 30) routinely

Topical fluorinated corticosteroids (with caution)

Use of an occlusive hydrocolloid patch with steroids (left on for 48 to 96 hours)

Intralesional triamcinolone acetonide, 3 to 5 mg per mL, for small lesions

Hydroxychloroquine ≤6.5 mg/kg per day. Pretreatment eye examinations and ophthalmologic monitoring are important as retinopathy has been reported. If hydroxychloroquine is ineffective, add quinacrine 100 mg t.i.d.

Hyperkeratotic CDLE lesions respond well to systemic etretinate (1 mg per kg body weight).

FOLLOW-UP (EVERY 6 MONTHS)

Review subjective visual complaints, slit-lamp and funduscopic test results, and visual acuity

Repeat visual testing if patients complain of difficulty in reading ("missing" words and letters) and demonstrate reproducible bilateral "fading" of Amsler grid squares.

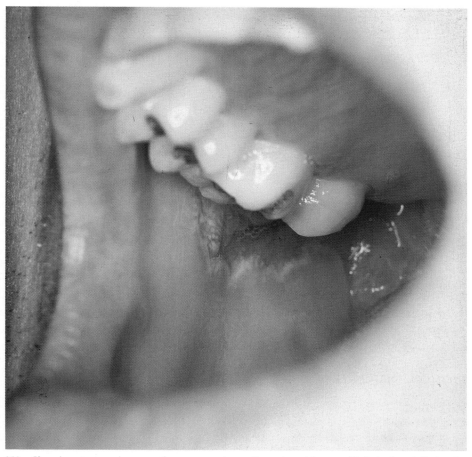

259 Chronic cutaneous lupus erythematosus   *An erythematous plaque with hyperkeratotic border (white area) is noted on the buccal mucosa.*

Chronic Cutaneous Lupus Erythematosus Panniculitis

This is a form of chronic cutaneous lupus erythematosus in which there are indolent, firm, circumscribed nodules on the face, scalp, breast, upper arms, thighs, and buttocks. Most patients also have typical lesions of discoid lupus erythematosus.

Synonym: lupus erythematosus profundus.

HISTORY

Duration of Lesions May precede or follow the onset of discoid lesions by several years.

Skin Symptoms Pain, slight tenderness

Systems Review In one series 35% of the patients had SLE

PHYSICAL EXAMINATION

Skin Findings
TYPE OF LESION
  Plaques, with or without grossly visible epidermal changes; these evolve into deep depressions

  Atrophic plaques (Figure 260)

  Ulcers may develop in the plaques or nodules
PALPATION Plaques or nodules are better felt than seen; the overlying skin may be normal or exhibit typical lesions of chronic discoid lupus erythematosus
SHAPE OF INDIVIDUAL LESION Platelike lesions or round nodules, linear plaques
ARRANGEMENT OF MULTIPLE LESIONS Scattered discrete lesions
DISTRIBUTION OF LESIONS Scalp, face, upper arms, trunk (especially the breasts), thighs, and buttocks

LABORATORY EXAMINATIONS

Dermatopathology
LIGHT MICROSCOPY *Site* Subcutaneous layer
Process Necrobiosis with fibrinoid deposits; later, hyalinization of the fat lobules; there may be considerable mucinous deposits and also rarely a severe vasculitis.
SPECIAL TECHNIQUES Special stains: mucin stains

Laboratory Examination of Blood In those patients with SLE there are typical hematologic and serologic abnormalities

SPECIAL EXAMINATIONS

Oblique Lighting In a completely darkened room, place a flashlight at the site of the lesion to detect subtle surface changes (elevation or depression)

DIFFERENTIAL DIAGNOSIS

Morphea, erythema nodosum, sarcoid, miscellaneous types of panniculitis

TREATMENT

Systemic Same as for chronic cutaneous lupus erythematosus, discoid type

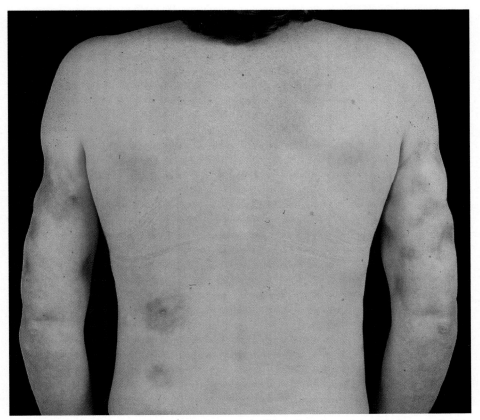

260   Chronic cutaneous lupus erythematosus panniculitis *Chronic panniculitis has resulted in large, sunken areas of overlying skin. Erythema and some atrophy of skin are seen.*

Scleroderma is a multisystem disorder characterized by inflammatory, vascular, and sclerotic changes of the skin and a variety of internal organs, especially the lungs, heart, and GI tract.

Synonyms: progressive systemic sclerosis, systemic sclerosis, systemic scleroderma.

EPIDEMIOLOGY AND ETIOLOGY

Age   Onset 30 to 50 years

Sex   Incidence in women 4 times greater than in men

Etiology   Unknown

Clinical Variant   CREST syndrome, i.e., *C*alcinosis cutis + *R*aynaud's phenomen + *E*sophageal dysfunction + *S*clerodactyly + *T*elangiectasia

HISTORY

Skin Symptoms   Raynaud's phenomenon with digital pain, coldness, rubor with pain and tingling.

Systems Review   Pain/stiffness of fingers, knees. Migratory polyarthritis. Heartburn, dysphagia especially with solid foods. Constipation, diarrhea, abdominal bloating, malabsorption, weight loss. Exertional dyspnea, dry cough.

PHYSICAL EXAMINATION

Skin, Hair, and Nail Findings

TYPES OF LESIONS   *Hands/feet Early:* Raynaud's phenomenon with triphasic color changes, i.e., pallor, cyanosis, rubor. Nonpitting edema of hands/feet. Painful ulcerations at fingertips, knuckles; heal with pitted scars. *Late:* sclerodactyly with tapering fingers (Figure 261), waxy shiny atrophic skin; flexion contractures; bony resorption results in loss of distal phalanges. Cutaneous calcification of fingers associated with drainage of white paste from ulcerations.

Face Early: periorbital edema. *Late:* edema and fibrosis result in loss of normal facial lines, masklike (Figure 261), thinning of lips, microstomia, radial perioral furrowing, small sharp nose.

Ulceration   Secondary to vascular occlusion, acrally (Figure 261)

Cutaneous Calcification   Occurs over bony prominences or any sclerodermatous site; may ulcerate and extrude white paste.

CREST Syndrome   Matlike telangiectasia (Figure 262), especially on face, neck, upper trunk, hands; also lips, oral mucous membranes, GI tract.

COLOR   Hyperpigmentation, generalized. In areas of sclerosis, postinflammatory hyper- and hypopigmentation.

PALPATION   *Early:* skin feels indurated, stiff. *Late:* tense, smooth, hardened, bound down. Leathery crepitation over joints, especially knees.

DISTRIBUTION OF LESIONS   *Early:* fingers, hands. *Late:* upper extremities, trunk, face, lower extremities

HAIR AND NAILS   Thinning/complete loss of hair on distal extremities. Loss of sweat glands with anhidrosis. Periungual telangiectasia with giant sausage-shaped capillary loops. Nails grow clawlike over shortened distal phalanges.

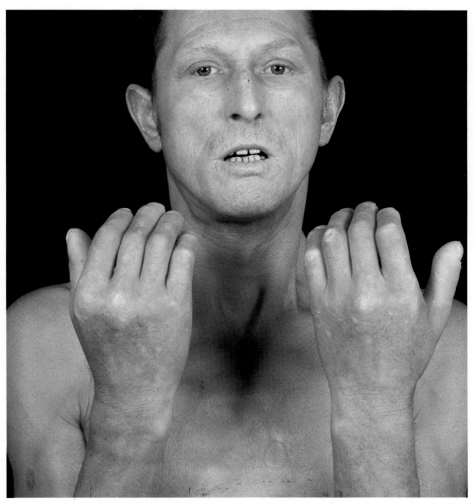

261　Scleroderma　*The connective tissue changes in the face result in loss of the normal facial lines producing a masklike appearance, a thinning of the lips, and a perioral furrowing (rhagades). The hands exhibits a sclerodactylia with tapering of the fingers and a waxy, shiny, atrophic skin. There are flexion contractures and ulceration of the skin overlying the bony prominences on the right hand.*

MUCOUS MEMBRANES   Sclerosis of sublingual ligament; uncommonly, painful induration of gums, tongue

General Examination
LUNG   Restricted movement of chest wall due to pulmonary fibrosis
MUSCULOSKELETAL SYSTEM   Carpal-tunnel syndrome. Muscle weakness.

DIAGNOSIS AND DIFFERENTIAL DIAGNOSIS

Diagnosis   Clinical diagnosis

Differential Diagnosis   Mixed connective tissue disease, eosinophilic fasciitis, scleromyxedema, lupus erythematosus, dermatomyositis, morphea, chronic graft-versus-host disease, lichen sclerosus et atrophicus, polyvinyl chloride exposure, adverse drug reaction (pentazocine, bleomycin)

LABORATORY AND SPECIAL EXAMINATIONS

Dermatopathology   *Early:* mild cellular infiltrate around dermal blood vessels, eccrine coils, subcutaneous tissue. *Late:* epidermis shows disappearance of rete ridges; paucity of blood vessels, thickening/hyalinization of vessel walls, narrowing of lumen; dermal appendages atrophied; sweat glands are situated in upper dermis; calcium in sclerotic, homogeneous collagen of subcutaneous tissue.

PATHOPHYSIOLOGY

Pathogenesis unknown. Primary event might be endothelial cell injury in blood vessels, the cause of which is unknown. Early in course, target organ edema occurs followed by fibrosis; cutaneous capillaries reduced in number; remainder dilate and proliferate, becoming visible telangiectasia. Fibrosis due to overproduction of collagen by fibroblasts.

COURSE AND PROGNOSIS

Course characterized by slow relentless progression of skin and/or visceral sclerosis; however, the 10-year survival is more than 50%. Renal disease leading cause of death; also cardiac and pulmonary involvement. Spontaneous remissions do occur. CREST syndrome progresses more slowly and has a more favorable prognosis; some cases do develop visceral involvement.

TREATMENT

Symptomatic. There is no effective treatment to halt the progression of the disease.

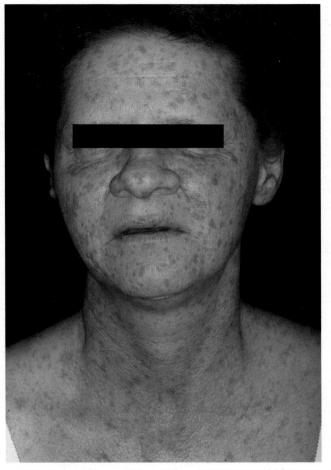

262　Scleroderma　*Illustrated are numerous matlike telangiectases, which can sometimes be very prominent in scleroderma.*

Raynaud's phenomenon (RP) is digital ischemia that occurs on exposure to cold and/or due to emotional stress. RP may be associated with other diseases, but when no etiology is found the term *Raynaud's disease (RD)* is used. RD is the most common cause of RP, and this précis will largely summarize RD. The various causes of RP include: *rheumatic disorders:* systemic scleroderma (85%), SLE (35%), dermatomyositis (30%), Sjögren's syndrome, rheumatoid arthritis, polyarteritis nodosa; *diseases with abnormal blood proteins:* cyroproteins, cold agglutinins, macroglobulins; *drugs:* β-adrenergic blockers, nicotine; *arterial diseases:* arteriosclerosis obliterans, thromboangiitis obliterans; *carpal-tunnel syndrome.*

EPIDEMIOLOGY

Incidence As high as 20% in young women!

Age Young adults, or at menopause

Sex Female

Occupation RP may occur in persons using vibratory tools (chain saw users), meat cutters, typists, and pianists.

Precipitating Factors Cold, mental stress, certain occupations (see above), smoking (see Treatment)

HISTORY

Relationship of Skin Changes to Other Factors Season (worse in winter in temperate climates), cold (meat cutters), previous treatment (drugs), occupation (using vibratory tools). Skin symptom: numbness, pain.

Systems Review Careful review is important to detect diseases in which RP is associated: arthralgia, fatigue, dysphagia, muscle weakness, etc.

PHYSICAL EXAMINATION

Skin

TYPES OF SKIN CHANGES

The episodic attack There is sharply demarcated blanching or cyanosis of the fingers or toes, extending from the tip to varying levels of the finger or toe. The finger distal to the line of ischemia is white or blue and cold (Figure 263); the proximal skin is pink and warm. When the digits are rewarmed, the blanching may be replaced by cyanosis because of slow blood flow; at the end of the attack the normal color or a red color reflects the reactive hyperemic phase. To recapitulate, the sequence of color changes is often: white → blue → red. Rarely the tip of the nose, earlobes, or the tongue may be involved. Blanching may occur in 1 or 2 digits or all the digits; often the thumb is spared. The feet are involved only 40% of the time.

Repeated or persistent vascular vasospasm Patients with RP often have a persistent vasospasm, rather than episodic attacks. Skin changes include trophic changes with development of taut, atrophic skin and shortening of the terminal phalanges—this is called *sclerodactyly.*

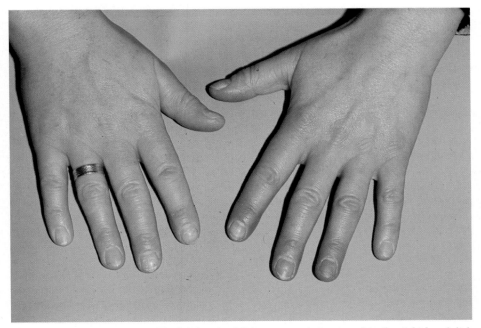

263 Raynaud's phenomenon   *The left hand exhibits a cyanosis compared to the right hand; it is especially seen in the nail bed. This is due to episodic attacks of digital ischemia on exposure to cold and, sometimes, to emotional stress.*

Acrogangrene is rare in RD (<1%). In RP associated with scleroderma, painful ulcers and fissures develop (Figure 264); sequestration of the terminal phalanges or the development of gangrene may lead to autoamputation of the fingertips.

Nails Pterygium, clubbing

LABORATORY EXAMINATIONS

Laboratory Examination of Blood
SEROLOGIC   ANA and other tests to rule out lupus erythematosus, immunoproteins

DIAGNOSIS

The vascular changes in RP are characteristic and when no other disease is discovered (see above) the diagnosis is RD.

PATHOGENESIS

The vasomotor tone is regulated by the sympathetic nervous system. The centers for vaso-motor tone are located in the brain, in the spinal cord, and in the peripheral nerves. The digital vessels are innervated only by sympathetic adrenergic, vasoconstrictor fibers. Vasodilatation occurs only on withdrawal of the sympathetic activity. It is conjectured that there may be a "local fault" in which blood vessels are abnormally sensitive to cold.

COURSE AND PROGNOSIS

RP may disappear spontaneously; it progresses in about 1 of 3 patients.

TREATMENT

Education regarding the use of loose-fitting clothing, avoiding cold and pressure on the fingers. Giving up smoking is necessary.

Drug therapy such as reserpine and nifedipine should be used only in patients who have severe RD.

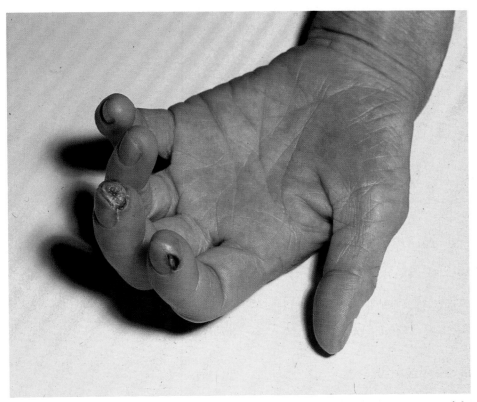

264 Acrogangrene *Persistent vasospasm of the arterials can sometimes lead to gangrene of the terminal digits, as illustrated in this patient.*

Hypersensitivity vasculitis (HV) encompasses a heterogeneous group of vasculitides associated with hypersensitivity to antigens from infectious agents, drugs, or other exogenous or endogenous sources, characterized pathologically by involvement of small blood vessels (principally venules) with segmental inflammation and fibrinoid necrosis. Clinically, skin involvement is characteristic of HV, manifested by "palpable purpura" in the skin; systemic vascular involvement occurs, chiefly in the kidney, muscles, joints, GI tract, and peripheral nerves.

Synonyms: allergic cutaneous vasculitis, necrotizing vasculitis.

EPIDEMIOLOGY AND ETIOLOGY

Age All ages

Sex Equal incidence in males and females

Etiology Idiopathic 50%

CLASSIFICATION

Exogenous Stimuli Proved or Suspected

Henoch-Schönlein purpura

Serum sickness/serum sickness-like reactions Sulfonamides, penicillin, serum

Other drug-induced vasculitides

Vasculitis associated with infectious diseases Hepatitis B virus, group A hemolytic streptococcus, *Staphylococcus aureus, Mycobacterium leprae*

Endogenous Antigens Likely Involved
Vasculitis associated with:

Neoplasms Lymphoproliferative disorders

Connective tissue diseases SLE, rheumatoid arthritis, Sjögren's syndrome

Other underlying diseases Cryoglobulinemia, paraproteinemia, hypergammaglobulinemic purpura

Congenital deficiencies of the complement system

Duration of Lesions Acute (days, as in drug-induced or idiopathic), subacute (weeks, especially urticarial types), chronic (recurrent over years)

Symptoms Pruritus, burning, pain, or no symptoms

Constitutional Symptoms Fever, malaise

Systems Review Symptoms of peripheral neuritis, abdominal pain, arthralgia, myalgia, kidney involvement (microhematuria), CNS involvement

PHYSICAL FINDINGS

Skin Findings
TYPE OF LESION "Palpable purpura" (Figure 265), petechiae. Nodules, vesicles, necrotic ulcers. Urticarial wheals (persist more than 24 hours) (urticaria perstans).
COLOR Purpuric lesions do not blanch (using a glass slide)
SHAPE Round, oval, annular, arciform
ARRANGEMENT Scattered, discrete lesions or dense and confluent (Figure 266)
DISTRIBUTION OF LESIONS Usually regional localization: lower third of legs, ankles,

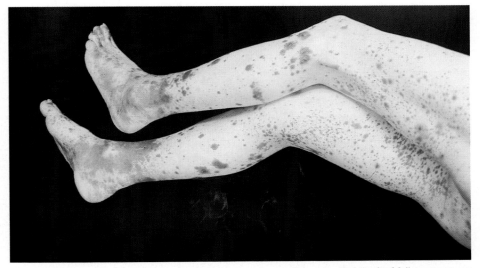

265 Necrotizing vasculitis *There are many purpuric papules, so-called "palpable" purpura, on the lower extremities. Some of these lesions are infarcted or vesicular.*

buttocks, arms. Stasis factor aggravates or precipitates lesions.

General Examination Should include search for underlying disease and organ involvement (kidney!)

DIAGNOSIS AND DIFFERENTIAL DIAGNOSIS

Diagnosis The American College of Rheumatology 1990 criteria for diagnosis of HV are as follows; a diagnosis of HV is made if at least 3 of these criteria are present:

CRITERION	DEFINITION
1. Age at disease onset >16 years	Development of symptoms after age 16
2. Medication at disease onset	Medication was taken at the onset of symptoms that may have been a precipitating factor
3. Palpable purpura	Slightly elevated purpuric rash over one or more areas of the skin; does not blanch with pressure and is not related to thrombocytopenia
4. Maculopapular rash	Flat and raised lesions of various sizes over one or more areas of the skin
5. Biopsy including arteriole and venule	Histologic changes showing granulocytes in a perivascular or extravascular location

HYPERSENSITIVITY VASCULITIS

Henoch-Schönlein purpura is a specific subtype of HV; the diagnosis is made if 2 of these 4 criteria are present:

CRITERION	DEFINITION
1. Palpable purpura	Slightly raised "palpable" hemorrhagic skin lesions, not related to thrombocytopenia
2. Age ≤20 at disease onset	Patient 20 years or younger at onset of first symptoms
3. Bowel angina	Diffuse abdominal pain, worse after meals, or the diagnosis of bowel ischemia, usually including bloody diarrhea
4. Wall granulocytes on biopsy	Histologic changes showing granulocytes in the walls of arterioles or venules

Differential Diagnosis An important differentiation is necrotizing vasculitis vs. infarcts associated with bacteremia. Biopsy may not be helpful in this differentiation. When faced with this dilemma in an acutely ill patient, antibiotic treatment is given, pending the result of the blood cultures. In the urticarial type the wheals are persistent (more than 24 hours) and show petechiae, while all other types of urticarial wheals disappear completely in several hours.

LABORATORY AND SPECIAL EXAMINATIONS

ESR Elevated

Serology Serum complement is reduced or normal in some patients, depending on associated disorders.

Urinalysis RBC casts, albuminuria

Dermatopathology Deposition of eosinophilic material (fibrinoid) in the walls of postcapillary venules in the upper dermis, and perivenular and intramural inflammatory infiltrate (neutrophils in those patients with hypocomplementemia, and lymphocytes or neutrophils with normal serum complement). Extravasated RBC and fragmented neutrophils (nuclear "dust") are also present. Frank necrosis of vessel walls. Intramural C3 and immunoglobulin deposition is seen with immunofluorescent techniques. In Henoch-Schönlein syndrome the immunoglobulins are predominantly IgA.

PATHOPHYSIOLOGY

The most frequently postulated mechanism for the production of necrotizing vasculitis is the deposition in tissues of circulating immune complexes. Initial alterations in venular permeability, which may facilitate the deposition of complexes at such sites, may be due to the release of vasoactive amines from platelets, basophils, and/or mast cells. Immune complexes may activate the complement system or may directly interact with Fc receptors on cell membranes. When the complement system is activated, the generation of anaphylatoxins C3a and C5a could degranulate mast cells. Also, C5a can attract neutrophils that could release lysosomal enzymes during phagocytosis of complexes and subsequently damage vascular tissue.

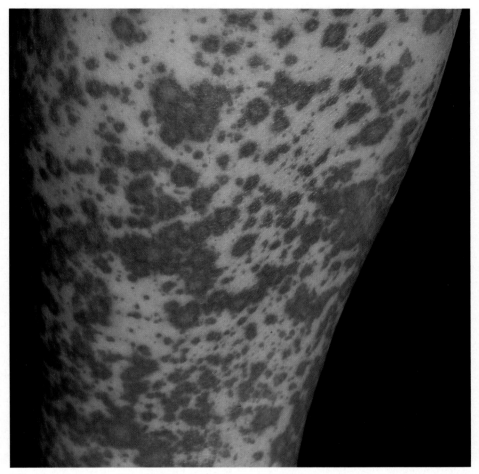

266 Necrotizing vasculitis *Striking, erythematous, purpuric papules and plaques, some of which are annular.*

COURSE AND PROGNOSIS

Depends on underlying disease. In the idiopathic variant, multiple episodes can occur over the course of years. Usually self-limited but irreversible damage to kidneys can occur.

TREATMENT

Treat underlying disease; antibiotics for patients in whom vasculitis follows bacterial infection. Systemic corticosteroids for patients with severe disease; cytotoxic immunosuppressives (cyclophosphamide, azathioprine). In exceptional cases: plasmapheresis may be tried. Lower legs: compressive bandages often have a beneficial effect.

Polyarteritis nodosa (PAN) is a multisystem, necrotizing vasculitis of small- and medium-sized muscular arteries characterized by its involvement of the renal and visceral arteries.

Synonyms: periarteritis nodosa, panarteritis nodosa.

EPIDEMIOLOGY AND ETIOLOGY

Age Mean age, 45

Sex Males:females, 2.5:1

Etiology Unknown

Clinical Variants *Cutaneous PAN* rare variant with symptomatic vasculitis limited to skin and at times peripheral nerves.

HISTORY

Systems Review *Chronic disease syndrome.* GI involvement: nausea, vomiting, abdominal pain, hemorrhage, perforation, infarction. CVS: congestive heart failure, pericarditis, conduction system defects, myocardial infarction. Paresthesias, numbness, *Cutaneous PAN:* Pain in nodules, ulcers, involved extremities; aching during flares, physical activity. Myalgia. Neuralgia, numbness, mild paresthesia.

PHYSICAL EXAMINATION

Skin Findings Occur in 15% of cases
TYPE OF LESION   Subcutaneous nodules which follow the course of involved arteries; may ulcerate (Figure 267). Palpable purpura. Violaceous macule, confluent with livedo reticularis pattern.
Cutaneous PAN: Inflammatory nodules (0.5 to 2.0 cm). Livedo reticularis (Figure 268), "starburst" livedo follows at site of cluster of nodular lesions. Ulcers may follow ischemia of nodules. Duration—days to months. Resolve with residual violaceous or postinflammatory hyperpigmentation.
COLOR   Nodules bright red to light pink; blue
PALPATION   Nodules often more palpable than visible. Tender.
DISTRIBUTION OF LESIONS   Palpable purpura: lower extremities. Nodules: usually bilateral. Lower legs > thighs. Other: arms > trunk > head/neck >buttocks

General Examination Elevated blood pressure
NEUROLOGIC EXAMINATION   CNS: cerebrovascular accident. Peripheral nerves: mixed motor/sensory involvement with mononeuritis multiplex pattern.
EYE   Hypertensive changes, ocular vasculitis, retinal artery aneurysm, optic disc edema/atrophy.

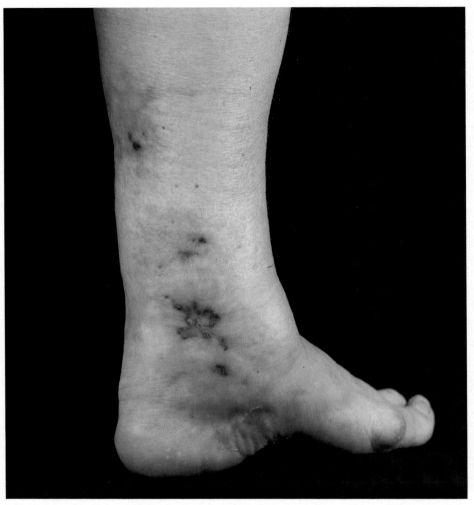

267   Polyarteritis nodosa   *There are nodular ulcerations occurring on the medial aspect of the lower leg. Scarring is present in the site of the previous lesions.*

DIAGNOSIS AND DIFFERENTIAL DIAGNOSIS

Diagnosis   ARA 1990 criteria for the classification of polyarteritis nodosa (traditional format)[1]

CRITERION	DEFINITION
1. Weight loss ≥4 kg	Loss of 4 kg or more of body weight since illness began, not due to dieting or other factors
2. Livedo reticularis	Mottled reticular pattern over the skin of portions of the extremities or torso
3. Testicular pain or tenderness	Pain or tenderness of the testicles, not due to infection, trauma, or other causes
4. Myalgias, weakness, or leg tenderness	Diffuse myalgias (excluding shoulder and hip girdle) or weakness of muscles or tenderness of leg muscles
5. Mononeuropathy or polyneuropathy	Development of mononeuropathy, multiple mononeuropathies, or polyneuropathy
6. Diastolic BP >90 mmHg	Development of hypertension with the diastolic BP higher than 90 mmHg
7. Elevated BUN or creatinine	Elevation of BUN >40.0 mg/dL or creatinine >1.5 mg/dL, not due to dehydration or obstruction
8. Hepatitis B virus	Presence of hepatitis B surface antigen or antibody in serum
9. Arteriographic abnormality	Arteriogram showing aneurysms or occlusions of the visceral arteries, not due to arteriosclerosis, fibromuscular dysplasia, or other noninflammatory causes
10. Biopsy of small or medium-sized artery containing PMN	Histologic changes showing the presence of granulocytes or granulocytes and mononuclear leukocytes in the artery wall

Differential Diagnosis   Other vasculitides

LABORATORY AND SPECIAL EXAMINATIONS

Dermatopathology   *Best yield biopsy of nodular skin lesion (deep wedge biopsy).* Polymorphonuclear neutrophils infiltrate all layers of vessel wall and perivascular areas. Later, infiltrates, mononuclear cells. Fibrinoid

[1] For classification purposes, a patient shall be said to have polyarteritis nodosa if at least 3 of these 10 criteria are present. The presence of any 3 or more criteria yields a sensitivity of 82.2% and a specificity of 86.6%. BP = blood pressure; BUN = blood urea nitrogen; PMN = polymophonuclear neutrophils.

necrosis of vessel wall with compromise of lumen, thrombosis, infarction of tissues supplied by involved vessel, ± hemorrhage. Skin pathology is identical in systemic and cutaneous PAN.

CBC   Commonly neutrophilic leukocytosis; rarely eosinophilia; anemia of chronic disease. ± Elevated ESR

Serology   Hepatitis B surface antigenemia in 30% of cases

Chemistry   Elevated creatinine, BUN

Arteriography   Aneurysms in small- and medium-sized muscular arteries of kidney/hepatic/visceral vasculature

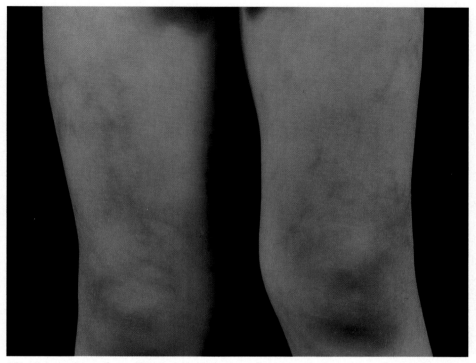

268 Polyarteritis nodosa *This is a livedo pattern. On biopsy lesions were polyarteritis nodosa.*

PATHOPHYSIOLOGY

Necrotizing inflammation of small- and medium-sized muscular arteries; may spread circumferentially to involve adjacent veins. Lesions segmental, tend to involve bifurcations of arteries. 30% of cases associated with hepatitis B antigenemia, i.e., immune complex formation.

COURSE AND PROGNOSIS

Untreated, very high morbidity and mortality characterized by fulminant deterioration or by relentless progression associated with intermittent acute exacerbations. Mortality from renal failure, bowel infarction and perforation, cardiovascular complications, intractable hypertension. Lesions may heal with scarring and further occlusion or aneurysmal dilatations. Effective treatment improves morbidity and mortality. *Cutaneous PAN:* chronic relapsing benign course.

TREATMENT

Combined therapy: prednisone, 1 mg per kg body weight per day and cyclophosphamide, 2 mg per kg per day

Cutaneous PAN: nonsteroidal anti-inflammatory agent; prednisone

POLYARTERITIS NODOSA

Wegener's granulomatosis is a distinct clinicopathologic entity, defined by a clinical triad of manifestations that includes involvement of the upper airways, lungs, and kidneys and by a pathologic triad consisting of necrotizing granulomas in the upper respiratory tract and lungs, vasculitis involving both arteries and veins, and glomerulitis.

EPIDEMIOLOGY AND ETIOLOGY

Age Mean age 40 years

Sex Males:females, 1.3:1

Etiology Unknown

Clinical Variants Variants limited to kidneys, i.e., glomerulitis occurs in 15% of cases

HISTORY

Systems Review Chronic disease syndrome. Fever. Paranasal sinus pain, purulent or bloody nasal discharge.

PHYSICAL EXAMINATION

Skin Findings Overall in 45% of patients, but in only 13% of patients at initial presentation.
TYPE OF LESION Ulcers most typical; resemble pyoderma gangrenosum. Papules, vesicles, palpable purpura (Figures 269*a* and 269*b*) as in necrotizing vasculitis, subcutaneous nodules, plaques, noduloulcerative lesions.
DISTRIBUTION OF LESIONS Most common on lower extremities. Also face, trunk, upper limbs.
MUCOUS MEMBRANES Oral ulcerations (Figure 270). Often first symptom

General Examination
EAR-NOSE-THROAT ±Nasal mucosal ulceration, crusting, blood clots; nasal septal perforation; saddle-nose deformity. Eustachian tube occlusion with serous otitis media; ±pain. External auditory canal: pain, erythema, swelling
RESPIRATORY TRACT Cough, hemoptysis, dyspnea, chest discomfort.
EYE 65%. Mild conjunctivitis, episcleritis, scleritis, granulomatous sclerouveitis, ciliary vessel vasculitis, retroorbital mass lesion with proptosis
NERVOUS SYSTEM Cranial neuritis, mononeuritis multiplex, cerebral vasculitis
KIDNEYS Focal/segmental glomerulonephritis

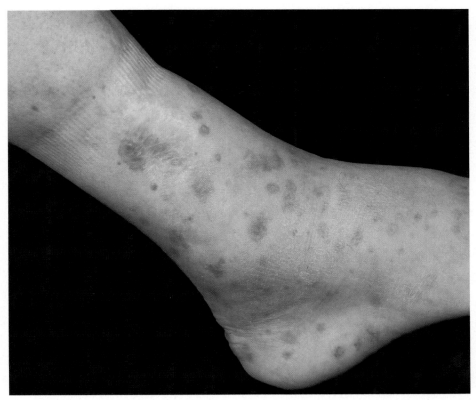

269a Wegener's granulomatosis *Typical areas of palpable purpura are seen on the lower leg and foot.*

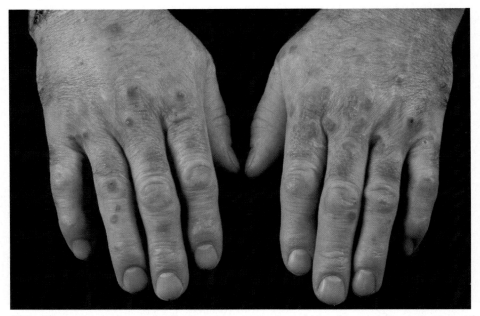

269b Wegener's granulomatosis *Erythematous, purpuric, non-blanching nodules on the dorsa of the fingers and hands.*

DIAGNOSIS AND DIFFERENTIAL DIAGNOSIS

Diagnosis ARA 1990 criteria for the classification of Wegener's granulomatosis (traditional format).[1]

CRITERION	DEFINITION
1. Nasal or oral inflammation	Development of painful or painless oral ulcers or purulent or bloody nasal discharge
2. Abnormal chest radiograph	Chest radiograph showing the presence of nodules, fixed infiltrates, or cavities
3. Urinary sediment	Microhematuria (>5 red blood cells per high-power field) or red cell casts in urine sediment
4. Granulomatous inflammation on biopsy	Histologic changes showing granulomatous inflammation within the wall of an artery or in the perivascular or extravascular area (artery or arteriole)

Differential Diagnosis Other vasculitides, Goodpasture's syndrome, tumors of the upper airway/lung, infectious/noninfectious granulomatous diseases (especially blastomycosis), midline granuloma, lymphomatoid granulomatosis (i.e., malignant lymphoma)

LABORATORY AND SPECIAL EXAMINATIONS

Dermatopathology *Ulcers, nodules:* necrotizing granulomas, multinucleated giant cells; ±necrotizing vasculitis of small arteries/veins. *Palpable purpura:* necrotizing vasculitis

Chemistry Impaired renal function

Urinanalysis Proteinuria, hematuria, RBC casts

Serology Rising titer of anticytoplasmic leukocytic antibodies (autoantibodies reacting with cytoplasm of granulocytes and monocytes) correlates with relapse.

X-Ray *Paranasal sinuses:* opacification, ±sclerosis. *Chest:* pulmonary infiltrates, nodules, consolidation, cavitation; upper lobes

PATHOPHYSIOLOGY

Immunopathogenesis unclear. Necrotizing vasculitis of small arteries and veins usually with intravascular or extravascular granuloma formation. Pulmonary involvement: multiple, bilateral, nodular infiltrates. Similar infiltrates in paranasal sinuses, nasopharynx.

COURSE AND PROGNOSIS

Untreated, usually fatal because of rapidly progressive renal failure. With adequate therapy, may in time undergo prolonged remission.

TREATMENT

Prednisone 1 mg per kg body weight per day combined with cyclophosphamide 2 mg per kg per day; taper prednisone during remission.

[1] For purposes of classification, a patient shall be said to have Wegener's granulomatosis if at least 2 of these 4 criteria are present. The presence of any 2 or more criteria yields a sensitivity of 88.2% and a specificity of 92.0%.

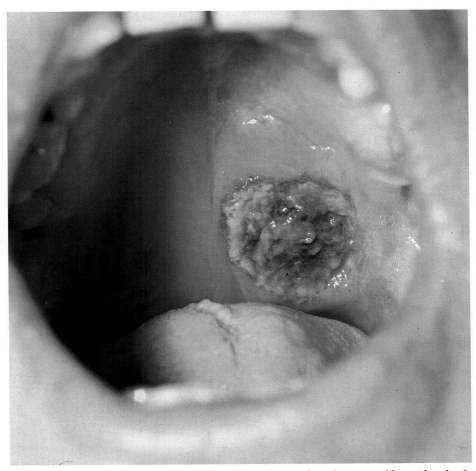

270 Wegener's granulomatosis *There is a very large ulcer on the palate covered by a sphacelus (a dense, necrotic membrane).*

Giant cell arteritis is a systemic granulomatous vasculitis of medium- and large-sized arteries, most notably the temporal artery and other branches of the carotid artery, characterized by headaches, fatigue, fever, anemia, and high ESR, in elderly patients.

Synonyms: temporal arteritis, cranial arteritis.

EPIDEMIOLOGY AND ETIOLOGY

Age Elderly, usually >55 years

Sex Females > males

Etiology Unknown. Probably via cell-mediated immunity.

Clinical Variants Temporal arteritis is a characteristic regional expression of giant cell arteritis affecting the temporal and other cranial arteries, which may or may not be accompanied by clinical symptoms of systemic involvement.

HISTORY

Systems Review *Fatigue.* Fever. Chronic disease syndrome. Headache usually bilateral. Scalp pain. *Claudication* of jaw/tongue while talking/chewing. Eye involvement: transient impairment of vision, ischemic optic neuritis, retrobulbar neuritis, persistent blindness. Systemic vasculitis: claudication of extremities, stroke, myocardial infarction, aortic aneurysms/dissections, visceral organ infarction.

Polymyalgia rheumatica syndrome: stiffness, aching, pain in the muscles of the neck, shoulders, lower back, hips, thighs.

PHYSICAL EXAMINATION

Skin Findings
TYPE OF LESION Superficial temporal arteries are swollen, prominent, tortuous, ±nodular thickenings (Figure 271). ±Erythema of overlying skin. Scalp gangrene, i.e., skin infarction with sharp, irregular borders; ulceration with exposure of bone (Figure 272). Scars at sites of old ulcerations. Postinflammatory hyperpigmentation over involved artery.

PALPATION *Tender.* Initially involved artery pulsates; later occluded with loss of pulsation.

DISTRIBUTION OF LESIONS Skin supplied by superficial temporal/occipital arteries in the temporal/parietal scalp

General Examination Findings in other organ systems related to tissue ischemia/infarction

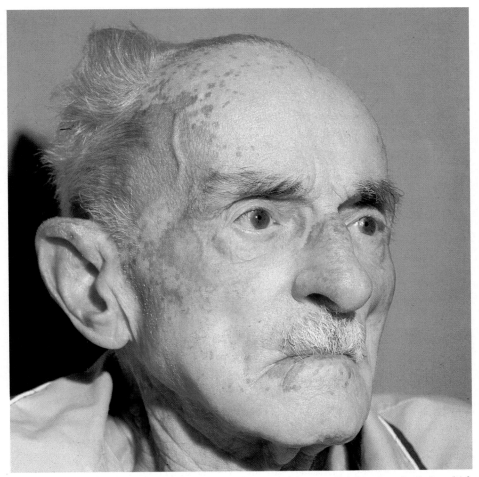

271   Giant cell arteritis   *There is an obvious involvement of the superficial temporal arteries which are swollen and tortuous.*

DIAGNOSIS AND DIFFERENTIAL DIAGNOSIS

Diagnosis   ARA 1990 criteria for the classification of giant cell (temporal) arteritis (traditional format):[1]

CRITERION	DEFINITION
1. Age at disease onset ≥50 years	Development of symptoms or findings beginning at age 50 or older
2. New headache	New onset or new type of localized pain in the head
3. Temporal artery abnormality	Temporal artery tenderness to palpation or decreased pulsation, unrelated to arteriosclerosis of cervical arteries
4. Elevated ESR	Erythrocyte sedimentation ≥50 mm/hour by the Westergren method
5. Abnormal artery biopsy	Biopsy specimen with artery showing vasculitis characterized by a predominance of mononuclear cell infiltration or granulomatous inflammation, usually with multinucleated giant cells

Differential Diagnosis   Other vasculitides

LABORATORY AND SPECIAL EXAMINATIONS

Dermatopathology   Biopsy tender nodule of involved artery ± overlying affected skin after Doppler flow examination. Lesions focal; section serially. Panarteritis with inflammatory mononuclear cell infiltrates within the vessel wall with frequent giant cell formation. Intimal proliferation with vascular occlusion, fragmentation of internal elastic lamina, extensive necrosis of intima and media.

CBC   Normochromic/slightly hypochromic anemia

ESR   Marked elevation

PATHOPHYSIOLOGY

Systemic vasculitis of multiple medium- and large-sized arteries. Symptoms secondary to ischemia.

COURSE AND PROGNOSIS

Untreated can result in blindness secondary to ischemic optic neuritis. Excellent response to adequate therapy. Remission following several years.

TREATMENT

Prednisone: intially 40.0 to 60.0 mg per day; taper when symptoms abate; continue 7.5 to 10.0 mg per day for 1 to 2 years

---

[1] For purposes of classification, a patient shall be said to have giant cell (temporal) arteritis if at least 3 of these 5 criteria are present. The presence of any 3 or more criteria yields a sensitivity of 93.5% and a specificity of 91.2%.

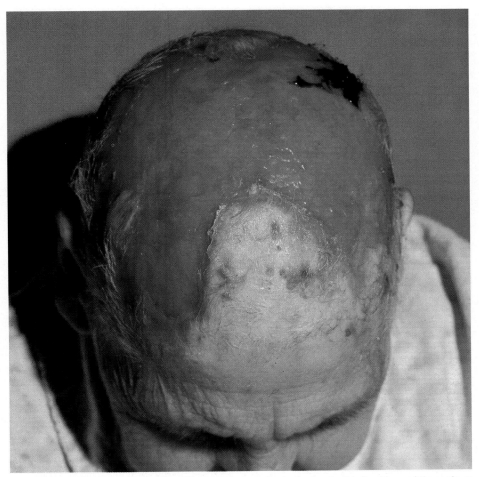

272   Giant cell arteritis   *Extensive ulceration in a patient who has had infarctions of the scalp as a result of vascular occlusion.*

Urticarial vasculitis is a multisystem disease characterized by cutaneous lesions resembling urticaria and biopsy findings of a leukocytoclastic vasculitis, accompanied by varying degrees of extracutaneous involvement.

Synonyms: hypocomplementemic vasculitis, urticaria perstans.

EPIDEMIOLOGY AND ETIOLOGY

Age Majority, 30 to 50 years

Sex Women:men, 3:1

Etiology Unknown

HISTORY

Systems Review *Lesions may be associated with itching, burning, stinging sensation/pain.* Fever (10 to 15%). Arthralgias ± arthritis in one or more joints (ankles, knees, elbows, wrists, small joints of fingers). Nausea, abdominal pain. Cough, dyspnea, hemoptysis. Pseudotumor cerebri. Cold sensitivity. Renal involvement: diffuse glomerulonephritis. May be cutaneous manifestation of SLE.

PHYSICAL EXAMINATION

Skin Findings

TYPE OF LESION Urticaria-like (i.e., edematous) lesions: raised, occasionally indurated, erythematous, circumscribed wheals (Figure 273); macular erythema; angioedema. Eruption occurs in transient crops, *usually lasting more than 24 and up to 72 hours,* changing shape slowly, ± resolve with purpura; hyperpigmentation. Less commonly: cold urticaria, Raynaud's phenomenon, palpable purpura, bullae, erythema multiforme-like lesions.

COLOR Erythematous. Resolving lesions, yellowish-green stain.
PALPATION Indurated. Blanch when pressed, but purpura remains.

General Examination Extracutaneous manifestations: joints (70%), GI tract (20 to 30%), CNS (>10%), ocular system (>10%), kidneys (10 to 20%), lymphadenopathy (5%)

DIAGNOSIS AND DIFFERENTIAL DIAGNOSIS

Diagnosis Clinical suspicion confirmed by skin biopsy

Differential Diagnosis Urticaria, serum sickness, other vasculitides, SLE, urticaria in acute hepatitis B infection

LABORATORY AND SPECIAL EXAMINATIONS

Dermatopathology Biopsy several early lesions. Features of leukocytoclastic vasculitis: perivascular infiltrate consisting primarily of neutrophils; leukocytoclasia; fibrinoid deposition in/around vessel walls; endothelial cell swelling; extravasation of RBC. In contrast, common urticaria exhibits dermal edema; sparse perivascular lymphohistiocytic infiltrate ± eosinophils.

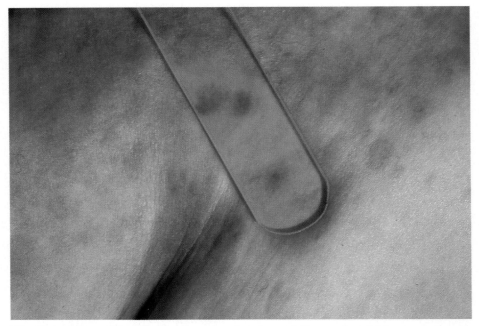

273　Urticarial vasculitis　*These erythematous papules and plaques do not blanch on diascopy and, in contrast to urticaria, persist for over 3 days.*

Urinanalysis　10% of patients—microhematuria, proteinuria

ESR　Elevated

Serologic Findings　Hypocomplementemia (70%); circulating immune complexes

PATHOPHYSIOLOGY

Thought to be an immune complex disease, similar to cutaneous vasculitis. Deposition of antigen-antibody complexes in cutaneous blood vessel walls leads to complement activation, resulting in neutrophil chemotaxis; collagenase, elastase released from neutrophils cause vessel wall and cell destruction.

COURSE AND PROGNOSIS

Most often is chronic but benign. Episodes recur over periods ranging from months to years. Renal disease occurs only in hypocomplementemic patients.

TREATMENT

First line　H_1 and H_2 blockers (doxepin [10.0 mg b.i.d. to 25.0 mg t.i.d.] + cimetidine [300 mg t.i.d.]/ranitidine [150 mg b.i.d.]) *plus* nonsteroidal anti-inflammatory agent (indomethacin [75 to 200 mg per day]/ibuprofen [1600 to 2400 mg per day]/naproxen [500 to 1000 mg per day])

Second line　Colchicine 0.6 mg b.i.d. or t.i.d. *or* dapsone 50 to 150 mg per day

Third line　Prednisone

Fourth line　Cytotoxic immunosuppressives (azathioprine, cyclophosphamide)

Cryoglobulinemia is the presence of serum immunoglobulin that precipitates at low temperature and redissolves at 37°C. It is associated clinically with Raynaud's phenomenon, vascular purpura, cold urticaria, acral hemorrhagic necrosis, bleeding disorders, vasculitis, arthralgia, neurologic manifestations, hepatosplenomegaly, and glomerulonephritis.

EPIDEMIOLOGY AND ETIOLOGY

Age, Sex That of associated disorders

Etiology That of associated disorders

CLASSIFICATION OF CRYOGLOBULINEMIA AND ASSOCIATED DISEASES

Cryoglobulins

TYPE I Monoclonal immunoglobulins (IgM, IgG, IgA, light chains). Cutaneous, vasomotor symptoms; renal/neurologic problems. Acral gangrene.

TYPE II Mixed cryoglobulins: a monoclonal immunoglobulin (usually IgM, less often IgG) with antibody activity against polyclonal IgG interacts and cryoprecipitates with the polyclonal IgG. Cutaneous, vasomotor symptoms, vascular purpura, Raynaud's phenomenon; renal/neurologic problems.

TYPE III Mixed polyclonal cryoglobulins containing one or more classes of immunoglobulins; probably represent immune complex disease in which the complexes form cryoprecipitates; occasionally mixed with complement and lipoproteins. Vascular purpura, Raynaud's phenomenon; renal/neurologic problems.

Associated Diseases

TYPES I, II Plasma cell dyscrasias such as multiple myeloma, Waldenström's macroglobulinemia, lymphoproliferative dis-

orders, asymptomatic "essential" cryoglobulinemia

TYPES II, III Autoimmune diseases: rheumatoid arthritis, SLE, and Sjögren's syndrome

TYPE III Autoimmune diseases, connective tissue diseases, wide variety of infectious diseases, i.e., hepatitis B virus infection, Epstein-Barr virus infection (infectious mononucleosis), cytomegalovirus infection, subacute bacterial endocarditis, leprosy, syphilis, β-hemolytic streptococcal infections

HISTORY

Systems Review Cold sensitivity, <50% of cases. Chills, fever, dyspnea, diarrhea may occur following cold exposure. Other organ system involvement: arthralgia, renal symptoms, neurologic symptoms, abdominal pain, arterial thrombosis

PHYSICAL EXAMINATION

Skin Findings

TYPE OF LESION Purpura often palpable, a common finding, occurs in crops precipitated by standing up; less commonly by cold. Livedo reticularis, acrocyanosis, and urticaria induced by cold, associated with purpura. Raynaud's phenomenon, ±severe with resultant gangrene of fingertips and toes.

DISTRIBUTION OF LESIONS Purpura: lower extremities with extension to thighs, abdo-

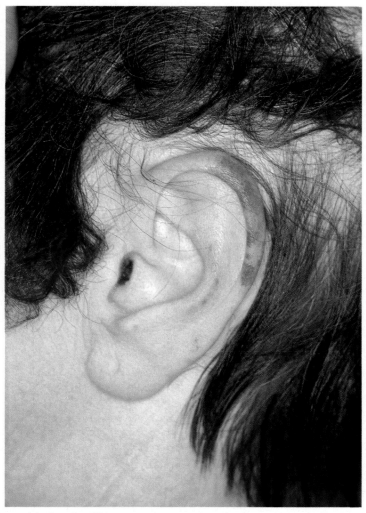

274   Mild cryoglobulinemia   *This purpura appeared on the first cold day in the fall.*

men. Hemorrhagic necrosis/ulceration: nose, ears (Figure 274), fingers, toes (Figure 275), legs. Livedo reticularis: extremities.

TYPE I Cryoglobulin present in large amounts; precipitation causes vessel occlusion; also associated with hyperviscosity. Higher incidence of Raynaud's phenomenon/distal skin necrosis.

TYPE II Leukocytoclastic vasculitis with mild Raynaud's phenomenon, purpura, arthralgia, glomerulonephritis.

TYPE III Overlaps Types I and II, showing both types of symptoms.

General Examination Usually noncontributory

DIAGNOSIS AND DIFFERENTIAL DIAGNOSIS

Diagnosis Clinical suspicion confirmed by detection of cryoglobulins

Differential Diagnosis Cold agglutinins, cryofibrinogenemia

LABORATORY AND SPECIAL EXAMINATIONS

Cryoglobulins Blood drawn into warmed syringe, removing RBC via warmed centrifuge. Plasma refrigerated in a Wintrobe tube at 4°C for 24 to 72 hours; then centrifuged and cryocrit determined. In Types I and II cryoglobulin levels high (75 mg per mL); Type III, low (<1 mg per mL)

Other Laboratory Findings Consistent with associated disorders

Dermatopathology *Type I* (monoclonal): dermal vessels contain intraluminal amorphous eosinophilic material, mainly precipitated cryoglobulin; inflammatory infiltrate usually absent. *Type II, III* (mixed): leukocytoclastic vasculitis, with or without intraluminal cryoprecipitate.

PATHOPHYSIOLOGY

Precipitation of cryoglobulins (when present in large amounts) causes vessel occlusion, also associated with hyperviscosity (Type I); immune complex deposition followed by complement activation and inflammation; platelet aggregation/consumption of clotting factors by cryoglobulins, causing coagulation disorder; small vessel thromboses and vasculitis produced by immune complexes (Types II and III).

COURSE AND PROGNOSIS

Cyclic eruptions usually induced by cold or fluctuations of activity of underlying disease. Prognosis depends on underlying disease; often guarded.

TREATMENT

Treat underlying disease. ±Plasmapheresis at 37°C.

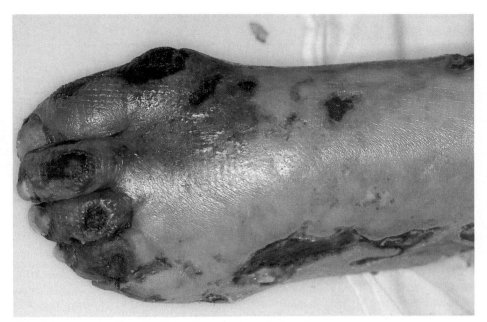

275   Severe cryoglobulinemia   *Extensive necrosis and ulcerations.*

Reiter's syndrome (RS) is an episode of peripheral arthritis of more than one month's duration occurring in association with urethritis and/or cervicitis, which is frequently accompanied by keratoderma blennorrhagicum, circinate balanitis, conjunctivitis, and stomatitis, that is to say, the classic triad of arthritis, urethritis, and conjunctivitis.

ETIOLOGY AND EPIDEMIOLOGY

Age Median, 22 years

Sex 90% of cases are males

Race Most common in Caucasians from northern Europe; rare in Orientals and African blacks.

Genetic Diathesis HLA-B27 occurs in up to 75% of Caucasians with RS, but in only 8% of normal whites. B27-negative patients have a milder course, with significantly less sacroiliitis, uveitis, and carditis.

Associated Disorders Incidence of RS appears to be increased in HIV-infected individuals.

Etiology Unknown

HISTORY

Incubation Period 1 to 4 weeks following enterocolitis. Urethritis and/or conjunctivitis usually first to appear, followed by arthritis.

History Malaise, fever. Dysuria, urethral discharge. Eyes: red, slightly sensitive. Arthritis: tendon/fascia inflammation results in pain over ischial tuberosities, iliac crest, long bones, rib; heel pain at site of attachment of plantar aponeurosis and/or Achilles tendon; back pain; joint pains

PHYSICAL EXAMINATION

Physical Findings Fever

Skin and Nail Findings
TYPE *Keratoderma blennorrhagicum (KDB):* early papules, vesicles, or macules which enlarge; centers of lesions become pustular and/or hyperkeratotic, crusted (Figure 276), i.e., resembling mollusk shells or ostraceous. Erosive patches resembling pustular psoriasis may occur, especially on shaft of penis, scrotum. *Circinate balanitis* (Figure 277): shallow erosions with serpiginous borders if uncircumcised; crusted and/or hyperkeratotic plaques if circumcised, i.e., psoriasiform
COLOR Erythematous
ARRANGEMENT Random; lesions may be scanty or numerous to the point of confluence.
DISTRIBUTION KDB: soles and palms. Scaling plaques: scalp, elbows, knees, buttocks
NAILS Small subungual pustules; extensive involvement may result in onycholysis and extensive subungual hyperkeratosis with erythema surrounding the nail
MUCOUS MEMBRANES *Urethra* Sterile serous or mucopurulent discharge
Mouth Erosive lesions on tongue or hard palate resembling circinate balanitis
Eyes Conjunctivitis (Figure 278), mild, evanescent, bilateral; anterior uveitis

Systemic Findings Arthritis: oligoarticular, involving up to 6 joints, asymmetrical;

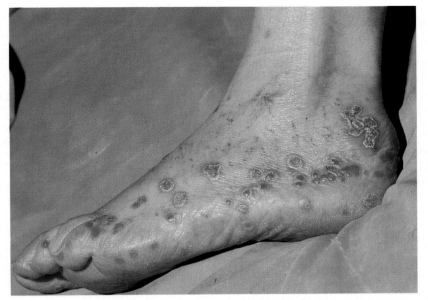

276 Reiter's syndrome, keratoderma blennorrhagicum *Red-to-brown papules, vesicles, pustules, with central erosion and confluence of lesions on the foot.*

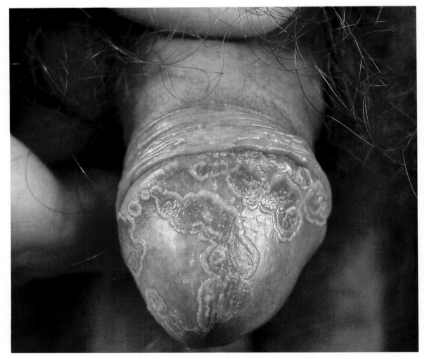

277 Reiter's syndrome, balanitis circinata *Illustrated in this patient is circinate balanitis with moist, well-demarcated erosions with slightly raised border.*

REITER'S SYNDROME   529

most commonly knees, ankles, small joints of feet, diffuse swelling of fingers and toes

DIAGNOSIS AND DIFFERENTIAL DIAGNOSIS

Diagnosis Clinical findings, ruling out other spondylo- and reactive arthropathies

Differential Diagnosis Psoriasis vulgaris with psoriatic arthritis, disseminating gonococcal infection, SLE, ankylosing spondylitis, rheumatoid arthritis, gout, Behçet's disease

PATHOPHYSIOLOGY

RS appears linked to two factors: *genetic factors,* i.e., HLA-B27 in up to 75% of Caucasians (8% incidence in normal whites); *enteric pathogens* such as *Salmonella enteritidis, S. typhimurium, S. heidelberg; Yersinia enterocolitica, Y. pseudotuberculosis; Campylobacter fetus, Shigella flexneri.* Two patterns are observed: the *epidemic form,* which follows venereal exposure, the most common type in the United States and the United Kingdom, and the *postdysenteric form,* the most common type of RS seen in continental Europe and North Africa.

LABORATORY AND SPECIAL EXAMINATIONS

Hematology Nonspecific findings: anemia, leukocytosis, thrombocytosis, elevated ESR

Culture Urethral culture negative for gonococcus

Serology ANA, rheumatoid factor negative. Rule out HIV infection.

Dermatopathology *Epidermis:* acutely, spongiosis, vesiculation; later, psoriasiform epidermal hyperplasia, spongiform pustules, parakeratosis. *Dermis:* perivascular neutrophilic infiltrate in superficial dermis; edema

COURSE AND PROGNOSIS

Only 30% of RS patients develop complete triad of arthritis, urethritis, conjunctivitis; 40% have only one manifestation, i.e., incomplete RS. Majority have self-limited course, with resolution in 3 to 12 months. RS may relapse over many years in 30%. Chronic deforming arthritis in 10 to 20%.

TREATMENT

Prevent articular inflammation/joint deformity: rest, nonsteroidal anti-inflammatory agents. Occasionally phenylbutazone or methotrexate or etretinate are indicated. Role of antibiotics to treat precipitating infection is unproven. In HIV-infected, zidovudine may improve RS.

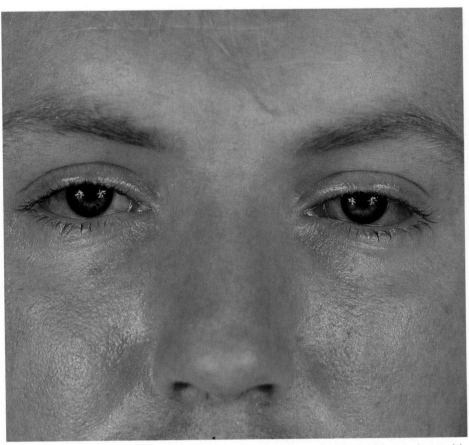

278　Reiter's syndrome, conjunctivitis　*Bilateral conjunctivitis associated with anterior uveitis.*

Pyoderma gangrenosum (PG) is a rapidly evolving, idiopathic, chronic and severely debilitating skin disease occurring most commonly in association with a systemic disease, especially chronic ulcerative colitis, and characterized by the presence of irregular, boggy, blue-red ulcers with undermined borders surrounding purulent necrotic bases.

EPIDEMIOLOGY AND ETIOLOGY

Etiology Unknown

HISTORY

Acute onset with painful hemorrhagic pustule or painful nodule either de novo or following minimal trauma.

PHYSICAL EXAMINATION

Skin Findings
TYPE OF LESION *Primary lesion:* deep-seated nodule or superficial hemorrhagic pustule. Breakdown of this lesion occurs with ulcer formation (Figure 279). *Ulcer borders:* irregular and raised, undermined, boggy, with perforations that drain pus. *Ulcer base:* purulent, hemorrhagic exudate; partially covered by necrotic eschar; ±granulation tissue (Figure 280). Pustules may be seen at the advancing border and in the ulcer base. Healing of ulcers results in thin, atrophic, ±cribriform scar. Pathergy, i.e., slight trauma initiating new PG lesion, noted at sites of minor trauma, biopsy sites, needle sticks.

COLOR *Ulcer border:* dusky red or purple. Halo of erythema spreads centrifugally at the advancing edge of ulcer.

PALPATION Primary nodule and ulcer are painful.

SHAPE OF INDIVIDUAL LESION Ulcer margin may be irregular or serpiginous.

ARRANGEMENT OF LESIONS Usually solitary. May form in clusters which coalesce.

DISTRIBUTION OF LESIONS Most common sites: lower extremities > buttocks > abdomen > face.

Mucous Membranes Rarely, aphthous stomatitis-like lesions; massive ulceration of oral mucosa and conjunctivae

General Examination Patient may appear ill.

Associated Systemic Diseases Up to 50% occur without associated disease. Remainder of cases associated with large- and small-bowel disease (Crohn's disease, ulcerative colitis), diverticulosis (diverticulitis), arthritis, paraproteinemia and myeloma, leukemia, active chronic hepatitis, Behçet's syndrome

DIAGNOSIS AND DIFFERENTIAL DIAGNOSIS

Diagnosis Clinical impression plus course of illness

Differential Diagnosis Progressive synergistic gangrene, ecthyma gangrenosum, atypical mycobacterial infection, clostridial infection, deep mycoses, amebiasis, bromoderma, pemphigus vegetans, stasis ulcers, Wegener's granulomatosis

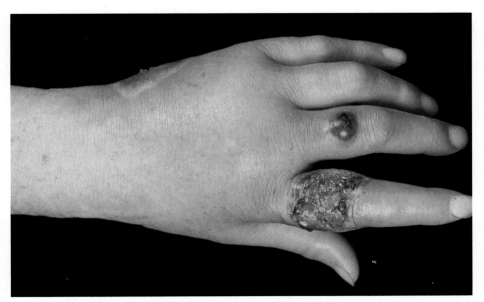

279   Pyoderma gangrenosum   *Hand, illustrating superficial hemorrhagic pustule and an ulcer with irregular, raised border and a purulent hemorrhagic exudate.*

LABORATORY AND SPECIAL EXAMINATIONS

CBC, ESR   Variably elevated

Dermatopathology   Not diagnostic

COURSE AND PROGNOSIS

Untreated, course may last months to years. Ulceration may extend rapidly within a few days, or slowly. Healing may occur centrally with peripheral extension. New ulcers may appear as older lesions resolve.

TREATMENT

With associated underlying disease: treat underlying disease.

For PG: high doses of oral corticosteroids or IV corticosteroid pulse therapy (1 to 2 g prednisolone per day) may be required. ±Intralesional triamcinolone. Sulfasalazine, sulfones, and cyclosporine have been shown to be effective in uncontrolled studies.

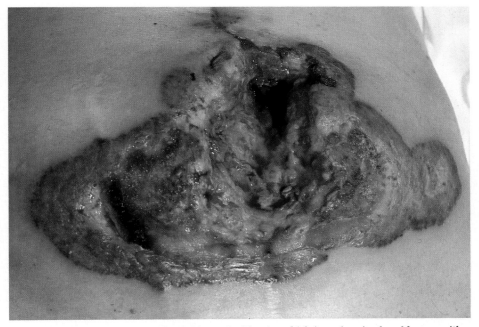

280 Pyoderma gangrenosum *Ulcer with a raised border which is undermined and boggy, with a purulent hemorrhagic exudate at the base.*

Pemphigus vulgaris (PV) is a serious, acute or chronic, bullous, autoimmune disease of skin and mucous membranes that is often fatal unless treated with immunosuppressive agents.

EPIDEMIOLOGY AND ETIOLOGY

Age 40 to 60 years

Sex Equal incidence in males and females

Etiology Autoimmune disorder

HISTORY

Duration of Lesions PV starts usually in oral mucosa, and months may elapse before skin lesions occur; these may be localized for 6 to 12 months, following which generalized bullae occur. Less frequently there may be a generalized, acute eruption of bullae from the beginning.

Skin Symptoms No pruritus; painful and tender mouth lesions may prevent adequate food intake. Skin lesions: burning, pain.

Constitutional Symptoms Weakness, malaise, weight loss (if prolonged mouth involvement)

Systems Review Epistaxis, hoarseness, dysphagia

PHYSICAL EXAMINATION

Skin Lesions
TYPES OF LESIONS Vesicles and bullae (Figure 281), flaccid (flabby), easily ruptured, and weeping, arising on normal skin. Extensive erosions that bleed easily, crusts particularly on scalp.

COLOR Skin-colored

SHAPE Round or oval

ARRANGEMENT Randomly scattered, discrete lesions (Figure 281)

DISTRIBUTION Localized (e.g., to mouth) or generalized with a random pattern (see Figure 281)

NIKOLSKY'S SIGN Dislodging of epidermis by lateral finger pressure in the vicinity of lesions, which leads to an erosion. Pressure on bulla leads to lateral extension of blister (Figure 282).

SITES OF PREDILECTION Scalp, face, chest, axillae, groin, umbilicus

Mucous Membranes Bullae rarely seen, erosions of mouth and nose, pharynx and larynx, vagina

DIFFERENTIAL DIAGNOSIS

Can be a difficult, subtle problem if only mouth lesions present. Biopsy of the skin and mucous membrane, direct immunofluorescence, and demonstration of circulating autoantibodies confirm a high index of suspicion.

LABORATORY AND SPECIAL EXAMINATIONS

Dermatopathology Light microscopy (select early small bulla or, if not present, margin of larger bulla or erosion): (1) loss of intercellular cohesion in lower part of epidermis, leading to (2) acantholysis (separation of keratinocytes) and to (3) bulla which is split just

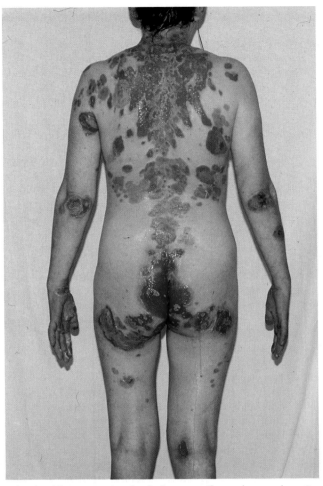

281 Pemphigus vulgaris *There are extensive lesions, mostly erosions and crusts, and no intact bullae.*

above the basal cell layer and contains separated, rounded-up (acantholytic) keratinocytes

Immunofluorescence (IF) Direct IF staining reveals IgG and often C3 deposited at the site of the primary lesion in *the intercellular substance of the epidermis.*

Serum Autoantibodies (IgG) detected by indirect immunofluorescence. Titer usually correlates with activity of disease process.

PATHOPHYSIOLOGY

A loss of the normal cell-to-cell adhesion in the epidermis occurs as a result of circulating antibodies of the IgG class; these antibodies bind to cell surface glycoproteins (pemphigus antigens) of the epidermis and induce acantholysis, probably by the activation of serine proteases.

COURSE

The disease inexorably progresses to death unless treated aggressively with immunosuppressive agents. The mortality has been markedly reduced since treatment has become available.

VARIANTS

Pemphigus Vegetans (PVeg) Usually confined to intertriginous regions, perioral area, neck and scalp. Granulomatous vegetating purulent plaques that extend centrifugally. Suprabasal acantholysis with intraepidermal abscesses containing mostly eosinophils. Pseudoepitheliomatous hyperplasia of the epidermis, exuberant granulation tissue with abscess formation. IgG autoantibodies as in PV. PV may evolve into PVeg and vice versa.

Pemphigus Foliaceus (PF) Most commonly on face, scalp, upper chest, and abdomen but may involve entire skin, presenting as exfoliative erythroderma. Superficial form of pemphigus with acantholysis in the granular layer of the epidermis. Bullae hardly ever present; lesions consist of erythematous patches and erosions covered with crusts. PF is also mediated by circulating autoantibodies to an intercellular (cell surface) antigen on keratinocytes, but PV and PF antigens differ. This explains the different sites of acantholysis and thus different clinical appearance of the two conditions.

Brazilian Pemphigus (Fogo Selvagem) A distinctive form of pemphigus foliaceus endemic to south central Brazil. Clinically, histologically, and immunopathologically the disease is identical to PF. Patients improve when moved to urban areas but relapse after returning to endemic regions. It is speculated that the disease is somehow related to an arthropod-borne infectious agent. More than 1000 new cases per year are estimated to occur in the endemic regions.

Pemphigus Erythematosus (PE) *Synonym:* Senear-Usher syndrome. A localized variety of PF largely confined to seborrheic sites. Erythematous, crusted, and erosive lesions in the "butterfly" area of the face, forehead, presternal, and interscapular regions. Despite clinical, histopathologic, and immunopathologic similarity to PF, PE may be unique, as patients have immunoglobulin and complement deposits at the dermoepidermal junction in addition to intercellular pemphigus antibody deposits in the epidermis and antinuclear antibodies, as is the case in lupus erythematosus. In addition, PE may be associated with thymoma and myasthenia gravis.

Drug-induced Pemphigus A PV- and PF/PE-like syndrome can be induced by D-penicillamine and less frequently by captopril and other drugs. In most, but not all, instances the eruption resolves after termination of therapy with the offending drug.

TREATMENT

Corticosteroids 2.0 to 3.0 mg per kg body weight of prednisone until cessation of new blister formation and disappearance of Nikolsky's sign. Then rapid reduction to about half the initial dose until patient is almost clear, followed by slow tapering of dose to minimal effective maintenance dose.

Concomitant Immunosuppressive Therapy Immunosuppressive agents are given concomitantly for their corticosteroid-saving effect:

Azathioprine, 2.0 to 3.0 mg per kg body weight until complete clearing; tapering of dose to 1.0 mg per kg. Azathioprine alone is continued even after cessation of corticosteroid treatment and may have to be continued for many months. Clinical freedom from disease and a negative pemphigus antibody titer for at least 3 months permits cessation of therapy.

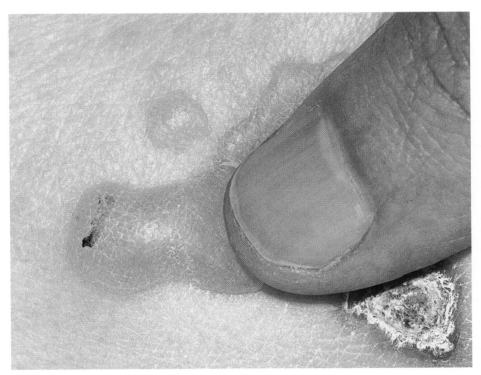

282 Pemphigus vulgaris *The bulla has been extended following pressure with the finger (Nikolsky's sign).*

Methotrexate, either p.o. or IM at doses of 25 to 35 mg per week. Dose adjustments are made as with azathioprine.

Cyclophosphamide, 100 to 200 mg daily with reduction to maintenance doses of 50 to 100 mg per day. Alternatively, cyclophosphamide "bolus" therapy with 1000 mg IV once a week or every 2 weeks in the initial phases, followed by 50 to 100 mg per day p.o. as maintenance.

Plasmapheresis, in conjunction with corticosteroids and immunosuppressives in poorly controlled patients, in the initial phases of treatment to reduce antibody titers.

Gold therapy, for milder cases. After an initial test dose of 10 mg IM, 25 to 50 mg of gold sodium thiomalate are given IM at weekly intervals to a maximum cumulative dose of 1 g.

Other measures: cleansing baths, wet dressings, topical and intralesional corticosteroids; antibiotics to combat bacterial infections. Correction of fluid and electrolyte imbalance.

Monitoring Clinical, for improvement of skin lesions and development of drug-related side effects. Laboratory monitoring of pemphigus antibody titers and for hematologic and metabolic indicators of corticosteroid- and/or immunosuppressive-induced adverse effects.

Bullous pemphigoid is an autoimmune disorder presenting as a chronic bullous eruption mostly in patients over 60 years of age.
Synonym: parapemphigus.

EPIDEMIOLOGY

Age   60 to 80 years or childhood

Sex   Equal incidence in males and females

HISTORY

Duration of Lesions   Often starts with a prodromal eruption (urticarial lesions) and evolves in weeks to months to bullae which may appear suddenly as a generalized eruption

Skin Symptoms   Initially, usually none except mouth lesions; occasionally moderate pruritus and tenderness or eroded lesions

Constitutional Symptoms   None, except in widespread, severe disease

PHYSICAL EXAMINATION

Skin Lesions
TYPES OF LESIONS   Bullae, large, tense, firm-topped; may arise in normal or erythematous skin. Erosions. Erythematous, urticarial-type lesions, not unlike the lesions in erythema multiforme (Figure 283).
SHAPE   Bullae are oval or round.
ARRANGEMENT   Arciform, annular, or serpiginous lesions are scattered and discrete.
DISTRIBUTION   Generalized or localized and randomly distributed
SITES OF PREDILECTION   Axillae; medial aspects of thighs, groins, abdomen; flexor aspects of forearms; lower legs (often first manifestation)

Mucous Membranes   Mouth, anus, vagina: less common and less severe and painful than in pemphigus (see page 536), the bullae less easily ruptured

DIAGNOSIS AND DIFFERENTIAL DIAGNOSIS

Diagnosis   Clinical, confirmed by histopathology and immunopathology

Differential Diagnosis   Histopathology and immunology permit a differentiation from pemphigus, erythema multiforme, or dermatitis herpetiformis.

DERMATOPATHOLOGY

Light Microscopy   Neutrophils in "Indian-file" alignment at dermoepidermal junction; neutrophils, eosinophils, and lymphocytes in papillary dermis; subepidermal bullae, with regeneration of the floor of the bulla

Electron Microscopy   Junctional cleavage, i.e., split occurs in lamina lucida of basement membrane

Immunopathology   IgG deposits along the basement membrane zone. Also C3, which may occur in the absence of IgG.

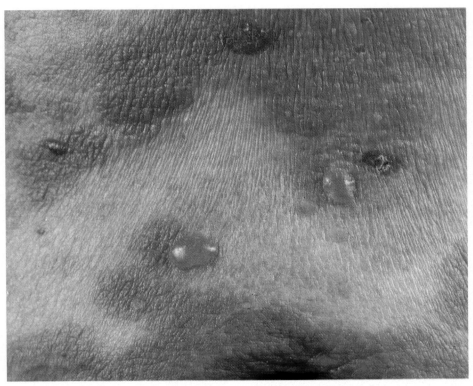

283 Bullous pemphigoid *Large tense bullae and erythematous urticarial-type lesions.*

Serum Circulating antibasement membrane IgG antibodies detected by indirect immunofluorescence in 70% of patients. Titers do not correlate with course of disease.

PATHOGENESIS

Interaction of autoantibody with bullous pemphigoid antigen on the surface of basal keratinocytes (extending into the lamina lucida of basement membrane) is followed by complement activation and attraction of neutrophils and eosinophils. Bullous lesion results from interaction of multiple bioactive molecules released by mast cells and eosinophils.

TREATMENT

Systemic prednisone with starting doses of 50 to 100 mg to clear, either alone or combined with azathioprine for maintenance; or azathioprine alone, 150 mg daily for remission induction and 50 to 100 mg for maintenance; in milder cases sulfones (dapsone), 100 to 150 mg per day. In very mild cases and for local recurrences, topical corticosteroid therapy may have a beneficial effect.

Sweet's syndrome (SS) is an uncommon, recurrent skin disease characterized by painful plaque-forming inflammatory papules and associated with fever, arthralgia, and peripheral leukocytosis. *Synonym:* acute febrile neutrophilic dermatosis.

EPIDEMIOLOGY AND ETIOLOGY

Age Majority 30 to 60 years

Sex Women > men

Etiology Unknown, possibly hypersensitivity reaction. In some cases associated with *Yersinia* infection.

HISTORY

Prodrome Febrile upper respiratory tract infection, GI symptoms (diarrhea), tonsillitis, influenza-like illness, 1 to 3 weeks prior to skin lesions

Systems Review Lesions tender/painful. Headache, arthralgia, general malaise.

PHYSICAL EXAMINATION

Skin Findings
TYPES OF LESIONS Papules or nodules which coalesce to form irregular, sharply bordered inflammatory plaques (Figure 284). Intense edema gives appearance of vesiculation. ±Tiny pustules. If associated with leukemia, bulbous lesions may occur and lesions may mimic pyoderma gangrenosum.
COLOR Red, bluish red
PALPATION *Lesions are tender.*
SHAPE OF INDIVIDUAL LESION As lesions evolve, central clearing may lead to annular or arcuate patterns.
ARRANGEMENT May present as single lesion or multiple lesions, asymmetrically distributed
DISTRIBUTION OF LESIONS Most commonly, face, neck, upper extremities; also lower extremities where lesions may be deep in the panniculus and thus mimic panniculitis or erythema nodosum. Truncal lesions uncommon. Widespread and generalized forms occur.

Mucous Membranes ±Conjunctivitis, episcleritis

General Examination Patient may appear ill.

DIAGNOSIS AND DIFFERENTIAL DIAGNOSIS

Diagnosis Clinical impression plus skin biopsy confirmation

Differential Diagnosis Erythema multiforme, erythema nodosum, prevesicular herpes simplex infection, pre-ulcerative pyoderma gangrenosum, bowel-bypass syndrome, urticaria, serum sickness, other vasculitides, SLE, panniculitis

LABORATORY AND SPECIAL EXAMINATIONS

CBC Leukocytosis with neutrophilia

ESR Elevated

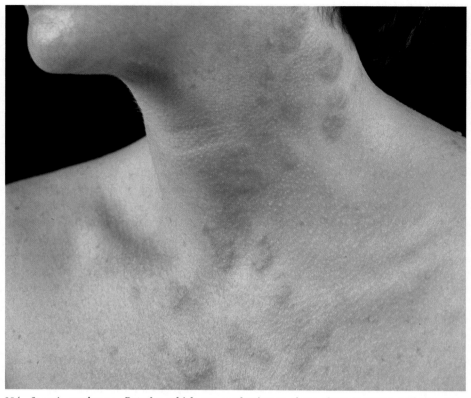

284 Sweet's syndrome *Papules which are coalescing to form sharp-bordered inflammatory plaques.*

Dermatopathology Epidermis usually normal but may show subcorneal pustulation. Edema of papillary body, dense leukocytic infiltrate with starburst pattern of lower dermis. Infiltrate: diffuse or perivascular, consisting of neutrophils with occasional eosinophils/ lymphoid cells. Leukocytoclasia leading to nuclear dust, but other signs of vasculitis absent. ±Neutrophilic infiltrates in subcutaneous tissue.

COURSE AND PROGNOSIS

Untreated, lesions enlarge over a period of days or weeks, and eventually resolve without scarring after weeks or months. Treated with oral prednisone, lesions resolve within a few days. Recurrences occur in 50% of patients, often in previously involved sites. Some cases follow *Yersinia* infection or are associated with acute myeloid leukemia, transient myeloid proliferation, various malignant tumors, ulcerative colitis, benign monoclonal gammopathy.

TREATMENT

Rule out sepsis. Prednisone 30 to 60 mg daily, tapering in 2 to 3 weeks; some but not all cases respond to dapsone, 100 mg per day, or to potassium iodide. Appropriate antibiotic therapy clears eruption in *Yersinia*-associated cases; in all other cases antibiotics ineffective.

Sarcoidosis is a chronic granulomatous inflammation in young adults, affecting diverse organs, but it presents primarily as skin lesions, eye lesions, bilateral hilar lymphadenopathy, and pulmonary infiltration.

EPIDEMIOLOGY AND ETIOLOGY

Age   Under 40 years (range, 12 to 70 years)

Sex   Equal incidence in males and females

Race   All races. In the United States and South Africa, much more frequent in blacks. Frequent in Scandinavia.

Other Factors   The disease occurs worldwide, and there is no clue as to the etiology. The disease can occur in families.

HISTORY

Duration of Lesions   Days (presenting as acute erythema nodosum) or months (presenting as papules or plaques on skin or pulmonary infiltrate discovered in routine chest radiography)

Skin Symptoms   Asymptomatic

Constitutional Symptoms   Fever, fatigue, weight loss, arrhythmia

Systems Review   Enlarged parotids, cardiac dyspnea, neuropathy, kidney stones, uveitis, arthralgia (with erythema nodosum)

PHYSICAL EXAMINATION

Skin Lesions
TYPE AND COLOR
   Brownish-purple infiltrated plaques (Figure 285)

Lupus pernio—violaceous, soft, doughy nodules on the nose, cheek, and earlobes

Multiple maculopapular lesions, 0.5 to 1.0 cm, yellowish-brown

"Scar sarcoidosis"—translucent purplered nodules occurring in an old scar

Note: Upon blanching with glass slide all cutaneous lesions of sarcoidosis reveal "apple-jelly" yellowish-brown color.

SHAPE   Annular, polycyclic (Figure 285), serpiginous
ARRANGEMENT   Scattered discrete lesions (maculopapular and nodular types) and diffuse infiltration (lupus pernio)
DISTRIBUTION   *Plaques*   Extremities, buttocks, trunk
Papular   Face (Figure 286), extremities
Lupus Pernio   Nose, cheeks, and earlobes
"Scar Sarcoidosis"   Anywhere
Erythema Nodosum   Legs
Scalp   May have scarring alopecia

Associations   In acute, bilateral hilar sarcoidosis, particularly in young women, the first clinical manifestation of sarcoidosis may be erythema nodosum (see page 478) and arthritis (Löfgren's syndrome). The Heerford syndrome describes patients with fever, parotid enlargement, uveitis, and facial nerve palsy.

RADIOGRAPHIC STUDIES

In 90% of patients: hilar lymphadenopathy, pulmonary infiltrate

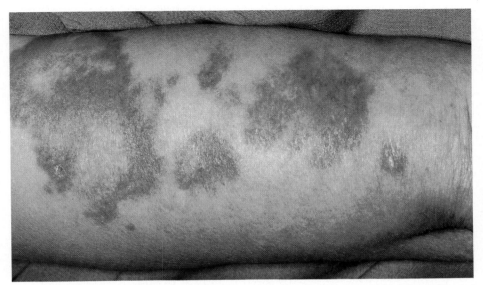

285   Sarcoidosis   *On the left arm are firm, irregularly demarcated, brownish-violet, infiltrated areas.*

DIAGNOSIS

Tissue biopsy of skin or lymph nodes is the best criterion for diagnosis of sarcoidosis.

LABORATORY AND SPECIAL EXAMINATIONS

Dermatopathology Site: dermis. Large islands of epithelioid cells with a few giant cells, and lymphocytes (so-called naked tubercles). Asteroid bodies in large histiocytes; occasionally fibrinoid necrosis.

Skin Tests Intracutaneous tests for recall antigens usually but not always negative. The Kveim-Stilzbach test (antigen prepared from sarcoid spleen injected intracutaneously) is of historical interest only.

Internal Organs Systemic sarcoidosis is verified radiologically by gallium scan and transbronchial, liver, or lymph-node biopsy.

Blood Chemistry
> Increase in serum angiotensin-converting enzyme (ACE)
>
> Hypergammaglobulinemia
>
> Hypercalcemia

TREATMENT

Systemic corticosteroids for active ocular disease, active pulmonary disease, cardiac arrhythmia, CNS involvement, or hypercalcemia

For skin lesions, topical corticosteroids under plastic dressings or intralesional triamcinolone acetonide. For extensive lesions, systemic corticosteroids or chloroquine.

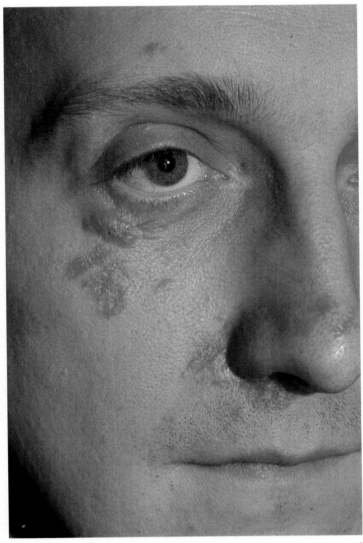

286   Sarcoidosis   *Yellowish-brown plaques and papules on the face. On diascopy these lesions exhibit a pale brownish-red color.*

Genetic, Metabolic, Endocrine, and Nutritional Diseases

Necrobiosis Lipoidica Diabeticorum

Necrobiosis lipoidica diabeticorum (NLD) is a cutaneous disorder often, but not always, associated with diabetes mellitus. The lesions are distinctive, sharply circumscribed, multicolored (red, yellow, brown) plaques occurring on the anterior and lateral surfaces of the lower legs.

EPIDEMIOLOGY

Incidence <1.0% of diabetics, >66% of patients with NLD have overt diabetes mellitus, and 90% of the remaining patients with NLD can be shown to develop an abnormal glucose tolerance with corticosteroids.

Age Young adults, early middle age, but not uncommon in juvenile diabetics

Sex Female:male ratio is 3:1, in both diabetic and nondiabetic forms.

Precipitating Factors A history of preceding trauma to the site can be a factor in the initial development of the lesions, and for this reason NLD is often present on the shins and over the bony areas of the feet. (A cowboy had extensive lesions on the thighs where the skin rubbed against the sides of the horse.)

HISTORY

Duration of Lesions Slowly evolving and enlarging over months

Skin Symptoms None, except pain in lesions that develop ulcers

Systems Review Diabetes may or may not be present at the time of onset of lesions; diabetes mellitus, however, develops in the majority of patients.

PHYSICAL EXAMINATION

Skin
TYPES OF LESIONS
>*Characteristic lesions:* early lesions are small and dusky red plaques, and as the lesions enlarge the center becomes atrophic and there is usually a raised brownish-red border; there are waxy yellow atrophic areas, in which many well-marked telangiectases are seen throughout the center of the lesion where the atrophy is most prominent (Figure 287).

>*Less common lesions:* skin-colored nodules, and, rarely, small annular lesions on the elbows without epidermal atrophy, and these closely mimic granuloma annulare or sarcoidosis.

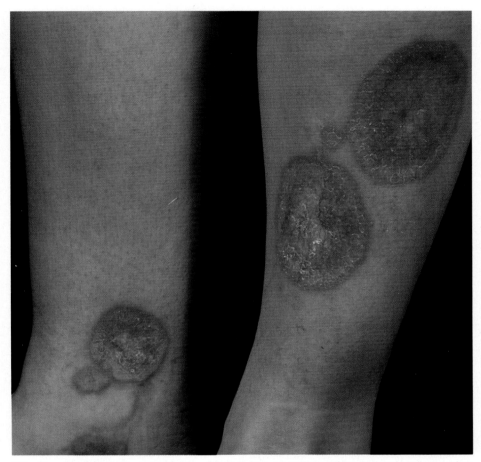

287   Necrobiosis lipoidica diabeticorum   *On both legs are rather striking lesions composed of an atrophic center, exhibiting delicate vessels traversing the area, and a raised, rolled border.*

Ulcers: shallow, painful, and slow-healing ulcers not infrequently develop.

Shape Serpiginous, irregularly irregular

Arrangement of Lesions Often symmetrical

Distribution of Lesions >80% occur on the legs and feet (shins, bony areas of the feet, heels); other areas include arms, trunk, or the face and scalp.

LABORATORY EXAMINATIONS

Dermatopathology
LIGHT MICROSCOPY *Site* Epidermis (atrophy) and dermis
Process In the lower dermis there is sclerotic collagen and obliteration of the bundle pattern, necrobiosis of connective tissue, and concomitant granulomatous infiltration. Fat-containing foam cells are often present, imparting the yellow color to the clinical lesion. There is a "microangiopathy" with thickening of the capillary walls with endothelial thickening, and focal deposits of PAS-positive material.
IMMUNOFLUORESCENCE Presence of immunoglobulins and complement (C3). Immune complexes may occur in the walls of the small blood vessels.
SPECIAL TECHNIQUES *Special stains:* fat stains
CHEMISTRY Evidence of frank diabetes or an abnormal glucose tolerance with corticosteroids

DIAGNOSIS AND DIFFERENTIAL DIAGNOSIS

Diagnosis The lesions are so distinctive that biopsy confirmation is not usually done.

Differential Diagnosis Sarcoid has been confused with the fully developed lesions on the leg, and small plaques of NLD on the arms can exactly mimic granuloma annulare.

PATHOGENESIS

The granulomatous inflammatory reaction is believed to be due to alterations in the collagen. The arteriolar changes in the areas of necrobiosis of the collagen have been thought by some to be precipitated by aggregation of platelets.

SIGNIFICANCE

The lesions are unsightly and patients are usually upset about the cosmetic appearance; the ulcers are painful but usually can be healed over time. NLD is regarded by most as an indication of latent diabetes in the majority of patients.

COURSE AND PROGNOSIS

The lesions are indolent and can enlarge to involve large areas of the skin surface unless treated. The severity of NLD is not related to the severity of the diabetes mellitus. Furthermore, control of the diabetes has no effect on the course of NLD.

TREATMENT

Intralesional triamcinolone usually limits the spread of the lesions; the resulting scar is more resistant to trauma and the risk of ulceration is less. Also potent topical corticosteroids under occlusion can be judiciously used. Resistant and painful ulcers can be excised and grafted.

Cholesterol embolism is the phenomenon of dislodgement of cholesterol crystals from an atheromatous abdominal aorta with centrifugal microembolization and resultant ischemic and infarctive cutaneous lesions.

EPIDEMIOLOGY AND ETIOLOGY

Age Middle-aged to elderly

Sex Males > females

Etiology Arteriosclerosis. Embolization of vessels by cholesterol crystals from atheromatous aorta. "Blue toe," "purple toe" syndrome: peripheral ischemia, livedo reticularis of sudden onset.

HISTORY

Pains in legs, buttocks, low back; myalgia

PHYSICAL EXAMINATION

Skin Findings
TYPE OF LESION Livedo reticularis (Figure 288*a*). Indurated nodules and plaques; may undergo necrosis, become crusted and ulcerate. Cyanosis and gangrene (Figure 288*b*).
COLOR Nodules/plaques: violaceous. Ulcers: erythematous halo
PALPATION Nodules/plaques: firm, painful
DISTRIBUTION OF LESIONS Livedo reticularis: lower abdomen/back, buttocks, legs, feet. Plaques/nodules: thighs, calves.

Systems Review Cholesterol embolism may occur in kidney, pancreas, spleen, GI tract, brain, liver, retina.

General Examination Patient often obese; arteriosclerotic vessels; ±reduction of pulses (femoral, popliteal, dorsalis pedis, posterior tibial)

DIAGNOSIS AND DIFFERENTIAL DIAGNOSIS

Diagnosis Clinical suspicion confirmed by arteriography. Deep skin biopsy

Differential Diagnosis Necrotizing vasculitis, polyarteritis nodosa, nodular vasculitis, septic emboli, warfarin necrosis, livedo reticularis syndromes

LABORATORY AND SPECIAL EXAMINATIONS

Laboratory Elevated serum lipids

Dermatopathology Deep skin and muscle biopsy specimen shows arterioles occluded by multinucleated foreign-body giant cells and fibrosis surrounding biconvex, needle-shaped clefts corresponding to the cholesterol crystal microemboli.

Arteriography Abdominal aorta: ulceration of atheromatous plaques

PATHOPHYSIOLOGY

Detachment of atheromatous plaque from large arterial vessels, e.g., aorta, and embolization of small arteries. Occurs spontaneously or after vascular surgery, arteriography, fibrinolysis, or anticoagulation.

COURSE AND PROGNOSIS

Acute onset; recurring episodes; prognosis guarded

TREATMENT

Symptomatic. Heparin, analgesics, excision of necrotic area, or amputation may be necessary

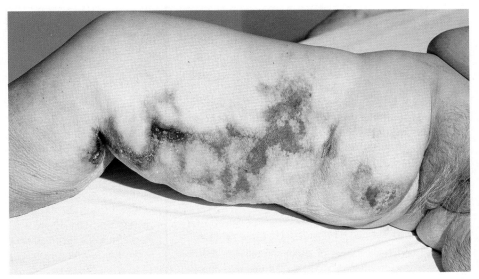

288*a* Cholesterol embolism *In a livedoid distribution there are infarcts.*

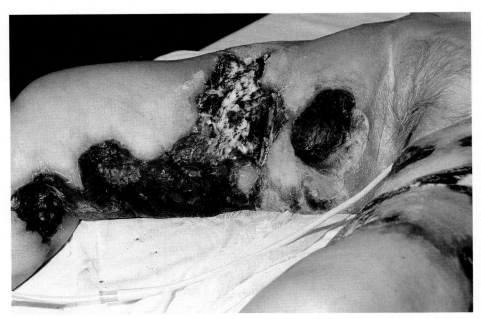

288*b* Cholesterol embolism *In a very short period of time the initial lesions have progressed to become much more extensive.*

CHOLESTEROL EMBOLISM

This autosomal dominant condition affects blood vessels, especially in the mucous membranes of the mouth and the GI tract. The disease is frequently heralded by recurrent epistaxis that appears often in childhood. The diagnostic lesions are small, pulsating, macular and papular, usually punctate, and vascular telangiectasia. There are frequent attacks of nasal and GI bleeding.

Synonym: Osler-Weber-Rendu disease.

EPIDEMIOLOGY

Age Epistaxis may appear in childhood but skin lesions begin after puberty, as can epistaxis.

HISTORY

Duration of Lesions The typical lesions (punctate red macules and papules) begin to appear after puberty but peak in the third or fourth decade.

Systems Review Recurrent epistaxis often in childhood; GI bleeding (12 to 50%); pulmonary arteriovenous (A-V) fistulae occur in 15% of patients; A-V fistulae may occur in the liver; aneurysms of the CNS

Family History Autosomal dominant

PHYSICAL EXAMINATION

Skin
TYPE OF LESION Macules or papules 3.0 mm in diameter which usually pulsate; can often be blanched
COLOR Red
SHAPE OF LESION Punctate (most frequent), stellate, or linear
ARRANGEMENT OF MULTIPLE LESIONS Symmetrical and scattered, nonpatterned

DISTRIBUTION OF LESIONS Upper half of the body; begin on the mucous membranes of the nose, later develop on the face (lips), mouth (tongue) (Figure 289), conjunctivae, trunk, upper extremities, palms (Figure 290) and soles, hands, fingers, and toes

Nails Nail beds of fingers and toes

Mucous Membranes Telangiectases appear in Kiesselbach's area of the nasal septum, on the tip and dorsum of the tongue, nasopharynx, and throughout the GI tract.

LABORATORY EXAMINATIONS

Laboratory Examination of Blood
HEMATOLOGIC Anemia from chronic blood loss

Dermatopathology
LIGHT MICROSCOPY *Site* Papillary dermis *Process* Capillaries and venules, irregularly dilated and lined by flattened endothelial cells

IMAGING

X-ray or CT or MRI of the chest to discover pulmonary A-V fistulae

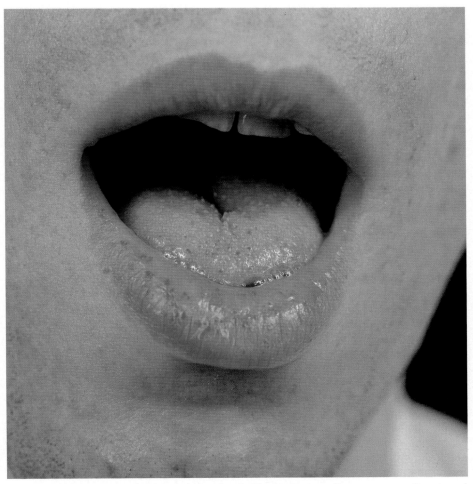

289   Hereditary hemorrhagic telangiectasia   *On the lips and tongue there are many discrete, red, tiny macular and papular lesions.*

DIAGNOSIS

Triad of (1) typical telangiectases on skin (fingers and palms) *and* mucous membranes (lips and tongue), (2) repeated GI hemorrhages, and (3) family history

PATHOGENESIS

There is a breakdown of the junction between the endothelial cells because of a lack of perivascular support (pericytes, smooth muscle, and elastic fibers). The abnormal telangiectatic capillaries rupture easily, and this is the basis for the repeated nasal and GI hemorrhages.

TREATMENT

Electrocautery of the abnormal vessels in Kiesselbach's plexus

Laser: the tunable dye laser may now be used to destroy the abnormal blood vessels in the various sites

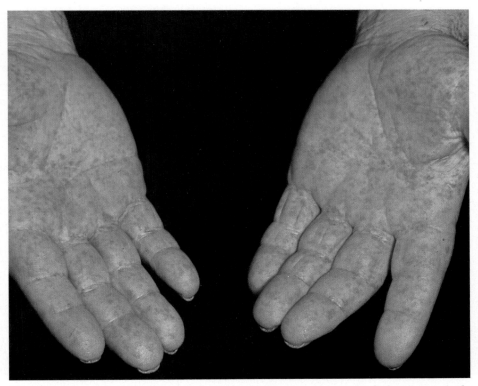

290   Hereditary hemorrhagic telangiectasia   *On the palms there are myriads of telangiectases in the form of tiny mats.*

Cushing's Syndrome (Hypercorticism)

This syndrome results from hyperactivity of the adrenal cortex or exogenous cortisol administration and is characterized by a rounded "moon" facies, plethora, truncal obesity, a buffalo hump, purplish striae, hirsutism, hypertension, and oligomenorrhea or amenorrhea. Hyperactivity of the adrenal cortex occurs principally as a result of bilateral adrenal hyperplasia secondary to stimulation by increased secretion of pituitary ACTH or by production of ACTH by nonendocrine tumors, especially pulmonary oat-cell carcinoma.

HISTORY

The history of fatigue, muscle weakness, and, often, psychiatric abnormalities is nonspecific, and the diagnosis is suspected on the basis of the physical findings.

PHYSICAL EXAMINATION

Appearance of Patient A plethoric obese person with a "classic" habitus which results from the redistribution of fat (Figure 291): buffalo hump, truncal obesity, and thin arms.

Skin Findings
Purple striae, mostly on the abdomen, similar to striae produced by topical application of corticosterioids

Hirsutism: facial hypertrichosis with pigmented hairs and often increased lanugo hairs on the face and arms

Easy bruising, ecchymoses

Acne: "steroid" monomorphous type with few or no comedones; occurs in patient's with Cushing's syndrome, resulting from excess exogenous steroid administration

General Examination Hypertension, hypertrophy of the clitoris. A careful medical examination is necessary to look for clues to the multiple causes of Cushing's syndrome, especially nonendocrine neoplasms: oat-cell carcinoma, carcinoid of the thymus, pancreatic carcinoma, bronchial adenoma.

LABORATORY EXAMINATIONS

Chemistry
Blood sugar: about 20% have diabetes mellitus and most have impaired carbohydrate tolerance

Elevated plasma and urinary cortisol levels are present except in iatrogenic Cushing's syndrome.

Imaging CT scan of the abdomen and the pituitary

DIAGNOSIS

This is difficult, and specialized tests are required; the patient, therefore, should be referred to an endocrinologist. Although the clinical appearance is characteristic, the diagnosis is confirmed by the demonstration of increased cortisol production and by doing a number of special tests, among which are those to demonstrate a failure to suppress endogenous cortisol secretion when dexamethasone is administered.

ETIOLOGY

Adrenal hyperplasia secondary to:

Pituitary ACTH hypersecretion: adenomas of the pituitary

ACTH production by nonendocrine tumors, especially oat-cell carcinoma

Exogenous corticosteroids

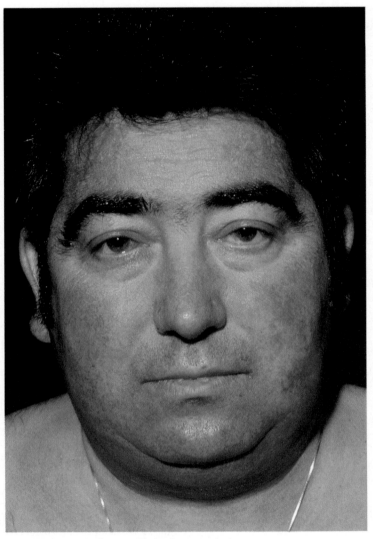

291 Cushing's syndrome *Plethoric moon facies.*

This syndrome, an autoimmune disease, is a triad of changes: hyperthyroidism, eye changes (principally proptosis), and, rarely, skin lesions (pretibial myxedema).

Synonym: Graves' disease.

EPIDEMIOLOGY

Incidence Relatively common

Age Third and fourth decades

Race Haplotypes: Caucasians—HLA-B8 and -DRw3; Japanese—HLA-Bw36; Chinese—HLA-Bw46

Sex Females > males

HISTORY

General Symptoms Nervousness, emotional lability, insomnia, tremors, especially in younger patients. Weight loss despite an increased appetite. Older patients more often have cardiac manifestations: dyspnea, palpitations, and angina pectoris.

Symptoms Relating to the Skin Pruritus, hyperhidrosis, heat intolerance

Family History There is an association with other autoimmune diseases: pernicious anemia, Hashimoto's thyroiditis.

PHYSICAL EXAMINATION

Appearance of Patient The patient appears anxious, is irritable and tremulous. There is often a persistent facial flush, palmar erythema, increased sweating on the palms and soles.

Skin Findings
GENERAL Warm, moist, soft, smooth as an infant's skin
REGIONAL Pretibial myxedema (Figure 292), rarely, preradial myxedema; present in about 5% of patients with Graves' disease, and in half of these it occurs during the active stage of the disease and in the other half it occurs after treatment of the Graves' disease.
TYPE OF LESION Nodules and confluent plaques with peau d'orange appearance, which may or may not be verrucous
COLOR Pink or skin-colored or purple
PALPATION Firm, plus nonpitting brawny edema in the normal skin (Figure 292)

Hair Scalp hair is fine and soft, with an altered texture. Diffuse alopecia is not uncommon; pretibial myxedema may show hypertrichosis.

Nails A special type of onycholysis (Plummer's nail) (see Appendix H) in which the free edge of the nail becomes undulated and curves upward. Clubbing of the nails, which may be associated with diaphyseal proliferation of the periosteum in the acral (Figure 292) and long bones; this is known as *thyroid acropachy.*

Thyroid Examination Asymmetric and lobular thyroid enlargement, often with the presence of a bruit

Eyes "Stare," lid lag, lid retraction—"frightened" appearance (Figure 292). Proptosis, periorbital swelling

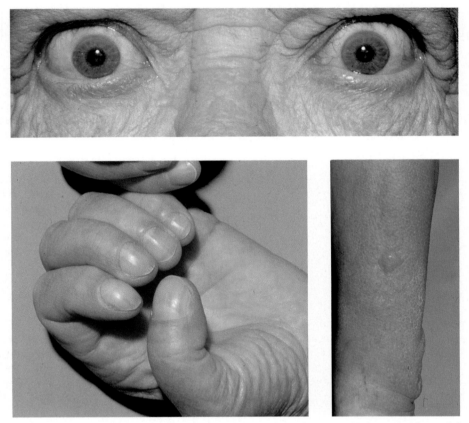

292 Hyperthyroidism *This composite photograph illustrates the proptosis, the acropathy, and the pink or flesh-colored papules, plaques, and nodules of pretibial myxedema.*

Cardiovascular Findings Atrial arrythmias, systolic murmurs

LABORATORY EXAMINATIONS

Dermatopathology
LIGHT MICROSCOPY Pretibial myxedema
Site Dermis; "edematous" separation of collagen bundles, stellate fibroblasts
Process Accumulation of hyaluronic acid and chondroitin sulfate in the lesions, and in the normal skin

Laboratory Examination of Blood
CHEMISTRY—THYROID TESTS

Increased radioactive iodine uptake, increased serum T4, increased T3, RT3U, and FT4I

Antithyroid antibodies

ETIOLOGY AND PATHOGENESIS

This is not settled, but it is thought that circulating thyroid stimulators in the serum, which are immunoglobulin antibodies (LATS, long-acting thyroid stimulators), are directed against the TSH receptor site and specifically stimulate the activity of the thyroid.

This syndrome results from a deficiency of thyroid hormone caused by an autoimmune reaction following inflammation of the thyroid (chronic lymphocytic thyroiditis or Hashimoto's thyroiditis). The skin changes reflect an accumulation of hydrophilic mucopolysaccharides in the dermis, thus the term *myxedema*.

EPIDEMIOLOGY

Age 40 to 60 years

Sex Females > males

HISTORY

Systems Review The early symptoms are slow in developing and are nonspecific and often overlooked, e.g., lethargy, cold intolerance, and constipation. Patients complain of dry hair, hair loss, dry skin, weight gain. The voice may become deeper.

PHYSICAL EXAMINATION

Appearance of Patient (Figure 293) Dull and listless facies, with puffiness of the eyelids. The nose is broadened and the lips are thick. There is a slowing down of bodily activity.

Skin Diffuse involvement of the entire skin
COLOR Pale skin due to increased concentration of water and mucopolysaccharides; carotenemia may be present, and the palms and soles appear yellow-orange.
PALPATION The skin is dry due to decreased sebum and sweat secretion. There is doughy induration. The boggy, nonpitting edema is not in dependent parts but more in acral parts.

Hair and Nails The hair is dry, coarse, and brittle; alopecia of the lateral one-third of the eyebrows is characteristic. Hair growth is slow in the scalp, beard, and sexual areas; there is an increase in the number of telogen hairs. The nails are brittle and grow slowly.

Mucous Membranes The tongue is large, smooth, red, and clumsy.

General Examination The thyroid is not usually palpable unless a goiter is present. There may be a decrease in heart rate. The relaxation phase of the deep tendon reflexes (ankle) is prolonged, a "hung-up" reflex—brisk contraction and slow relaxation time.

LABORATORY EXAMINATIONS

Dermatopathology
LIGHT MICROSCOPY *Site* Papillary dermis, around hair follicles and blood vessels
Process Accumulation of chondroitin sulfate and hyaluronic acid with separation of the collagen bundles
LABORATORY EXAMINATION OF BLOOD
Chemistry
Thyroid tests, decreased T3 and T4, with marked elevation of TSH in primary hypothyroidism. Also the TSH has a subnormal response to administration of thyroid-releasing hormone, and this confirms the diagnosis of primary hypothyroidism.

Elevation of serum cholesterol

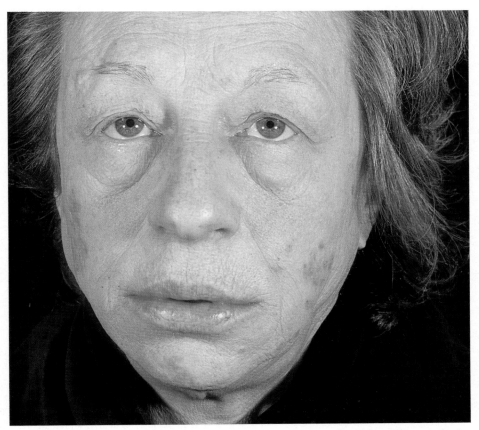

293 Hypothyroidism *This patient has many of the typical features of hypothyroidism: a cold, dry, pale skin; absence of hair in the lateral third of the eyebrows; and a puffiness of the face and lips due to the accumulation of water and mucopolysaccharides in the dermis. The hair is dry, coarse, and brittle. The nose is broadened, the tongue is large, smooth, red, and clumsy, and there is a drooping of the eyelids. The face lacks expressiveness and is the most pathognomonic of any of the features.*

DIAGNOSIS

Subclinical hypothyroidism may be present in patients with vitiligo vulgaris, especially in women over 50 years. There are also several diseases in which there are circulating autoantibodies, including SLE, pernicious anemia, Sjögren's syndrome, and rheumatoid arthritis, and these diseases as well as primary hypothyroidism are associated with increased specific HLA haplotypes.

PATHOGENESIS

The circulating antithyroid antibodies cause primary hypothyroidism by the action of the antibodies that block the TSH receptor. Carotenemia results from a reduction in the conversion of beta-carotene to vitamin A. The pale color of the skin is due to the water content and the mucopolysaccharides in the skin which change the refraction of incident light.

TREATMENT

Synthetic levothyroxine, p.o. once daily

HYPOTHYROIDISM, PRIMARY (MYXEDEMA)

Scurvy is an acute or chronic disease of infancy and of middle and old age caused by dietary deficiency of ascorbic acid. The disorder is characterized principally by anemia, hemorrhagic manifestations in the skin (ecchymoses and perifollicular hemorrhage) and in the musculoskeletal system (hemorrhage into periosteum and muscles), and changes in the gums (loosening of teeth, bleeding gums).

EPIDEMIOLOGY

Age In infancy and childhood, from processed milk with no added citrus fruit or vegetables in diet; in middle or old age, edentulous single persons who live alone, cook for themselves, and do not eat salads and uncooked vegetables

Precipitating Factors Pregnancy, lactation, and thyrotoxicosis increase requirements of ascorbic acid; alcoholism

HISTORY

There may be a history of lassitude, weakness, arthralgia, and myalgia, but the diagnosis is suspected by the purpura and perifollicular hemorrhages and by the history of lack of intake of ascorbic acid, e.g., food faddists may boil orange juice to sterilize it and this destroys ascorbic acid; dietary deficiency due to alcoholism.

PHYSICAL EXAMINATION

Appearance of Patient Lethargic and weak

Skin
TYPES OF LESIONS
Ecchymoses of arms and legs (inner thighs) (Figure 294)

Follicular, hyperkeratotic papules with hemorrhage (Figure 294), especially on the backs of the lower legs (almost pathognomonic)

Hemorrhages into the muscles and arms with secondary phlebothrombosis

Periosteal hemorrhages of long bones causing painful swellings and epiphyseal separation (infancy and childhood)

Nails Splinter hemorrhages

Mucous Membranes Bleeding of the gums (Figure 295) which are swollen, purple, and spongy (a late clinical finding; the skin lesions occur much earlier)

LABORATORY AND SPECIAL EXAMINATIONS

Laboratory Examination of Blood
PLATELET ASCORBIC ACID LEVELS Accurately correlate with the clinical state and are available in most of the larger medical laboratories

HEMATOLOGIC Moderate to severe normocytic, normochromatic anemia resulting from bleeding into tissues. Positive capillary fragility test

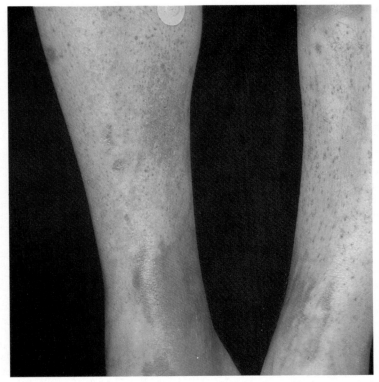

294   Scurvy   *Legs showing ecchymoses. Also there are follicles plugged by horny material showing hemorrhages.*

DIFFERENTIAL DIAGNOSIS

Arthritis, hemorrhagic diseases, and gingivitis are the most confusing problems in differential diagnosis; the skin lesions are almost pathognomonic.

ETIOLOGY AND PATHOGENESIS

Humans cannot synthesize ascorbic acid, which is required in the peptidyl hydroxylation of procollagen. Failure of hydroxylation of collagen leads to its instability and the triple helix required for normal tissue structure cannot be formed. This defective collagen synthesis is the basis for the capillary fragility.

COURSE AND PROGNOSIS

Unless treated, scurvy is fatal

TREATMENT

Ascorbic acid, 100 mg 3 to 5 times daily until 4 g are given, then 100 mg per day is curative in days to weeks.

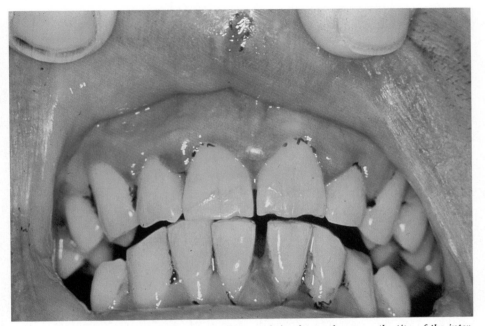

295 Scurvy *Gums showing reddening, swelling, and tiny hemorrhages on the tips of the inter-dental papillae.*

Acrodermatitis enteropathica (AE) is a genetic disorder of zinc absorption, presenting in infancy, characterized by a triad of acral dermatitis (face, hands, feet, anogenital), alopecia, and diarrhea; nearly identical clinical findings occur in other individuals with *acquired zinc deficiency (AZD)* due either to dietary deficiency or failure of intestinal absorption.

EPIDEMIOLOGY AND ETIOLOGY

Age *AE:* in infants bottle-fed with bovine milk, days to few weeks. In breast-fed infants, soon after weaning. *AZD:* older individuals

Etiology *AE:* autosomal recessive trait resulting in failure to absorb zinc. *AZD:* secondary to reduced dietary intake of zinc, malabsorption (regional enteritis, following intestinal bypass surgery for obesity), increased urinary loss (nephrotic syndrome), hypoalbuminemic states, penicillamine therapy, high catabolic states (trauma, burns, surgery), hemolytic anemias, adolescents who eat dirt, prolonged parenteral nutrition without supplemental zinc

Predisposition *AZD:* pregnancy, growing child, or adolescent

HISTORY

Skin Findings
TYPE OF LESION   Patches and plaques of dry, scaly, eczematous skin. Perlèche. Evolve to vesiculobullous, pustular, erosive, and crusted lesions (Figure 296). Dermatitis: palmar/digital creases; paronychia, fissures on fingertips. Annular lesions with collarette scaling. Lesions become secondarily infected with *Candida albicans, Staphylococcus aureus.* Impaired wound healing.
COLOR   Initially pink. Later, brightly erythematous

DISTRIBUTION OF LESIONS   Initially, face (particularly perioral), scalp, anogenital area (Figure 296). Later, hands (Figure 297) and feet, flexural regions, trunk
HAIR AND NAILS   Diffuse alopecia, graying of hair. Paronychia, nail ridging, loss of nails
MUCOUS MEMBRANES   Oral: red, glossy tongue, superficial aphthous-like erosions, oral candidiasis, perlèche. Photophobia

General Examination   Irritable, depressed mood. Failure of growth

DIAGNOSIS AND DIFFERENTIAL DIAGNOSIS

Diagnosis   Clinical diagnosis confirmed by zinc blood levels

Differential Diagnosis   Atopic dermatitis, seborrheic dermatitis, mucocutaneous candidiasis, glucagonoma.

LABORATORY AND SPECIAL EXAMINATIONS

CBC   Anemia

Chemistry   Low serum/plasma zinc levels

Urine   Reduced urinary zinc excretion

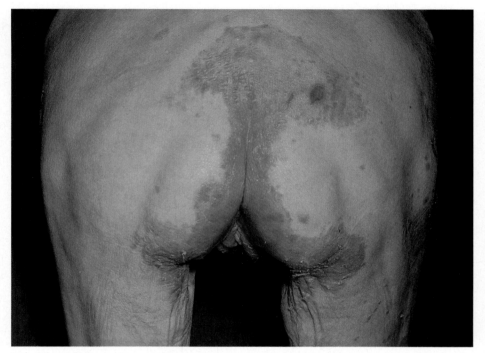

296 Zinc deficiency *There are plaques of dry, scaly, eczematous skin around the buttocks. The lesions often become secondarily infected with* Candida albicans.

Dermatopathology Intraepidermal clefts and blisters with acantholysis.

PATHOPHYSIOLOGY

In AE, patients do not absorb enough zinc from the diet. The specific ligand involved in basic transport mechanisms for zinc which might be abnormal in AE is not known. The defect appears to be somewhere in the early stages of zinc nutriture where zinc is presented to the intestinal brush border. This defect can be overcome by increased zinc supply in the diet. It is also not known how zinc deficiency leads to skin and other lesions.

COURSE AND PROGNOSIS

Before it was known that AE is due to a deficient zinc uptake from the diet it was usually fatal in infancy or early childhood. Patients failed to thrive and suffered from severe candidal and bacterial infections. Following zinc replacement: severe infected and erosive skin lesions heal within 1 to 2 weeks; diarrhea ceases and irritability and depression of mood improve within 24 hours.

TREATMENT

Dietary or IV supplementation with zinc salts with 2 to 3 times the RDA restores normal zinc status in days to weeks.

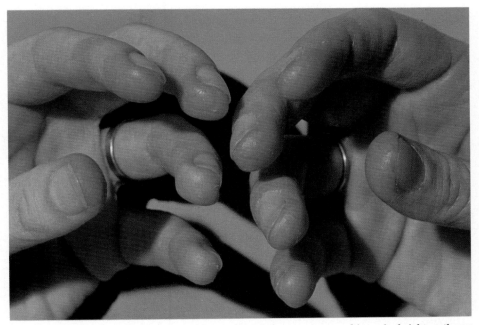

297 Zinc deficiency *Hands. The fingers are enlarged, there are paronychia and a bright erythema on the terminal phalanges.*

Pancreatic panniculitis is characterized clinically by painful erythematous nodules occurring at any site, frequently accompanied by arthritis and polyserositis, associated with either pancreatitis or pancreatic carcinoma, and histologically by a lobular panniculitis.

EPIDEMIOLOGY AND ETIOLOGY

Age Middle-aged to elderly

Sex Male > females

Etiology Associated with chronic pancreatitis or carcinoma of the pancreas

HISTORY

Alcoholism, abdominal pain, weight loss, recent-onset diabetes mellitus. Lesions are quite tender.

PHYSICAL EXAMINATION

Skin Findings
TYPE OF LESION Papules, nodules (Figure 298), and plaques. Following biopsy of lesion, liquified fat drains from lesion.
COLOR Erythematous
PALPATION Lesions tender, warm. ±Fluctuant (Figure 298)
DISTRIBUTION OF LESIONS Occur at any site; however, predilection for legs and buttocks.

General Examination Pleural effusion, ascites, arthritis (especially ankles)

DIAGNOSIS AND DIFFERENTIAL DIAGNOSIS

Diagnosis Clinical diagnosis confirmed by histologic examination of an adequate biopsy including subcutaneous tissue.

Differential Diagnosis Erythema nodosum, subacute nodular migratory panniculitis (Villanova's disease), lupus erythematosus panniculitis, poststeroid panniculitis, relapsing febrile nonsuppurative nodular panniculitis (α-antitrypsin deficiency), Sweet's syndrome

LABORATORY AND SPECIAL EXAMINATIONS

CBC Eosinophilia

Chemistry Hyperlipasemia, hyperamylasemia

Urine Increased amylase, lipase

Dermatopathology Lobular panniculitis with necrosis of lipocytes and varying degrees of calcification. Foci of granular basophilic degeneration of lipocytes occur in lobular area, leading to loss of nuclear staining and formation of ghostlike fat cells with thick walls and no nuclei. ±Calcification. Polymorphic lobular infiltrate surrounds foci of necrosis. Contiguous lobules may be spared.

PATHOPHYSIOLOGY

Breakdown of subcutaneous fat caused by enzymes (amylase, trypsin, lipase) released to the circulation from the diseased pancreas.

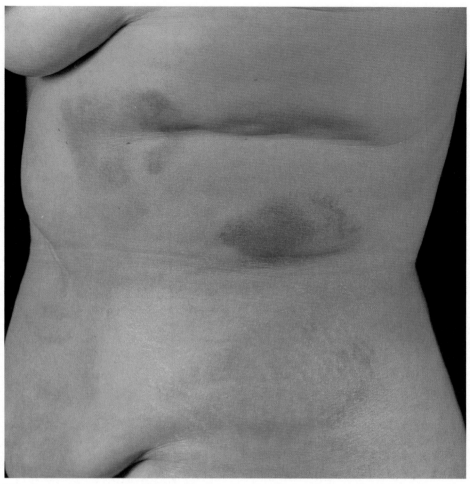

298　Pancreatic panniculitis　*Erythematous, tender, fluctuant nodules on the abdomen.*

COURSE AND PROGNOSIS

Depends on pancreatic disease. Crops of painful lesions recur.

TREATMENT

Directed at treatment of underlying pancreatic disorder.

Pseudoxanthoma Elasticum

Pseudoxanthoma elasticum (PXE) is a serious hereditary disorder of connective tissue that involves the elastic tissue in the skin, blood vessels, and eyes. The principal skin manifestations are a distinctive peau d'orange surface pattern resulting from closely grouped clusters of yellow (chamois-colored) papules in a reticular pattern on the neck, axillae, and other body folds. The effects on the vascular system include GI hemorrhage, hypertension occurring in young persons and resulting from involvement of renal arteries, and claudication. Ocular manifestations (''angioid'' streaks and retinal hemorrhages) can lead to blindness.

EPIDEMIOLOGY

Incidence 1:160,000

Age of Onset 20 to 30 years

Heredity Autosomal recessive and autosomal dominant

Classification The studies of Pope recognize four genetic types—two dominant and two recessive: Type I recessive and dominant are the most common; these have vascular and retinal changes. Type II dominant and recessive are rarer and have minimal systemic involvement.

HISTORY

History The asymptomatic skin lesions, which may at first be overlooked, may develop in early childhood and usually do before the age of 30 but may not appear until old age. Decrease of visual acuity in a young person may be the first clue to the disease.

Systems Review Symptoms relating to multisystem involvement such as cardiac disease, hematemesis and melena, symptoms associated with hypertension, claudication

PHYSICAL EXAMINATION

Skin
TYPE OF LESION Small (2.0 to 3.0 mm) papules or larger plaques, often with telangiectasia

COLOR OF LESIONS Yellow, chamois-colored

PALPATION The skin is soft and lax and hangs in folds.

ARRANGEMENT OF MULTIPLE LESIONS Reticulated or linear, furrows between individual plaques

DISTRIBUTION OF LESIONS Sides of the neck (Figure 299), axillae, abdomen, groin, perineum, and thighs

MUCOUS MEMBRANES Lesions may be present on the soft palate, inside the lips, rectum, and vagina.

General Examination Decrease of peripheral pulses

Ophthalmologic Examination Fundoscopic changes noted are: angioid streaks (Figure 300) which are slate-gray, wider than blood vessels, and extend across the fundus, radiating from the optic disc; retinal hemorrhages are common.

GENETIC, METABOLIC, ENDOCRINE, AND NUTRITIONAL DISEASES

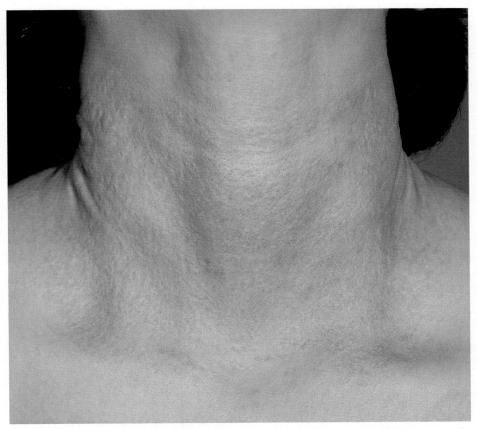

299　Pseudoxanthoma elasticum　*Pebbled (peau d'orange), infiltrative, yellowish lesions on the neck that have a chamois color.*

LABORATORY AND SPECIAL EXAMINATIONS

Dermatopathology
LIGHT MICROSCOPY *Site* Reticular dermis
Process Elastic tissue changes (swelling and irregular clumping) can be seen as a faintly basophilic staining in tissue with routine stains; with special stains, elastic tissue is seen as characteristic curled and "chopped-up"-appearing clumps. There is also extensive calcium deposition by the elastic fibers.

Imaging X-ray: extensive calcification of the peripheral arteries of the lower extremities

DIAGNOSIS

By the skin lesions, which are distinctive, but the diagnosis of PXE is confirmed by biopsy. The ophthalmologic findings are also characteristic but may be noted also in Paget's disease of bone.

ETIOLOGY AND PATHOGENESIS

The biochemical defect is not known but there are abnormalities of both collagen and elastic tissue.

SIGNIFICANCE

An important syndrome to recognize early in life so the complications (especially the eye and vascular involvement) can be monitored. Loss of central vision develops in over two-thirds of the patients with angioid streaks.

COURSE AND PROGNOSIS

The course is inexorably progressive.

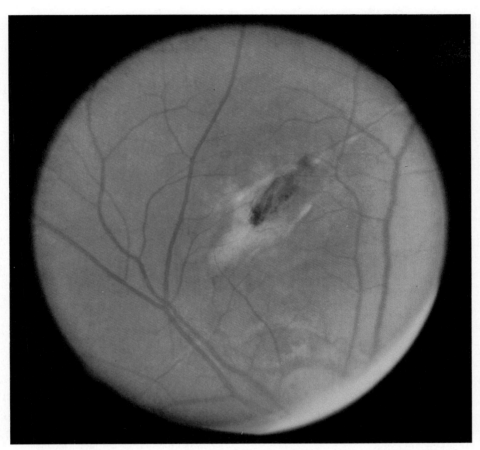

300   Pseudoxanthoma elasticum   *Angioid streaks in the eye. These streaks, which are wider than blood vessels, are extending across the fundus in a distribution more or less radial from the optic disc.*

Tuberous sclerosis is an autosomal dominant disease arising from a genetically programmed hyperplasia of ectodermal and mesodermal cells and manifested by a variety of lesions in the skin, CNS (hamartoma), heart, kidney, and other organs. The principal early manifestations are the triad of seizures, mental retardation, and congenital white spots (macules). Facial angiofibromata are pathognomonic but do not appear until the third or fourth year.

EPIDEMIOLOGY

Incidence In institutions, 1:100 to 1:300; in general population, 1:20,000 to 1:100,000

Age Infancy

Sex Equal incidence

Race All races

Inheritance Autosomal dominant

HISTORY

Onset of Lesions
White macules are present at birth or appear in infancy (80% occur by 1 year of age, 100% appear by the age of 2 years)

Other skin lesions: angiofibromata (>20% are present at 1 year of age, 50% occur by age of 3 years)

Systems Review
Seizures (infantile spasms) 86%; the earlier the onset of seizures the worse the mental retardation

Mental retardation (49%)

PHYSICAL EXAMINATION

Skin 96% incidence of skin lesions

TYPES OF LESIONS
Hypomelanotic macules (present in >80% of patients)—"off-white"; 1 or many, usually more than 3

Papules/nodules on the face (adenoma sebaceum or angiofibromas) (present in 70%)—red and skin-colored, but these appear after infancy (<20% at 1 year of age)

Plaques representing connective tissue nevi ("shagreen" patch) (present in 40%)—skin-colored

Periungual papules or nodules—ungual fibromas present in 22%, arise late in childhood and have the same pathology (angiofibroma) as the facial papules

SHAPE AND SIZE OF WHITE MACULES
Polygonal or "thumbprint," 0.5 to 2.0 cm (Figure 301)

Lance ovate or "ash-leaf" spots (Figure 302), 3.0 to 4.0 cm (1.0 to 12.0 cm)

Tiny white spots or "confetti," 1.0 to 2.0 mm

DISTRIBUTION OF LESIONS
White macules occur on the trunk (56%), lower extremities (32%), upper extremities (7%), head and neck (5%)

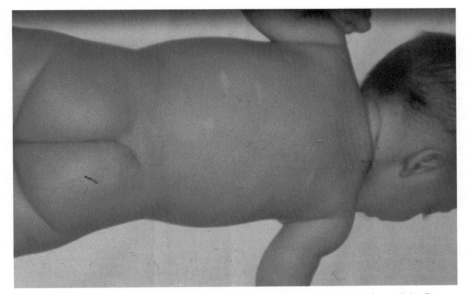

301   Tuberous sclerosis   *White macules in a black child. These are the shape of an ash leaflet or are polygonal and were present at birth.*

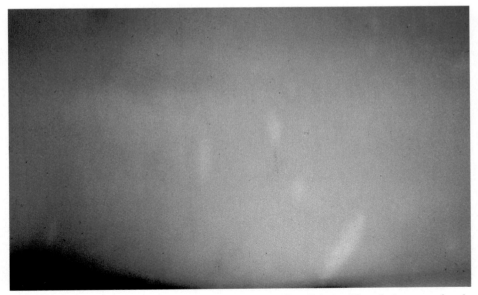

302   Tuberous sclerosis   *White macules viewed with the Wood's lamp. These lesions were barely perceptible in this white child until the skin was examined with the Wood's lamp. There are polygonal (thumb-print) and ash-leaf-shaped macules.*

Angiofibromatous papules and nodules occur on the face (Figure 303*a*) and around the toe- and fingernails

"Shagreen" patches occur on the back or buttocks

Hair Depigmented tufts of hair present at birth

Associated Systems CNS (tumors producing seizures), eye (gray or yellow retinal plaques, 50%), heart (benign rhabdomyomas), hamartomas of mixed-cell type (kidney, liver, thyroid, testes, and GI system)

LABORATORY EXAMINATIONS

Dermatopathology
LIGHT MICROSCOPY *White Macules* Decreased number of melanocytes, decreased melanosome size, decreased melanin in melanocytes and keratinocytes
Angiofibromata Dermal fibrosis, capillary dilatation, absence of elastic tissue
Brain "Tubers" are gliomas.

Special Techniques
DOPA REACTION Decreased melanin formation
TRANSMISSION ELECTRONMICROSCOPY Decreased size and decreased melanin in the melanosomes
ELECTROENCEPHALOGRAPHY Abnormal

IMAGING

Skull X-ray Multiple calcific densities

CT Scan Ventricular deformity and tumor deposits along the striothalamic borders

SPECIAL EXAMINATIONS

Illumination (allow for dark adaptation) Wood's lamp examination should always be used to detect white macules with a decreased melanin pigmentation (Figure 302). This examination is essential for light-skinned persons, as white spots will be detected.

DIAGNOSIS AND DIFFERENTIAL DIAGNOSIS

The diagnosis may be difficult or impossible in an infant or child if white macules are the only cutaneous finding. Dermatologists usually do not have any difficulty in identifying the type of leukoderma that is present in tuberous sclerosis. Nevus depigmentosus may, however, be a confounding lesion, as the white macules in tuberous sclerosis and nevus depigmentosus contain a normal number of melanocytes. Other white macules (in vitiligo and piebaldism) contain few or no melanocytes. The angiofibromata of the face are almost pathognomonic but do not appear until late infancy or, in some patients, until 3 to 4 years of age; for this reason this sign is not as valuable as the white macules which are present early in infancy.

The "shagreen" patch can be confused with a connective tissue nevus.

Even when typical white "ash-leaf" or "thumbprint" macules are present it is necessary to confirm the diagnosis. Confetti spots (Figure 303*b*) are virtually pathognomonic. A pediatric neurologist can then evaluate the patient with a study of the family members and by obtaining various types of imaging as well as electroencephalography. It should be noted that mental retardation and seizures may be absent.

ETIOLOGY AND PATHOGENESIS

Genetic alterations of ectodermal and mesodermal cells with hyperplasia, with a disturbance in embryonic cellular differentiation

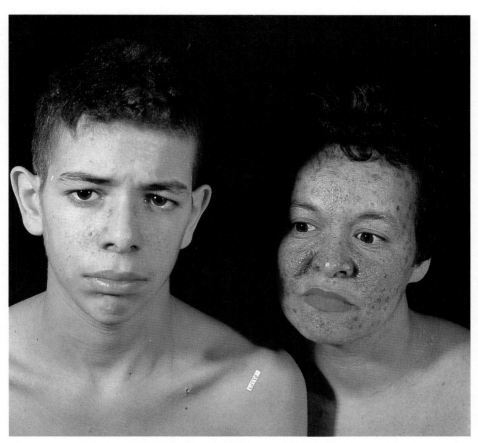

303a Tuberous sclerosis *Mother and son. Angiofibromata on the face, more severe in the mother. These lesions do not appear until approximately age 4.*

SIGNIFICANCE

A serious autosomal disorder that causes major problems: in behavior, because of mental retardation, and in therapy, to control the serious seizure problem present in many patients.

COURSE AND PROGNOSIS

In severe cases, 30% die before the fifth year of life, and 50% to 75% before reaching adult age. Malignant gliomas are not uncommon.

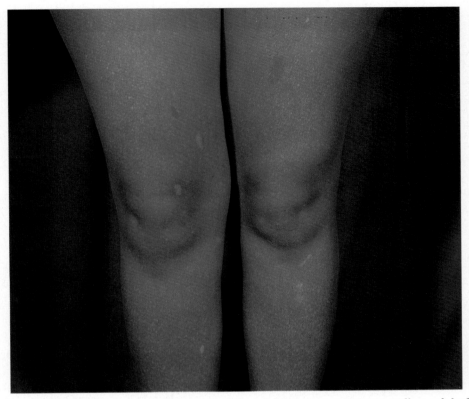

303b Tuberous sclerosis *Myriads of confetti-like hypopigmented macules as well as ash-leaf*
spots are seen on the legs.

TUBEROUS SCLEROSIS

Neurofibromatosis (NF) is an autosomal dominant trait manifested by changes in the skin, nervous system, bones, and endocrine glands. These changes include a variety of congenital abnormalities, tumors, and hamartomas. Two forms of NF are now recognized: (1) classical von Recklinghausen's NF, termed NF1 and first described in 1882, and (2) central, or acoustic, NF, termed NF2. Both types have café-au-lait macules and neurofibromas, but only NF2 has *bilateral* acoustic neuromas (unilateral acoustic neuromas are a variable feature of NF1). An important diagnostic sign present only in NF1 is pigmented hamartomas of the iris (Lisch nodules).

EPIDEMIOLOGY

Incidence   NF1, 1:4,000; NF2, 1:50,000

Race   All races

Sex   Males slightly more than females

Heredity   Autosomal dominant, the gene for NF1 is on chromosome 17 and that for NF2 on chromosome 22.

HISTORY

Duration of Lesions   Café-au-lait (CAL) macules are not usually present at birth but appear during the first three years; neurofibromata appear during late adolescence.

Skin Symptoms   Neurofibromata may be tender to firm; pressure causes pain.

Systems Review   Clinical manifestations in various organs related to pathology: hypertensive headache (pheochromocytomas), pathologic fractures (bone cysts), mental retardation, brain tumor (astrocytoma), short stature, precocious puberty (early menses, clitoral hypertrophy)

PHYSICAL EXAMINATION

Appearance of Patient   Patients not uncommonly consult physician only because of the physical disfigurement.

SKIN   *Type of Lesion*
   CAL macules: Light- or dark-brown *uniform* melanin pigmentation. Lesions vary in size from multiple "frecklelike" tiny macules (Figure 304) <2.0 mm to very large >20 cm brown macules. The common size, however, is 2.0 to 5.0 cm. Tiny frecklelike lesions in the axillae are highly characteristic (Figure 305). A few CAL macules (3 or less) may be present in 10 to 20% of the normal population.
   Nodules: Skin-colored, pink, or brown (Figure 304); pedunculated; soft or firm; "buttonhole sign"—invagination with the tip of the index finger is pathognomonic.

Plexiform neuromas: Drooping, soft, doughy; may be massive involving entire extremity, the head, or a portion of the trunk

Palpation   Nodules are very soft and compressible.

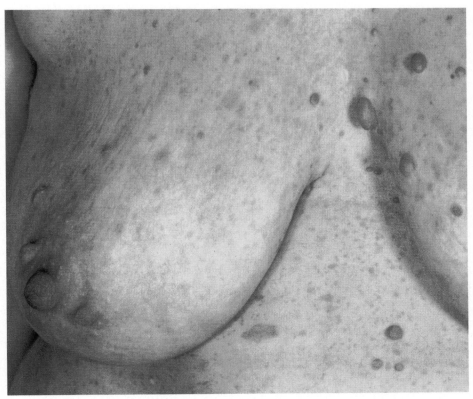

304　Neurofibromatosis (von Recklinghausen's disease)　*On the trunk are many flesh-colored or violaceous papules and nodules. These appeared during late childhood. There are also café-au-lait macules and many frecklelike macules which appeared during infancy.*

Distribution of Lesions Randomly distributed but may be localized to one region (segmental NF1). The segmental type may be heritable or a localized hamartoma; therefore, to do genetic counseling it is necessary to rule out the heritable type by a complete study, including eye examination and family history.

Other Physical Findings

EYE Pigmented hamartomas of the iris (Lisch nodules) begin to appear at age 5 and are present in 20% of children with NF before the age of 6 years; they can be found in 95% of patients after the age of 6 in NF1, but Lisch nodules are not present in NF2. These are visible only with slit lamp examination and appear as "glassy," transparent, dome-shaped, yellow-to-brown papules up to 2.0 mm. They do not correlate with the severity of the disease.

MUSCULOSKELETAL Cervicothoracic kyphoscoliosis, segmental hypertrophy

ADRENAL PHEOCHROMOCYTOMA Elevated blood pressure and episodic flushing

PERIPHERAL NERVOUS SYSTEM Elephantiasis neuromatosa (gross disfigurement from neurofibromatosis of the nerve trunks)

CENTRAL NERVOUS SYSTEM Optic glioma, acoustic neuroma (rare in NF1 and unilateral, bilateral in NF2), astrocytoma, meningioma, neurofibroma

LABORATORY EXAMINATIONS

Dermatopathology More than 10 *melanin macroglobules* per 5 high-power fields in "split" dopa preparations. The melanin macroglobules can also be seen in routine H&E sections. These do not occur in Albright's syndrome.

SPECIAL EXAMINATIONS

Wood's Lamp Examination Skin: in white persons with pale skin, the CAL macules are more easily visualized with Wood's lamp examination.

DIAGNOSIS AND DIFFERENTIAL DIAGNOSIS

Diagnosis Two of the following criteria:

1. Multiple CAL macules, >6 lesions with a diameter of 1.5 cm in adults and >5 lesions or with a diameter of 0.5 cm or more in children younger than 5 years

2. Multiple freckles in the axillary and inguinal regions

3. Based on clinical and histologic grounds, 2 or more neurofibromas of any type, or 1 plexiform neurofibroma

4. Sphenoid wing dysplasia or congenital bowing or thinning of long bone cortex, with or without pseudoarthrosis

5. Bilateral optic nerve gliomas

6. Two or more Lisch nodules on slit lamp examination

7. First-degree relative (parent, sibling, or child) with NF1 by the above criteria

Differential Diagnosis The CAL macules present in Albright's syndrome (polyostotic fibrous dysplasia) are impossible to differentiate clinically from the CAL macules in neurofibromatosis. Other criteria listed above in Diagnosis are required to establish a diagnosis of neurofibromatosis.

ETIOLOGY AND PATHOGENESIS

Action of an abnormal gene on cellular elements derived from the neural crest: melanocytes, Schwann cells, endoneurial fibroblasts

SIGNIFICANCE

It is important to establish the diagnosis in order to do genetic counseling and to follow patients for development of malignancy. Also, neurofibromatosis support groups help with social adjustment in severely affected persons.

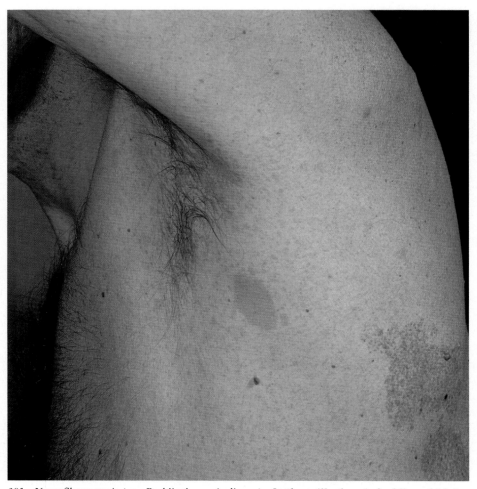

305   Neurofibromatosis (von Recklinghausen's disease)   *In the axilla there is freckling which is a
characteristic feature, almost pathognomonic for this disease. Also on the left side of the
patient there is a large nevus spilus, which is thought by some to be more frequently seen in
von Recklinghausen's neurofibromatosis than in the normal population.*

COURSE AND PROGNOSIS

There is a variable involvement of the organs
affected over time, from only a few pigmented
macules to marked disfigurement with thousands of nodules, segmental hypertrophy, and
plexiform neuromas. The mortality rate is
higher than in the normal population, principally because of the development of neurofi-
brosarcoma during adult life. Serious complications are relatively infrequent.

MANAGEMENT

An orthopedic physician should manage the
two major bone problems: kyphoscoliosis and
tibial bowing. The plastic surgeon can do re-
constructive surgery on the facial assymetry.
The language disorders and learning disabilities should be evaluated by psychologic assessment. Close follow-up annually should be
mandatory to detect sarcomas which may arise
within plexiform neuromas.

Xanthomas

Cutaneous xanthomas are yellow-brown, pinkish, or orange macules (xanthoma striatum), papules (xanthoma papuloeruptivum), plaques (xanthelasma palpebrarum), nodules (xanthoma tuberosum), or infiltrations in tendons (xanthoma tendineum). Xanthomas are histologically characterized by accumulations of xanthoma cells—macrophages containing droplets of lipids. A xanthoma may be a symptom of a general metabolic disease, a generalized histiocytosis, or a local cell dysfunction. The following classification is based on this principle: (1) xanthomas due to hyperlipoproteinemia (hyperlipidemia) and (2) normolipoproteinemic xanthomas. Of the latter group only the normolipoproteinemic xanthelasmata of the eyelids are common enough to be discussed in this book. Although the hyperlipoproteinemic xanthomas are relatively rare, they are important for two reasons: (1) they may be the first symptom of a serious metabolic disease; (2) they may be regarded as an experiment of nature which may enable us to study the pathogenesis of atherosclerotic disease.

The causes of hyperlipoproteinemia may be divided into primary, in most cases genetically determined, and secondary, those caused by severe hyperthyroidism, biliary cirrhosis, grossly deranged diabetes, and a number of still rarer conditions.

In 1972 Fredrickson and Lees considerably furthered the study of hyperlipoproteinemias by dividing them into five phenotypes, depending upon the distribution of the lipoprotein classes. Lipids, which are insoluble in water, are transported in the blood and bound in various proportions to proteins, resulting in so-called lipoproteins (see Table A).

From Table A it can be calculated that a hypercholesterolemia may be caused by an excess of LDL as well as by an excess of VLDL. However, in the first case the triglycerides are normal; in the second case cholesterol *and* triglycerides are elevated. It is important to recognize this because a hypercholesterolemia caused by LDL has more serious consequences than one caused by VLDL.

APOPROTEINS

The lipids, which are insoluble in water, are coated with proteins which have three functions: (1) causing water solubility, (2) fixing lipoproteins to cellular receptors, (3) exercising enzymatic activity.

The sources of the lipids and apoproteins are the gut and the liver. Lipids and apoproteins interact in two cascades: one originates from the chylomicrons from the gut and the other from the VLDL synthesized in the liver. The principal apoprotein of the chylomicrons is apoprotein $\beta48$, of the VLDL the apoproteins B100, E, and C11. During the transformation of VLDL via IDL (floating β, VLDL remnant) to LDL, apoproteins E and C11 are lost.

In the past decade it has been recognized that Fredrickson's phenotypes are symptoms of genetic metabolic diseases with distinct and different pathogeneses (Tables B and C).

GENETIC, METABOLIC, ENDOCRINE, AND NUTRITIONAL DISEASES

Table A Common Abnormal Lipoprotein Patterns in Hyperlipoproteinemia

TYPE	LIPOPROTEIN ABNORMALITIES	APPEARANCE OF PLASMA*	USUAL CHANGES IN LIPID CONCENTRATIONS
I	Massive chylomicronemia VLDL normal, LDL, HDL normal or decreased	Cream layer on top, clear below	C normal, TG ↑ ↑
II^a	LDL increased, VLDL normal	Clear	C ↑ , TG normal
II^b	LDL increased, VLDL increased	May be slightly turbid	C ↑ , TG ↑
III	Presence of β-VLDL	Usually turbid, often with faint cream layer	C ↑ , TG ↑ ↑
IV	VLDL increased	Usually turbid no cream layer	C normal, TG ↑ ↑
V	Chylomicrons present, VLDL increased	Cream layer on top, turbid below	C ↑ , TG ↑ ↑

*After standing at 4°C for 18 hours or more.

Note: VLDL = very low-density pre-β-lipoproteins; LDL = low-density (beta) lipoproteins; HDL = high-density (alpha) lipoproteins; C = cholesterol; TG = triglycerides; β-VLDL = IDL = inter-mediate-density lipoproteins, floating β.

Source: Modified from Fredrickson DS: Plasma lipid abnormalities and cutaneous and subcutaneous xanthomas, in *Dermatology in General Medicine,* 2nd ed. Edited by TB Fitzpatrick et al. New York, McGraw-Hill, 1979, p 1120

Table B Classification of Genetic Lipoprotein Disturbances

1. Familial hypercholesterolemia (FH): type II^a
2. Familial dyslipoproteinemia (FD): type III
3. Familial combined hyperlipoproteinemia (FCL): types 11$^{a\ or\ b}$, or IV
4. Familial hypertriglyceridemia (FHT): type IV/V
5. Familial lipoproteinlipase deficiency (FLD) (very rare): type I

Table C Relation of the Type of Xanthomatosis to the Various Phenotypes of Lipoprotein Disturbance and Their Nosologic Cause

Xanthelasma palpebrarum	Normolipemic or FH, FD
Xanthoma tendineum	FH (type II^a)
Xanthoma tuberosum	FD, FHT, FH (if homozygous) (types III, IV, II^a)
Xanthoma papuloeruptivum	FD, FHT, FLD (types II, IV/V, I)
Xanthochromia and xanthoma striatum palmare	FD (type III)

Xanthelasma palpebrarum *may* or *may not* be associated with hyperlipoproteinemia.

EPIDEMIOLOGY AND ETIOLOGY

Age Over 50 years; when in children or young adults, it is associated with FH or FD.

Sex Either

Incidence Most common of all xanthomas

Significance May be an isolated finding unrelated to hyperlipoproteinemia, but sometimes there is an elevation of LDL. When the LDL is markedly elevated, it is a sign of FH or FD.

HISTORY

Duration of Lesions Months, with slow enlargement from tiny spot

Skin Symptoms None

PHYSICAL EXAMINATION

Skin Lesions (Figure 306)
TYPE Plaques, soft
COLOR Yellow-orange
SHAPE Polygonal
DISTRIBUTION Localized to eyelids

DIFFERENTIAL DIAGNOSIS

Quite typical but early lesions can be confused with milia, conglomerates of senile closed comedones, or syringomata, and biopsy may be necessary in small lesions.

LABORATORY EXAMINATION

Cholesterol estimation in plasma, if enhanced screening for type of hyperlipoproteinemia.

PROGNOSIS

If due to hyperlipoproteinemia, complication with atherosclerotic cardiovascular disease may be expected.

TREATMENT

Excision or applications of trichloroacetic acid are the treatments of choice; however, recurrences are not uncommon.

SIGNIFICANCE

In a larger proportion of the patients with xanthelasmata palpebralia no metabolic disturbances are found. In others, xanthelasmata palpebralia are a sign of familial hyperlipoproteinemia FH or FD. When total lipids and total cholesterol content of the serum are within normal limits, no further lipid analysis is necessary.

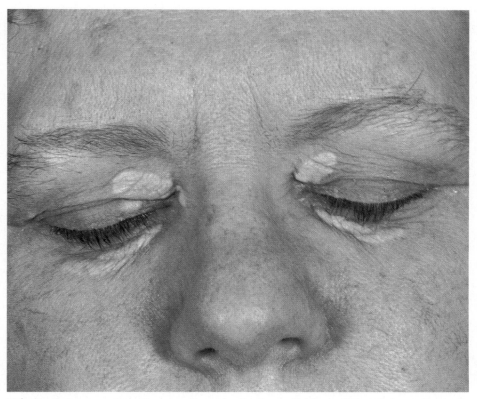

306 Xanthelasmata palpebralia (normolipemic) *On the medial part of the inferior and superior eyelids there are longitudinal, yellowish-brown, slightly elevated infiltrations. This was the sole site of xanthomata on this patient.*

Xanthoma Tendineum

Xanthomata tendinea are yellow or skin-colored subcutaneous tumors that move with the extensor tendons (Figure 307). They are a symptom of familial hypercholesterolemia (FH) which presents as a type 11^a hyperlipoproteinemia. This condition is autosomal recessive, with a different phenotype in the heterozygote and homozygote. In the heterozygote the xanthomata appear in adult life as do the cardiovascular complications. In the homozygote the xanthomata appear in early childhood, the cardiovascular complications in early adolescence; the elevation of the LDL content of the plasma is extreme. These patients rarely attain ages above 20 years.

FH is caused by a defect in the LDL receptors on the cell membrane localized in the coated pits on this membrane. This defect is partial in the heterozygotes, total in the homozygotes. Due to this defect the cholesterol-rich LDL is insufficiently cleared from the blood, which again results in an insufficient checking of the endocellular cholesterol synthesis. Recent investigations have shown that different deletions on the DNA cause different defects in the LDL receptors.

TREATMENT

A diet low in cholesterol and saturated fats is necessary but insufficient. This should be supplemented with a bile acid sequestrant, cholestyramine, and an HMG CoA reductase inhibitor (simvastine, pravastine). In this way the production of LDL receptors is stimulated. This stimulation is impossible in homozygous patients, due to the total absence of LDL receptors. Here heroic measures such as portacaval shunt or liver transplantation have to be considered.

Xanthoma Tuberosum

This comprises yellowish nodules located especially on the elbows (Figure 308) and knees originating by confluence of concomitant eruptive xanthomata. They are to be found in patients with FD, FHT, and FLD. In homozygous patients with FH the tuberous xanthomata are flatter and skin-colored. They are not accompanied by eruptive xanthomata.

TREATMENT

Of the underlying condition.

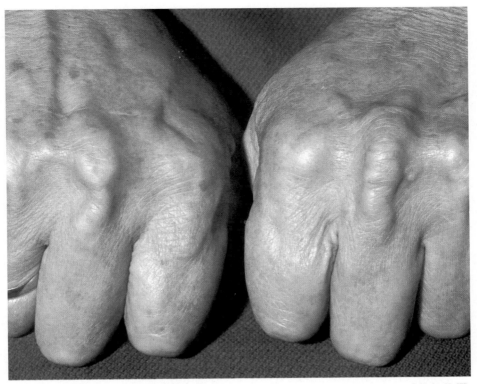

307 Xanthomata tendinae in hyperlipoproteinemia, type II^a   *On the extensor tendons of digits II, III, and IV there are subcutaneous tumors, varying from round to longitudinal.*

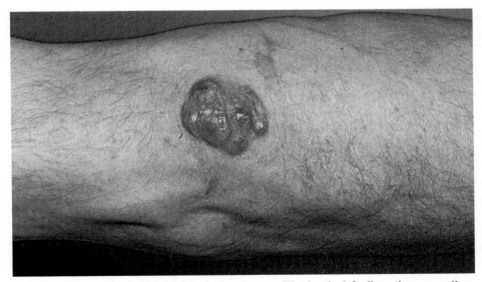

308 Xanthomata tuberosa in hyperlipoproteinemia, type III   *On the left elbow there are yellow-violet tumors, 3.0 cm in diameter. There was no arterial sclerotic arteriovascular disease.*

Xanthoma Papuloeruptivum (Eruptive Xanthoma)

These discrete inflammatory-type papules "erupt" suddenly and in showers, appearing typically on the buttocks.

ETIOLOGY

A sign of FHT, FD, and the very rare FLD (exogenous hyperchylomicronemia) and a diabetes out of control

HISTORY

Lesions appear suddenly.

PHYSICAL EXAMINATION

Skin Lesions

TYPE

Papules, discrete

Nodules represent confluent papules

COLOR   Yellow center with red halo

SHAPE   Dome-shaped

ARRANGEMENT

Scattered discrete lesions in a localized region (e.g., buttocks) (Figure 309)

"Tight" clusters may become confluent to form "tuberoeruptive" xanthomata

DISTRIBUTION

Papules: buttocks, elbows, knees, back, or anywhere

"Tuberoeruptive" lesions: elbows

TREATMENT

React very favorably on a low-caloric and low-fat diet

Xanthoma Striatum Palmare

Xanthoma striatum palmare presents as yellow-orange, flat or elevated infiltrations of the volar creases of palms and fingers. This is highly characteristic for FD. FD is characterized by a type III phenotype of lipoprotein disturbance due to the presence of chylomicron- and VLD-remnants in the plasma (IDL, β-VLDL, with an enhanced ratio of cholesterol/triglycerides). These particles are present in the plasma due to defective binding in the liver. The deficient binding is caused by an hereditary abnormality in the E apoprotein, which is responsible for the binding of the VLDL remnants in the liver. Investigation on the molecular-genetic level has shown a variation in alleles causing different types of apoprotein E patterns.

Next to the highly characteristic xanthomata striata palmare (Figure 310), FD also presents with tuberous xanthoma (page 592), eruptive xanthoma, and xanthelasma palpebrarum (page 590).

Patients with FD are prone to atherosclerotic cardiovascular disease, especially ischemia of the arteries of the legs and coronary vessels.

TREATMENT

Patients with FD react very favorably to a diet low in fats and carbohydrates. If necessary this may be supplemented with clofibrate, an aryloxylid derivative, which inhibits the VLDL synthesis in the liver.

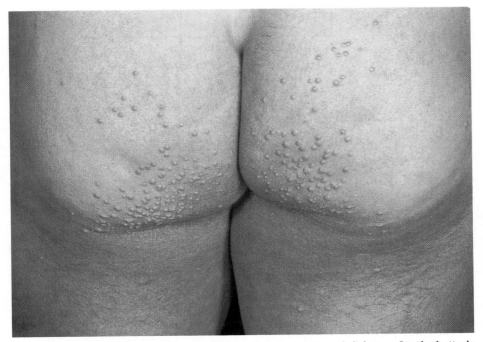

309 Xanthomata papuloeruptiva in type IV hyperlipoproteinemia and diabetes *On the buttocks there are disseminated, discrete, yellow papules, 1.0 to 3.0 mm in diameter. There are similar papules on the arms and trunk.*

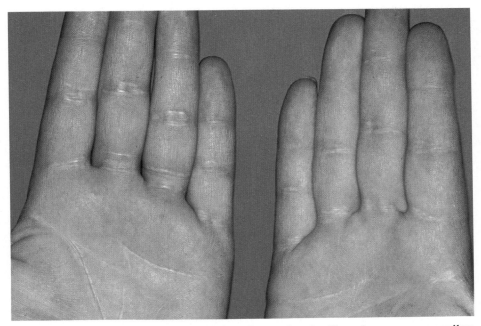

310 Xanthomata striata palmaria in type III hyperlipoproteinemia *The palmar creases are yellow and there are yellow streaks in the metacarpophalangeal and interphalangeal joints. There was no arteriosclerotic cardiovascular disease.*

Drug Reactions

Drug Eruptions Due to Hypersensitivity Mechanisms

Drug eruptions can mimic virtually all the morphologic expressions in dermatology and must be first on the differential diagnosis in the appearance of a sudden symmetrical eruption.

Drug eruptions are caused by immunologic or nonimmunologic mechanisms and are provoked by systemic or topical administration of a drug. The majority are based on a hypersensitivity mechanism and may be of types I, II, III, or IV. The nonimmunologic drug eruptions are caused by (1) idiosyncrasy *sensu strictirori*—reactions due to hereditary enzyme deficiencies; (2) cumulation, such as melanosis due to gold or amiodarone; (3) irritancy of a topically applied drug; (4) an individual idiosyncrasy to a topical or systemic drug; (5) mechanisms not yet known; and (6) reactions due to the combination of a drug with ultraviolet irradiation (photosensitivity). All may have toxic (T) or immunologic (allergic) (A) pathology.

Photosensitivity after systemic administration

Phenothiazines	A + T
Chlorpromazine	
Promethazine	
Sulfanilamides	A + T
Oral antidiabetics	
Sulfanilureum derivatives	
Demethylchlortetracycline	T
Doxycycline	T
Other tetracyclines more rarely	
Nalidixic acid	T
Amino hydrochloride	T

Photosensitivity after topical application

Phenothiazines	A + T
Sulfonamides	A + T
A number of halogenated salicylanilides	A
Bithionol	A
Psoralens	T
Musk ambrette	A

EPIDEMIOLOGY AND ETIOLOGY

Age Occur at any age

Sex More common in females

Incidence Reactions in the skin are the most common manifestations of drug sensitivity; affect 3.0% of hospitalized patients in the United States—about half are minor

Most Frequent Types

EXANTHEMATOUS (See Figures 311 and 312) Penicillin, ampicillin, barbiturates, phenylbutazone, gold, quinidine, sulfonamides, allopurinol, phenytoin

URTICARIA (See page 452) Penicillins, salicylates, erythromycin, carbamazepine

PHOTOSENSITIVITY (See pages 226 and 228) Sulfonamide diuretics and antidiabetics, phenothiazines, nalidixic acid, tetracycline, demethylchlortetracycline, vinblastine, carbamazepine, nonsteroidal anti-inflammatory agents

FIXED DRUG (See Figure 313) Phenolphthalein, barbiturates, phenacetin, sulfonamides, tetracycline, griseofulvin, food dyes

PURPURA (NONTHROMBOCYTOPENIC) Thiazides, carbromal, type II (cytotoxic) reactions

BULLOUS Barbiturates, iodides, sulfonamides, penicillin

SERUM SICKNESS Penicillin, salicylates, sulfonamides, barbiturates

ERYTHEMA MULTIFORME SYNDROME (See page 474) Sulfonamides, phenytoin, barbiturates, phenylbutazone, penicillin carbamazepine

OTHER LESS FREQUENT TYPES Acneform, toxic epidermal necrolysis, necrotizing vasculitis, erythema nodosum, lichenoid

HISTORY

Duration of Lesions Usually appear within first week except in reactions due to ampicillin and other semisynthetic penicillins, when eruptions may be delayed. In patients with fixed drug reaction, lesions recur at the identical site whenever drug is readministered.

Skin Symptoms Pruritus—mild, severe, or absent. Pain at sites of erosions

PHYSICAL EXAMINATION

Skin Lesions

TYPE

Maculopapular (morbilliform or scarlatiniform)

Urticarial wheal

Vesicular and bullous

Purpuric macules or papules (vasculitis)

COLOR *Exanthematous Eruptions* Bright "drug" red

Fixed Drug Eruptions Dusky red or violaceous, often bullous

SHAPE Round, oval, polycyclic, annular, iris-shaped

ARRANGEMENT Scattered discrete lesions

DISTRIBUTION Isolated single lesion (fixed drug) or generalized, sun-exposed areas

SITES OF PREDILECTION *Fixed Drug* Legs, hands, glans penis, oral mucosa, vulva

Exanthematous Trunk, may be generalized

Urticaria Generalized, hands and feet, lips, eyelids

Mucous Membranes Commonly involved in erythema multiforme major and fixed reactions

DIAGNOSIS

Detailed history with list of all medications taken by mouth or by injection, and proprietary preparations for headache, sleep, cold, constipation, pain, etc.

No laboratory tests are available at present that can establish the diagnosis; RAST correlates well with skin-test reactivity in penicillin-sensitive patients

COURSE

Progression may continue for a while, but in most cases the eruption disappears within days after the offending drug is stopped.

TREATMENT

Systemic corticosteroids are frequently used for severe reactions, although their efficacy has not been proved.

Antihistamines are helpful in some urticarial drug eruptions

An exanthematous drug eruption is an adverse hypersensitivity reaction to an ingested or parenterally administered drug, characterized by a cutaneous eruption which mimics a measleslike viral exanthem.

Synonyms: morbilliform drug eruption, maculopapular eruption.

EPIDEMIOLOGY AND ETIOLOGY

Incidence Most common type of cutaneous drug reaction

Age Less common in very young

Etiology *Drugs with high probability of reaction* (3 to 5%): penicillin and related antibiotics, carbamazepine, allopurinol, gold salts (10 to 20%). *Medium probability:* sulfonamides (bacteriostatic, antidiabetic, diuretic), nitrofurantoin, hydantoin derivatives, isoniazid, chloramphenicol, erythromycin, streptomycin. *Low probability* (1% or less): pyrazolon derivatives, barbiturates, benzodiazepines, phenothiazines, tetracyclines

HISTORY

Mononucleosis Up to 100% of patients with Epstein-Barr or cytomegalovirus mononucleosis syndrome given ampicillin or amoxicillin develop an exanthematous drug eruption.

HIV Infection 50 to 60% of HIV-infected patients who receive sulfa drugs (i.e., trimethoprim-sulfamethoxazole) develop eruption.

Drug History Increased incidence of reactions in patients on allopurinol given ampicillin/amoxicillin.

Prior Drug Sensitization Patients with prior history of exanthematous drug eruption will most likely develop a similar reaction if rechallenged with same drug. 10% of patients sensitive to penicillins given cephalosporins will exhibit cross-drug sensitivity and develop eruption. Patients sensitized to one sulfa-base drug (bacteriostatic, antidiabetic, diuretic) may cross-react with another category of the drug.

Onset *Early reaction:* In a previously sensitized patient, eruption starts within 2 or 3 days of administration of drug. *Late reaction:* Sensitization occurs during administration or after completing course of drug; peak incidence at ninth day after administration. However, drug eruption may occur at any time between the first day and 3 weeks after the beginning of treatment. Reaction to penicillin can begin 2 or more weeks after drug discontinued.

Systems Review ±Fever. Usually quite pruritic

PHYSICAL EXAMINATION

Vital Signs ±Elevated temperature

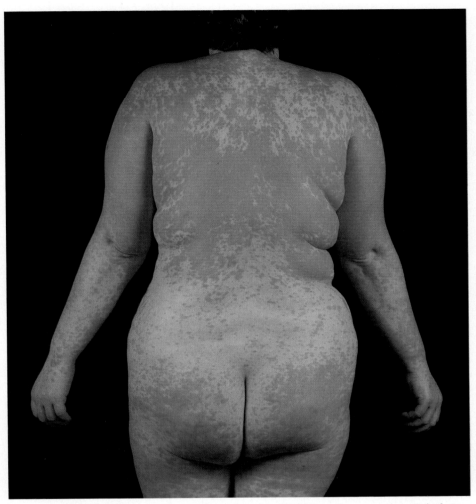

311 Exanthematous drug eruption *On the trunk and extremities can be seen a symmetrical, morbilliform, erythematous eruption. Some of the lesions have become confluent. This eruption was caused by ampicillin.*

Skin Findings

TYPE OF LESION Macules and/or papules, few mm to 1 cm in size (Figure 311). Purpura may be seen in lesions of lower legs. May progress to generalized exfoliative dermatitis, especially if drug not discontinued. Scaling and/or desquamation may occur with healing.

COLOR Bright or *"drug" red*. Resolving lesions have hues of tan and purple.

ARRANGEMENT OF MULTIPLE LESIONS Macules and papules frequently become confluent.

DISTRIBUTION OF LESIONS Symmetrical (Figure 312). Almost always on trunk and extremities. Confluent lesions in intertriginous areas, i.e., axilla, groin, inframammary area. Palms and soles variably involved. In children, may be limited to face and extremities. Eruption may be accentuated in striae. May spare face, nipple, periareolar area, surgical scar.

MUCOUS MEMBRANES ±Enathem on buccal mucosa

General Examination Findings associated with indication for drug administration

DIAGNOSIS AND DIFFERENTIAL DIAGNOSIS

Diagnosis Clinical diagnosis

Differential Diagnosis Viral exanthem, secondary syphilis, atypical pityriasis rosea

LABORATORY AND SPECIAL EXAMINATIONS

Dermatopathology Perivascular lymphocytes and eosinophils

PATHOPHYSIOLOGY

Exact mechanism unknown. Probably delayed hypersensitivity

COURSE AND PROGNOSIS

Eruption fades when drug discontinued. Occasionally fades even though drug is continued. Eruption usually recurs with rechallenge, although not always.

TREATMENT

Discontinue implicated drug. Symptomatic treatment; oral antihistamine to alleviate pruritus.

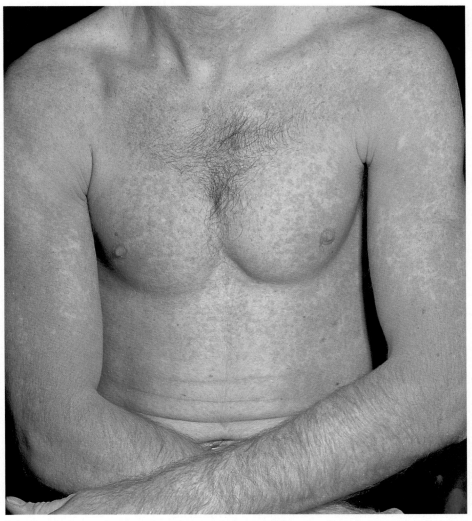

312　Exanthematous drug eruption　*Symmetrical, morbilliform, erythematous eruption. Some of the lesions have become confluent. This eruption was caused by phenytoin.*

Fixed Drug Eruption

A fixed drug eruption (FDE) is an adverse cutaneous reaction to an ingested drug, characterized by the formation of a solitary, but at times multiple, plaque, bulla, or erosion; if the patient is rechallenged with the offending drug, the FDE occurs repeatedly at the identical skin site (i.e., fixed) within hours of ingestion.

ETIOLOGY AND EPIDEMIOLOGY

Etiology The drugs most commonly reported to cause FDE include: barbiturates, phenacetin, pyrazolon derivatives (i.e., phenylbutazone), phenolphthalein, sulfonamides, tetracyclines. The list of drugs causing FDE uncommonly includes many commonly used medications.

HISTORY

Skin Symptoms Usually asymptomatic. May be pruritic or burning. Painful when eroded. Patients give a history of an identical lesion occurring at the identical location. FDE may be associated with a headache for which the patient takes a barbiturate-containing analgesic, with constipation for which the patient takes a phenolphthalein-containing laxative, or with a cold for which the patient takes an over-the-counter medication containing a yellow dye. The offending "drug" in food dye-induced FDE may be difficult to identify, i.e., yellow dye in Galliano liqueur or phenolphthalein in maraschino cherries or quinine in tonic water. Patients note a residual area of postinflammatory hyperpigmentation between episodes.

PHYSICAL EXAMINATION

Skin Findings
TYPE   The characteristic early lesion is a sharply demarcated erythema, round or oval in shape, occurring within hours after ingestion of the offending drug. Most commonly, lesions are solitary (Figure 313) but may be multiple. Size varies from a few millimeters up to 10 to 20 cm in diameter. Frequently, the edematous plaque evolves to become a bulla and then an erosion.

COLOR   Initially erythema, then dusky-red to violaceous (Figure 313). After healing, dark brown with violet hue postinflammatory hyperpigmentation.

PALPATION   Eroded lesions, especially on genital or oral mucosa, are quite painful.

ARRANGEMENT   When multiple, random.

DISTRIBUTION   The genital skin is the most commonly involved site.

Mucous Membranes FDE may occur within the mouth or on the conjunctiva.

DIAGNOSIS AND DIFFERENTIAL DIAGNOSIS

Diagnosis Made on clinical grounds. Readministration of the drug is helpful but should be avoided. Sometimes a patch test with the drug at the site of the lesion is positive.

Differential Diagnosis *Solitary FDE:* recurrent herpetic lesions. *Multiple FDEs:* erythema multiforme, toxic epidermal necrolysis. *Oral mucosal FDE:* aphthous stomatitis, primary herpetic gingivostomatitis, erythema multiforme.

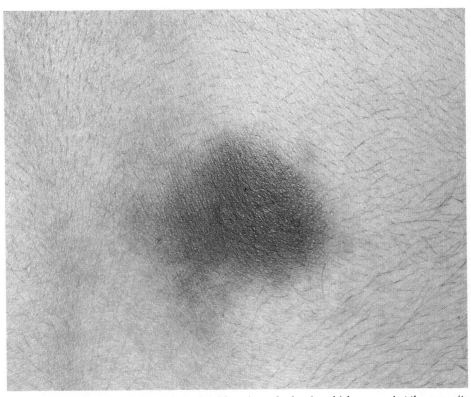

313 Fixed drug eruption *A violet macule with an irregular border which occurred at the same site at irregular intervals for 5 months. The patient was taking an antipyrine-containing analgesic.*

LABORATORY AND SPECIAL EXAMINATIONS

Dermatopathology Similar to findings in erythema multiforme: dyskeratosis, basal vacuolization, dermal edema, perivascular and interstitial lymphohistiocytic infiltrate, at times with eosinophils. Subepidermal vesicles and bullae with overlying epidermal necrosis. Between outbreaks, the site of FDE shows marked pigmentary incontinence with melanin in macrophages in upper dermis.

PATHOGENESIS

Unknown

COURSE AND PROGNOSIS

FDE resolves within a few weeks of withdrawing the drug. Recurs within hours following ingestion of a single dose of the drug.

TREATMENT

Identify and withhold the offending drug. Symptomatic treatment of lesion(s).

FIXED DRUG ERUPTION

Skin necrosis from warfarin is a rare reaction usually occurring between the third and tenth day of anticoagulation therapy with the warfarin derivatives, manifested by sharply demarcated, purpuric cutaneous infarction.

EPIDEMIOLOGY AND ETIOLOGY

Incidence Rare

Age Middle-aged to elderly

Sex Females > males

Etiology Idiosyncratic reaction. If warfarin inadvertently readministered, reaction recurs.

HISTORY

Lag Time Reaction appears within 3 to 10 days of initiation of warfarin therapy

Systems Review Indications for warfarin use: history of venous thrombosis, atrial fibrillation ± embolization, prophylaxis and treatment of pulmonary embolism

PHYSICAL EXAMINATION

Skin Findings
TYPE OF LESION Large painful erythematous plaque(s). Quickly evolve to well-demarcated, deep-purple-to-black, geographic areas of necrosis (Figure 314). Hemorrhagic bullae, large erosions may complicate infarcts. Later, deep tissue sloughing (Figure 315) and ulceration if lesions are not debrided and grafted.
COLOR Initial deep erythema; violaceous infarcted plaque
PALPATION Lesions are quite tender and painful

SHAPE OF INDIVIDUAL LESION Usually geographic
ARRANGEMENT OF MULTIPLE LESIONS Often single. Many present as two lesions, one on either breast
DISTRIBUTION OF LESIONS Areas of abundant subcutaneous fat: breasts, buttocks, abdomen, thighs, calves

General Examination Findings for indications for warfarin administration. Otherwise, unremarkable

DIAGNOSIS AND DIFFERENTIAL DIAGNOSIS

Diagnosis Clinical diagnosis

Differential Diagnosis Differentiate from heparin necrosis, which occurs at site of subcutaneous heparin injection. Hematoma in overly anticoagulated patient, synergistic gangrene (Meleney's ulcer)

LABORATORY AND SPECIAL EXAMINATIONS

Dermatopathology Epidermal necrosis, thrombosis and occlusion of most blood vessels, scanty inflammatory response

Coagulation Studies Usually within normal limits; may be associated with hereditary or acquired protein C deficiency.

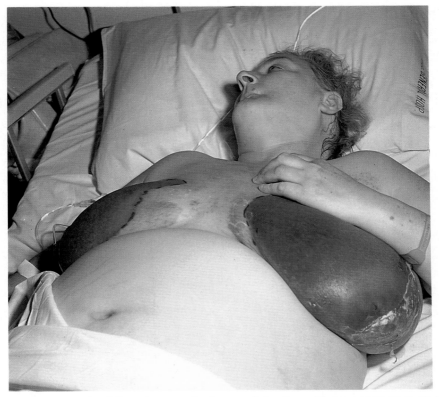

314　Warfarin necrosis　*Bilateral areas of cutaneous infarction with pigmented areas on the breasts surrounded by an area of erythema. The patient had been taking warfarin for 5 days when the lesions appeared.*

PATHOPHYSIOLOGY

Pathogenesis of thrombus formation in vessels of dermis and subcutaneous fat is unknown.

TREATMENT

Treat as a third degree thermal burn. Early debridement and grafting.

COURSE AND PROGNOSIS

If area of necrosis is large in an elderly debilitated patient, may be life-threatening.

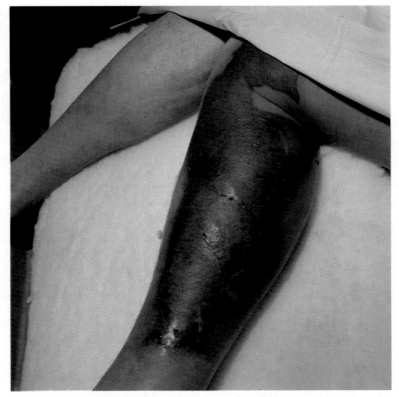

315   Warfarin necrosis   *Large demarcated area of cutaneous infarction with epidermal sloughing. The patient had thrombophlebitis and was on warfarin for 8 days.*

Photosensitivity in Systemic Disease*

Porphyria Cutanea Tarda

Porphyria cutanea tarda (PCT), as the name implies, occurs mostly in adults rather than children. *Patients do not present with photosensitivity* but with complaints of "fragile skin," vesicles, and bullae, particularly on the dorsa of the hands, especially following minor trauma; the diagnosis is confirmed by the presence of an orange-red fluorescence in the urine when examined with Wood's lamp. PCT is distinct from variegate porphyria (VP) and acute intermittent porphyria (AIP) in that patients with PCT do not have acute life-threatening attacks (abdominal pain, peripheral autonomic neuropathy, and respiratory failure). Furthermore the drugs that induce PCT (ethanol, estrogens, and chloroquine) are fewer than the drugs that induce VP and AIP (see "Variegate Porphyria," on page 616).

EPIDEMIOLOGY AND ETIOLOGY

Age 30 to 50 years, rarely in children; females on oral contraceptives (18 to 30 years of age), males on estrogen therapy for prostate cancer (>60 years of age)

Sex Equal in males and females

Heredity Most PCT patients have so-called *PCT-symptomatic* (not hereditary) induced by drugs, especially alcohol, or chemicals (e.g., hexachlorobenzene fungicide). PCT-hereditary—possibly these patients actually have VP, but this is not yet resolved.

Chemicals and Drugs that Induce PCT Ethanol, estrogens, hexachlorobenzene (fungicide), chlorinated phenols, iron, tetrachlorodibenzo-*p*-dioxin. High doses of chloroquine may lead to clinical manifestations in "latent" cases (low doses are used as treatment).

Other Predisposing Factors Diabetes mellitus (25%)

HISTORY

Duration of Lesions No acute skin changes but gradual onset, and patients may present with bullae on the hands and feet and have a suntan in midsummer!

Symptoms Pain from erosions in easily traumatized skin ("fragile skin")

Systems Review In VP there is autonomic neuropathy with acute abdominal pain and peripheral neuropathy. In erythropoietic protoporphyria and PCT there can be hepatic disease. Associated diseases may lead to multisystem alterations (see Differential Diagnosis).

*See also Section 12.

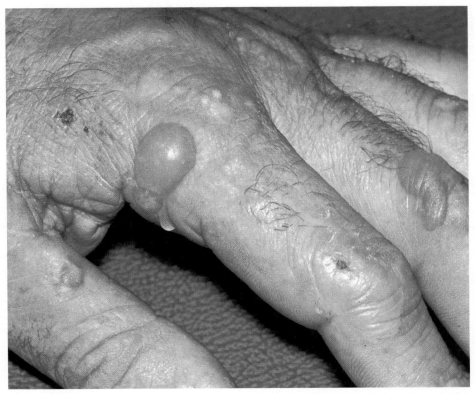

316　Porphyria cutanea tarda　*On the extensor surfaces of both hands, predominantly on the fingers, there are bullae with clear fluid. There are also collapsed bullae on the thumb, and on the second metacarpophalangeal joint are two small white papules of hard consistency (milia). On the index finger there is a pink atrophic scar.*

Classification of Porphyria

	ERYTHROPOIETIC PORPHYRIAS		HEPATIC PORPHYRIAS		
	CONGENITAL ERYTHROPOIETIC PORPHYRIA	ERYTHROPOIETIC PROTOPORPHYRIA	PORPHYRIA CUTANEA TARDA	VARIEGATE PORPHYRIA	INTERMITTENT ACUTE PORPHYRIA
Inheritance	Autosomal recessive	Autosomal dominant	Autosomal dominant (familial form)	Autosomal dominant	Autosomal dominant
Signs and symptoms:					
Photosensitive cutaneous lesions	Yes	Yes	Yes	Yes	No
Attacks of abdominal pain, neuropsychiatric syndrome	No	No	No	Yes	Yes
Laboratory abnormalities:					
Red blood cells:					
Uroporphyrin	+++	N	N	N	N
Coproporphyrin	++	+	N	N	N
Protoporphyrin	(+)	+++	N	N	N
Urine:					
Porphobillinogen	N	N	N	(+++)	(+++)
Uroporphyrin	+++	N	+++	+	++
Feces:					
Protoporphyrin	+	++	N	+++	N

N, normal; +, above normal; ++, moderately increased; +++, markedly increased; (+++), frequently increased; (+), increased in some patients

PHYSICAL EXAMINATION

Skin Lesions

TYPE

Bullae: tense bullae on normal-appearing skin (Figure 316)

Erosions: in the sites of the vesicles and bullae, erosions slowly heal to form pink atrophic scars at sites of erosions

Milia (Figure 316), 1.0 to 5.0 mm

Hypertrichosis (may be the presenting complaint)

Scleroderma-like induration (Figure 317)

Purple-red suffusion ("heliotrope") of central facial skin (Figure 318), especially periorbital areas

Brown hypermelanosis, diffuse, on exposed areas (uncommon)

PHOTOSENSITIVITY IN SYSTEMIC DISEASE

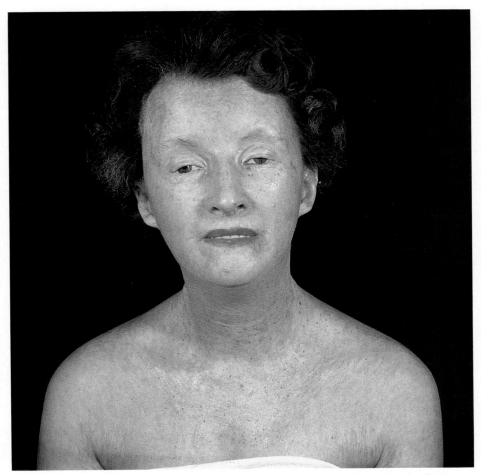

317 Porphyria cutanea tarda   *Well-demarcated, shiny, sclerodermoid plaques on the chest.*

DISTRIBUTION (See Figure XV)

Dorsa of hands (Figure 316) and feet (toes), nose (vesicles, bullae, and erosions)

Scleroderma-like changes (Figure 317), diffuse or circumscribed, waxy yellowish-white areas on exposed areas of face, neck, and trunk, sparing the doubly clothed area of the breast in females

Hypertrichosis: dark-brown or black hair on the temples and cheeks and, in severe disease, on the trunk and extremities

DIFFERENTIAL DIAGNOSIS

"Pseudo-PCT" Drugs (sulfonamides, nalidixic acid, furosemide, naproxen, tetracycline) and hemodialysis combine to form a distinctive syndrome with blisters and erosions indistinguishable from PCT; only the absence of the defect in porphyrin metabolism excludes PCT. *Epidermolysis bullosa acquisita,* which has the same clinical picture (increased skin fragility, easy bruising, and light-provoked bullae) and some of the histology (subepidermal bullae with little or no dermal inflammation).

Variegate porphyria (VP) See page 616.

Conditions associated with PCT-like syndromes Hepatoma, SLE, hemodialysis for renal failure, sarcoidosis, Sjögren's syndrome. May occasionally resemble dyshidrotic eczema

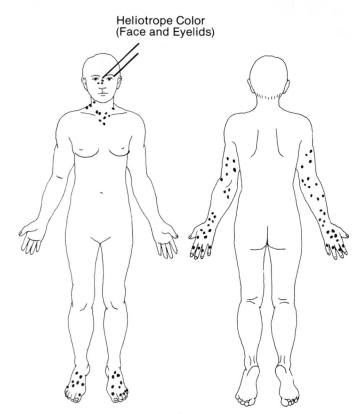

Heliotrope Color
(Face and Eyelids)

Figure XV   Porphyria cutanea tarda

PHOTOSENSITIVITY IN SYSTEMIC DISEASE

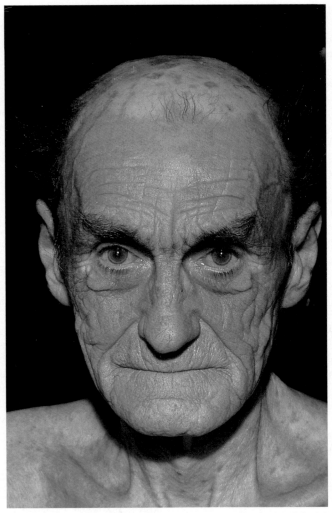

318   Porphyria cutanea tarda   *Purple-red suffusion ("heliotrope") of central facial skin, most pronounced in the periorbital areas; hypermelanosis in sun-exposed areas.*

LABORATORY EXAMINATION

Dermatopathology

SITE   Epidermis and papillary dermis, blood vessels

PROCESS   Bullae, subepidermal with "festooned" (undulating base). PAS reveals thickened vascular walls.

IMMUNOFLUORESCENCE   IgG and other immunoglobulins at the dermoepidermal junction and in and around blood vessels, in the sun-exposed areas of the skin. Thickening of vessel walls is due to multiple reduplications of vascular basement membrane and deposits of immunoglobulins and fibrin.

CELLS   Paucity of an inflammatory infiltrate

LABORATORY EXAMINATIONS OF BLOOD, STOOL, AND URINE

Blood Chemistry

Increased plasma iron (33 to 50%) (there is increased hepatic iron in Kupffer cells and hepatocytes)

Blood glucose increased in those patients with diabetes mellitus (25% of patients)

Porphyrin Studies in PCT

Increased uroporphyrin (I isomer, 60%) in urine and plasma

Increased isocoproporphyrin (type III) and 7-carboxylporphyrin in the feces

No increase in δ-aminolevulinic acid or porphobilinogen in the urine

Wood's lamp examination of the urine. To enhance the orange-red fluorescence, add a few drops of 10% hydrochloric acid.

It is important to obtain levels of porphyrins in the stool to rule out VP, which has markedly elevated fecal protoporphyrin as the diagnostic hallmark.

Liver Biopsy
Reveals porphyrin fluorescence

PATHOPHYSIOLOGY

In some patients there is a reduction in the liver of the enzyme uroporphyrin decarboxylase (UROGEND) which catalyzes decarboxylation of the 4 acetate groups to methyl groups. This reduction of UROGEND may occur in familial or nonfamilial PCT.

TREATMENT

Avoid ethanol, stop drugs that could be inducing PCT, such as estrogen, and eliminate exposure to chemicals (chlorinated phenols, tetrachlorodibenzo-p-dioxin). In some patients complete avoidance of ethanol ingestion will result in a clinical and biochemical remission and in depletion of the high level of iron stores in the liver. Phlebotomy is done by removing 500 mL of blood at weekly or biweekly intervals until the hemoglobin is decreased to 10 g. Clinical and biochemical remission occurs within 5 to 12 months after regular phlebotomy. Relapse within a year is uncommon (5 to 10%).

Chloroquine is used to induce remission of PCT in patients where phlebotomy is contraindicated because of anemia. Since chloroquine can exacerbate the disease and, in higher doses, may even induce hepatic failure in these patients, this treatment requires considerable experience. However, long-lasting remissions and, in a portion of patients, clinical and biochemical "cure" can be achieved. Presently, the most efficient therapeutic approach to the treatment of PCT is a combination of phlebotomy (3 to 4 sessions) followed by low-dose chloroquine therapy.

Variegate porphyria is a serious autosomal dominant disorder of heme biosynthesis characterized by skin lesions (vesicles and bullae, skin fragility, milia, and scarring of the dorsa of the hands and fingers), acute attacks of abdominal pain and neuropsychiatric manifestations, and increased excretion of porphyrins; especially characteristic are high levels of protoporphyrin in the feces.

Synonym: porphyria variegata

EPIDEMIOLOGY

Race All races; especially common in white South Africans (3/1000) (the disease was imported in 1688 by one female Dutch settler). It is increasingly recognized in Europe (Finland) and the United States

Age Second to fourth decade

HISTORY

Change with Seasons Skin lesions occur during the summer season but may persist throughout the winter; lesions result from exposure to sunlight.

Skin Symptoms Painful erosions, skin fragility

Constitutional Symptoms None

Systems Review Acute attacks of abdominal pain, constipation, nausea and vomiting, muscle weakness, seizures, confusional state, psychiatric symptoms (depression, coma); rarely, cranial nerve involvement, bulbar paralysis, sensory loss, and paresthesias

PHYSICAL EXAMINATION

Skin
TYPE OF LESION
  Vesicles, or more commonly bullae (Figure 319)

  Erosions, milia

  Sclerosis (scleroderma-like changes)

  Scars (pink, atrophic)

COLOR
  Periorbital heliotrope hue

  Diffuse melanoderma on exposed areas

ARRANGEMENT Scattered, discrete lesions
DISTRIBUTION Localization to dorsa of hands, fingers, and feet (Figure 319) (exposed areas)

Hair Hirsutism (especially in sunny climates)

Miscellaneous Findings Neurologic, especially peripheral neuropathy

LABORATORY AND SPECIAL EXAMINATIONS

Dermatopathology
SITE Dermoepidermal interface and dermis
PROCESS Subepidermal bullae formation (festooning); PAS-positive, diastase-resistant depositions in and around blood vessels of the upper dermis

General Laboratory Examination
PORPHYRINS See Table A.
Plasma Distinctive plasma fluorescence with emission maximum at 626 nm

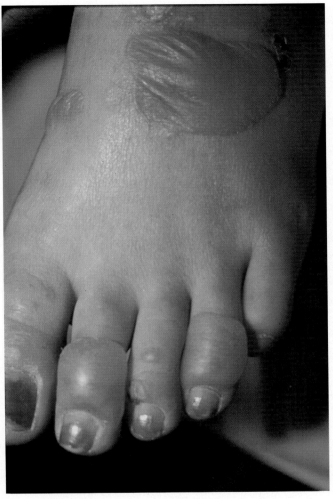

319 Variegate porphyria *Bullae on the dorsa of the feet in exposed areas.*

Urine Increased porphobilinogen during acute attacks

Stools High protoporphyrin

Wood's Lamp Examination Pink-orange fluorescence of urine

ETIOLOGY AND PATHOPHYSIOLOGY

The basic metabolic defect is accentuated by ingestion of certain drugs (sulfonamides, barbiturates, phenytoin, estrogens, alcohol, and others) (see Table B), with the resultant precipitation of acute attacks of abdominal pain and neuropsychiatric disorders (delirium, seizures, personality changes). There is an enzyme defect resulting in a reduction of protoporphyrin oxidase, with accumulation of protoporphyrinogen in the liver, which is excreted in the bile and is nonenzymatically converted to protoporphyrin; this accounts for the high fecal protoporphyrin.

COURSE

Lifetime disease with onset after puberty and peak incidence in second to fourth decade; skin manifestations not provoked by drugs that precipitate abdominal and neuropsychiatric symptoms, except for estrogens, which provoke cholestatic hepatitis, diverting porphyrin from the bile to the blood, with resulting increased porphyrin deposition in the skin.

PROGNOSIS

Good, if exacerbating factors are avoided (certain drugs, alcohol, infection). Rarely, death can occur following ingestion or injection of drugs (e.g., barbiturates) that induce increased amounts of cytochrome P450 and create a demand for increased synthesis of heme.

TREATMENT

None; oral beta-carotene may or may not control the skin manifestations but has no effect on porphyrin metabolism or the important systemic manifestations.

PHOTOSENSITIVITY IN SYSTEMIC DISEASE

Table A. Laboratory Differential Diagnosis of Hepatic Porphyrias

	PORPHYRIA CUTANEA TARDA	VARIEGATE PORPHYRIA
Urine tests		
During acute attacks		
PBG	N	++
URO	++	++
COPRO	+	++
Between acute attacks		
PBG	N	N
URO	++	N
COPRO	+	N
Ratio URO/COPRO	>1	<+
Stool tests		
COPRO	++	++
PROTO	+	++
URO	+	N

Abbreviations: N, normal; +, mild elevation; ++, marked elevation

Table B. Drugs Hazardous to Patients with Variegate Porphyria

Anesthetics: barbiturates and halothane
Anticonvulsants: hydantoins, carbamazepine, ethosuximide, methsuximide, phensuximide, primidone
Antimicrobial agents: chloramphenicol, griseofulvin, novobiocin, pyrazinamide, sulfonamides
Ergot preparations
Ethyl alcohol
Hormones: estrogens, progestins, oral contraceptive preparations
Imipramine
Methyldopa
Minor tranquilizers: chlordiazepoxide, diazepam, oxazepam, flurazepam, meprobamate
Pentazocine
Phenylbutazone
Sulfonylureas: chlorpropamide, tolbutamide
Theophylline

This hereditary metabolic disorder of porphyrin metabolism is unique among the porphyrias in that porphyrins or porphyrin precursors are not excreted in the urine. Also, erythropoietic proto-porphyria (EPP) is characterized by an acute sunburnlike photosensitivity, in contrast to the other common porphyrias (porphyria cutanea tarda or variegate porphyria) in which obvious acute photosensitivity is not a presenting complaint.

Synonym: erythrohepatic protoporphyria.

EPIDEMIOLOGY AND ETIOLOGY

Age Acute photosensitivity begins early in childhood; rarely, late onset in early adulthood

Sex Equal in males and females

Race All ethnic groups including blacks

Heredity Autosomal dominant

Incidence Not uncommon, series reported from Europe (in the Netherlands, 1:100,000), United Kingdom, and the United States

HISTORY

Duration of Onset of Lesions Stinging and itching may occur within a few minutes of sunlight exposure, later erythema and edema appear after 1 to 8 hours

Seasonal Changes Photosensitivity is less common in the winter months in temperate areas.

Symptoms Burning or "stinging" sensation within minutes may be the only abnormality. Children may choose not to go out in the direct sunlight after a few painful episodes, which may cause serious sociopsychologic problems. Symptoms occur when exposed to sunlight through window glass.

Systems Review Biliary colic, even in children

PHYSICAL EXAMINATION

Skin Changes in Acute Reactions to Sunlight Exposure Bright red erythema, later edema (swelling of hands especially), urticaria (less common), purpura [especially on the nose (Figure 320) and tips of ears]. Vesicles or bullae rarely occur. These changes appear within 1 to 8 hours and subside after several hours or days without obvious scarring.

Skin Changes Following Chronic Recurrent Exposures Shallow, often linear scars, especially on the nose and dorsa of the hands ("aged knuckles"). Diffuse wrinkling of the skin of the face (nose, around the lips, cheeks) with obvious thickening of the skin and a waxy color (Figure 321). Crusted, erosive lesions may occur on the nose and lips. Absence of sclerodermoid changes, hirsutism, or hyperpigmentation.

General Medical Findings

Hemolytic anemia with hypersplenism (rare)

Cholelithiasis (12%), even in children. Stones contain large amounts of proto-porphyrin.

Liver disease may result from massive dep-

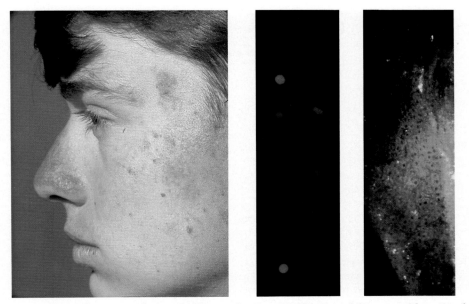

320   Erythropoietic protoporphyria   *Diffuse, erythematous infiltration of the nose, with scattered atrophic scars on the side of the face. In the center there are fluorescent erythrocytes containing protoporphyrin. On the right is a portion of the liver which exhibits a bright red fluorescence due to the presence of protoporphyrin.*

osition of protoporphyrin in the hepatocytes (Figure 320); fatal hepatic cirrhosis is not uncommon.

LABORATORY AND SPECIAL EXAMINATIONS

Porphyrin Studies   Increased protoporphyrin in RBC, plasma, and stools but no excretion in the urine. Decreased activity of the enzyme, ferrochelatase, in the bone marrow, liver, and in skin fibroblasts.

Liver Function   Tests for liver function are indicated. Liver biopsy has demonstrated portal and periportal fibrosis and deposits of brown pigment in hepatocytes and Kupfer cells. With electron microscopy, needlelike crystals have been observed. About 20 patients have been reported with cirrhosis and portal hypertension.

Special Examination for Fluorescent Erythrocytes   RBC in a blood smear exhibit a characteristic *transient* fluorescence (see Figure 320) when examined with a fluorescent microscope with a mercury or tungsten-iodide lamp which contains 400 nm radiation.

Dermatopathology
SITE   Upper dermis
PROCESS   Marked eosinophilic homogenization and thickening of the blood vessels in the papillary dermis; there is an accumulation of an amorphous, hyaline-like eosinophilic substance in and around blood vessels.

Radiography   Gallstones may be present.

PATHOPHYSIOLOGY

The specific enzyme defect occurs at the step in porphyrin metabolism in which protoporphyrin is converted to heme by the enzyme, ferrochelatase. This leads to an accumulation of protoporphyrin which is highly photosensitizing.

DIAGNOSIS AND DIFFERENTIAL DIAGNOSIS

In EPP there is photosensitivity but no "rash," only an exaggerated sunburn response which appears much earlier than ordinary sunburn erythema. Also the skin changes occur behind window glass. Finally there are virtually no photosensitivity disorders in which the symptoms appear so rapidly (minutes after exposure to sunlight). Porphyrin examination establishes the diagnosis with elevated free protoporphyrin levels in the RBC and in the stool. The fecal protoporphyrin is most consistently elevated.

COURSE AND PROGNOSIS

EPP persists throughout life, but the photosensitivity may become less apparent in late adulthood. Liver cirrhosis may become manifest in adults.

TREATMENT

There is no treatment for the basic metabolic abnormality, but symptomatic relief of the photosensitivity can be achieved in many patients with oral beta-carotene in divided doses of 180 mg daily. Therapeutic levels of carotenoids are achieved in 1 to 2 months. This treatment brings about an amelioration of the photosensitivity but does not completely eliminate the problem of photosensitivity. Patients on beta-carotene can remain outdoors longer by a factor of 8 to 10 but still burn if exposures are too long. Nevertheless many patients can participate in outdoor sports for the first time. There is no toxicity with prolonged treatment with beta-carotene.

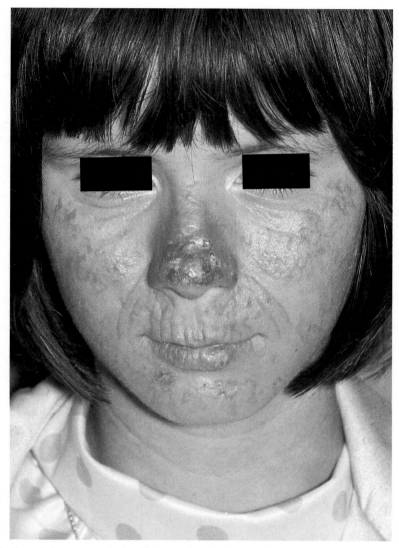

321 Erythropoietic protoporphyria   *The nose, lower lip, and chin show erythematous, in part erosive and crusted, lesions in a 15-year-old female. On both cheeks are erythematous lesions. The nose and cheeks, in addition, show a few small, slightly depressed scars and peculiar waxy thickening of the skin. Linear scars are present between the nose and mouth.*

Xeroderma pigmentosum (XP) is an autosomal recessive disease with photosensitivity, photophobia, *early* onset of frecklelike pigmented macules (lentigines) strictly limited to the sun-exposed areas of skin, and *later* development of skin cancers exclusively in the sun-exposed areas. Following chronic exposure to the sun there is a marked alteration of the skin (dermatoheliosis) consisting of keratoses, telangiectasia, atrophy, and lentigines. XP patients also have a cellular hypersensitivity to ultraviolet radiation (UVR) and to certain chemicals, which results from a defect in the repair of DNA damage. There is a deficiency in the initiation of excision repair of pyrimidine dimers and other photoproducts. In some patients there are also severe progressive neurologic changes. There are at least nine molecular forms of XP (complementation groups plus a variant). Recently, the defective genes in complementation groups A and B have been cloned.

EPIDEMIOLOGY

Incidence 1:250,000 in the United States; higher in Japan, Egypt, and Lebanon

Age Infancy or early childhood

Race XP has been reported in all races

Sex Equal incidence in males and females

HISTORY

Onset and Development

SKIN In about 50% of cases there is a history of an acute sunburn reaction; the sunburn erythema may persist for days, in contrast to a normal sunburn, which disappears in a few days; the other patients appear to have normal sunburn reactivity. Frecklelike macules (lentigines) appear on the exposed areas by age 1 year in 50% of the patients, and in almost all patients by age 15. Solar keratoses develop at an early age, and the epithelial skin cancers (basal cell or squamous cell) appear by the eighth year of life. The skin has a fully developed dermatoheliosis similar to a ''farmer's skin'' by the end of childhood: dry and leathery.

Most important are the series of malignancies that develop, including melanoma, epithelial cancers, fibrosarcoma, and angiosarcoma. There is about a 1000-fold increase in the frequency of basal cell carcinoma, squamous cell carcinoma, and cutaneous malignant melanoma.

NEUROLOGIC SYSTEM A progressive neurologic degeneration occurs in 40% of the patients, either in infancy or by the second decade. There is a wide range of abnormalities: severe progressive mental retardation, spasticity, seizures. The most common neurologic abnormalities are progressive sensorineural deafness and diminished to absent deep tendon reflexes.

EYE The eye is involved with frequency equal to the skin, and it is a prominent feature of the disease. Most striking is the photophobia with redness of the eyes due to conjunctival injection; later there is severe keratitis and vascularization leading to blindness. Ectropion is common and epithelial cancers and melanomas of the eyelids or anterior eye may develop.

Family History Autosomal recessive, consanguinity is common. Parents (obligate heterozygotes) are clinically normal.

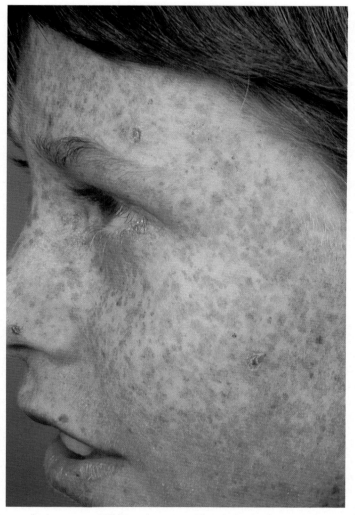

322　Xeroderma pigmentosum　*Mild involvement with a few solar keratoses but marked freckle-like lentigines on the face and lips of a white Dutch child.*

PHYSICAL EXAMINATION

Appearance of Patient Depends on the severity of involvement of the skin and the extent of sun exposure and the degree of DNA-repair deficiency. The patient may appear severely scarred with marked poikilodermatous dermatoheliosis, or those well protected from sun exposure since early childhood may exhibit only a few lentigines and telangiectasia in the exposed areas.

Skin

TYPES OF LESIONS　(Figures 322 and 323) A mix of dark-brown macules, telangiectasia, guttate hypomelanotic macules and warty solar keratosis, basal cell carcinoma and squamous cell carcinoma.

DISTRIBUTION OF LESIONS　The skin changes occur exclusively on the habitually exposed areas (face, neck, forearms and dorsa of arms, legs in females) and also in the areas covered with a single layer of thin clothing (such as a blouse or cotton shirt); the "double-covered" areas are spared (breasts of females, bathing trunk areas of males and females).

MUCOUS MEMBRANES Telangiectasia can occur on the lips and the lingual mucous membrane; primary squamous cell carcinomas can occur on the tip of the tongue.

LABORATORY EXAMINATIONS

Dermatopathology

LIGHT MICROSCOPY Same changes as noted in dermatoheliosis (see page 214)

ELECTRON MICROSCOPY Abnormal melanocytes with changes in melanosomes, melanin macroglobules are numerous.

SPECIAL EXAMINATIONS

Cultured cells from XP patients exhibit a striking inhibition of growth following exposure to UVR, and cellular recovery is considerably delayed. In one type of XP defect, present in 80% of XP patients, there is a deficiency of the initiation of excision repair acting on pyrimidine dimers. In the other group (called XP "variants"), which comprises about 2%, the fibroblasts exhibit a defect in "S" phase DNA replication following irradiation with UVR. Cell fusion studies permit a separation of the excision repair-deficient types into eight groups: A–H.

DIAGNOSIS AND DIFFERENTIAL DIAGNOSIS

Some young patients with severe freckling or with multiple lentigines syndrome (LEOPARD syndrome, see page 644) could be regarded as having XP, but at this age these patients do not have a history of acute photosensitivity, which is always present in XP, even in infancy. Also there is no dermatoheliosis (telangiectasia, atrophy, or guttate hypomelanosis), which is present in XP even in childhood.

In addition, there can occur skin cancers (squamous cell and basal cell carcinoma, malignant melanoma, fibrosarcoma, angiosarcoma).

PATHOGENESIS

There are now known to be 9 molecular defects as the basis for the clinical syndrome of XP. There are 8 complementation groups and a variant form. The latter has a normal excision repair but has defective postreplication repair. The genes involved in complementation groups A and B have recently been cloned.

SIGNIFICANCE

XP is a very serious disease that requires constant attention from the first moment of diagnosis, not only to prevent exposure to UVR but to closely monitor the patient for the detection of skin malignancies, especially melanoma. Antenatal diagnosis is possible by amniocentesis, measuring UV-induced unscheduled DNA synthesis in cultured amniotic fluid cells. There is as yet no laboratory test that can detect XP heterozygotes in the parents.

COURSE AND PROGNOSIS

Metastatic melanoma and squamous cell carcinoma are the most frequent causes of death and over 60% die by age 20. Some patients with mild involvement, however, may live beyond middle age. Early diagnosis and careful protection from sun exposure may prolong life substantially.

MANAGEMENT

Patients with XP need to be followed by a dermatologist every 3 months, not only to detect malignancies early but to constantly educate

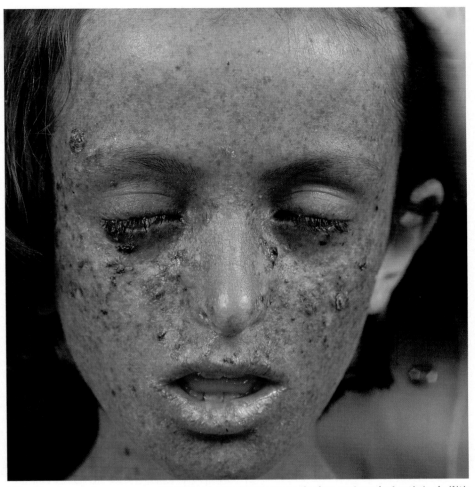

323 Xeroderma pigmentosum *Myraids of solar keratoses on the face and marked actinic cheilitis in a child from North Africa.*

the patient (and the parents!) in effective sun protection and in the early recognition of skin cancers.

Topical Potent sunblocks worn daily, even in winter in northern latitudes. Avoidance of daylight between the hours of 1000 and 1500. Protective hats, clothing, and sunglasses with side shields should always be used throughout the year. An ophthalmologist should also follow the patient; soft contact lenses are usually necessary. Vision can be restored with corneal transplants.

Systemic Oral retinoids have now been shown to reduce the number of new epithelial cancers that develop over time. The limitation of this therapy is the dose-related irreversible calcification of ligaments and tendons.

The Future A gene has been cloned from mice, XPAC, which confers protection against UVR when transferred into cells from patients with XP group A, the most common and most serious form of XP; and recently a human gene XPAC has been cloned. This correcting gene is located on the long arm of chromosome 9 (9q34.1).

Pellagra (Italian *pelle agra*, "rough skin") is a syndrome with a characteristic dermatitis, stomatitis and glossitis, GI disturbances, especially diarrhea, and neurologic and psychiatric disorders. The cause is a deficiency of niacin, either in the diet or as a result of isoniazid therapy, or due to the presence of a carcinoid tumor.

CLASSIFICATION

Dietary deficiency: starvation, alcoholism

Drug therapy: isoniazid therapy (the drug replaces niacinamide in coenzyme I)

Rare: Hartnup disease, carcinoid syndrome

Associated diseases: cirrhosis of the liver, carcinoid in which the dietary tryptophan is diverted to form 5-hydroxytryptamine

HISTORY

History   The skin changes are usually preceded by prodromal GI symptoms, and the diagnosis of pellagra is difficult in the absence of the skin changes.

Skin Symptoms   Pruritus and burning

Constitutional Symptoms   Fatigue, weakness, anorexia, weight loss, malaise

Systems Review
GI   Dysphagia and burning of the esophagus, nausea, vomiting, diarrhea (often bloody)
CNS   Impairment of memory, apathy, confusion, paranoid psychosis

PHYSICAL EXAMINATION

Appearance of Patient   The patient appears chronically ill and weak.

Skin
TYPE OF LESION   An acute and chronic "sunburn type" reaction: erythema, vesicles and bullae (Figure 324), and, later, development of a scaling and thickened leathery skin with fissuring; in this latter stage it is

referred to as "goose skin" (Figure 325). The involvement of the anogenital area with a moist dermatitis is part of an associated riboflavin deficiency.

DISTRIBUTION OF LESIONS   Sharply limited to the exposed areas of the face, neck, dorsal areas of the hands, arms, and feet. The hands are most characteristic, with a "glove" or "gauntlet" pattern, and on the feet a "boot" pattern, rarely above the malleoli. On the face there is a "butterfly" pattern, and on the neck what is called "Casal's necklace," covering a broad band, as a collar, entirely around the neck in perfect symmetry.

MUCOUS MEMBRANES   There is a scarlet stomatitis and scarlet-red tongue.

DIAGNOSIS AND DIFFERENTIAL DIAGNOSIS

Diagnosis   As there is no laboratory test, the diagnosis of pellagra is based on the characteristic dermatosis and the response to therapy with niacin.

Differential Diagnosis   Phototoxic drug sensitivity

ETIOLOGY AND PATHOGENESIS

Although pellagra responds quickly to low doses of niacin (10 mg per day), it is now regarded as a *mixed* deficiency of both trytophan and available niacin in the diet.

TREATMENT

Niacinamide, 100 to 300 mg in divided doses, plus vitamin B complex, as well as a high-protein diet of 100 to 150 g per day

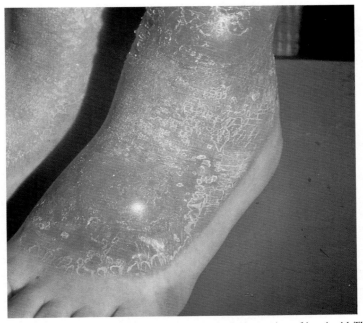

324   Pellagra *This condition was induced by prolonged adminstration of isoniazid. These lesions are erythematous, edematous, and confined to the exposed areas of the dorsa of the feet.*

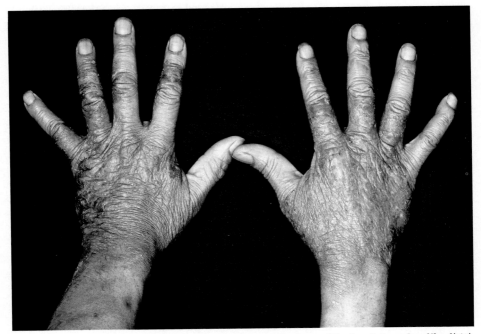

325   Pellagra *Marked thickening and pigmentation of the dorsa of the hands in a glovelike distribution. The term* pellagra *literally means rough skin. These changes are the result of exposure to sun in a patient with this nutritional deficiency.*

PELLAGRA

Pigmentary Disorders

Vitiligo

Vitiligo, a specific type of acquired leukoderma, is an idiopathic, patterned, circumscribed hypomelanosis of skin and of hair in which other causes of leukoderma have been excluded. The disease is important principally because of the social stigma associated with vitiligo in brown- and black-skinned persons. Vitiligo may be an autoimmune disease, since it is associated with other autoimmune diseases: diabetes mellitus, pernicious anemia, and Addison's disease.

EPIDEMIOLOGY AND ETIOLOGY

Age of Onset Infancy to old age; peak incidence is 10 to 30 years

Race Occurs in white, brown, or black persons with equal frequency. Apparent prevalence in darker-skinned persons because in those people the disease is more cosmetically disfiguring.

Skin Phototypes (SPT) Mostly SPT IV, V, and VI

Sex Reported female predominance may be spurious, especially in India where vitiligo can be a considerable disfigurement and can affect eligibility for marriage because vitiligo mimics leprosy.

Incidence 1.0% (reported as 1.0 to 8.8%)

Etiology Unknown. Family history in 30% of patients

Geography The prevalence appears greater in southern sunny climates, but this is due to exaggerated contrast of tanned skin with the white spots.

HISTORY

Onset and Duration of Lesions The white spots usually gradually appear and remain for life, with about 30% of patients reporting some limited spontaneous repigmentation.

Precipitating Factors Trauma, as with cuts, suture sites, etc.; this is called the *Koebner* or *isomorphic phenomenon* and is frequently observed. Emotional stress is often mentioned by patients (e.g., grief over lost partner) as a cause.

Skin Symptoms Rarely, vitiligo macules may be erythematous with a raised border and with itching; this "inflammatory" vitiligo has no special significance.

Systems Review See General Examination, below.

Other Findings in the History Premature graying (<20 years of age), history of halo nevi or alopecia areata

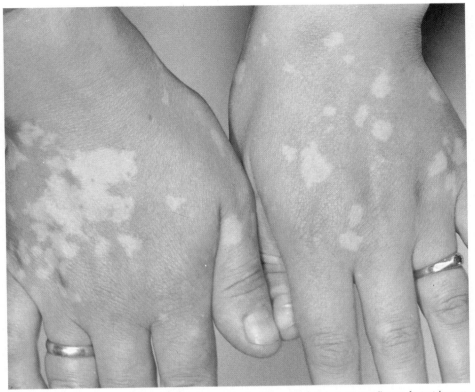

326   Vitiligo   *On the dorsa of the hands, irregularly disseminated, in part confluent, hypopigmented macules; similar lesions on the feet and hands.*

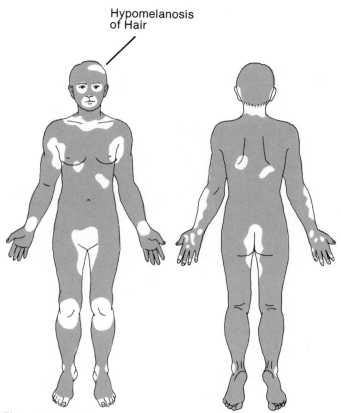

Hypomelanosis
of Hair

Figure XVI   Vitiligo

PHYSICAL EXAMINATION

Skin Findings

TYPE OF LESION   White macules varying in size from 1.0 mm to large areas of the body

COLOR   "Snow" white is typical, but newly developing lesions may be "off-white" or even a light tan

SHAPE OF INDIVIDUAL LESION   Oval, geographic patterns (Figure 326); the borders may often be scalloped. There may be linear patterns or artifactual-type areas (as under a neck pendant); these represent the isomorphic, or Koebner, phenomenon.

DISTRIBUTION OF LESIONS   (See Figure XVI)
Focal type: isolated macules in one site.
Segmental: unilateral, quasidermatomal.
Generalized (Figure 327): multiple discrete macules, often strikingly symmetrical (in fact, mirror image) and at sites of repeated trauma, such as the bony prominences (malleoli, tip of the elbow, necklace area in females).

Hair   Pigmented or white hairs may be present in a vitiligo macule.

Mucous Membranes   Rarely present in the mouth (gums)

Eye   Iritis in 10%, but may not be symptomatic; retinal changes consistent with healed chorioretinitis in up to 30% of patients.

General Examination   Search for thyroid disease (Figure 328) (up to 30% in females), diabetes mellitus, pernicious anemia, Addison's disease, syndrome of polyendocrinopathy with mucocutaneous candidiasis.

PIGMENTARY DISORDERS

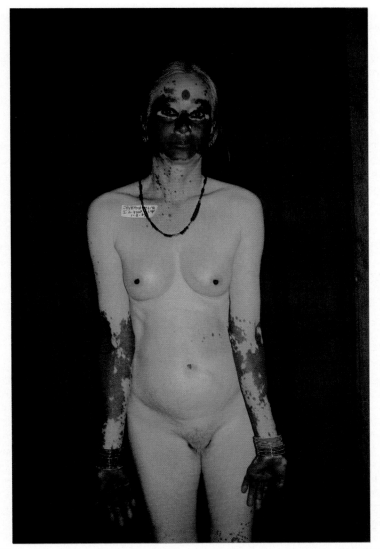

327   Vitiligo   *This striking photograph shows extensive white depigmentation occurring in a patient who has normally brown skin. The remaining brown skin can be seen on the face, the nipples, and the forearms.*

DIAGNOSIS AND DIFFERENTIAL DIAGNOSIS

Diagnosis Characteristic symmetrical white macules without any other skin change located in the typical sites.

Differential Diagnosis Lupus erythematosus, pityriasis alba, tinea versicolor, piebaldism, chemical leukoderma, leprosy, nevus depigmentosus, tuberous sclerosis, leukoderma with metastatic melanoma, postinflammatory hypomelanosis

LABORATORY EXAMINATIONS

Dermatopathology

SITE Epidermis. Melanocytes are absent in fully developed vitiligo macules, but at the margin of the white macules there may be melanocytes present and a few lymphocytes. Progressive destruction of melanocytes, possibly by cytolytic T cells.

Laboratory Examination of Blood

SEROLOGIC ANA and other special tests for lupus erythematosus; adrenal autoantibodies in 50% of patients who have Addison's disease

HEMATOLOGIC Normal, except in patients with pernicious anemia (obtain complete blood study including indices)

CHEMISTRY TSH (radioimmunoassay). Addison's disease: there may be a low FBS, low sodium and high potassium, and an elevated BUN. FBS should be done to exclude diabetes mellitus.

SPECIAL EXAMINATIONS

Wood's Lamp Examination It is essential to examine patients with a light skin color with the Wood's lamp to detect all the areas of vitiligo.

Eye An examination by an ophthalmologist is necessary before therapy.

PATHOPHYSIOLOGY

An immune process is the most probable mechanism of destruction of melanocytes, as there are several autoimmune disorders that occur with vitiligo: thyroiditis, adrenal insufficiency, and pernicious anemia, based on an autoimmune mechanism. An immune hypothesis would involve an aberration of immune surveillance that results in destruction of melanocytes; the primary event would be damage to melanocytes with the release of antigen and subsequent autoimmunization (probably in a genetically predisposed individual).

COURSE AND PROGNOSIS

The course of vitiligo is unpredictable; lesions may remain stable for years or progress rapidly. About 30% of patients have some degree of spontaneous repigmentation but rarely to a cosmetically acceptable degree. In rare instances the total melanin pigmentation is lost, except for the eyes.

SIGNIFICANCE

Vitiligo, or "leukoderma" as it is more familiarly known in many parts of the world, is a serious social problem. In India, because of the social ostracism, the sufferer often cannot marry or get employment. Similar but less severe social problems exist for other brown or black peoples and for white persons who tan well (SPT III and IV) and who therefore exhibit the contrast of the white vitiligo macules with the normal brown tanned skin.

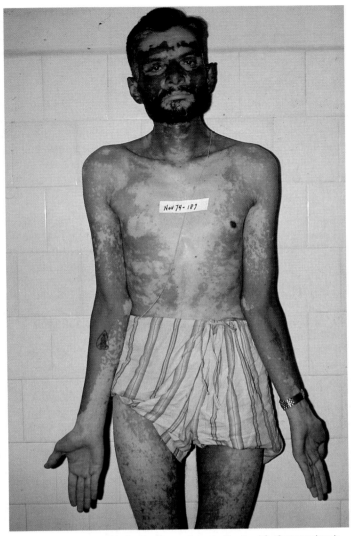

328   Vitiligo   *Extensive leukoderma in a patient with thyrotoxicosis.*

TREATMENT

The treatment of vitiligo is best managed by a dermatologist who, depending on (1) concern about the disfigurement by the patient and (2) the age of the patient, may choose topical PUVA photochemotherapy or oral PUVA pho-tochemotherapy. In patients with extensive loss of *normal* pigmentation, "bleaching" the normal skin to make it totally white is a very satisfactory method of treatment. This is accomplished with topical preparations of monobenzylether of hydroquinone.

Albinism is a heritable disorder that affects skin, hair, and eyes. It principally involves the synthesis of melanin but also includes some alterations of the pathways of the CNS. Albinism can affect the eyes, *ocular albinism* (X-linked recessive), or the eyes and skin, *oculocutaneous albinism* (OCA). In OCA, the disorder is autosomal recessive, with dilution of normal amounts of skin, hair, and melanin pigment; nystagmus and iris translucency are always present, and there is a reduction of visual acuity, sometimes severe enough to cause blindness.

EPIDEMIOLOGY

Incidence   The general incidence is 1:20,000

Age   Present at birth

Race   There is no special predilection in any one skin color. Hermansky-Pudlak syndrome (OCA and a platelet disorder) is seen in Hispanics from Puerto Rico, in persons of Dutch origin, and in East Indians from Madras.

Classification of Oculocutaneous Albinism   There are 10 types of OCA, based on (1) the level of tyrosinase in the plucked hair bulb (ty-positive and ty-negative), (2) hair color (yellow, red, platinum), and (3) associated problems such as platelet abnormalities and ceroid storage disease (Hermansky-Pudlak syndrome, HPS) or defects in immunity (Chédiak-Higashi syndrome, CHS).

HISTORY

Duration   Patients with albinism early in life avoid the sun because of repeated sunburns, especially as toddlers.

Systems Review   *HPS:* epistaxis, gingival bleeding, excessive bleeding after childbirth or tooth extraction, fibrotic restrictive lung disease

Family History   There may be no family history of albinism in the autosomal recessive or X-linked recessive types.

Social History   Albinos live an essentially normal life, except for problems with vision and, in lower latitudes, the development of skin cancers and dermatoheliosis. There is a national volunteer group of albinos called NOAH (National Organization for Albinism and Hypomelanosis—Noah, builder of the ark in the Old Testament, was thought to be an albino). The volunteer group assists albinos in various ways, especially in dealing with vision problems: obtaining driver's license, etc. Many albinos appear to be musicians and to be high achievers (Rev. W. A. Spooner, Head of New College, Oxford, was an albino and famous for his "spoonerisms").

PHYSICAL EXAMINATION

Appearance of Patient   "Poring" (eyes half closed, squinting) when in sunlight

Skin   "Snow"-white, fair, cream, light tan

Hair   White (ty-neg), yellow cream, or light brown (ty-pos) (Figure 329), red, platinum

Eyes   Iris translucency, nystagmus

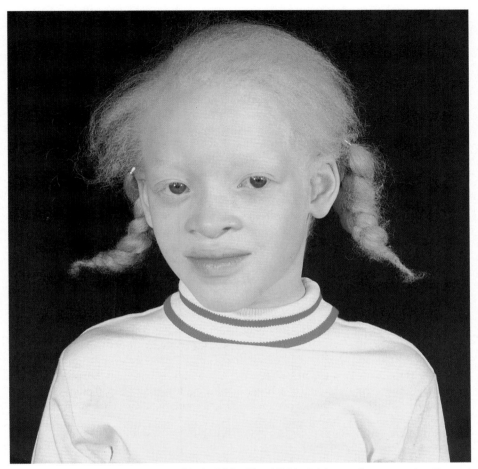

329 Albinism, oculocutaneous, in a black child *The child had iris translucency and yellow-red hair (ty-pos albinism).*

LABORATORY AND SPECIAL EXAMINATIONS

Dermatopathology

LIGHT MICROSCOPY Melanocytes are present in the skin and hair bulb in all types of albinism. The dopa reaction of the skin and hair is markedly reduced or absent in melanocytes of the skin and hair, depending on the type of albinism (ty-neg or ty-pos).

ELECTRON MICROSCOPY Melanosomes are present in melanocytes in all types of albinism but, depending on the type of albinism, there is a reduction of the melanization of melanosomes, with many being completely unmelanized (stage I) in ty-neg albinism. Melanosomes in the albino melanocytes are transferred in a normal manner to the keratinocytes.

Laboratory Examination of Blood

HEMATOLOGIC Morphologic, chemical, and functional defects of platelets in HPS type of albinism

Tyrosine Hair Bulb Test (ty-neg and ty-pos)

Hair bulbs are incubated in tyrosine solutions for 12 to 24 hours and develop new pigment formation from normal and ty-pos patients, but no new pigment formation is present in ty-neg albinism. For details of methods, see Witkop CJ et al: Albinism, Chapter 119 in *The Metabolic Basis of Inherited Disease,* 6th ed, edited by C Scriver et al. New York, McGraw-Hill, 1989.

DIAGNOSIS

White persons with fair skin (skin phototype I), blond hair, and blue eyes may mimic albinos but they do not have iris translucency or nystagmus. Some persons with albinism who have a constitutive black or brown skin color may have a dilution of their skin color from black to a light brown and have the capacity to tan; also they may have brown irides but will still have iris translucency. Therefore, iris transclucency and the presence of other eye

findings in the fundus are the pathognomonic signs of albinism.

ETIOLOGY AND PATHOGENESIS

The defect in melanin synthesis has recently been shown to result from absence of the activity of the enzyme, tyrosinase. Tyrosinase is a copper-containing enzyme that catalyzes the oxidation of typrosine to dopa and the subsequent dehydrogenation of dopa to dopaquinone. Recent cloning of complementary DNAs (cDNAs) encoding tyrosinase has made it possible to directly characterize the mutations in the tyrosinase gene responsible for deficient tyrosinase activity in type 1A albinism. Two different missense mutations, one from each parent, result in amino acid substitutions within one of the two copper-binding sites.

SIGNIFICANCE

Albinism is an important disease to recognize early in life, in order to start prophylactic measures to prevent dermatoheliosis and skin cancer.

COURSE

Albinos with ty-pos OCA form melanin pigment in the hair, skin, and eyes during early life, the hair becoming cream, yellow, or light brown, and the eye color changing from light gray to blue, hazel, or even brown.

PROGNOSIS

Albinos living in central Africa who are unprotected develop squamous cell carcinomas early in life, and this significantly shortens their life span; few survive to the age of 40 years because of metastasizing squamous cell carcinoma. Dermatoheliosis and basal cell carcinomas are frequent in albinos living in

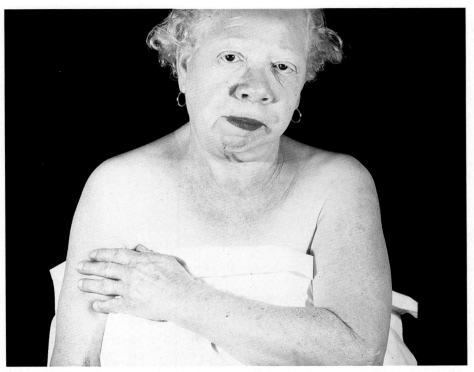

330 Albinism, oculocutaneous, in a black woman *This patient grew up in Boston, but she has extensive dermatoheliosis and basal cell carcinomas.*

temperate climates (Figure 330). Melanomas occur in albinos, as do melanocytic nevi, and are usually amelanotic (nonpigmented).

MANAGEMENT

Skin A lifetime program beginning in infancy including:

Daily application of topical, potent, broad-spectrum sunblocks, including lip sunblocks

Avoidance of sun exposure in the high solar intensity season during the hours of 1000 to 1500

Yearly examination by a dermatologist to detect skin changes: skin cancers and dermatoheliosis

Use of topical tretinoin for dermatoheliosis and for its possible prophylactic effect against sun-induced epithelial skin cancers

Systemic Beta-carotene (30 to 60 mg t.i.d.) imparts a more normal color to the skin and may possibly have some protective effect on the development of skin cancers, although this has been proved only in mice.

Melasma is an acquired, light- or dark-brown hyperpigmentation that occurs in the exposed areas, most often on the face, and results in part from, and is exacerbated by, exposure to sunlight. Melasma occurs principally in women of child-bearing age, although up to 10% of cases may be seen in men. Melasma may be idiopathic or associated with pregnancy, with ingestion of contraceptive hormones, or possibly with certain medications such as diphenylhydantoin.

Synonym: chloasma.

EPIDEMIOLOGY

Incidence Common, especially among persons with brown skin color and who are taking contraceptive regimens and who live in sunny areas. During the early clinical trials of estrogen-synthetic progesterone combinations, which were done in the Caribbean in brown-skinned Hispanic women, melasma occurred in 20% of the patients.

Age Young adults

Race Melasma is more apparent or more frequent in persons with brown constitutive skin color (people from Asia, the Middle East, India, South America).

Sex Females >> males; about 10% of patients with melasma are men

Geography More apparent or more frequent in sunny areas of the world, especially in the Caribbean and in countries bordering on the Mediterranean

Precipitating Factors Sun exposure + pregnancy or oral contraceptives, diphenylhydantoin; cosmetics probably do not play a role

HISTORY

Duration of Lesions The pigmentation usually evolves quite rapidly over weeks, particularly following exposure to high-intensity sunlight.

Relationship of Melasma to Other Factors Season (more apparent in summer months in northern latitudes), medications (following or during ingestion of oral contraceptives), menses (during premenstrual period a darkening of preexisting melasma may sometimes occur), pregnancy

Family History There is often a family history, but no kindreds have been studied to determine the Mendelian pattern.

PHYSICAL EXAMINATION

Skin See Figure 331.
TYPE OF LESION Completely macular hyperpigmentation, the hue and intensity depending largely on the skin phototype of the patient
COLOR OF LESION Light- or dark-brown or even black

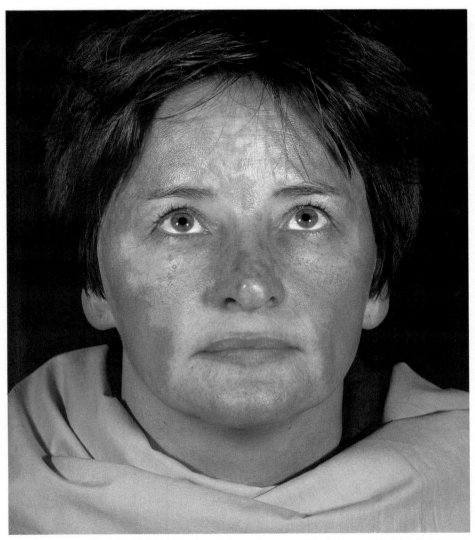

331   Melasma   *Note the solid macular hyperpigmentation on the cheeks and the blotchy pigmentation on the nose and forehead.*

ARRANGEMENT OF LESIONS   Most often symmetrical

SHAPE AND BORDER OF INDIVIDUAL LESIONS   The pattern follows the areas of exposure, and the lesions have serrated, irregular, and geographic borders.

DISTRIBUTION OF LESIONS   Two-thirds on central part of the face: cheeks, forehead, nose, upper lip, and chin; a smaller percentage involve the malar or mandibular areas of the face.

LABORATORY AND SPECIAL EXAMINATIONS

Dermatopathology
LIGHT MICROSCOPY *Site* Epidermis
Process Stimulation of melanocytic activity with an increase in number of melanocytes and in the production and transfer of melanosomes to the keratinocytes in the epidermis

Illumination (Allow for dark adaptation)
PARTIALLY DARKENED ROOM This permits the examiner to better visualize the pigment change, as the contrast is markedly accentuated.
WOOD'S LAMP EXAMINATION In order to detect all areas of melasma in persons with light skin color, it is essential to use the Wood's lamp. In these patients there can be seen a marked accentuation of the hyperpigmented macules. This contrast is not so clearly accentuated in patients with normal brown or black skin.

DIFFERENTIAL DIAGNOSIS

A patient with *vitiligo* can sometimes be erroneously diagnosed as having melasma, the physician regarding the uninvolved dark tanned *normal* skin on the face as abnormal brown melasma; this normal hyperpigmented skin sits in the center of the abnormal "snow-white" vitiligo skin. *Postinflammatory hypermelanotic macules* on the face may be brown but do not have sharp margins and are not located in the special sites where melasma occurs: upper lip, malar areas, etc.

PATHOGENESIS

The pathogenesis of melasma is not known. There are some clinical observations that would implicate female hormones. Estrogen preparations alone, however, given to postmenopausal women do not cause melasma, despite sun exposure. However, pregnancy causes melasma, and combinations of estrogen and progestational agents, as used for contraception, are the most frequent cause of melasma. There is, therefore, a hormonal basis for melasma but the mechanism is not yet known.

SIGNIFICANCE

While this is a strictly cosmetic problem, it is very disturbing to both males and females, especially persons with brown skin color and good tanning capacity, skin phototype V. For a discussion of how to determine skin phototype (SPT I to VI) see page 210.

COURSE AND PROGNOSIS

Melasma may disappear spontaneously over a period of months following delivery or after cessation of contraceptive hormones. Melasma may or may not return with each pregnancy.

TREATMENT

Topical Weak (3%) hydroquinone in solution used in combination with topical tretinoin is reasonably effective and at present the therapy of choice. The bleaching effect is not observed until treatment has been given for several weeks. Under no circumstances should monobenzylether of hydroquinone or the other ethers of hydroquinone (monomethyl- or monoethyl-) be used in the treatment of melasma as these drugs can lead to a permanent loss of melanocytes with the development of a disfiguring spotty leukoderma. Also for the treatment to be effective at all, it is essential that the patient use, every morning, an *opaque* sunblock containing titanium dioxide and/or zinc oxide; the action spectrum of pigment darkening extends into the visible, and even the potent (with high SPF) transparent sunscreens are completely ineffective in blocking visible radiation.

The term *LEOPARD* is a mnemonic for seven features of this hereditary cardiocutaneous syndrome which has as its principal visible manifestation, generalized lentigines (dark brown macules). The seven features in the mnemonic are: *L*—lentigines, *E*—EKG abnormalities, *O*—ocular hypertelorism, *P*—pulmonic stenosis, *A*—abnormal genitalia, *R*—retardation of growth (dwarfism), *D*—deafness.

EPIDEMIOLOGY

Incidence Rare

Age Infants

HISTORY

Duration of Lesions The lesions start during infancy and increase to a peak in adult life and then remain stable for life.

Skin Symptoms None

Family History Autosomal dominant

PHYSICAL EXAMINATION

Skin
TYPE OF LESION Macule, portions of which may be slightly raised
SIZE OF LESIONS 2.0 to 3.0 mm but may be >15 mm in the mouth
COLOR OF LESIONS Dark-brown or black
SHAPE OF INDIVIDUAL LESION Round or oval
ARRANGEMENT OF MULTIPLE LESIONS There is no pattern.
DISTRIBUTION OF LESIONS Uncountable numbers of pigmented macules (Figure 332) are scattered all over the body, including both the exposed and also the unexposed areas, such as scalp, genitalia, palms, and soles.

Mucous Membranes Lips

General Examination Nerve deafness, pulmonic stenosis with EKG changes, gonadal or ovarian hypoplasia, reduced stature, ocular hypertelorism

LABORATORY EXAMINATIONS

Dermatopathology
LIGHT MICROSCOPY *Site* Epidermis
Process Hyperplasia of melanocytes and increase in melanin in the melanocyte, elongation of the rete ridges

DIAGNOSIS AND DIFFERENTIAL DIAGNOSIS

The pigmentary lesions are striking and not observed in any other condition except generalized lentigines, where they appear without any of the other manifestations of LEOPARD syndrome—this may be a forme fruste of LEOPARD syndrome. In Peutz-Jeghers syndrome there are usually only acral, perioral, and oral pigmented macules. Multiple frecklelike lesions occur in the atrial myxoma syndrome.

SIGNIFICANCE

The pigmentary changes may be the most important part of the syndrome as they can be very disfiguring.

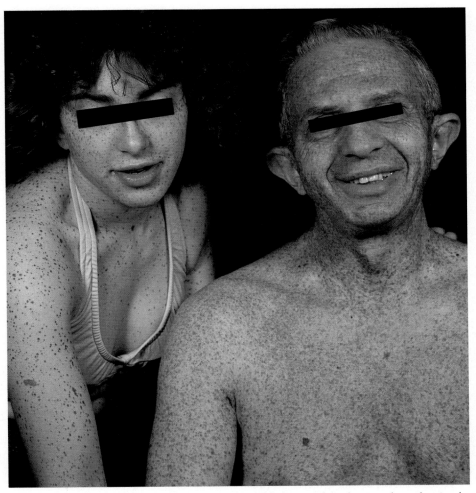

332 LEOPARD syndrome *Father and daughter both have pulmonic stenosis and extensive freckle-like lentigines in the exposed and unexposed areas. Some lesions are larger than 2.0 to 3.0 mm.*

COURSE AND PROGNOSIS

An essentially normal life ensues.

TREATMENT

Topical hydroquinone-containing preparations can lead to a reduction in the number of pigmentary lesions.

LEOPARD SYNDROME

Addison's Disease

Addison's disease is a syndrome resulting from adrenocortical insufficiency caused by infections (e.g., tuberculosis) or as an autoimmune disease. The disease is insidious and is characterized by generalized brown hyperpigmentation, slowly progressive weakness, fatigue, anorexia, nausea, and, frequently, GI symptoms: vomiting and diarrhea. Suggestive laboratory changes include a low serum sodium, high serum potassium, and elevation of the blood urea nitrogen; the diagnosis is confirmed by specific tests of adrenal insufficiency.

EPIDEMIOLOGY

Incidence 4 : 100,000

Age All ages

Sex Equal

HISTORY

History Characterized by an insidious onset of progressive hyperpigmentation in which the patients state that their summer tan did not fade during the winter, or that friends comment that they are "getting darker." Weakness is a prominent symptom, first after stress and then chronic weakness, fatigue, and weight loss. The disease may become manifest after physical or metabolic stress.

Systems Review Nausea, vomiting, and diarrhea are frequent complaints. There may be orthostatic hypotension with dizziness and syncope.

PHYSICAL EXAMINATION

Appearance The patient may appear completely normal except for a generalized brown hyperpigmentation.

Skin There is increased brown melanin hyperpigmentation in those areas where it nor-

mally occurs (see Distribution, below) (Figure 333). It is therefore the *change* in the intensity of the pigmentation in these areas or the *development of new areas* of pigmentation, e.g. gingival or buccal mucous membrane, that is significant. The intensity of the pigmentation is related to skin phototype; but even light-skinned persons (SPT I and II) can develop marked pigmentation.

Distribution Pigmentation occurs in areas that are *normally* hyperpigmented: around the eyes, gingival and buccal mucous membrane, tongue, nipples, creases of the palms, over bony prominences, in the linea nigra (abdomen), axillae, and anogenital areas in males and females. Pigmentation also develops in new scars, as after surgery.

Hair and Nails There are often linear streaks of pigmentation in the nail plate (a normal finding in brown and black persons). Gray scalp hair may darken as the disease progresses. Axillary hair may be decreased or absent.

Mucous Membranes Brown or blue-black spotty pigmentation of the gingival and buccal mucosa (a normal finding in most black- and brown-skinned persons) and the dorsum of the tongue

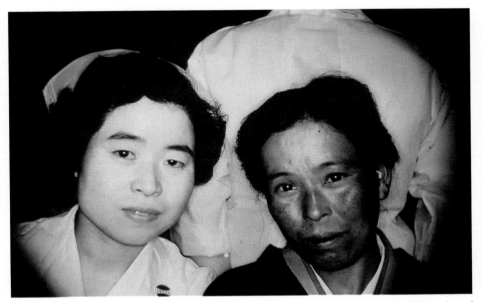

333   Addison's disease   *Japanese patient in whom tuberculosis was the etiology of the adrenal insufficiency. Note the striking contrast in the skin color of a normal Japanese female nurse compared to the diffuse brown hyperpigmentation in the patient with Addison's disease.*

LABORATORY AND SPECIAL EXAMINATIONS

Dermatopathology
LIGHT MICROSCOPY Increased melanin in melanocytes, melanophages in the dermis

Laboratory Examination of Blood
SEROLOGY Adrenal autoantibodies in 50% of patients

CHEMISTRY There may be a low FBS, low sodium and high potassium, and elevated BUN.

Wood's Lamp Examination There is a marked enhancement of pigmentation.

DIAGNOSIS AND DIFFERENTIAL DIAGNOSIS

Diagnosis The presenting problem may not be the change in skin pigmentation but only abdominal symptoms: vague abdominal pain and diarrhea. If abnormal generalized pigmentation can be documented and the patient has GI complaints, it is necessary to obtain special ACTH stimulation tests. The laboratory diagnosis may be impossible in the early phases of the disease. Even the specialized tests, such as ACTH stimulation to measure the adrenal reserve, may be within the normal range and need to be repeated later.

Differential Diagnosis Hemochromatosis, porphyria cutanea tarda, chronic renal failure, hepatic cirrhosis, functioning benign endocrine tumors such as chromophobe adenomas that produce ACTH and associated peptides (Nelson's syndrome), metastatic cancers (especially lung), carcinoid, Whipple's intestinal lipodystrophy, vitamin B_{12} deficiency, chemotherapy (doxorubicin, busulfan, bleomycin, systemic 5-fluorouracil), systemic scleroderma

ETIOLOGY

At the present time the majority of patients with Addison's disease do not have tuberculosis of the adrenal as they did in the past, but idiopathic atrophy, probably based on an autoimmune mechanism. Rarely, patients may have adrenal insufficiency as part of a polyglandular syndrome (usually beginning in childhood) with, in addition to adrenal insufficiency, hypoparathyroidism, chronic mucocutaneous moniliasis, alopecia areata, and vitiligo.

PATHOGENESIS

The brown hyperpigmentation results from the melanogenic action of increased blood levels of pituitary peptides. The pigmentation is not due to ACTH itself: for every ACTH molecule cleaved from its pituitary precursor, a molecule of beta-lipotrophin (LPH) and gamma-melanotrophin (MSH) is also cleaved; the beta-MSH sequence is contained in the beta-LPH and the alpha-MSH sequence within the ACTH. The increased secretion of these peptides is the result of a decrease or absence of the cortisol-hypothalamic-pituitary feedback regulation, or arises from pituitary chromophobe adenoma or a metastatic cancer producing peptides (Figure 334).

SIGNIFICANCE

A diffuse, increased brown melanin hyperpigmentation of recent onset must always be thoroughly investigated, as the treatment of Addison's disease can be life-saving. Adrenal crises, in fact, can be fatal and may be precipitated by trauma (auto accidents, surgery) or severe illness.

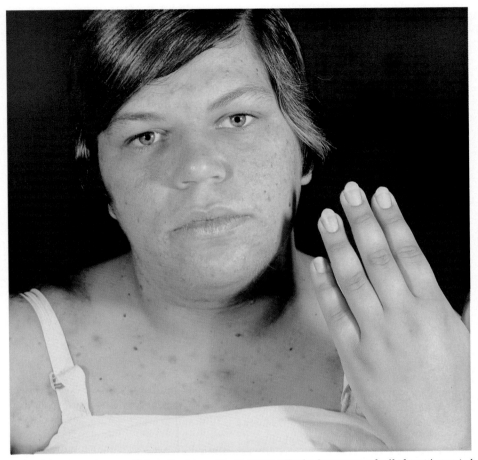

334 Nelson's syndrome   *This patient is a skin phototype II who became markedly hyerpigmented as the result of a functioning tumor of the pituitary. The patient had a chromophobe adenoma which excreted large amounts of ACTH and associated peptides.*

COURSE AND PROGNOSIS

The disease is inexorably progressive unless treated with hormone replacement; with treatment there is a normal life expectancy.

TREATMENT

Hormone replacement with prednisone plus fludrocortisone for mineralocorticoids

Amiodarone Photosensitivity (Ceruloderma)

Amiodarone is a very effective drug for the treatment of ventricular tachycardia and must be given continuously over long periods. Amiodarone induces, in over 75% of patients after 40-g cumulative dose, a low-grade or minimal photosensitivity and, in a small number (8%) of patients, a striking slate-gray hyperpigmentation (ceruloderma) limited to the light-exposed areas. Other side effects include: pulmonary fibrosis, pneumonitis, hepatotoxicity, thryoid disturbances, neuropathy, and myopathy.

EPIDEMIOLOGY

Incidence Amiodarone-induced ceruloderma develops after 20 months of therapy and 160 g. Amiodarone ceruloderma occurs in about 8% of patients, usually those with skin phototypes I and II.

HISTORY

History Some patients gradually develop pigmentary changes without a true photosensitivity, i.e., it is apparently a ''subclinical'' photosensitivity. In others a typical sunburn reaction is not noted but instead a dusky-red erythema on the face and dorsa of the hands; symptoms develop within 30 minutes to 2 hours after first exposure to the sun and the reaction fades within 1 to 2 days. Other patients have severe erythematous, papular lesions—the severity is related to the duration and intensity of solar exposure.

Skin Symptoms Pruritus, burning, stinging

PHYSICAL EXAMINATION

Skin Findings
TYPE OF LESION
  Dusky-red erythema and, later, blue-gray

dermal melanosis (Figure 335) in exposed areas (face and hands)
  ''Phototoxic''-type erythema (rare)

Systems Review Patients may develop pulmonary fibrosis, pneumonitis, neuropathy, myopathy, hepatotoxicity.

LABORATORY EXAMINATIONS

Dermatopathology There is a perivascular infiltrate of lymphocytes and histiocytes in the dermis. Brown granular pigment is noted in the histiocytes, endothelial cells, and large amounts in the macrophages throughout the dermis. The pigment occurs as electron-dense, compact, and lamellated granules in lysosomes present in the perivascular histiocytes.

Peripheral Blood Electron microscopy reveals increased number of lamellated granules in WBC; these can also be seen in pulmonary and hepatic tissue.

DIAGNOSIS

With a history of amiodarone ingestion and the typical ceruloderma there is no problem in diagnosis.

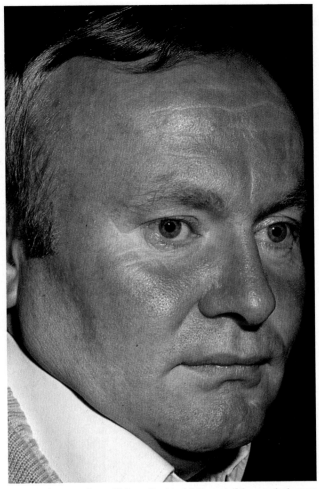

335 Amiodarone hyperpigmentation *This patient exhibits a striking amiodarone-induced, dusky-red, erythematous pigmentation of the face. The blue color (ceruloderma) is due to the deposition of melanin in the dermis, contained in macrophages.*

ETIOLOGY AND PATHOGENESIS

Amiodarone is incorporated into cell membranes, which then absorb UVA (the action spectrum) and induce a phototoxic injury to erythrocytes, macrophages, and lymphocytes.

COURSE AND PROGNOSIS

The low-grade photosensitivity disappears 12 to 24 months after the drug is discontinued. The long period results from the gradual elimination of the photoactive drug from the lysosomal membranes.

Minocycline, a tetracycline derivative, is an antibiotic frequently used for long periods in the treatment of acne vulgaris. This antibiotic is also not uncommonly used for other diseases with skin lesions, such as pyoderma gangrenosum. Following high-dose (100 to 200 mg daily) and long-term (1 to 3 years) therapy, a blue-gray pigmentation (ceruloderma) develops in acne scars as well as in isolated areas on the legs and feet, the hard palate, and around the eyes. The lesions are circumscribed (Figure 336), very rarely generalized, and diffuse ceruloderma may occur. Gray-green discoloration of the teeth can occur. A black discoloration of the thyroid has been found at operation. The pigmentation is not melanin. The brown pigment, located in the dermal macrophages, is iron-containing pigment; on analysis with electron microscopy and x-ray micro-analysis the pigment is shown to be contained in sidersomes that are composed of iron and sulfur.

DIFFERENTIAL DIAGNOSIS

Circumscribed acquired blue-gray pigmentation can occur with a number of heavy metals (topical mercury, topical silver, gold at the site of injection), oral quinacrine, chloroquine, oral bismuth, oral amiodarone. History of exposure to a specific drug is usually quite easily established.

COURSE

The ceruloderma from minocycline gradually disappears over a period of months after the drug is stopped.

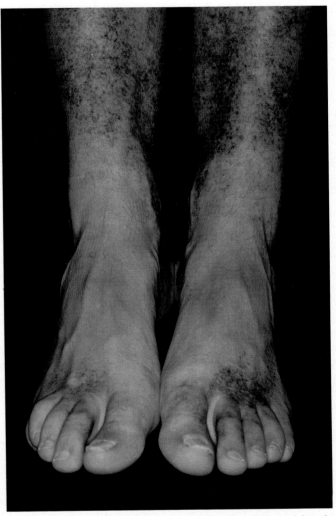

336 Minocycline pigmentation *The blue-gray pigmentation (ceruloderma) has developed in circumscribed areas on the legs and feet. The brown pigment is iron-containing and is not melanin. This patient had received high doses of minocycline (300 mg per day) for over 10 months.*

Melanoma Precursors and Primary Cutaneous Melanoma

Cutaneous Melanoma and Precursors

Of all the cancers, melanoma of the skin represents the greatest challenge in what we have called "preventive detection": finding early curable primary tumors, thereby preventing metastatic disease and death. Melanoma of the skin in white persons is now not a rare tumor in the United States—32,000 new primary melanomas will develop in 1991, and 6500 deaths will occur.

In males ages 30 to 49 melanoma is the second most prevalent cancer (the first being cancer of the testis), and in slightly older males (ages 50 to 59) melanoma is the fourth most prevalent cancer, exceeded only by bladder, lung, and rectal cancer (in that order). Primary melanoma of the skin is therefore a disease affecting the young and middle-aged. Mortality rates of primary melanoma for single years from 1976 to 1987 rose at the rate of 3% per year for men and 1% for women. Easy accessibility to physicians is especially important in primary melanoma because curability is directly related to the size and depth of invasion of the tumor.

Even with a rising mortality there has been an encouraging increase in the detection of early stage 1 melanoma, with very high five-year survival rates (approaching 98%) for thin (<0.76 mm) primary melanoma and an 83% rate for all stages. The trend over the past 3 decades illustrates the dramatic increased survival of melanoma patients: in 1960–1963 the overall five-year survival for melanoma was 60%, and by 1977–1983 this had increased to 80%. At the present time, the most critical tool for conquering this disease is the identification of early "thin" melanomas by clinical examination. In most instances, early melanoma can be recognized by three physical characteristics: *color, contour,* and *size* of the lesion.

Total skin examination for melanoma and its precursors should be routinely done. Special stress should be given to: the back above the waist; legs, between the knees and ankles in women; the scalp; toes and soles of black- or brown-skinned persons; skin around body orifices (mouth, anus, vulva).

Classification of Cutaneous Malignant Melanoma and Precursors

A. *Melanoma*
  1. Superficial spreading melanoma
  2. Nodular melanoma
  3. Lentigo maligna melanoma
  4. Acral lentiginous melanoma
  5. Desmoplastic melanoma
  6. Melanoma of the mucous membranes
B. *Precursors of Cutaneous Melanoma*
  1. Congenital nevomelanocytic nevus (giant *or* small)
  2. Clark's (dysplastic) melanocytic nevus
  3. Lentigo maligna
  4. Melanoma in situ

All melanomas show an initial radial and subsequent vertical growth phase. The prognostic difference between the clinical types relates mainly to the duration of the radial growth phase, which may last from years to decades in lentigo maligna melanoma, from months to 2 years in superficial spreading melanoma, and may be very short in nodular melanoma. Since metastasis occurs only infrequently during the radial growth phase, detection of melanoma (i.e., "thin" melanomas) during this phase is essential.

The Clark Melanocytic Nevus (Dysplastic Melanocytic Nevus)

Clark melanocytic nevi (CMN) are a special type of acquired, circumscribed, pigmented lesions that represent disordered proliferations of variably atypical melanocytes. CMN arise de novo or as part of a compound melanocytic nevus. CMN differ from common acquired nevi, are clinically distinctive, and have characteristic histologic features. CMN are regarded as potential precursors of superficial spreading melanoma and also as markers of persons at risk for developing primary malignant melanoma of the skin.

EPIDEMIOLOGY

Prevalence CMN occur in almost every patient with familial cutaneous melanoma and in 30 to 50% of patients with sporadic (nonfamilial) primary melanomas of the skin. CMN are, moreover, present in 5.0% of the general white population.

Race White persons. Data on persons with brown or black skin are not available; CMN are rarely seen in the Japanese population.

Age Children and adults

Sex Equal in males and females

Transmission Autosomal dominant

HISTORY

Duration of Lesions CMN usually arise later in childhood than common acquired nevomelanocytic nevi, appearing first in late childhood, just before puberty. New lesions continue to develop over many years in affected persons; in contrast, common acquired nevomelanocytic nevi do not appear after middle age and disappear entirely in older persons. CMN are thought not to undergo spontaneous regression at all or at least much less than common acquired nevomelanocytic nevi.

Precipitating Factors Exposure to sunlight is regarded by some as an inducing agent for CMN; nevertheless CMN are not infrequently observed in completely covered areas such as the scalp and anogenital areas.

Skin Symptoms Asymptomatic

Family History Autosomal dominant trait; in the familial setting, family members can develop melanoma without the presence of CMN.

PHYSICAL EXAMINATION

See Comparative Clinical Features, page 658

LABORATORY EXAMINATION

Dermatopathology Hyperplasia and proliferation of melanocytes in a single file, "lentiginous" pattern in the basal cell layer either as spindle cells or epithelioid cells, and as irregular and dyshesive nests.

1. Melanocytes are "atypical," larger than normal size, exhibiting both pleomorphism of nuclei and cell bodies, and hyperchromasia of nuclei.
2. Increased number of melanocytes with tendency for dyshesive and irregular

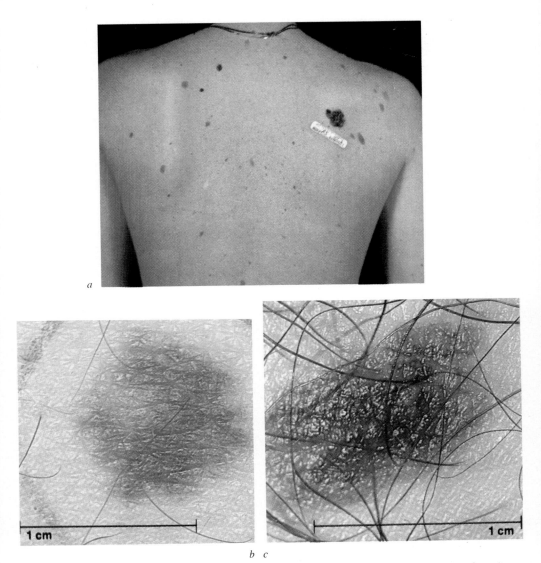

337a–c Malignant melanoma—Clark's melanocytic nevus (dysplastic melanocytic nevus syndrome)
(a) *This 28-year-old woman gave a history of a rapidly growing (3 to 6 months), asymptomatic lesion on her right scapular area. Her mother had melanoma and both mother and siblings had many dark "moles." Diagnosis: (1) Superficial spreading melanoma, level IV, 4.75 mm. (2) Regional nodes—of 32 removed, 1 was positive. (3) Dysplastic nevus syndrome with family history of melanoma. Primary lesion and many dark "moles" on back.*
(b) *Round, essentially macular, lesions in which the slightly elevated area is present at 12:00 o'clock. The elevation is detectable only by oblique lighting. Note striking variegation of color with tan, brown, and pink areas. (c) This lesion is more obviously elevated in the central portion. Note "pebbly" surface. Both lesions have indistinct and irregular borders. [From* Dermatologic Capsule and Comment 7(4), 1985, *with permission.]*

THE CLARK MELANOCYTIC NEVUS (DYSPLASTIC MELANOCYTIC NEVUS)   657

	CLARK'S NEVUS (DYSPLASTIC MELANOCYTIC NEVUS)	COMMON ACQUIRED NEVOMELANOCYTIC NEVUS
Number	One or many (Figure 337a). Dozens or uncountable, especially in familial melanoma	One or many, average in white males is 12 to 15; 30% have no nevi
Distribution	Mostly on the trunk (Figure 337a), arms, legs; rarely on the face. Exposed and covered areas	Exposed areas of trunk and extremities
Type*	Macules with only slightly elevated portions, especially in the center	Small lesions (junctional nevi) are macules; compound nevi are uniformly elevated papules or nodules
Size*	May be up to 15 mm or larger (Figures 337b and 337c). *Pigmented lesions >6 mm are Clark's nevi or congenital nevomelanocytic nevi*	Most lesions, despite elevation are rarely >10 mm in diameter
Shape	Round (Figure 337b), oval, or ellipsoid (Figure 337c)	Round, oval, papillomatous
Border of Lesion*	Indistinct margin (Figure 337b) with normal skin	Sharply demarcated
	Irregularly irregular (Figure 337b)	Regular
Color*	Brown [dark (Figure 337c) or medium], tan, pink, or red	Brown (medium or dark), tan
Pattern	Irregular display or variegation (Figures 337b and 337c)	Uniform or orderly pattern

*Type, size, border, and color are distinctive features.

nesting; "bridging" between rete ridges by melanocytic nests; spindle-shaped melanocytes are oriented parallel to skin surface.

3. Lamellar fibroplasia and concentric eosinophilic fibrosis (not a constant feature)

4. Proliferation of blood vessels (not a constant feature)

5. Sparse or dense lymphocytic infiltrate (not a constant feature)

Association Most CMN arise in contiguity with a compound melanocytic nevus (rarely junctional nevus) that is centrally located, i.e., CMN often have extension of intraepidermal melanocytic hyperplasia beyond the shoulder

of the dermal nevus component; some CMN may not have a dermal nevus component.

SPECIAL EXAMINATIONS

Wood's Lamp Examination This will markedly accentuate the epidermal hyperpigmentation of the individual lesions.

DIAGNOSIS AND DIFFERENTIAL DIAGNOSIS

Diagnosis The diagnosis of CMN is made by clinical recognition of typical distinctive lesions; one of these lesions should be excised for histologic confirmation of the diagnosis of

CMN. The clinicopathologic correlations are now well documented. Siblings, children, and parents should also be examined for CMN once the diagnosis is established in one family member.

Differential Diagnosis Of the clinical lesions: congenital nevomelanocytic nevi, common acquired nevomelanocytic nevi, superficial spreading malignant melanoma, melanoma in situ, lentigo maligna, Spitz's nevus

ETIOLOGY AND PATHOGENESIS

The gene locus is 1p36 of the short arm of chromosome 1. The abnormal clone of melanocytes can be activated by exposure to sunlight. Immunosuppressed patients (renal transplantation) with dysplastic nevi have a higher incidence of melanoma.

SIGNIFICANCE

Anatomic association (in contiguity) of dysplastic nevi has been observed in 36% of sporadic primary melanomas, in about 70% of familial primary melanomas, and in 94% of melanomas with familial melanoma and dysplastic nevi. The lifetime risks of developing primary malignant melanoma are estimated to be:

General population	0.8%
Familial dysplastic nevus syndrome with 2 blood relatives with melanoma	100.0%
All other patients who have dysplastic nevi	18.0%

TREATMENT AND FOLLOW-UP

Surgical excision of lesions with minimal margins. Laser or other types of physical destruction should never be used as they do not permit histopathologic verification of diagnosis. The following guidelines for selection of lesions to be excised are suggested:

- Lesions that are changing (increase in size, change in pigmentation pattern, changes in shape and/or border)
- Lesions that cannot be closely followed by the patient by self-examination (on the scalp, genitalia, upper back)

Patients with dysplastic nevi in the familial melanoma setting need to be carefully followed (every 3 to 6 months) for changes in existing dysplastic nevi or for the development of new CMN. Polaroid prints of lesions that cannot be easily seen (e.g., on the back, scalp, anogenital area) should be given to the patient in order that any changes can be observed by a second person. Patients should be given color-illustrated pamphlets that depict the clinical appearance of CMN, malignant melanoma, and common acquired nevomelanocytic nevi.

Congenital nevomelanocytic nevi (CNN) are pigmented lesions of the skin usually present at birth; rarely CNN can develop and become clinically apparent during infancy. CNN may be any size from very small to very large. CNN are benign neoplasms composed of cells called *nevomelanocytes,* which are derived from melanoblasts. All CNN, regardless of size, may be precursors of malignant melanoma.

EPIDEMIOLOGY

Age Present at birth (congenital). Some CNN become visible after birth ("tardive"), usually within the first 3 to 12 months of life, "fading in" as a relatively large lesion over a period of weeks. Large nevomelanocytic nevi (i.e., >1.5 cm) that are historically "acquired" should be regarded as tardive CNN.

Sex Equal prevalence in males and females

Race All races

Prevalence Present in 1.0% of white newborns—majority <3.0 cm in diameter. Larger varieties of CNN are present in 1:2000 to 1:20,000 newborns. Lesions ≥9.9 cm in diameter have a prevalence of 1:20,000 and giant CNN (occupying a major portion of a major anatomic site) occur in 1:500,000 newborns.

PHYSICAL EXAMINATION

Small and Large CNN CNN have a rather wide range of clinical features, but the following are typical:

TYPE OF LESION CNN usually distort the skin surface to some degree and are, therefore, a plaque with or without coarse hairs (Figure 338).

BORDERS Sharply demarcated or merging imperceptibly with surrounding skin; regular or irregular contours

PALPATION Large lesions may be "wormy" or soft but are not normally firm except in desmoplastic types of CNN (rare).

SURFACE May or may not have altered skin surface ("pebbly," mammillated, rugose, cerebriform, bulbous, tuberous, or lobular). These surface changes are more frequently observed in lesions that extend into the reticular dermis (so-called deep CNN).

COLOR Light- or dark-brown. When examined with a 10× magnification lens (under oil) a fine speckling of a darker hue with a lighter surrounding brown hue is seen; often the pigmentation is follicular. A "halo" similar to the type that is observed in leukoderma acquisitum centrifugum (so-called halo nevus) may occur.

SIZE Small or large (Figure 339). Nevomelanocytic nevi ≥1.5 cm in diameter should be regarded as probably CNN when history is not available; dysplastic melanocytic nevi must, however, be excluded.

SHAPE Oval or round

DISTRIBUTION OF LESIONS Isolated, discrete lesion in any site. Fewer than 5% of CNN are multiple. Multiple lesions are more common in association with large CNN. Numerous small CNN are very rare, except in patients with giant CNN in whom there may be numerous small CNN on the trunk and extremities away from the site of the giant CNN.

Very Large ("Giant") CNN Giant CNN of the head and neck may be associated with involvement of the leptomeninges with the same

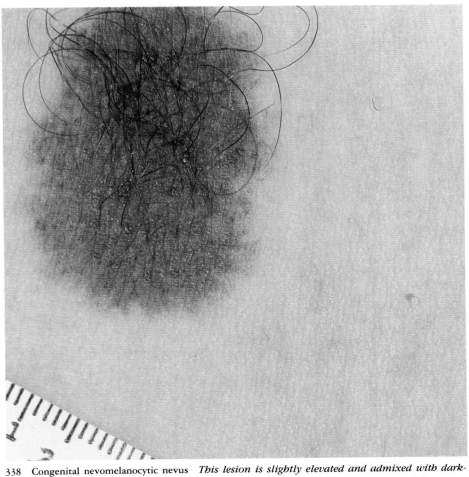

338 Congenital nevomelanocytic nevus *This lesion is slightly elevated and admixed with dark-brown papules throughout. There are coarse terminal hairs limited to areas of the nevus.*

pathologic process; this presentation may be asymptomatic or be manifested by seizures, focal neurologic defects, or obstructive hydrocephalus.

NUMBER OF LESIONS   While small CNN usually occur as single lesions (95%), giant CNN often present as a single very large lesion and multiple smaller lesions.

TYPE OF LESION   Usually a plaque with at least some surface distortion, often with focal nodules and papules on a background of a raised plaque, often with coarse, usually dark, hair (Figure 339).

SIZE   Entire segments of the trunk, extremities, head, or neck

SHAPE   Oval or round, bizarre shapes. Borders may be regular or irregular.

DISTRIBUTION OF LESIONS   Present on any region of the body and localized or widespread

CONGENITAL NEVOMELANOCYTIC NEVUS

DIFFERENTIAL DIAGNOSIS

Common acquired nevomelanocytic nevi, dysplastic melanocytic nevi, Mongolian spot, nevus of Ota, congenital blue nevus, nevus spilus, Becker's nevus, pigmented epidermal nevi, and café-au-lait macules should be considered in the differential diagnosis of CNN. Small CNN are virtually indistinguishable clinically from common acquired nevomelanocytic nevi except for size—lesions >1.5 cm may be presumed to be either CNN or Clark's dysplastic melanocytic nevi. Without a good history it may not be possible to ascertain the age of onset of a nevomelanocytic nevus <1.5 cm in diameter.

LABORATORY AND SPECIAL EXAMINATIONS

Histopathology

Nevomelanocytes occur as well-ordered clusters ("thèques") in the epidermis, and in the dermis as sheets, nests, or cords. *A diffuse infiltration of strands of nevomelanocytes in the lower one-third of the reticular dermis and subcutis is, when present, highly specific for CNN.*

Small and large CNN: Unlike the common acquired nevomelanocytic nevus, the nevomelanocytes in CNN tend to occur in the skin appendages (eccrine ducts, hair follicles, sebaceous glands) and in nerve fascicles and/or arrectores pilorum muscles, blood vessels (especially veins), and lymphatic vessels, and extend into the lower two-thirds of the reticular dermis and deeper.

Very large or giant CNN: A similar histopathology to small and large CNN but the nevomelanocytes may extend into the muscle, bone, dura mater, and cranium.

ETIOLOGY AND PATHOGENESIS

Congenital and acquired nevomelanocytic nevi are presumed to occur as the result of a developmental defect in neural crest-derived melanoblasts. This defect probably occurs after 10 weeks in utero but before the sixth uterine month; the occurrence of the "split" nevus of the eyelid is an indication that nevomelanocytes migrating from the neural crest are in place in this site before the eyelids have split (24 weeks).

COURSE AND PROGNOSIS

By definition CNN appear at birth, but varieties of CNN may arise during infancy (so-called tardive CNN). The life history of CNN is not documented, but CNN have been observed in elderly persons, an age when acquired nevomelanocytic nevi have disappeared.

Very large or giant CNN: The lifetime risk for development of melanoma in large CNN has been estimated to be at least 6.3%; in 50% of patients who develop melanoma in large CNN, the diagnosis is made between ages 3 to 5 years.

Small CNN: The lifetime risk of developing malignant melanoma is 1 to 5%.

MANAGEMENT

Small Nevi Nevi <1.5 cm that are not known to be present at birth should be assumed to be acquired and be managed according to the appearance and growth pattern.

Large Nevi Nevi >1.5 cm that are not obviously dysplastic melanocytic nevi should be managed as CNN when the history is not available.

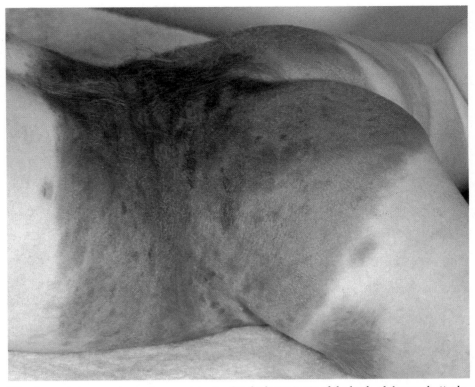

339 Congenital nevomelanocytic nevus (giant) *On the lower parts of the back, abdomen, buttocks, and thighs is an extensive, brown-colored lesion, and scattered throughout the lesion are darker-colored areas. There are also a large number of similar but much smaller lesions present on parts of the trunk, extremities, and scalp.*

Alternatives

Prophylactic excision (small typical stable CNN can probably be safely removed up to age 10 years)

Periodic follow-up for life, or

Patient's parents or patient advised to see physician only if a change (color, pattern, size) in the lesion

TREATMENT

Surgical excision is the only acceptable method

Small and large CNN:

Excision, with full-thickness skin graft, if required

Swing flaps, tissue expanders for large lesions

Giant CNN: Risk of development of melanoma is significant even in the first 3 to 5 years of age, and, therefore, giant CNN should be removed as soon as possible. Individual considerations are necessary (size, location, degree of loss of function or amount of mutilation). New surgical techniques utilizing the patient's own normal skin grown in tissue culture can now be used to facilitate removal of very large CNN. Also, tissue expanders can be utilized.

Lentigo maligna melanoma is the least common of the three principal melanomas of white persons [superficial spreading melanoma (SSM), nodular melanoma (NM), and lentigo maligna melanoma (LMM)] and occurs in older persons on the most sun-exposed areas, the face and forearms. LMM is the only melanoma about which there is general agreement that sunlight is a major etiologic factor. Lentigo maligna (LM), a flat (macular) intraepidermal neoplasm and the precursor or evolving lesion of LMM, develops focal papular and nodular areas that signal invasion into the dermis; the lesion is then called LMM.

EPIDEMIOLOGY AND ETIOLOGY

Age   Median age is 65 for LMM.

Sex   Incidence in males and females is equal.

Race   Very rare in brown- (e.g., Asiatics, East Indians) or black-skinned (African-Americans) peoples. Highest incidence in whites with skin phototypes I, II, III

Incidence   5 to 10% of primary cutaneous melanoma

Predisposing Factors   Same factors as in sun-induced nonmelanoma skin cancer (squamous cell carcinoma and basal cell carcinoma): older population, outdoor occupations (farmers, sailors, construction workers)

HISTORY

LMM very slowly evolves from LM over a period of several years, sometimes 20 years.

PHYSICAL EXAMINATION

Skin Lesions
TYPE   *Lentigo Maligna*   Uniformly flat, macule (Figure 340, on right side of photo)
Lentigo Maligna Melanoma   Flat with focal areas of papules (Figure 340, on left side of photo) and nodules
COLOR   *Lentigo Maligna*   Striking variations in hues of brown and black, appears like a "stain," haphazard network of black on a background of brown
Lentigo Maligna Melanoma   Same as LM plus gray areas (indicate focal regression) and blue areas indicate dermal pigment (melanocytes or melanin). Papules or nodules may be blue, black, or pink.
SIZE   *Lentigo Maligna*   3.0 to 20.0 cm or larger
Lentigo Maligna Melanoma   Same as LM
SHAPE   *Lentigo Maligna and Lentigo Maligna Melanoma*   Irregular borders, often with a notch, "geographic" shape with inlets and peninsulas
DISTRIBUTION   *Lentigo Maligna and Lentigo Maligna Melanoma*   Single isolated lesion on the sun-exposed areas: forehead, nose, cheeks (Figure 341), neck, forearms, and dorsa of hands
OTHER SKIN CHANGES IN AREAS OF TUMOR Sun-induced changes: solar keratosis, freckling, telangiectasia, thinning of the skin

General Medical Examination   Search for regional lymphadenopathy

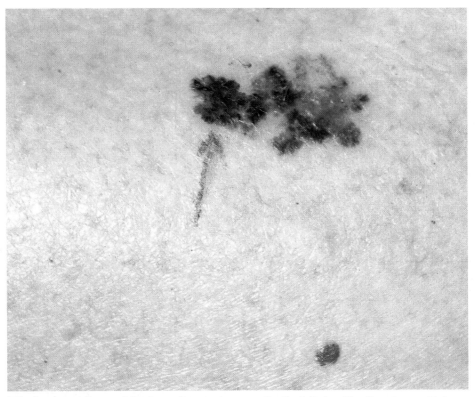

340   Lentigo maligna and lentigo maligna melanoma *On the left shoulder there is a serpiginous macule composed of two different lesions. The lesion on the right is variegated and brown-black (lentigo maligna); on the left side (arrow) the lesion is slightly elevated (papular) and almost exclusively black—this is the melanoma portion of the lesion.*

DIAGNOSIS AND DIFFERENTIAL DIAGNOSIS

LMM and LM are quite unique dark flat lesions, with focal elevations (papules and nodules) in LMM. Seborrheic keratoses may be dark but are exclusively papules or plaques and have a characteristic stippled surface often with a verrucous component, i.e., a "warty" surface which, when scratched, exhibits fine scales; also "horn cysts" can often be seen. Solar lentigo, although macular, does not exhibit the intensity or variegation of brown, dark brown, and black hues seen in LM.

LABORATORY AND SPECIAL EXAMINATIONS

Biopsy

Excision biopsy for lesions 5.0 to 10.0 mm

Excision biopsy for facial lesions 10.0 to 15.0 mm

Dermatopathology See Figure E-1 in Appendix

PATHOPHYSIOLOGY

In contrast to SSM and NM, which appear to be related to intermittent high-intensity sun exposure and occur on the intermittently exposed areas (back and legs) and in young or middle-aged adults, LM and LMM occur on the face and neck and dorsa of the forearms or hands; furthermore, LM and LMM occur most always in persons with evidence of heavily sun-damaged skin (telangiectasia, marked freckling, atrophy and solar keratosis, basal cell carcinoma).

PROGNOSIS

Summarized in Table E-1 in Appendix

TREATMENT

1. Excise with 1.0-cm or greater margin beyond the clinically visible lesion provided the flat component does not involve a major organ.
2. Excise down to or including the fascia or to the underlying muscle where fascia is absent. Graft is needed. Margin width greater than 1.0 cm is determined by location; a greater margin should be obtained if technically possible.
3. No node dissection recommended unless nodes are clinically palpable.

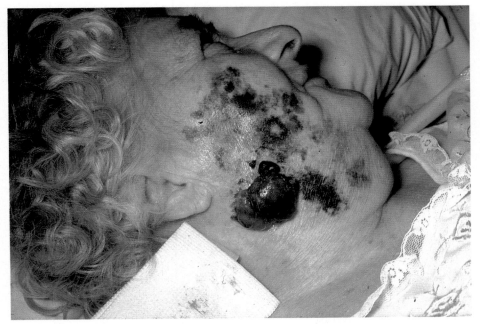

341   Lentigo maligna and lentgo maligna melanoma   *This photograph illustrates the entire spectrum of lentigo maligna melanoma which developed over a period of 40 years, starting as a small dark spot. On the upper cheek are strictly macular, brown and dark-brown lesions (this is lentigo maligna). On the angle of the jaw there are blue-black, papular lesions which are melanoma and a large polypoid nodule which is a deeply invasive melanoma.*

The term *desmoplasia* refers to connective tissue proliferation and when applied to malignant melanoma describes a few different clinical presentations; however, each has a similar microscopic pathology, characterized by (1) a dermal fibroblastic component with only minimal or absent melanocytic proliferation at the dermoepidermal junction or (2) nerve-centered superficial malignant tumors with or without an atypical intraepidermal melanocytic component or (3) other lesions in which the tumor appears to arise in lentigo maligna or, rarely, in acral lentiginous melanoma or superficial spreading melanoma. Also desmoplastic melanoma (DM) growth patterns have been noted in recurrent malignant melanoma.

EPIDEMIOLOGY

Age Median age at diagnosis 56 years (range, 4th to 9th decades)

Sex More common in women

Race Skin phototypes I to III

Incidence Rare

Etiology As most, but not all, lesions are seen on the sun-damaged skin of the head and neck, ultraviolet radiation exposure has been implicated in its pathogenesis, just as it has in superficial spreading melanoma, lentigo maligna melanoma, and nodular melanoma.

Predisposing and Risk Factors DM occurs most frequently on the head and neck, in a distribution similar to lentigo maligna/lentigo maligna melanoma.

HISTORY

Duration of Lesion Months to many years. DM is commonly misdiagnosed clinically as a dermatofibroma or neurofibroma.

Skin Symptoms Asymptomatic. Early and slowly growing lesions are often overlooked by the patient, even though visible on the face and neck.

PHYSICAL EXAMINATION

Skin Lesion

TYPE *Macule* Early lesions may appear as a variegated lentiginous macule (Figure 342), at times with small blue-gray dermal nodules. The lesions may actually arise in lentigo maligna melanoma.

Papule/Nodule (Figure 342) May appear as a dermal nodule, with or without any epidermal involvement

COLOR Tumors commonly lack any melanin pigmentation. When melanin is principally contained in malignant melanocytes in the dermis, DM may be gray to blue.

SIZE Because of delay in correct diagnosis, DM may be several centimeters in diameter.

PALPATION Early lesions often cannot be palpated. Older nodular lesions are firm, like a dermal scar or dermatofibroma.

SHAPE Borders, when epidermal involvement is present as in lesions arising in lentigo maligna melanoma, are irregular.

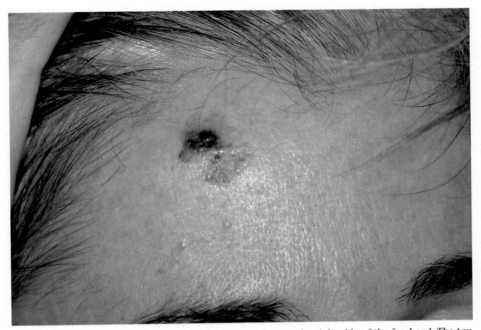

342 Desmoplastic melanoma *Solitary pigmented lesion on the right side of the forehead. The tan area is flat, and there is a blue-gray nodule arising in the tan lesion. The clinical diagnosis of this lesion would be lentigo maligna melanoma.*

DISTRIBUTION ON BODY 85% of DM occurs on the head and neck, and the majority of these on the face (Figure 342), but lesions also occur rarely on the trunk and in acral areas.

DIAGNOSIS AND DIFFERENTIAL DIAGNOSIS

Diagnosis It is essential to obtain an adequate biopsy; punch biopsies can be misleading.

Differential Diagnosis
CLINICAL DIFFERENTIAL DIAGNOSIS Basal cell carcinoma, blue nevus, cellular blue nevus, Spitz (spindle cell) nevus, metastatic melanoma to skin

HISTOLOGIC DIFFERENTIAL DIAGNOSIS Pigmented malignant schwannoma, blue nevus, malignant melanoma arising in a blue nevus, cellular blue nevus, dermatofibroma, neurofibroma, scar, desmoplastic Spitz nevus, lentigo maligna melanoma

LABORATORY AND SPECIAL EXAMINATIONS

Dermatopathology
EPIDERMIS Atypical junctional melanocytic proliferation, either individual or focal nests, occurs, resembling lentigo maligna.

DERMIS S-100 positive spindle-shaped cells embedded in matrix collagen which widely separates the spindle cell nuclei. Spindle cells may have non-membrane-bound melanosomes and premelanosomes. Small aggregates of lymphocytes are commonly seen at periphery of DM. Neurotropism is characteristic, i.e., fibroblast-like tumor cells around or within endoneurium of small nerves. DM often has a thickness of 2.0 mm. Often, DM is seen with a background of severe solar damage to the dermis.

PATHOPHYSIOLOGY

DM may be a variant of lentigo maligna melanoma in that most lesions occur on the head and neck, in patients with sun-damaged skin. DM is more likely to recur locally and metastasize than lentigo maligna melanoma, however.

COURSE AND PROGNOSIS

Diagnosis of DM is often delayed because of the bland clinical appearance. There are mixed views about the prognosis of DM. In one series following primary excision of DM, approximately 50% of patients experienced local recurrence, usually within 3 years of excision; some patients experienced multiple recurrences. Lymph node metastasis occurs less often than local recurrence. In one series 20% developed metastases, and DM was regarded as a more aggressive tumor than lentigo maligna melanoma.

TREATMENT

Aggressive surgical treatment, including parotidectomy, for lesions on the cheek.

Superficial spreading melanoma (SSM) is one of two major cancers [SSM and nodular melanoma (NM)] that arise in melanocytes of persons with white skin. It arises most frequently on the upper back and occurs as a moderately slow-growing lesion over a period of years. SSM has a distinctive morphology: a uniformly elevated, flattened lesion (plaque), usually with a strikingly variegated brown, blue-gray color pattern, and an irregularly irregular border.

EPIDEMIOLOGY

Age   30 to 50 (median, 37 years)

Sex   Slightly higher incidence in females

Race   In world surveys (4800 patients) white-skinned persons overwhelmingly predominate. Only 2% were brown- or black-skinned. Furthermore, brown and black persons have melanomas usually occurring on the extremities; half of brown or black persons have primary melanoma arising on the sole of the foot.

Incidence   SSM constitutes 70% of all melanomas arising in white persons. Melanoma accounts for about 5% of all skin cancers, but new cases increase each year by 7%.

Predisposing and Risk Factors   Four important risk factors are, in order of importance:

1. Presence of precursor lesions (Clark's dysplastic melanocytic nevus, congenital melanocytic nevus)
2. Family history of melanoma in parents, children, or siblings
3. Light skin color with inability to tan and ease of sunburning (skin phototypes I and II)
4. Excessive sun exposure, especially during preadolescence

Especially increased incidence in young urban professionals, with a frequent pattern of intermittent, intense sun exposure (''weekenders'') or winter holidays near the equator.

History   Evolves over a period of 1 to 5 years

PHYSICAL EXAMINATION

Skin Lesions
TYPE   Flattened papule, becoming plaque (Figure 343), then developing one or more nodules

COLOR   Dark brown, black (Figure 344), with admixture of pink, gray, and blue-gray hues—with marked variegation and haphazard pattern. White areas indicate regressed portions.

SIZE   Mean diameter 8.0 to 12.0 mm. Early lesions, 5.0 to 8.0 mm; late lesions, 10.0 to 25.0 mm

SHAPE   Asymmetrical (one half unlike the other), oval with irregularly irregular borders (Figures 343 and 344) and often with one or more indentations (notches) (Figure 343).

DISTRIBUTION ON BODY   Isolated, single lesions; multiple primaries are rare.

Sites of Origin
   Back (males and females) (Figure 344)

   Legs (females, between knees and ankles)

   Anterior trunk and legs in males

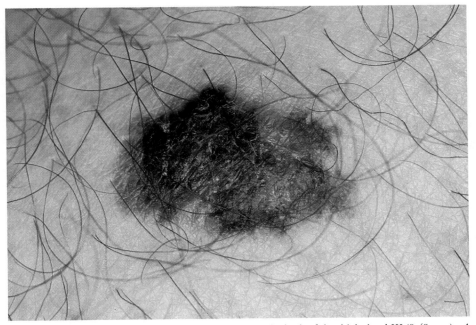

343 Superficial spreading melanoma arising de novo on the back of the thigh, level III (0.49 mm) *A classical presentation: there is a pigmented plaque in which all of the borders of the lesion are elevated with a central thicker portion. The lesion has the 5 cardinal features of a superficial spreading melanoma: asymmetry, border irregular and scalloped, color mottled, diameter large, elevation present with surface distortion (see Appendix F).*

Relatively fewer lesions on covered areas: swim suit, bra

General Medical Examination Search for lymph nodes

DIAGNOSIS AND DIFFERENTIAL DIAGNOSIS ("ABCDE")

The five cardinal features of SSM are:

A, for asymmetry

B, border is irregular and scalloped

C, color is mottled, haphazard display of brown, black, gray, pink

D, diameter is large—greater than the tip of a pencil eraser (6.0 mm)

E, elevation is almost always present with surface distortion, subtle or obvious, and assessed by side-lighting of lesion

LABORATORY AND SPECIAL EXAMINATIONS

Biopsy

Total excisional biopsy with narrow margins—optimal biopsy procedure, where possible (see Appendix E)

Incisional or punch acceptable when total excisional biopsy cannot be performed or when lesion is large, requiring extensive surgery to remove the entire lesion

Wood's Lamp Examination Desirable for defining borders

Dermatopathology See Figure E-2 in Appendix.

PATHOPHYSIOLOGY

The pathophysiology of SSM is not yet understood. Certainly, in some considerable number of SSM, sunlight exposure is a factor, and both SSM and NM are related to occasional bursts of recreational sun exposure during a susceptible period (15 to 20 years) in early adult life of persons with inability to tan. The gene for melanoma is located on chromosome 23. It is possible that severe sunburn in youth could alter the gene. About 10% of the 32,000 new melanomas each year occur in high-risk families. The rest of the cases may occur sporadically among people without a specific genetic risk. Persons at high risk inherit the gene in a mutated form of a normal gene that controls melanocytic proliferation.

COURSE AND PROGNOSIS

Left untreated, SSM develops deep invasion (vertical growth) over months to years. Prognosis is summarized in Table E-1 in Appendix. Melanoma is responsible for about 6500 deaths per year; this is 3 times the number of deaths from other skin cancers.

TREATMENT AND FOLLOW-UP

See Appendix E.

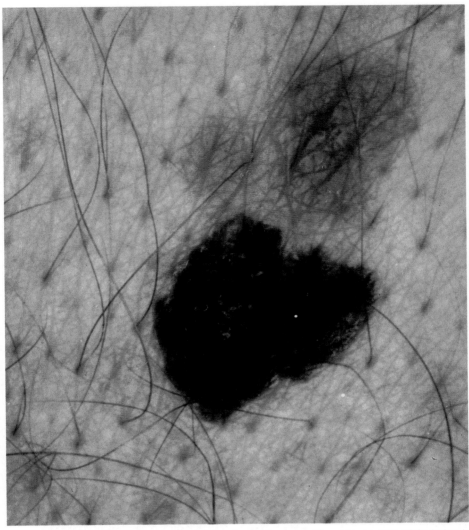

344 Superficial spreading melanoma arising in a dysplastic nevus *The upper portion of the lesion is a dysplastic nevus, and on the lower portion is a blue-black plaque which is the superficial spreading melanoma. The melanoma had a thickness of 1.2 mm. This occurred on the upper back in a 34-year-old internist who died 36 months following the discovery of this lesion.*

Nodular melanoma (NM) is the one type of primary melanoma that arises quite rapidly (4 months to 2 years) from normal skin or from a melanotic nevus as a nodular (vertical) growth without an adjacent epidermal component, as is always present in superficial spreading melanoma (SSM) and lentigo maligna melanoma (LMM).

EPIDEMIOLOGY AND ETIOLOGY

Age Median age is 50 years.

Sex Equal incidence in males and females

Race NM occurs in all races, but in the Japanese it occurs 8 times more frequently (27%) than SSM (3%).

Incidence NM constitutes 15 to 30% of the melanomas in the United States.

Predisposing and Risk Factors Four important risk factors, in order of importance: *presence of precursor lesions* (Clark's dysplastic melanocytic nevus, congenital nevomelanocytic nevus); *family history* of melanoma in parents, children, or siblings; *light skin color* with inability to tan and ease of sunburning; *excessive sun exposure*, especially during preadolescence. Especially increased incidence in young urban professionals with a frequent pattern of intermittent intense sun exposure ("weekenders," or winter holidays near the equator).

HISTORY

Evolution over 6 to 18 months

PHYSICAL EXAMINATION

Skin Lesions
TYPE Uniformly elevated "blueberry"-like nodule (Figures 345 and E-3) or ulcerated or "thick" plaque; may become polypoid

COLOR Uniformly dark blue (Figure 345) or "thundercloud" gray; polypoid lesions may appear pink (amelanotic) with trace of brown.

SIZE 1.0 to 3.0 cm (early lesions) but may grow much larger if undetected

SHAPE Oval or round, usually with smooth, not irregular, borders as in all other types of melanoma

DISTRIBUTION ON BODY Same as SSM. In the Japanese, NM occurs on the extremities (arms and legs).

General Medical Examination Always search for nodes.

DIAGNOSIS AND DIFFERENTIAL DIAGNOSIS

NM can be confused with *hemangioma* (long history), *pyogenic granuloma* (short history—weeks), and are sometimes almost indistinguishable from *pigmented basal cell carcinoma* (only biopsy settles this), and blue nevus (present for life). A "blueberry"-like nodule of recent origin (6 months to 1 year) should be excised or, if large, an excision biopsy is mandatory for histologic diagnosis.

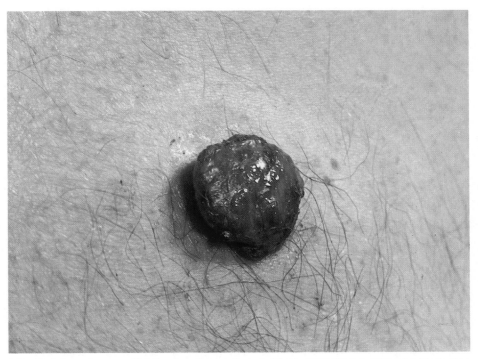

345 Nodular melanoma *This is a mushroom-shaped, 1.5 cm, partially red, otherwise black, firm tumor, round and sharply demarcated.*

LABORATORY EXAMINATIONS

Biopsy

Total excisional biopsy with narrow margins—optimal biopsy procedure, where possible (see Appendix E)

Incisional or punch acceptable when total excisional biopsy cannot be performed or when lesion is large, requiring extensive surgery to remove the entire lesion.

Dermatopathology

See Figure E-3 in Appendix.

PATHOPHYSIOLOGY

Both SSM and NM occur in approximately the same sites (upper back in males, lower legs in females) and presumably the same pathogenetic factors are operating in NM as were described in SSM (page 672). The reason for the high frequency of NM in the Japanese is not known.

PROGNOSIS

Summarized in Table E-1 in Appendix.

TREATMENT AND FOLLOW-UP

See Appendix E.

Acral Lentiginous Melanoma

This rare tumor occurs as a flat pigmented lesion on the soles, palms, and subungual regions. Acral lentiginous melanoma (ALM) is the most common melanoma in persons with brown and black skin, and occurs rarely in persons with white skin.

EPIDEMIOLOGY AND ETIOLOGY

Age Median age is 65

Sex Male:female ratio, 3:1

Race The best data are on American blacks and Japanese brown-skinned persons, and the incidence of melanoma is about one-seventh that of white persons. ALM is the principal melanoma in the Japanese and in American and African blacks. ALM accounts for 50 to 70% of melanomas in Japanese.

Incidence 7 to 9% of all melanomas; in whites, 2 to 8%

Predisposing Factors There are pigmented lesions on the soles of African blacks that are regarded by some as precursor lesions. Subungual melanoma is the most frequent type of ALM in white persons, but trauma has not been proved to be a factor.

HISTORY

ALM is slow growing (about 2.5 years). The tumors occur on the volar surface (palm or sole) and in their radial growth phase may appear as a gradually enlarging "stain": brown-black or bluish, and occupying relatively large areas (8.0 to 12.0 cm) of the sole especially. ALM subungual (thumb or great toe) melanoma appears first in the nail bed and involves, over a period of 1 to 2 years, the nail matrix, eponychium, and nail plate.

PHYSICAL EXAMINATION

Skin Lesion (Volar or Plantar—Palm or Sole)
TYPE Macular lesion in the radial growth phase with focal papules and nodules developing during the vertical growth phase
COLOR Marked variegation of color including brown, black, blue (Figure 346), depigmented pale areas
SIZE 3.0 to 12.0 cm
SHAPE Irregularly irregular borders like lentigo maligna melanoma (Figure 346)
DISTRIBUTION Soles, palms, fingers, and toes

Skin Lesion (Subungual)
TYPE Subungual macule beginning at the nail matrix, extending to involve the nail bed and nail plate. Papules, nodules, and destruction of the nail plate may occur in the vertical growth phase.
COLOR Dark brown or black pigmentation that may involve the entire nail. Often the nodules or papules are unpigmented. Amelanotic melanoma is often overlooked for weeks to months.
DISTRIBUTION Thumb or great toe

General Medical Examination Search for regional lymphadenopathy

DIAGNOSIS AND DIFFERENTIAL DIAGNOSIS

ALM (volar type) is not infrequently regarded as a "plantar wart" and treated as such. Examination with Wood's lamp may reveal extensive, barely visible pigmentation far beyond what appears to be the borders when viewed with normal light.

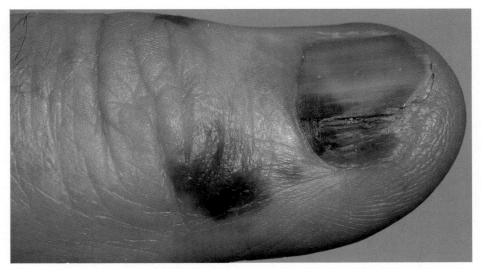

346 Acral lentiginous melanoma *The lesion involves the dorsum of the skin of the thumb and the nail bed. It is characterized by a macular, lateral growth component with irregular borders and variegation of color.*

ALM (subungual) is usually considered to be traumatic bleeding under the nail and, in fact, subungual hematomas may persist for over 1 year, but usually the whole pigmented area moves gradually forward. With the destruction of the nail plate the lesions are most often regarded as "fungal infection." When nonpigmented tumor nodules appear, these are diagnosed as a pyogenic granuloma.

LABORATORY AND SPECIAL EXAMINATIONS

Dermatopathology The histologic diagnosis of the radial growth phase of the volar type of ALM may be difficult and may require large incisional biopsies to provide for multiple sections. There is usually an intense lymphocytic inflammation at the dermoepidermal junction. Characteristic large melanocytes with prominent dendrites along the basal cell layer may extend as large nests into the dermis, as along eccrine ducts.

PATHOPHYSIOLOGY

There is no clear understanding as to why ALM is so much rarer in white people than in brown or black people. The pigmented macules that are frequently seen on the soles of African blacks could be comparable to Clark's dysplastic melanocytic nevi.

PROGNOSIS

The volar type of ALM can be deceptive in its clinical appearance, and "flat" lesions may be quite deeply invasive. Survival rates (five years) are less than 50%.

The subungual type of ALM has a better five-year survival rate, 80%, than ALM (volar type). There are so few patients that the data are probably not accurate. Poor prognosis of ALM (volar type) may be related to inordinate delay in the diagnosis.

TREATMENT

Subungual ALM and volar type ALM: amputation [toe(s), finger(s)] and regional node dissection and/or regional perfusion with chemotherapeutic agents such as melphalan (L-phenylalanine mustard).

Malignant Melanoma Arising in a Preexisting Nevocellular Nevus

The lifetime risk of developing a malignant melanoma in a *giant* congenital nevus cell nevus (GCNN) (so-called garment nevus or bathing-trunk nevus) (Figure 347) is at least 6.3%, and these melanomas often appear before the age of 5 years. GCNN are lesions that cover large areas of the body.

Based on the detection of congenital nevi in association with melanoma using histology and a careful history, there is a significantly increased risk for developing melanoma in persons with small congenital nevus cell nevi (SCNN). This risk is as high as 21-fold based on history, and 3- to 10-fold based on histology. Fifteen percent of 134 patients with primary cutaneous melanoma stated that the melanoma arose in a congenital nevus. Of 234 primary melanomas, 8.1% had nevus cell nevi with congenital features (Figure 348). The expected association of SCNN and melanoma is less than 1 in 171,000 based on chance alone. Therefore, all SCNN should be considered for prophylactic excision at puberty if there are no atypical features (variegated color and irregular borders); SCNN with atypical features should be excised immediately.

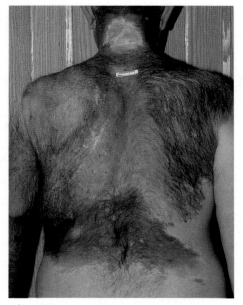

347 Melanoma arising in a giant congenital nevomelanocytic nevus *In this 63-year-old man a primary malignant melanoma developed in the nuchal area.*

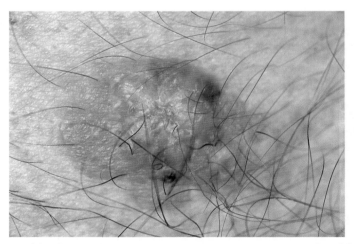

348 Melanoma arising in a small congenital nevus *A 2.0-cm, tan lesion with a 1.0-cm central nodule with pinks, grays, blues, and browns within it. The lesion was on the anterior pectoral area of a 40-year-old white man.*

Precancerous Lesions and Cutaneous Carcinomas

The two principal serious nonmelanoma cancers are squamous cell carcinoma (SCC) and basal cell carcinoma (BCC). Both are invasive into the dermis, and SCC can become metastatic. Certain types (e.g., SCC induced by ionizing radiation or by inorganic trivalent arsenic) can be aggressive and are probably responsible for the mortality from this cancer. BCC in certain locations (nasolabial areas, around the eyes, and in the posterior auricular sulcus) can become deeply invasive and pose a major therapeutic challenge. Invasive SCC of the vulva is induced by human papillomavirus; it is an increasingly common disorder in women under 40 years of age and, while not a highly aggressive tumor, can be associated with carcinoma of the anogenital area, with cancer of the cervix, and with cancer of the bladder.

Oral Leukoplakia

The term *leukoplakia* is a clinical not a histologic designation and describes (in the mouth) a sharply defined, white, macular or slightly raised area which cannot be rubbed off and which remains after the irritation (e.g., tobacco smoking) has been stopped for several weeks. *Candida* infection may be a secondary invader. Leukoplakia must be biopsied to detect the presence of atypical keratinocytes.

EPIDEMIOLOGY

Age 40 to 70 years

Sex Males:females 2:1

Etiology or Predisposing Factors
Smoking (cigarette, cigar, and pipe), oral snuff (smokeless tobacco), alcohol, human papillomavirus (HPV 11 and 16)

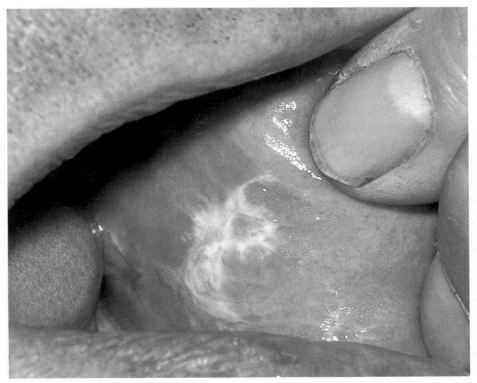

349   Oral leukoplakia   *On the inner side of the left cheek is a white, slightly elevated plaque of firm consistency. It has an irregular margin. The surface is rough. An improperly fitted denture presses against the lesion.*

HISTORY

Duration of Lesions Years

Skin Symptoms None

PHYSICAL EXAMINATION

Mucous Membrane Lesions
TYPE Small or large plaque; homogeneous or "speckled"; ulceration may be present.
COLOR Gray-white
PALPATION Moderately rough or leathery
SHAPE AND SIZE Angular. Size varies from a small (2.0 cm) to very large (4.0 cm) plaque.
SITES OF PREDILECTION Buccal mucosa (Figure 349), retrocommissural mucosa, tongue, hard palate, sublingual region, and gingiva

DIFFERENTIAL DIAGNOSIS

Lichen planus, oral lesion of chronic discoid lupus erythematosus, oral hairy leukoplakia, condyloma acuminatum, bite "callus"

DERMATOPATHOLOGY

Site Epidermis

Process Neoplastic. Dysplasia of keratinocytes with keratinization of single cells, abnormal mitosis, increased nuclear/cytoplasmic ratio, cell and nuclear pleomorphism, enlarged and/or multiple nucleoli

PATHOPHYSIOLOGY

A premalignant lesion arising from chronic irritation or inflammation. Certain types carry a high risk for developing malignancy: (1) leukoplakia that is speckled (with gray and white patches) rather than homogeneous, (2) leukoplakia in certain sites—floor of the mouth and central surface of the tongue. Pipe and cigar smoking can produce *leukokeratosis nicotina palati,* which rarely becomes malignant.

PROGNOSIS

About 10% of leukoplakic lesions can progress to malignancy, and the frequency of this event is related to the site of occurrence. Leukoplakia on the buccal mucosa is almost always found to be benign. On the other hand, leukoplakia on the floor of the mouth is serious, with over 60% showing either carcinoma in situ or invasive squamous cell carcinoma; these patients must be carefully followed. Also, clinically speckled gray and white patches are more likely to develop carcinoma. Oral mouth cancer is clearly related to cigarette smoking, alcohol, oral snuff, and certain dietary factors (especially, high carotenoids may be protective).

TREATMENT

Careful follow-up is important, and all lesions should be biopsied to exclude dysplasia or frank carcinoma. Lesions with dysplasia can be treated with cryosurgery. Recent studies have shown that oral beta-carotene may cause a partial regression of leukoplakia. Leukoplakia that shows in situ carcinoma or invasive carcinoma must be surgically excised.

Radiation dermatitis is defined as skin changes resulting from exposure to ionizing radiation. There are *reversible effects*: erythema, epilation, suppression of sebaceous glands, and pigmentation which lasts for weeks to months to years; and *irreversible effects*: acute and chronic radiation dermatitis, radiation-induced cancers.

TYPE OF EXPOSURE

Result of therapy (for cancer, formerly used for acne and psoriasis), accidental, or occupational (e.g., formerly in physicians, dentists)

TYPES OF REACTIONS

Acute   Temporary erythema which lasts 3 days and then the main erythema which reaches a peak in 2 weeks (Figure 350*a*); pigmentation appears about day 20; a late erythema can also occur beginning on day 35 to 40 and this lasts 2 to 3 weeks. Permanent scarring may result.

Chronic   Following *fractional* but relatively intensive therapy with total doses of 3000 to 6000 rad there develops an epidermolytic reaction in 3 weeks. This is repaired in 3 to 6 weeks and scars and hypopigmentation develop; there is loss of all appendages and atrophy of the epidermis and dermis. During the next 2 to 5 years the atrophy increases; there is hyper- and hypopigmentation, superficial venules become telangiectatic. Ulceration is rare except by accidental exposure or error in doses. *Very small doses at infrequent intervals (monthly or weekly) or relatively large doses.* This occurs mostly in occupational exposure and affects the hands, feet, and face. There is a destruction of the fingerprint pattern, xerosis, scanty hair, atrophy of sebaceous and sweat glands, development of keratoses (Figure 350*b*). Persistent painful ulcers may appear.

Generalized Exanthems   These occur beyond the irradiated area and usually follow deep x-ray therapy for internal cancers, given through multiple ports. There may be fever and a dermatosis mimicking erythema multiforme, or urticaria.

PHYSICAL EXAMINATION

Skin Lesions   See Figures 350*a* and *b*.
TYPE   See above descriptions of acute and chronic radiation dermatitis
SHAPE
  Sharp borders, rectangular, square (when result of therapy)
  Diffuse involvement (when result of prolonged, repeated exposures, as on the hands)
DISTRIBUTION
  Hands and fingers (in professional personnel, dentists, or physicians)
  Any site of previous therapy with ionizing radiation

Nails   Longitudinal striations (in chronic— following repeated exposures)

DERMATOPATHOLOGY (CHRONIC RADIATION DERMATITIS)

Site   Epidermis and dermis

We acknowledge the contribution of Profs. F. Urbach and A. Wiskemann.

PRECANCEROUS LESIONS AND CUTANEOUS CARCINOMAS

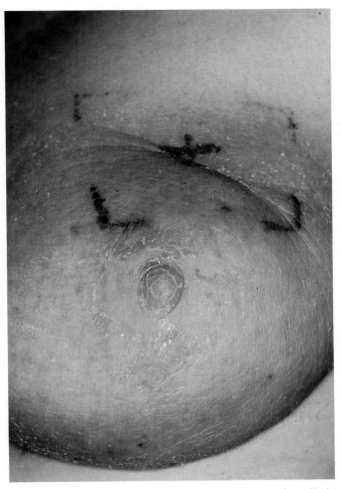

350a   Radiodermatitis, acute   *Localized area of erythema and edema in the radiation portal occurring at the end of course of radiotherapy for breast cancer.*

RADIATION DERMATITIS

Atrophy of epidermis, with loss of hair follicles, sebaceous glands, and alteration of sweat glands

Hyalinization, loss of nuclei, fusion of collagen and elastic tissue

Vessel changes including telangiectatic dilatation and fibrous thickening of the arterial wall resulting in endarteritis obliterans

COURSE, PROGNOSIS, AND TREATMENT

Chronic radiation dermatitis is permanent, progressive, and irreversible. Squamous cell carcinoma (SCC) may develop in 4 to 39 years, with a median of 7 to 12 years, almost exclusively from the chronic repeated type of exposures. SCC always develops within the area of radiodermatitis, never in normal skin. SCC appears usually on three sites: hands, feet, rarely the face. The tumors are often multiple and metastasize late in about 25%; despite extensive surgery (excision, grafts, etc.) the prognosis is poor, recurrences are common. In recent years there has been about an equal incidence of SCC and basal cell carcinomas. Basal cell carcinomas appear mostly in patients formerly treated with x-ray for acne vulgaris and acne cystica or epilation (tinea capitis).

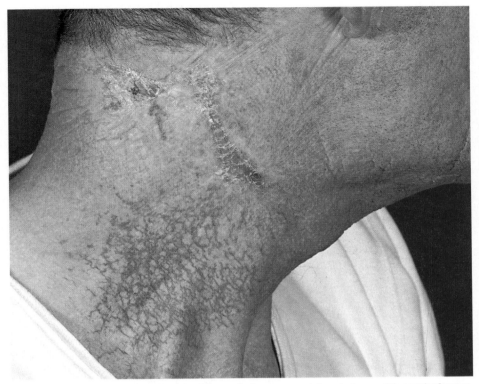

350b Radiodermatitis   *The right side of the neck shows many telangiectases with a reticular pattern. The skin is atrophic. Near the scalp is a scaling crusted patch; after removal of this crust a superficial ulcer became apparent. Just below the lower mandibula is a somewhat linear, erythematous, slightly indurated scaling lesion.*

Basal cell carcinoma (BCC) is the most common type of skin cancer, and the majority of lesions are readily controlled by various surgical techniques or cryotherapy. Small, well-circumscribed BCC in nonrisk areas may also be treated by curettage and electrocoagulation. Serious problems, however, may occur with BCC arising in certain locations on the face: around the eyes, in the nasolabial folds, around the ear canal, or in the posterior auricular sulcus. In these sites the tumor may invade deeply.

EPIDEMIOLOGY AND ETIOLOGY

Incidence USA: 500 to 1000 per 100,000, higher in the sunbelt; 400,000 new patients annually

Age Over 40 years

Sex Males more than females

Race Rare in brown- and black-skinned persons

Predisposing Factors White-skinned persons with poor tanning capacity (skin phototypes I and II) and albinos are highly susceptible to develop BCC with prolonged sun exposure. Previous therapy with x-ray for facial acne greatly increases the risk of BCC, even in those persons with good ability to tan (skin phototypes III and IV). In the *basal cell nevus syndrome,* BCC occurs in both sun-exposed skin and areas protected from the sun. The *basal cell nevus syndrome* is an autosomal dominant disorder (see page 696).

PHYSICAL EXAMINATION

Skin Lesions

TYPE Papule or nodule, translucent or "pearly." Ulcer (often covered with a crust) with a rolled border (rodent ulcer) (Figure 351).

COLOR Pink or red; fine telangiectasia can be seen with the aid of a hand lens. Pigmented BCC may be brown to blue or black (Figure 352).

PALPATION Hard, firm; cystic lesions may occur, however.

SHAPE Round, oval, depressed center ("umbilicated")

DISTRIBUTION Isolated single lesion (Figure 353); multiple lesions are not infrequent (Figure 354). Search carefully for danger sites: medial and lateral canthi, nasolabial fold.

Variants

SCLEROSING (SCLERODERMIFORM OR MORPHEA-LIKE) BCC (See Figure 355) In this infiltrating type of BCC there is an excessive amount of fibrous stroma. The lesion therefore appears as a whitish, sclerotic patch with ill-defined borders and only occasional pearly papules at the periphery. Histologically, fingerlike strands of tumor extend far into the surrounding tissue, and excision therefore requires wide margins.

SUPERFICIAL MULTICENTRIC BCC (See Figure 356) These superficial lesions are usually multiple, occur on the trunk, and often have no relation to sun exposure. They appear as erythematous, slightly scaly plaques, often but not always with a fine, rolled, pearly border. These lesions can mimic psoriasis, seborrheic keratosis, Bowen's disease, tinea corporis.

PIGMENTED BCC These may occur in skin phototypes IV and V and are easily con-

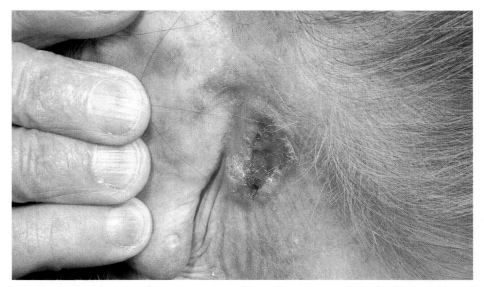

351 Basal cell carcinoma, rodent ulcer type *A solitary ulcer (diameter 2.5 cm) with firm, elevated border and an occasional crust. The site of this lesion is precarious because the initial treatment must be definitive. The best treatment is the Mohs microscopically controlled excision.*

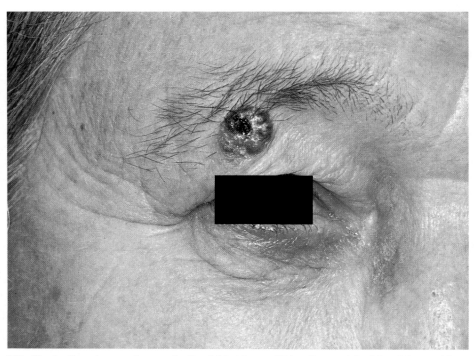

352 Basal cell carcinoma, pigmented *On right upper eyelid is a firm nodule, 2.5 × 2.5 cm, with an irregular surface and ulceration in the center. Color: brownish black, translucent. These lesions may be virtually indistinguishable from a nodular melanoma.*

BASAL CELL CARCINOMA

fused with primary malignant melanoma, especially nodular melanoma.

DIAGNOSIS

Serious BCC occurring in the danger sites are readily detectable by careful examination with good lighting, a hand lens, and careful palpation.

DERMATOPATHOLOGY

Site Epidermis and dermis

Process Proliferating atypical basal cells (large, oval, deep-blue staining on H&E, but with little anaplasia and infrequent mitoses) with variable amounts of stroma

TREATMENT

Excision with primary closure, skin flaps, or grafts. Cryosurgery and electrosurgery are options.

For lesions in the danger zones (nasolabial area, around the eyes, in the ear canal, in the posterior auricular sulcus, and in the sclerosing BCC) microscopically controlled surgery (Mohs surgery) is the best approach. Radiation therapy is an acceptable alternative but should be given only when disfigurement may be a problem with surgical excision (e.g., eyelids or large lesions in the nasolabial area).

Cryosurgery, curettage, and electrosurgery

PRECANCEROUS LESIONS AND CUTANEOUS CARCINOMAS

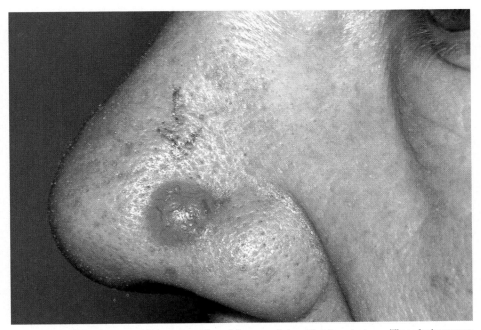

353   Basal cell carcinoma, nodular type   *Firm, 1.5-cm nodule with telangiectases. These lesions may be virtually indistinguishable from dermal nevomelanocytic nevi.*

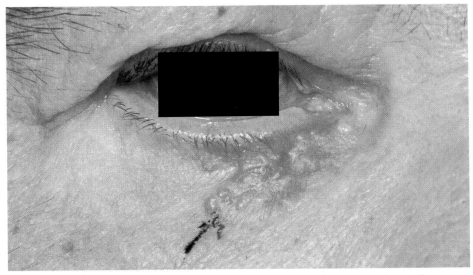

354   Basal cell carcinoma, nodular type   *Clusters of firm, skin-colored, translucent nodules over an area of 7.0 to 20.0 mm, some of which have become confluent.*

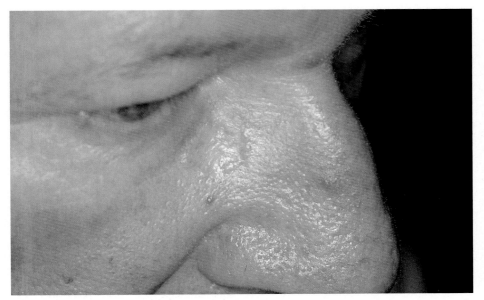

355 Basal cell carcinoma, cicatrizing *Just below the inner canthus of the right eye is a barely visible, slightly white, very slightly elevated, firm lesion which is better felt than seen. Histologically there are fingerlike projections of cancerous cells into the dermis and subcutaneous tissue layers. This lesion is best treated by Mohs microscopically controlled surgery.*

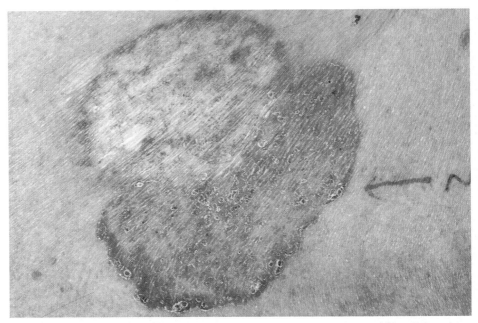

356 Basal cell carcinoma, superficial multicentric type *On the back, a plaque of 6.0 × 5.0 cm merging with an atrophic macule. The plaque shows a reticular red infiltration with a slightly elevated, firm, scaling border with a pearl-like aspect. The right-hand lesion is white, atrophic, with telangiectases and a red border.*

BASAL CELL CARCINOMA

This autosomal dominant disorder affects skin (multiple basal cell carcinomas and palmoplantar pits) and has a variable expression of abnormalities in a number of systems, including bones, soft tissue, eyes, CNS, and endocrine organs.

EPIDEMIOLOGY

Incidence Frequency not known but the condition is not rare.

Age The basal cell carcinomas may begin in late childhood, although several abnormalities are congenital.

Race Mostly white but also occurs in African-Americans and Asians.

Sex Equal incidence

Precipitating Factors There appear to be more basal cell carcinomas on the sun-exposed areas of the skin, but they can occur in covered areas also.

HISTORY

Duration of Lesions The basal cell carcinomas begin to appear singly in childhood or early adolescence and continue to appear throughout life; there may be thousands of skin cancers.

Systems Review Congenital anomalies include undescended testes, hydrocephalus, blindness from coloboma, cataracts, glaucoma.

Family History Autosomal dominant with variable penetrance

PHYSICAL EXAMINATION

Appearance of Patient There may be hundreds of lesions. Characteristic facies, with frontal bossing, broad nasal root, and hypertelorism

Skin
PRINCIPAL LESIONS Basal cell carcinomas (translucent, 1.0- to 10.0-cm papules and nodules with and without ulcers) that are skin colored or pigmented. Invasive tumors are not uncommon. Tumors on the eyelids, axillae, and neck tend to be pedunculated.
ARRANGEMENT Bilateral, symmetrical
DISTRIBUTION OF LESIONS Face (Figure 357), neck, trunk, axillae, usually sparing scalp and extremities
PALMOPLANTAR LESIONS (See Figure 358) Present in 50% and these pits are pinpoint to several millimeters in size and 1.0 mm deep. There may be hundreds of lesions especially on the lateral surfaces of the palms, soles, and fingers. The pits are the result of premature shedding of the horny layer. There may rarely be a basal cell carcinoma at the bottom of the pit, and there are almost always telangiectases at the bottom of the pit.
EXTRACUTANEOUS LESIONS *Bone* Mandibular jaw cysts, which are multiple and may be unilateral or bilateral odontogenic keratocysts. Other bone lesions include defective dentition, bifid or splayed ribs, pectus excavatum, short fourth metacarpals, scoliosis, and kyphosis.
Eye Strabismus, hypertelorism, dystopia canthorum, and congenital blindness

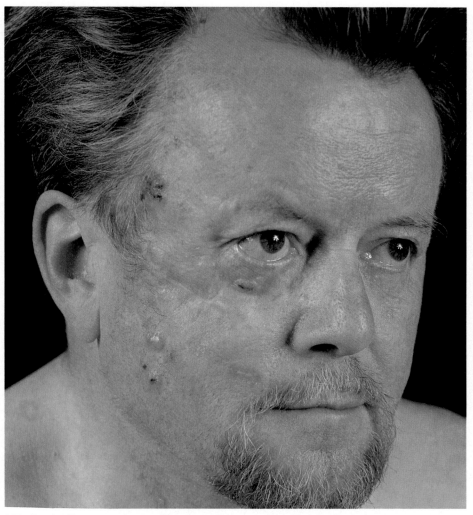

357 Basal cell nevus syndrome *There are a large number of basal cell carcinomas, especially on the right side of the face. There is also frontal bossing.*

Central Nervous System Agenesis of the corpus callosum, medulloblastoma; mental retardation is rare.

Other Neoplasms Fibrosarcoma of the jaw, ovarian fibromas, teratomas, and cystadenomas

LABORATORY EXAMINATIONS

Dermatopathology
LIGHT MICROSCOPY All types of basal cell carcinomas: solid, adenoid, cystic, keratotic, superficial, and fibrosing

IMAGING

Lamellar calcification of the falx is a useful diagnostic sign.

DIAGNOSIS

The disease is often discovered by oral surgeons or dentists and the patient referred to a dermatologist who detects the palmar pits and observes the characteristic facies.

ETIOLOGY AND PATHOGENESIS

Chromosome abnormalities, increased chromosome breakage, and deletions of some chromosomes have been observed.

SIGNIFICANCE

The large number of skin cancers create a lifetime problem of vigilance on the part of the patient and the physician. The multiple excisions can cause considerable scarring.

COURSE AND PROGNOSIS

The tumors continue throughout life and the patient must be carefully followed to detect early lesions in order to prevent disfiguring scars.

TREATMENT

Surgical excision and Mohs surgery for cancers in certain locations. Small lesions can be treated with electrocautery.

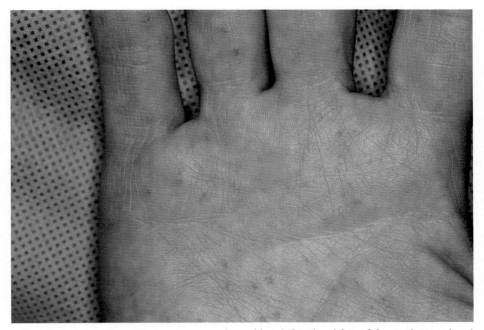

358 Basal cell nevus syndrome *Palmar surface of hand showing 1.0- to 2.0-mm depressed, red lesions, i.e., palmar pits.*

Squamous Cell Carcinoma of Skin and Mucous Membranes

Squamous cell carcinoma (SCC) is a malignant tumor of epithelial keratinocytes (skin and mucous membrane). SCC arises as a result of exogenous carcinogens [sunlight exposure, ingestion of arsenic, exposure to ionizing radiation (x-rays and gamma rays), and other etiologies].

EPIDEMIOLOGY AND ETIOLOGY

Incidence   Continental USA: 12 per 100,000 white males; 7 per 100,000 white females; 1 per 100,000 blacks. Hawaii: 62 per 100,000 whites

Race   Persons with white skin and poor tanning capacity (skin phototypes I and II). Brown- or black-skinned persons can develop SCC from numerous etiologic agents other than sunlight exposure.

Age   Over 55 years

Sex   Males > females, but SCC can occur more frequently on the legs in females.

Geography   SCC induced by sunlight exposure is most common in geographic areas that have many days of sunshine annually and are inhabited by fair-skinned individuals. Penile SCC accounts for approximately 20% of SCC in developing countries; however, in the United States, penile SCC accounts for only 1% of all SCC.

Occupation   Persons (usually male) working outdoors—farmers, sailors, telephone linemen, construction workers, dock workers. Industrial workers exposed to chemical carcinogens (nitrosureas, polycyclic aromatic hydrocarbons)

CLASSIFICATION OF INTRAEPITHELIAL (IN SITU) SCC

1. Solar (actinic) keratosis (see page 220)
2. Ionizing radiation-induced keratoses
3. Arsenical keratoses
4. Bowen's disease
5. Tar keratosis
6. Xeroderma pigmentosum (see page 624)
7. Squamous intraepidermal neoplasia, including vulvar intraepithelial neoplasms, bowenoid papulosis
8. Erythroplasia of Queyrat

PREDISPOSING FACTORS IN ADDITION TO SUNLIGHT EXPOSURE

Human papillomavirus (induction of carcinoma of the anogenital area and periungal skin); the types of HPV linked to carcinomas in these areas are HPV 16, 18, 31, 33, and 35. *Immunosuppression* (a major factor in rapidly promoting SCC and BCC in the sun-exposed sites of the skin of renal transplant patients on immunosuppressive drugs); *topical nitrogen mustards* (for the treatment of mycosis fungoides, can induce cutaneous SCC); *oral PUVA photochemotherapy* (can lead to promotion of SCC in patients who are skin phototypes I and

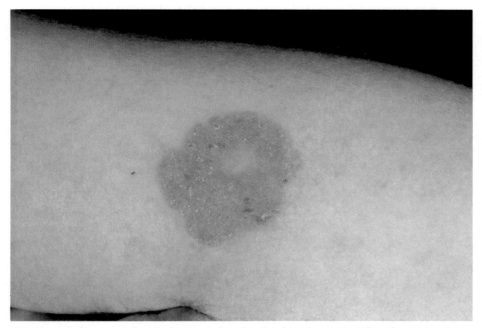

359 Bowen's disease *A sharply demarcated, scaly, often hyperkeratotic and erythematous plaque (as shown here on the arm), macule, or papule. The lesion arises de novo and can arise in any site including the penis, where it is called erythroplasia of Queyrat.*

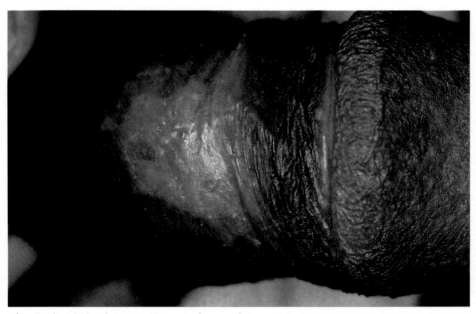

360 Erythroplasia of Queyrat (Bowen's disease of the penis) *Solitary, well-circumscribed plaque with areas of erosion. Lesion was in a 70-year-old uncircumcised black male.*

SQUAMOUS CELL CARCINOMA OF SKIN AND MUCOUS MEMBRANES 701

II and those patients with psoriasis who have had previous exposure to ionizing radiation, including grenz rays); *chronic ulcers* (of any etiology); *discoid lupus erythematosus* (a rare event); *industrial carcinogens* (pitch, tar, crude paraffin oil, fuel oil, creosote, lubricating oil); *arsenic* (inorganic trivalent arsenic as a medication in the past, as Fowler's solution used as a tonic and for the treatment of psoriasis; nowadays arsenic is present in the drinking water).

BOWEN'S DISEASE AND ERYTHROPLASIA OF QUEYRAT

Bowen's disease is a solitary lesion (Figure 359) on the exposed (induced by solar radiation) and on the unexposed (related to ingestion of inorganic trivalent arsenic) skin. The lesion appears as a slowly enlarging erythematous macule with a sharp border and little or no infiltration. There is usually slight scaling and some crusting. There is not a fine threadlike border as is seen in superficial basal cell carcinoma.

When this lesion occurs, usually in uncircumcised men, on the glans penis (Figure 360), coronal sulcus, or inner surface of the prepuce, it is known as *erythroplasia of Queyrat,* although it is identical clinically and histologically to Bowen's disease. The lesions of erythroplasia of Queyrat, however, are believed to metastasize more frequently (up to 30% in one series) than Bowen's disease on the glabrous skin.

HISTORY

Slowly evolving—any isolated, keratotic, eroded papule or plaque in a suspect patient that persists for over a month is carcinoma until proved otherwise.

PHYSICAL EXAMINATION

Skin Lesions (Sun-Induced)

TYPE   Indurated papule, plaque, or nodule; adherent thick keratotic scale; lesion often eroded, crusted, or ulcerated. In situ SCC appears as red, well-demarcated plaques with fine scale.

COLOR   Erythematous (Bowen's disease)

PALPATION   Hard

SHAPE   Polygonal, oval, round, or umbilicated

DISTRIBUTION   Isolated lesion or multiple discrete lesions. Exposed areas. Sun-induced keratotic and/or ulcerated lesions: especially on the face [cheeks, nose, lips (Figure 361)], tips of the ears, preauricular area, scalp (in bald men), dorsa of the hands (Figure 362) and forearms, trunk, shins (females)

MISCELLANEOUS OTHER SKIN CHANGES   Evidence of chronic sun exposure, which is termed *dermatoheliosis*: telangiectasia, freckling, dry scaly atrophic skin, small hypopigmented macules

OTHER PHYSICAL FINDINGS   Regional lymphadenopathy (35% in SCC arising in the lip or mouth)

Skin Lesions (Not Sun-Induced)

SCC of the penis arising in erythroplasia of Queyrat (Figure 363)

SCC of the lip may arise in areas of leukoplakia, and 90% occur on the lower lip

SCC arising in radiation-damaged skin may grow rapidly

SCC arising in a burn scar may be concealed under the scar

SCC arising in arsenical keratoses (Figure 364)

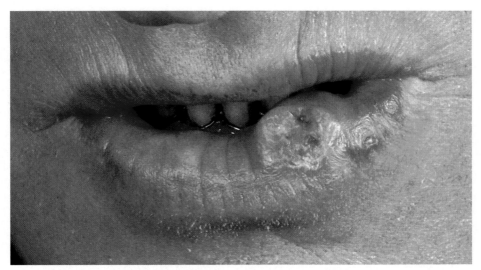

361 Squamous cell carcinoma *An elevated ulcerating nodule on the left lower lip. No lymphadenopathy. These lesions are induced by tobacco smoking (pipe and cigar), but the most common etiology is prolonged exposure to solar radiation.*

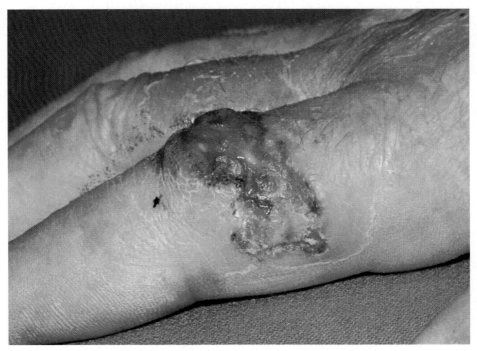

362 Squamous cell carcinoma *Ulcerations, 1.5 × 2.0 cm, with a serpiginous elevated border and a red granulating floor. (On the dorsal side of the phalanx of finger III, redness with a scaling border.) The ulcer was freely movable in relation to the bone. No enlargement of regional lymph nodes.*

SQUAMOUS CELL CARCINOMA OF SKIN AND MUCOUS MEMBRANES

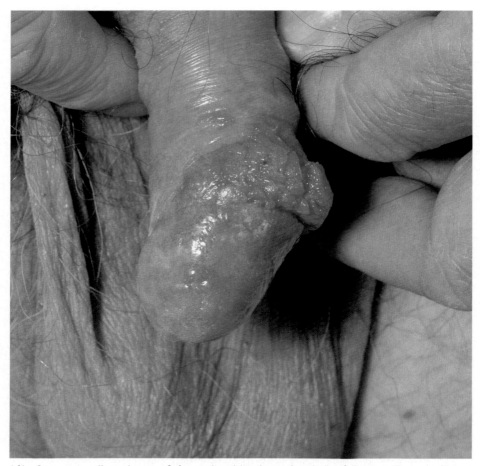

363 Squamous cell carcinoma of the penis arising in erythroplasia of Queyrat (Bowen's disease)
Glistening, velvety, red plaque of squamous cell carcinoma in situ on the glans penis and prepuce with a fungating squamous cell carcinoma arising within it.

DIAGNOSIS AND DIFFERENTIAL DIAGNOSIS

As stated previously, any persistent nodule or ulcer but especially when these occur in sun-damaged skin, in an area of radiodermatitis, or in an old burn scar must be examined for SCC. In situ SCC: nummular eczema, Paget's disease, superficial multicentric BCC.

DERMATOPATHOLOGY

Site Epidermis and dermis, and in deeper lesions subcutaneous tissue

Process Proliferating anaplastic cells that extend in broad masses into the dermis and subcutaneous tissue.

PRECANCEROUS LESIONS AND CUTANEOUS CARCINOMAS

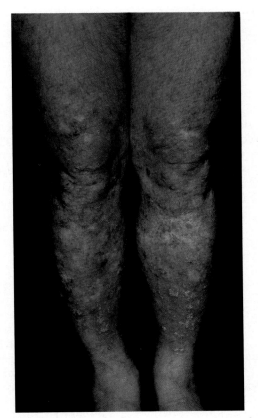

364　Arsenical keratoses and squamous cell carcinomas　*On the lower legs, from the knee down, are numerous verrucous papules and plaques. There are also squamous cell carcinomas which consist of erythematous, scaling, crusted lesions that slowly increase in size.*

TREATMENT

The choice of surgery or radiation depends on the size, shape, and localization of the tumor, and the decision should be made by a team approach of the surgeon and the radiotherapist. Microscopically controlled surgery is best for many lesions.

PROGNOSIS

SCC has an overall remission rate after therapy of 90%. Those tumors that are induced by ionizing radiation, or following inorganic trivalent arsenic, or in an old burn scar are more likely to metastasize. SCC in patients with arsenical ingestion can develop primary SCC of the lung and the bladder. There is some debate about the aggressiveness of sun-induced SCC, but the mortality is believed by most to be very low.

Merkel Cell Carcinoma (Trabecular Carcinoma)

This is a malignant solid tumor thought to be derived from a specialized epithelial cell, the Merkel cell: a nondendritic, nonkeratinizing, "clear" cell present in the basal cell layer of the epidermis, free in the dermis, and around hair follicles as the hair disk of Pinkus. The tumor may be solitary or multiple and occurs on the head and on the extremities. There is a high rate of recurrence following excision but, more important, it spreads to the regional lymph nodes in more than 50% of the patients and can be disseminated to the viscera and CNS.

EPIDEMIOLOGY

Incidence Rare, <500 reported patients

Age 15 to 90 years, mean age 65

HISTORY

Duration of Lesions Slowly growing

Skin Symptoms Asymptomatic

Systems Review Negative

PHYSICAL EXAMINATION

Skin Findings
TYPE OF LESION Papule or nodule (Figure 365)
Color Pink, red-to-violet
Palpation Firm
SHAPE OF INDIVIDUAL LESION Dome-shaped
ARRANGEMENT OF MULTIPLE LESIONS Scattered lesions in one region, such as the scalp or an extremity
DISTRIBUTION OF LESIONS Head and neck (50%), extremities (35%, mostly the lower), trunk (10%)

General Examination Search for lymph nodes (involved in over 50% of patients but not always palpable)

LABORATORY AND SPECIAL EXAMINATIONS

Dermatopathology
LIGHT MICROSCOPY *Site* Arises in the dermis; sparing of the epidermis. The tumor cells form trabeculae extending down into the subcutaneous tissue.
Process Neoplastic proliferation
Cell Types May resemble lymphoma, carcinoma, oat-cell carcinoma, sweat gland carcinoma, or neuroblastoma
SPECIAL TECHNIQUES *Special Stains* The cells contain variable numbers of granules which darken with silver nitrate stains. They contain neuron-specific enolase and low-molecular-weight cytokeratins.
Transmission Electron Microscopy Cytoplasmic organelles, 80 to 180 nm, which are round, with a dense core, similar to those present in normal Merkel cells. The cells also contain characteristic perinuclear filament whorls.

DIFFERENTIAL DIAGNOSIS

These firm, solid tumors are confusing to the clinician who must consider the diagnoses of *squamous cell carcinoma, desmoplastic melanoma, amelanotic melanoma,* or *metastatic cancer.* The histologic diagnosis is that of a small cell malignant tumor and includes, among others, *metastatic (lung) oat-cell carci-*

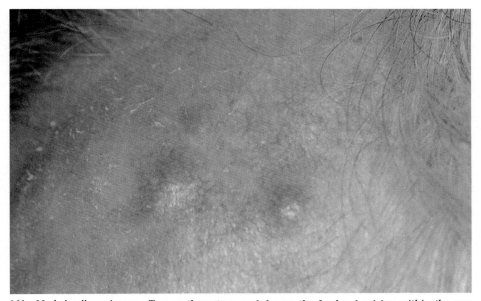

365　Merkel cell carcinoma　*Two erythematous nodules on the forehead arising within the scar from an earlier excision of the lesion, representing recurrence.*

noma, which is especially confounding because this tumor also contains neuroendocrine granules and neurofilaments and stains for neuron-specific enolase.

PATHOPHYSIOLOGY

The Merkel cell is thought to be of neuroendocrine origin but, at least in the mouse, has been shown to be within the epidermis before neurites have reached the epithelium. It functions as a specific, slowly adapting, sensory (touch) receptor in the epidermis and dermis, contains neuroendocrine features such as dense core granules, and shows immunoreactivity for neuroendocrine peptides and low-molecular-weight cytokeratins.

SIGNIFICANCE

These tumors are unpredictable and the patient must be carefully followed and appropriate treatments done, as outlined under Treatment.

COURSE

Recurrence rates are high, with a 5-month average for local recurrence. Patients are followed monthly for the first 6 months, every 3 months for the next 2 years, and then biannually.

PROGNOSIS

The mortality rate is 18%.

TREATMENT

Excision by Mohs surgery and prophylactic regional node dissection are advocated because of the high rate of regional metastases. In one series, *even without a local recurrence,* a large number of patients (60%) developed regional nodal metastases, and in those patients with local recurrence 86% developed regional node metastases. Therefore the excision should be followed by prophylactic radiotherapy to the nodal areas.

Cutaneous Lymphomas, Histiocytoses, and Mastocytosis

Adult T-Cell Leukemia/Lymphoma

Adult T-cell leukemia/lymphoma (ATL/L) is a neoplasm of the helper T-cell, caused by human T-cell lymphotrophic virus-I (HTLV-I), manifested by skin infiltrates, hypercalcemia, visceral involvement, lytic bone lesions, and abnormal lymphocytes on the peripheral smears.

EPIDEMIOLOGY AND ETIOLOGY

Age   Average age of onset 35 to 55 years

Sex   Male > female

Race   Japanese, blacks

Etiology   HTLV-I, a human retrovirus. Malignant cells are T-helper cells phenotypically, but T-suppressor cells functionally.

Transmission   Sexual intercourse; perinatally; exposure to blood or blood products (same as HIV)

Geography   Southwestern Japan (Kyushu); Africa; Caribbean Islands; southeastern United States

HISTORY

Systems Review   Fever, weight loss, abdominal pain, diarrhea, pleural effusion, ascites, cough, sputum

PHYSICAL EXAMINATION

Skin Findings
TYPE OF LESION   Lesions occur in 50% of ATL/L. Single to multiple papules/nodules (Figures 366a and 366b) ± purpura; large plaques ± ulceration; generalized erythroderma; poikiloderma; papulosquamous lesions; diffuse alopecia
COLOR   Erythematous, violaceous, brown
PALPATION   Firm lesions
DISTRIBUTION OF LESIONS   Trunk > face > extremities

General Examination
ABDOMEN   Hepatomegaly (50%), splenomegaly (25%)
LYMPH NODES   Lymphadenopathy (75%) sparing mediastinal lymph nodes

DIAGNOSIS AND DIFFERENTIAL DIAGNOSIS

Diagnosis   Characteristic clinical findings, seropositivity to HTLV-I, confirmation of integration of HTLV-I proviral DNA in the cellular DNA of the ATL/L cells.

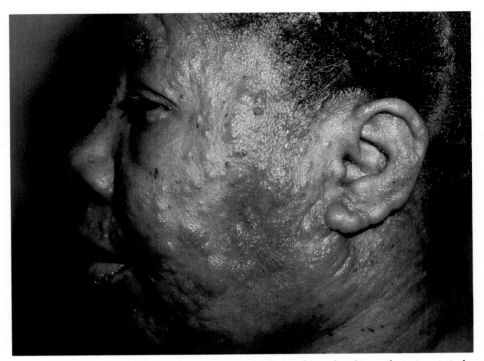

366a   Adult T-cell leukemia/lymphoma   *Multiple, confluent, skin-colored to erythematous papules and nodules seen on the face and ear. These infiltrative lesions appeared over a 3-month period. (Courtesy of Joseph C. Kvedar, M.D.)*

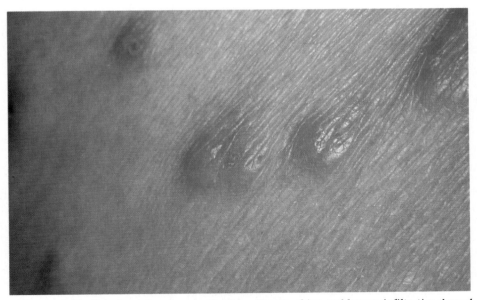

366b   Adult T-cell leukemia/lymphoma   *Multiple, discrete, shiny, red-brown infiltrative dermal nodules. (Courtesy of Y. Hori, M.D.)*

ADULT T-CELL LEUKEMIA/LYMPHOMA

Differential Diagnosis Cutaneous T-cell lymphoma (mycosis fungoides), Sézary's syndrome

LABORATORY AND SPECIAL EXAMINATIONS

Hematology WBC ranges from normal to 500,000. Peripheral blood smear—polylobulated lymphocytic nuclei, resembling Sézary cells

Dermatopathology Perivascular and/or diffuse infiltrates with large abnormal lymphocytes in the upper to middermis; epidermis often spared. Alternatively, dense intradermal infiltration and Pautrier's microabscesses, composed of many large abnormal lymphocytes, ± giant cells

Chemistry Hypercalcemia: 25% at time of diagnosis of ATL/L; >50% during clinical course

Serology Seropositive (ELISA, Western blot) to HTLV-I; in IVDU, up to 30% have dual retroviral infection with both HTLV-I and HIV

PATHOPHYSIOLOGY

Hypercalcemia felt to be due to osteoclastic bone resorption.

COURSE AND PROGNOSIS

Approximately 1 in 1500 individuals seropositive to HTLV-I go on to develop ATL/L. Course may be smoldering or chronic for prolonged period (abnormal lymphocytosis, skin infiltrates, modest bone marrow involvement), interrupted by an acute crisis. Mean survival with acute crisis in hypercalcemic patients, 12.5 weeks (range, 2 weeks to >1 year); if normocalcemic, 50 weeks. Therapeutic response—limited if at all. Cause of death: opportunistic infections, disseminated intravascular coagulation

TREATMENT

Combination chemotherapy

Obtain HTLV-I serology of family members, sexual partners. If seropositive, should not donate blood.

Cutaneous T-cell lymphoma (CTCL) is a term that applies to T-cell lymphoma first manifested in the skin, but, as the neoplastic process involves the entire lymphoreticular system, the lymph nodes and internal organs become involved in the course of the disease. CTCL is a malignancy of helper T cells.

Synonym: mycosis fungoides.

EPIDEMIOLOGY AND ETIOLOGY

Age 50 years (range, 5 to 70 years)

Sex Male:female ratio 2:1

Incidence Two per 1,000,000 population (about 200 deaths per year in the United States).

Etiology Human T lymphotrophic virus (HTLV) in some patients

HISTORY

Duration of Lesions Months to years, often preceded by nonspecific diagnoses such as psoriasis, nummular dermatitis, and "large plaque" parapsoriasis

Skin Symptoms Pruritus, often intractable, but may be none

Constitutional Symptoms Fever (in late tumor stage)

Systems Review Negative except in late stages with visceral organ involvement

PHYSICAL FINDINGS

Skin Findings
TYPE OF LESION
   Plaques, scaling (Figure 367) or not scal-

ing, large (>3.0 cm), at first superficial, much like "eczema" or psoriasis or mimicking a "mycosis," and later becoming thicker or "infiltrated" (Figure 368)

Nodules and tumors with or without ulcers

COLOR Different shades of red
SHAPE Round, oval, arciform, annular (Figure 369), concentric, bizarre
ARRANGEMENT Randomly distributed discrete plaques, nodules, and tumors, or diffuse involvement with erythroderma (Sézary's syndrome) and palmoplantar keratoderma
DISTRIBUTION Often spares exposed areas (in early stages). No typical distribution pattern, random localization.

General Examination Careful examination for lymphadenopathy

Sézary's Syndrome This is a leukemic form of CTCL consisting of (1) erythroderma, (2) lymphadenopathy, (3) elevated WBC (>20,000) with a high proportion of so-called Sézary cells, (4) hair loss, and (5) pruritus.

DIAGNOSIS AND DIFFERENTIAL DIAGNOSIS

Diagnosis In the early stages the diagnosis of CTCL is a problem. Clinical lesions may be typical but histologic confirmation may not be possible for years despite repeated biopsies.

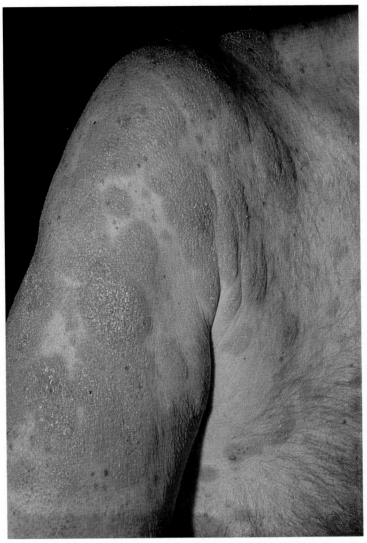

367   Mycosis fungoides (CTCL) plaque stage   *Psoriasiform lesions that are "infiltrated" on palpation. This patient was initially diagnosed as having psoriasis and was treated for a few years with UVB phototherapy.*

One-micron-thick sections may be helpful. For early diagnosis, cytophotometry (estimation of aneuploidy and polyploidy) and estimation of the indentation of pathologic cells (nucleocontour index) are helpful. Fresh tissue should be sent for analysis of cellular makeup by the use of monoclonal antibodies. Lymphadenopathy and the detection of abnormal circulating T cells in the blood appear to correlate well with *internal* organ involvement, and surgical staging is often not necessary. See TNM classification (Table A).

Differential Diagnosis High index of suspicion is needed in patients with atypical or refractory psoriasis, eczema, and poikiloderma atrophicans vasculare. Repeated biopsies are necessary. CTCL often mimics psoriasis in being a scaly plaque and disappearing with sunlight exposure.

LABORATORY AND SPECIAL EXAMINATIONS

Repeated and multiple (3) biopsies often necessary to finally establish the diagnosis.

Dermatopathology
SITE   Epidermis and dermis

1. Mycosis cells: T cells with hyperchromatic, irregularly shaped nuclei. Mitoses vary from rare to frequent.
2. Microabscesses in the epidermis (containing "mycosis" cells).
3. Bandlike and patchy infiltrate in upper dermis of atypical lymphocytes (mycosis cells) extending to skin appendages. Abnormal T cell can be identified by electron microscopy (and by experienced investigators somtimes even by light microscopy): typically convoluted nucleus.
4. Monoclonal-antibody techniques identify most mycosis cells as helper/inducer T cells.

Hematologic Eosinophilia, 6 to 12%, could increase to 50%. Buffy coat: abnormal circulating T cells (Sézary type) and increased white blood count (20,000). Bone marrow examination is not helpful.

Chemistry Lactic dehydrogenase isoenzymes 1, 2, 3 increased in erythrodermic stage

Chest X-Ray Search for hilar lymphadenopathy.

Liver-Spleen Scan To identify any focal areas

CT Scan To search for retroperitoneal nodes in patients with extensive skin involvement, lymphadenopathy, or tumors in the skin

COURSE AND PROGNOSIS

The course is quite unpredictable until a histologic diagnosis is made; i.e., a clinical diagnosis of suspicious CTCL (pre-CTCL) may be present for years. Once histologic diagnosis is made, the course of the disease varies with the source of the patient material studied: at the National Institutes of Health in the United States there was a median survival rate of 5 years from the time of the histologic diagnosis, while in Europe a less malignant course is seen; and, similarly, it would appear that, in office practice, there is a prolonged course (sometimes 10 to 15 years). After histologic diagnosis is made, everyone agrees that prognosis is much worse when (1) tumors are present (mean survival, 2.5 years), (2) there is lymphadenopathy (mean survival, 3 years), (3) more than 10% of the skin surface is involved with pretumor stage CTCL, and (4) there is a generalized erythroderma. Patients under 50 have twice the survival rate of patients over 60.

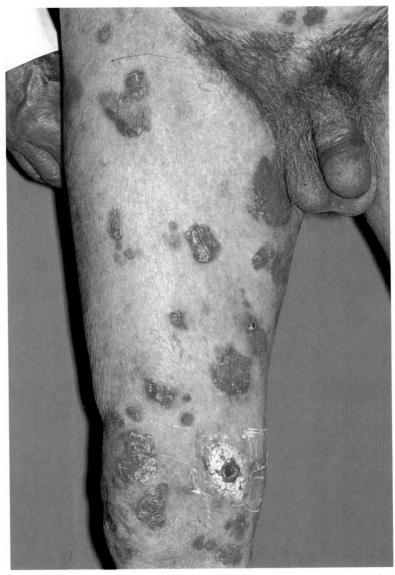

368   Mycosis fungoides (CTCL)   *Infiltrated scaling plaques with ulceration in one lesion. This patient was originally treated for psoriasis.*

TREATMENT (SEE TABLE B)

If the pre-CTCL stage, in which the histologic diagnosis is not established, PUVA photochemotherapy is the least harmful effective treatment. For histologically proved plaque-stage disease with no lymphadenopathy and with no circulating abnormal T cells, PUVA photochemotherapy is also the method of choice. Also used at this stage are topical chemotherapy with nitrogen mustard in an ointment base (10 mg%) and total electron-beam therapy, singly or in combination. If isolated tumors should develop, these should be treated with local x-ray or electron-beam therapy. For extensive plaque stage with multiple tumors, or in patients with lymphadenopathy or abnormal circulating T cells, electron-beam plus chemotherapy is probably the best combination, for now; randomized controlled studies of various combinations are now in progress. Also, extracorporeal PUVA photochemotherapy is being evaluated in patients with Sézary's syndrome.

Table A   TNM Classification of Mycosis Fungoides (MF) As Adopted for the U.S. National Cancer Institute Workshop on Cutaneous T-Cell Lymphomas (1979)

T: Skin	T_0	Clinically and/or histologically suspicious lesions
	T_1	Limited plaques, papules, or eczematous patches covering less than 10% of the skin surface
	T_2	Generalized plaques, papules, or erythematous patches covering more than 10% of the skin surface
	T_3	Tumors (1 or more)
	T_4	Generalized erythroderma (Sézary's)
N: Lymph nodes	N_0	No clinically abnormal peripheral nodes, pathology negative for MF
	N_1	Clinically abnormal peripheral lymph nodes, pathology negative for MF
	N_2	No clinically abnormal peripheral lymph nodes, pathology positive for MF
	N_3	Clinically abnormal peripheral lymph nodes, pathology positive for MF
B: Blood	B_0	Less than 5% atypical circulating lymphocytes
	B_1	Greater than 5% atypical circulating lymphocytes (Sézary's)
M: Visceral organs	M_0	No visceral organ involvement
	M_1	Histologically proven visceral involvement

Table B   Staging System for Cutaneous T-Cell Lymphomas

STAGE	T	N	M
IA	T_1	N_0	M_0
B	T_2	N_0	M_0
IIA	T_{1-2}	N_1	M_0
B	T_3	N_{0-1}	M_0
III	T_4	N_{0-1}	M_0
IVA	T_{1-4}	N_{2-3}	M_0
B	T_{1-4}	N_{0-3}	M_1

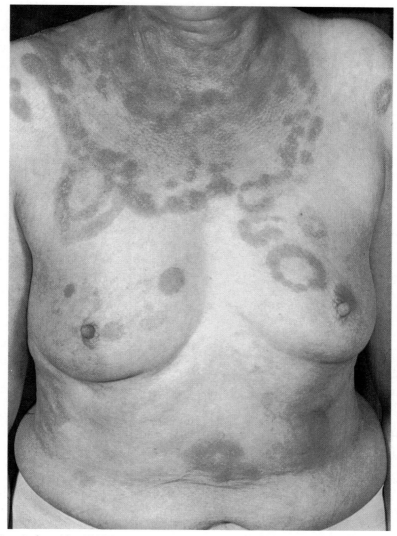

369   **Mycosis fungoides (CTCL)** *Annular, serpiginous, red, scaling plaques on the trunk. For 4 years, this patient had a red scaling eruption on the face, trunk, and extremities, which was diagnosed as an atypical psoriasis, responding poorly to corticosteroids and anthralin.*

This syndrome is a rare special variant of cutaneous T-cell lymphoma (CTCL) (mycosis fungoides) characterized by generalized or universal erythroderma, peripheral lymphadenopathy, and cellular infiltrates of atypical lymphocytes (Sézary cells) in the skin and in the blood.

EPIDEMIOLOGY

Age Over 60

Sex Male > females

HISTORY

Duration of Lesions The disease may arise de novo or, less commonly, result from extension of a preexisting circumscribed CTCL.

Skin Symptoms Pruritus, intense and generalized

PHYSICAL EXAMINATION

Appearance of Patient Sick, shivering, and scared

Skin
COLOR Red; the syndrome has been called the "red man syndrome" by French dermatologists
DISTRIBUTION OF LESIONS Generalized or involving the entire skin surface (universal) (Figure 370)

Hair Alopecia

General Examination Generalized lymphadenopathy

LABORATORY EXAMINATIONS

Dermatopathology
LIGHT MICROSCOPY *Site* Epidermis and dermis
Process Cell proliferation
Cell Types In the upper dermis there is a dense infiltration of lymphocytes, histiocytes, and varying numbers of Sézary cells. The Sézary cell is virtually indistinguishable from the so-called mycosis cell when viewed by either light microscopy or electron microscopy. In the epidermis there are Pautrier's microabscesses, containing Sézary cells, and other cells of the dermis. The lymph nodes may contain nonspecific inflammatory cells (dermatopathic lymphadenopathy) or there can be a complete replacement of the nodal pattern by Sézary cells. The cell infiltrates in the viscera in CTCL are the same as are present in the skin. However, a large number of Sézary cells is not absolutely specific for Sézary's syndrome, as these atypical lymphocytes can occur in nonspecific exfoliative dermatitis.
SPECIAL TECHNIQUES Transmission electron microscopy: the Sézary cells contain many infoldings of the nuclear membrane, with fingerlike projections in the nucleoplasm.

Laboratory Examination of Blood
HEMATOLOGIC There may be a moderate leukocytosis or a normal WBC. The buffy coat contains from 15 to 30% atypical lymphocytes (Sézary cells).

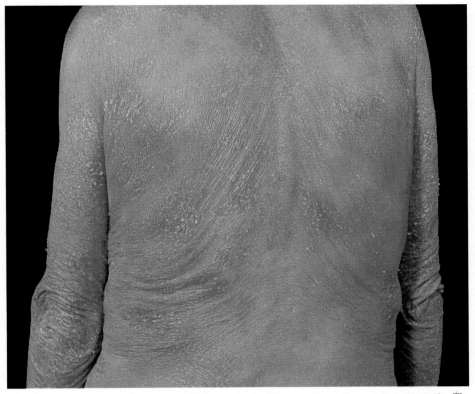

370 Sézary's syndrome *The entire trunk is involved with an erythematous, scaling dermatits. The patient had generalized lymphadenopathy and the buffy coat contained 38% atypical lymphocytes (Sézary cells).*

DIAGNOSIS AND DIFFERENTIAL DIAGNOSIS

Diagnosis The three features are: erythroderma, generalized lymphadenopathy, and presence of increased numbers of atypical lymphocytes in the buffy coat.

Differential Diagnosis Exfoliative dermatitis of unknown etiology can mimic Sézary's syndrome and can even have elevation of Sézary cells in the buffy coat. Adult T-cell leukemia/lymphoma (see page 708).

COURSE AND PROGNOSIS

The course without treatment is progressive and patients die from opportunistic infections in months, not years.

TREATMENT

Systemic Chemotherapy is effective in some patients.

Phototherapy PUVA photochemotherapy is effective for the erythroderma but does not induce remission of lymph node involvement. Extracorporeal PUVA photochemotherapy is the most recent promising treatment, but its efficacy in remission induction and maintenance is not yet known because there has not been long-term follow-up.

Lymphomatoid granulomatosis (LG) is a multisystem disease involving predominantly the skin, lungs, central nervous system, and kidneys, with characteristics of both inflammatory and neoplastic processes, combining the angiodestructive and granulomatous features of Wegener's granulomatosis with the cellular atypicality of lymphoma.

EPIDEMIOLOGY AND ETIOLOGY

Age Peak incidence, third to sixth decade

Sex Males > females

Etiology Considered to be a pleomorphic T-cell lymphoma

HISTORY

Cough, dyspnea, chest pain, ±hemoptysis

PHYSICAL EXAMINATION

Skin Findings Present in 40 to 50% of cases
TYPE OF LESION Macules, papules, nodules (Figure 371), plaques, annular plaques with central clearing, vesicles. Ulceration. Ichthyosis, alopecia, necrobiosis lipoidica-like lesions.
COLOR Initially, erythematous
PALPATION Soft to firm, ulcers with soggy borders
DISTRIBUTION OF LESIONS Gluteal areas, lower legs, head and neck. In the face LG presents as lethal midline granuloma with massive destruction of soft tissue.

General Examination Should include chest x-ray, endoscopy of upper digestive and respiratory tracts; CT scan and MRI of CNS

DIAGNOSIS AND DIFFERENTIAL DIAGNOSIS

Diagnosis Clinical suspicion confirmed by biopsy findings

Differential Diagnosis Wegener's granulomatosis, polymorphic reticulosis (a form of lymphomatoid granulomatosis localized to upper aerodigestive tract)

LABORATORY AND SPECIAL EXAMINATIONS

Chest X-Ray Transient alveolar or interstitial infiltrates and effusions; progress to nodular, masslike densities; ±cavitation of nodules

EKG Myocardial ischemia

Dermatopathology Angiocentric and angiodestructive granulomatous infiltrate with pleomorphic and highly atypical lymphoreticular cells having immunophenotypical markers of T cells; often massive necrosis.

PATHOPHYSIOLOGY

There is increasing evidence that LG is a malignant T-cell lymphoma.

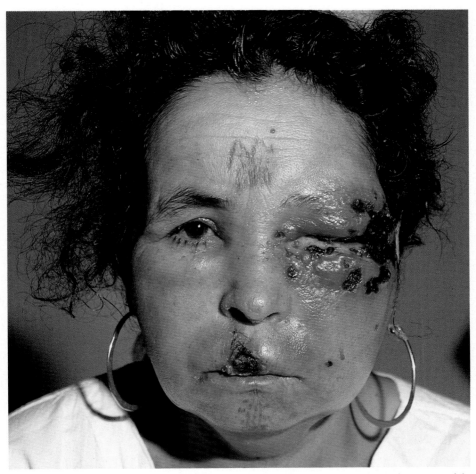

371 Lymphomatoid granulomatosis   *Papules, nodules, and tumors are seen on the face; some of the lesions have central ulceration accompanied by marked facial edema.*

COURSE AND PROGNOSIS

Frequently, LG presents in skin before clinically manifest in other organ systems (20% of cases). Skin most common site (40 to 50%) of extrapulmonary involvement, followed by brain and kidneys. Prognosis: poor, with 65 to 90% mortality reported.

TREATMENT

Early treatment of LG with prednisone and cyclophosphamide may transiently halt progression.

Langerhans Cell Histiocytosis (Histiocytosis X)

Langerhans cell histiocytosis (LCH) is an idiopathic group of disorders characterized histiologically by proliferation and infiltration of tissue by Langerhans cell-type histiocytes which fuse into multinucleated giant cells and form granulomas with eosinophils. LCH is characterized clinically by lytic bony lesions and cutaneous findings which range from soft tissue swelling to eczema- and seborrheic dermatitis-like changes and ulceration.

Synonyms: type II histiocytosis, nonlipid reticuloendotheliosis, eosinophilic granulomatosis.

CLASSIFICATION OF LCH

The disorders of xanthohistiocytic proliferation involving histiocytes, foam cells, and mixed inflammatory cells are divided into Langerhans cell (histiocytic X) (LCH) and non-Langerhans cell (non-histiocytic X) histiocytoses. LCH is classified as follows (see Table A):

Table A   Staging of LCH*

A. Localized LCH
    1. Bone (one or two adjacent lesions)
    2. Lymph node
    3. Skin

B. Disseminated LCH
    1. Bone, multifocal
    2. Bone and soft tissue or soft tissues alone (except skin and isolated lymph node)
    3. Organ dysfunction (liver, lungs, hemopoietic system)

---

*Histiocyte Society

Unifocal LCH   Most commonly manifested by a single osteolytic bony lesion. Skin and soft tissue lesions not so uncommon (known as eosinophilic granuloma).

Multifocal LCH   Similar to unifocal LCH; however, bony lesions are multiple and interfere with function of neighboring structures.

Multifocal LCH involves skin (second most frequently involved organ), soft tissue, lymph nodes, lungs, and pituitary.

Letterer-Siwe Syndrome (LSS)   The most aggressive of multifocal LCH forms, with skin involvement and infiltration of various organs causing organomegaly, thrombocytopenia.

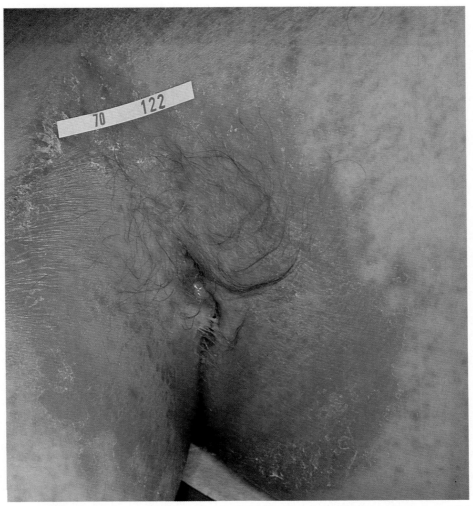

372　Multifocal Langerhans cell histiocytosis　*In the axilla there is a central ulceration surrounded by scaling, inflammatory lesions which was a superinfection with* Candida albicans. *Biopsy of the ulcer revealed histiocytosis X; the patient also had Langerhans cell histiocytosis involvement of the vertebrae.*

ETIOLOGY AND EPIDEMIOLOGY

Age
UNIFOCAL LCH   Most commonly, childhood and early adulthood

MULTIFOCAL LCH   Most commonly, childhood

LSS   More commonly, first few years; also, adult form occurs.

Sex   Males > females

Etiology   Unknown

Incidence   Rare

HISTORY

Unifocal LCH   Systemic symptoms uncommon. Pain and/or swelling over underlying bony lesion. Disruption of teeth with mandibular disease, fracture, otitis media due to mastoid involvement; recalcitrant ulcer on oral mucosa or genital region. Often, lesions are asymptomatic and diagnosed on radiographs for unrelated disorders.

Multifocal LCH   Erosive lesions are exudative, pruritic, or painful, with poor response to local treatments. Moist scalp lesions may have offensive odor. Associated disorders include otitis media caused by destruction of temporal and mastoid bones, proptosis due to orbital masses, loose teeth with infiltration of maxilla or mandible, anterior and/or pituitary dysfunction with involvement of sella turcica. Sellar involvement associated with growth retardation. Diabetes insipidus occurs secondary to hypothalamic or pituitary involvement. Triad of lytic skull lesions, proptosis, and diabetes insipidus: *Hand-Schüller-Christian disease*. Lung involvement associated with chronic cough, pneumothorax.

LSS   Child is systemically ill with a course that resembles a systemic infection or malignancy. Hepatomegaly, petechiae and purpura, generalized skin eruption.

PHYSICAL EXAMINATION

Skin Findings
UNIFOCAL LCH   *Type*
1. Swelling over bony lesion, over long or flat bone, tender
2. Cutaneous/subcutaneous nodule, yellowish, may be tender and break down, occurring anywhere
3. Sharply marginated ulcer, usually in genital and perigenital region or oral mucous membrane (gingiva, hard palate). Necrotic base, draining, tender.

MULTIFOCAL LCH   *Type*   As in unifocal LCH; in addition, regionally localized (head) or generalized eruptions. Papulosquamous, seborrheic dermatitis-like, eczematous dermatitis-like lesions; sometimes vesicular; lesions may be purpuric, necrotic; areas may coalesce with loss of epidermis; may become heavily crusted. Intertriginous lesions (Figure 372) may be exudative and become secondarily infected and ulcerate. Mandibular and maxillary bone involvement may result in loss of teeth (Figure 373). Ulceration of vulva.

Palpation   Area overlying bony lesions may be tender; papulosquamous eruption usually rough due to crusting; removal of crusts occurs easily and leaves erosions and punched-out, flat ulcers.

Distribution   Tumorous swelling: calvarium, sphenoid bone, sella turcica, mandible, long bones of upper extremities. Papulosquamous eruptions on scalp, face, and trunk, particularly abdomen and buttocks (Figure 374). Skin lesions can be discrete and localized or disseminated and generalized. Ulcers: vulva, gingiva. Eczema- and seborrhea-like changes seen on scalp and in intertriginous areas; erosions occur in groin, axillae, retroauricular, neck.

General Findings
UNIFOCAL LCH   Pain and swelling over affected bony lesion, painful ulcer

MULTIFOCAL LCH   Bony lesions occur in cal-

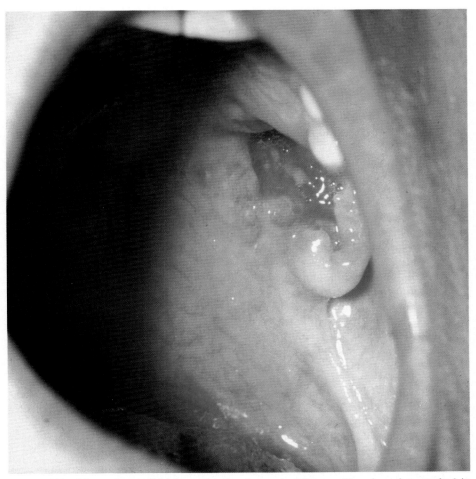

373 Multifocal Langerhans cell histiocytosis *Involvement of the maxillary bone has resulted in loss of the teeth and ulceration.*

varium, sphenoid bone, sella turcica, mandible, long bones of upper extremities, and vertebrae.

LSS Hepatosplenomegaly, lymphadenopathy, involvement of lungs and other organs, bone marrow; thrombocytopenia

DIAGNOSIS AND DIFFERENTIAL DIAGNOSIS

Diagnosis All forms of LCH require confirmation of diagnosis by biopsy (skin, bone, or soft tissue/internal organs). Since skin is the organ most frequently involved after the bone, skin biopsies have great diagnostic significance (see Histopathology below).

Differential Diagnosis

UNIFOCAL LCH Rule out other causes of lytic bony lesion

MULTIFOCAL LCH Infectious and neoplastic disorders

LSS Infectious and neoplastic disorders

LABORATORY AND SPECIAL EXAMINATIONS

Radiographic Findings

UNIFOCAL LCH Single osteolytic lesion in a long or flat bone (in children, calvarium, femur; in adults, rib)

MULTIFOCAL LCH Osteolytic lesions in calvarium, sphenoid bone, sella turcica, mandible, vertebrae, and/or long bones of upper extremities. Chest: diffuse micronodular and interstitial infiltrate in midzones and bases of lungs with sparing of costophrenic angles; later, honeycomb appearance, pneumothorax. Extent of osseous involvement established by bone scanning.

LSS Scans show organomegaly

Histopathology Constant histologic feature of LCH is proliferation of Langerhans cells that have abundant pale eosinophilic cytoplasm with indistinct cell borders, a folded, indented, kidney-shaped nucleus with finely dispersed chromatin, and small inconspicuous nucleoli. For diagnostic purposes Langerhans cells in LCH have to be recognized by morphologic, ultrastructural (Birbeck granules), histochemical, and immune-histochemical markers (see Table B).

PATHOPHYSIOLOGY

The proliferating Langerhans cell appears to be primarily responsible for the clinical manifestation. The stimulus for the proliferation is unknown.

COURSE AND PROGNOSIS

Unifocal LCH Benign course with excellent prognosis for spontaneous resolution

Multifocal LCH Spontaneous remissions possible. Prognosis poorer at extremes of age and with extrapulmonary involvement.

LSS Commonly fulminant and fatal. Spontaneous remissions uncommon. Current staging on scoring systems for evaluation of prognosis are based on number of organs involved, presence or absence of organ dysfunction, and age. The worst prognosis is in the very young with multifocal LCH and organ dysfunction.

TREATMENT

Unifocal LCH Curettage with or without bony chip packing. Low-dose (300 to 600 rad) radiotherapy. Extraosseous soft tissue lesions: surgical excision or low-dose radiotherapy

---

Table B Diagnosis in LCH*

Presumptive diagnosis	Clinical histopathologic
Diagnosis (2 or more criteria)	ATPase+
	S-100 protein+
	Alpha-D mannosidase+
	Peanut agglutinin+
Definite diagnosis	CD1a+
	Birbeck granules

---

*Histiocyte Society

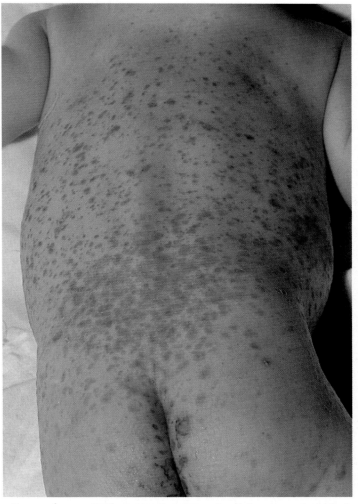

374 Letterer-Siwe syndrome *Erythematous papules and nodules, some of which show purpura and have become confluent, crusted, and ulcerated, on the trunk of a young child.*

Multifocal LCH   Diabetes insipidus and growth retardation treated with vasopressin and human growth hormone. Low-dose radiotherapy to bony lesions. Systemic treatment with corticosteroids, or vinblastine and methotrexate reserved for aggressive cases. Topical corticosteroids for discrete cutaneous lesions.

Cutaneous lesions respond best to PUVA or topical nitrogen mustard.

LSS   Only a few controlled studies of chemotherapy exist. The use of vinblastine results in complete or partial remission in 55%.

Mastocytosis is associated with an abnormal accumulation of mast cells within the skin and at various systemic sites, which, because of pharmacologically active substances, is manifested clinically by local cutaneous and systemic symptoms.

EPIDEMIOLOGY AND ETIOLOGY

Classification

Generalized cutaneous mastocytosis Urticaria pigmentosa (UP), telangiectasia macularis eruptiva perstans (TMEP), diffuse cutaneous mastocytosis (DCM)

Mastocytoma (M) Often solitary

Systemic mastocytosis (SM)

Mast cell "leukemia" Malignant mastocytosis

Age M and UP: onset between birth and 2 years of age (55%); adult-onset UP rarely associated with SM.

HISTORY

History Stroking lesion causes it to itch. Various drugs are capable of causing mast cell degranulation and release of pharmacologically active substances which exacerbate symptoms: alcohol, dextran, polymyxin B, morphine, codeine. Flushing episode may be accompanied by headache, dyspnea/wheezing, diarrhea, syncope.

Systems Review Tachycardia, hypotension, syncope. Headaches, nausea, vomiting, diarrhea (±alcohol exacerbated); malabsorption; portal hypertension. Bone pain. Neuropsychiatric symptoms (malaise, irritability). Rhinorrhea, wheezing. *Systemic mastocytosis: Up to half of patients may not have any skin findings;* weight loss, weakness, episodes of flushing, headache, diarrhea.

PHYSICAL EXAMINATION

Skin Findings

TYPE OF LESION *M* Macular-to-papular-to-nodular lesions (Figure 375), skin-color-to-yellow-to-tan-pink, which become raised and erythematous (urticate) when gently stroked (Darier's sign); in some patients, lesions become bullous. Often solitary; may be multiple.

UP Skin-color-to-slightly-tan macules to slightly raised papules/nodules (Figure 376). Positive Darier's sign. In infants, urticating wheals may become bullous. Dermographism. Bright-red flushing occurring spontaneously, following rubbing skin, after ingestion of alcohol or mast cell degranulation agents.

TMEP At first glance, frecklelike macules (Figure 377) with fine telangiectasia in long-standing lesion; urticate with gentle stroking. Dermographism

DCM Yellowish, thickened appearance of skin; "doughy." Smooth with scattered elevation, resembling leather, "pseudoxanthomatous mastocytosis"; skin folds exaggerated especially in axilla/groin. Large bullae may occur following trauma or spontaneously. DCM may present as erythroderma.

COLOR Skin-color-to-tan

DISTRIBUTION OF LESIONS *UP* Less than 10 to >100, widespread symmetrical distribution

TMEP Hundreds of lesions, centripetal, trunk > extremities; lesions may be confluent.

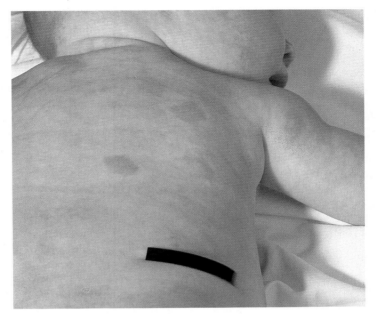

375 Mastocytosis, mastocytoma *Multiple, discrete mastocytomas in an infant. Two lesions are seen: a slightly indurated plaque on the back; erythematous urticaria lesions have developed from these brown plaques after being rubbed vigorously (Darier's sign).*

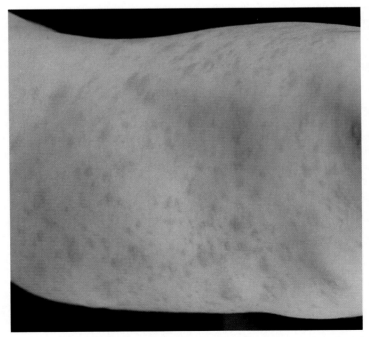

376 Mastocytosis, urticaria pigmentosa *Multiple, poorly defined, brown macules on the trunk. Some of the lesions show urtication which has occurred following rubbing.*

THE MASTOCYTOSIS SYNDROMES

General Examination

DCM, SM ±Hepatosplenomegaly

DIAGNOSIS AND DIFFERENTIAL DIAGNOSIS

Diagnosis Clinical suspicion, positive Darier's sign, confirmed by skin biopsy

Differential Diagnosis *M:* juvenile xanthogranuloma, Spitz nevus. *Flushing:* carcinoid syndrome. *UP, DCM, TMEP:* histiocytosis X, secondary syphilis, papular sarcoid, generalized eruptive histiocytoma, non-X histiocytosis of childhood

LABORATORY AND SPECIAL EXAMINATIONS

CBC Systemic mastocytosis: anemia, leukocytosis, eosinophilia

Urine Patients with extensive cutaneous involvement may have increased 24-hour urinary histamine excretion, 2 to 3 times normal (36 ± 15 μg).

Bone Scan and Imaging Define bone involvement and small bowel involvement

Dermatopathology Epidermis is normal. Accumulation of normal-looking mast cells in dermis. Mast cell infiltrates may be sparse (spindle-shaped mast cells) or densely aggregated (cuboidal shape) and have a perivascular or nodular distribution. Mast cells have metachromatically stained (Giemsa's or toluidine blue) granules either intracytoplasmic or extracellular. Pigmentation due to increased melanin in basal layer.

PATHOPHYSIOLOGY

Mast cells contain several pharmacologically active substances that are associated with the clinical findings in mastocytosis: histamine (urticaria, GI symptoms), prostaglandin D_2 (flush, cardiovascular symptoms, GI symptoms), heparin (bleeding at biopsy site), neutral protease/acid hydrolases (patchy hepatic fibrosis, bone lesions).

COURSE AND PROGNOSIS

Most cases of solitary mastocytoma and generalized UP in children resolve spontaneously. Adults with onset of UP or TMEP with extensive cutaneous involvement have a higher risk for development of systemic mastocytosis than do infants in whom SM is rare. In young children acute and extensive degranulation may be life-threatening (shock).

TREATMENT

Avoidance of drugs that may cause mast cell degranulation and histamine release: alcohol, dextran, polymyxin B, morphine, codeine, scopolamine, *d*-tubocurarine. Antihistamines, both H_1 and H_2. Disodium cromoglycate 200 mg q.i.d. may ameliorate pruritus, whealing, flushing, diarrhea, abdominal pain, and disorders of cognitive function. UP resolves after PUVA treatment but tends to recur. The same applies to topical corticosteroids under occlusion.

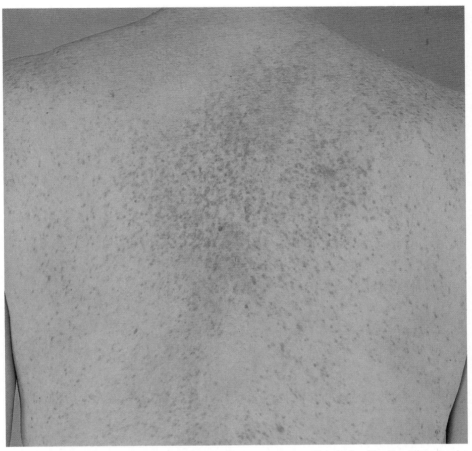

377 Mastocytosis, telangiectasia macularis eruptiva perstans type   *Hundreds of lentigo-like macules are seen on the back of this adult. If vigorously rubbed, these lesions will show urtication and become erythematous, raised, and pruritic.*

Skin Signs of Systemic Cancers

Acanthosis Nigricans

Acanthosis nigricans (AN) is a diffuse velvety thickening and hyperpigmentation of the skin, chiefly in axillae and other body folds, the etiology of which may be related to factors of heredity, endocrine disorders, obesity, drug administration, and, in one form, malignancy.

EPIDEMIOLOGY AND ETIOLOGY

Classification

Type 1—Hereditary benign AN No associated endocrine disorder

Type 2—Benign AN Various endocrine disorders associated with insulin resistance: insulin-resistant diabetes mellitus, hyperandrogenic states, acromegaly/gigantism, Cushing's disease, glucocorticoid therapy, diethylstilbestrol/oral contraceptive, growth hormone therapy, hypogonadal syndromes with insulin resistance, Addison's disease, hypothyroidism

Type 3—Pseudo-AN Complication of obesity; more commonly seen in patients with darker pigmentation. Obesity produces insulin resistance.

Type 4—Drug-induced AN Nicotinic acid in high dosage, stilbestrol in young males, oral contraceptives

Type 5—Malignant AN Paraneoplastic, usually adenocarcinoma; less commonly, lymphoma

Age Type 1: onset during childhood or puberty

Etiology Dependent on associated disorder

HISTORY

Usually insidious onset, first visible change is darkening of pigmentation.

PHYSICAL EXAMINATION

Skin Findings

TYPE OF LESION Darkening of pigmentation, skin appears dirty. As skin thickens, appears velvety; skin line further accentuated; surface becomes rugose, mammillated. *Type 3:* Velvety patch on inner, upper thigh at site of chafing; often has many skin tags in body folds, especially axillae (Figure 378), groins. *Type 5:* Hyperkeratosis and hyperpigmentation more pronounced. Hyperkeratosis of palms/soles, involvement of oral mucosa and vermilion border of lips.
COLOR Accentuation of normal pigmentation
PALPATION Velvety feel
DISTRIBUTION OF LESIONS Most commonly, axillae, neck (back, sides); also groins, anogenitalia, antecubital fossa, knuckles, submammary, umbilicus

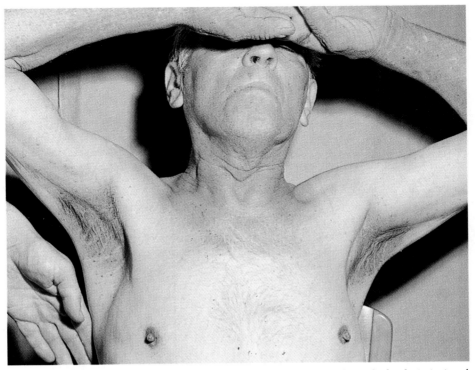

378 Acanthosis nigricans *The skin of the neck and axillae shows the typical velvety-textured, brown changes.*

MUCOUS MEMBRANES Oral mucosa, uncomely velvety texture with delicate furrows. *Type 5:* Mucous membranes and mucocutaneous junctions commonly involved; warty papillomatous thickenings periorbitally, periorally.

General Examination Examine for underlying endocrine disorder in benign AN and search for malignancy in malignant AN.

DIAGNOSIS AND DIFFERENTIAL DIAGNOSIS

Diagnosis Clinical diagnosis

Differential Diagnosis Confluent and reticulated papillomatosis (Gougerot-Carteaud syndrome). (The finding of abundant *Pityrosporum orbiculare* may support this diagnosis.)

LABORATORY AND SPECIAL EXAMINATIONS

Dermatopathology Papillomatosis, hyperkeratosis; epidermis thrown into irregular folds, showing varying degrees of acanthosis.

PATHOPHYSIOLOGY

Epidermal changes may be caused by hypersecretion of pituitary peptide, or nonspecific growth-promoting effect of hyperinsulinemia.

COURSE AND PROGNOSIS

Type 1: Accentuated at puberty, and, at times, regresses when older. *Type 3:* May regress subsequent to significant weight loss. *Type 4:* Resolves when causative drug discontinued. *Type 5:* AN may precede other symptoms of malignancy by 5 years; removal of malignancy may be followed by regression of AN.

Cowden's disease (named after the propositus) is a heritable cancer syndrome with variable expressivity in a number of systems in the form of multiple hamartomatous neoplasms of ectodermal, mesodermal, and endodermal origin. There is a special susceptibility for breast and thyroid cancers, and the skin lesions, which are adnexal tumors (tricholemmomas), are important markers, as they portend the onset of the breast and thyroid cancers.

EPIDEMIOLOGY

Incidence There are fewer than 100 patients reported to date, but the disease is probably more common than the published reports would indicate.

Age 4 to 75 years (median age, 40 years)

Race Mostly white, but there are reports in Japanese and in blacks.

Sex Males > females

HISTORY

History The skin lesions, which may appear first in childhood but develop over time, are tricholemmomas and are important because they often precede the onset of breast cancers in females.

Systems Review In addition to breast cancer (20.0%), which is often bilateral, and thyroid cancer (8.0%), there are various internal hamartomas: thyroid goiter, fibrocystic disease of the breast, GI polyposis, and, rarely, carcinoma of the colon, prostate, and uterus. The CNS may be involved: mental retardation, seizures, neuromas, ganglioneuromas, and meningiomas of the ear canal.

Family History Autosomal dominant

PHYSICAL EXAMINATION

Appearance of Patient The tricholemmomas may be quite extensive and disfiguring.

Skin

TYPE OF LESIONS

Tricholemmomas, skin-colored, pink (Figure 379), or brown papules having the appearance of warts or benign appendage tumors. These occur on the central area of the face, perioral areas, lips near the angles of the mouth, and on the ears.

Translucent punctate keratoses of the palms and soles

Hyperkeratotic, flat-topped papules on the dorsa of the hands and forearms

Lipomas and angiomas (rare)

Mucous Membranes These lesions are important and quite characteristic: *papules of the gingival, labial, and palatal surfaces;* they are whiter than the surrounding mucosa and often coalesce, giving a "cobblestone" appearance. *Papillomas of the buccal mucosa and the tongue.* Squamous cell carcinoma of the tongue and basal cell carcinoma of the anal area may occur.

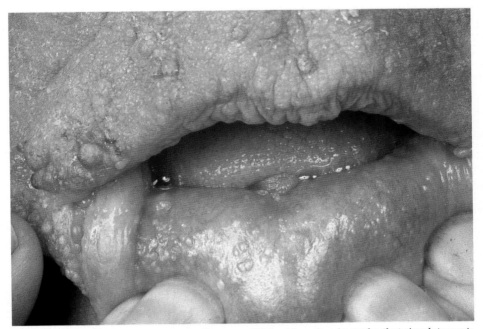

379 Cowden's syndrome *On the upper lip are multiple, skin-colored papules that simulate warts or benign appendage tumors; these are tricholemmomas. On the mucosal surface of the lower lip there are clusters of flat-topped papules that have a slightly lighter color than the surrounding mucosa.*

LABORATORY AND SPECIAL EXAMINATIONS

Dermatopathology

LIGHT MICROSCOPY The tricholemmomas show evidence of differentiation toward the outer root sheath cells of the hair follicles. Multiple biopsies may be necessary to obtain the characteristic histology. In one series only 29 of 53 (54%) facial lesions were diagnostic of tricholemmoma. The oral lesions are relatively acellular fibromas.

IMAGING

X-ray (mammography)

DIAGNOSIS

The tricholemmomas may be regarded by the examiner as one of a variety of benign papules or warts on the face; the striking lesions on mucous membranes of the mouth may be the special clue to obtaining a biopsy of the facial lesions, to establish the diagnosis of tricholemmoma.

SIGNIFICANCE

It is important to establish the diagnosis of Cowden's syndrome so that these patients can be carefully followed to detect breast and thyroid cancers.

COURSE

Tumors may continue to develop throughout life.

TREATMENT

Bilateral prophylactic mastectomy for females has been advocated.

COWDEN'S SYNDROME

Glucagonoma Syndrome

Glucagonoma syndrome is a rare but well-described clinical entity caused by excessive production of glucagon in an alpha-cell tumor of the pancreas, characterized by superficial migratory necrolytic erythema (MNE) with central blisters or erosions that crust and heal with hyperpigmentation, a beefy-red tongue, and angular cheilitis.

EPIDEMIOLOGY AND ETIOLOGY

Age Middle aged to elderly

Etiology Most cases associated with hyperglucagonemia; however, pathogenesis of MNE is not known.

HISTORY

Skin rash unresponsive to conventional therapy. Weight loss, abdominal pain.

PHYSICAL EXAMINATION

Skin Findings
TYPE OF LESION Inflammatory plaques enlarge with central clearing, resulting in geographic areas which become confluent. Borders show vesiculation to bulla formation, crusting, and scaling.
ARRANGEMENT Gyrate, circinate, arcuate, annular
DISTRIBUTION OF LESIONS Flexures, intertriginous areas (Figure 380), perioral (Figure 381), perigenital. Fingertips red, shining, erosive.
MUCOUS MEMBRANES Glossitis, angular cheilitis. Blepharitis.

General Examination Wasting, malnutrition.

DIAGNOSIS AND DIFFERENTIAL DIAGNOSIS

Diagnosis Clinical findings confirmed by skin biopsy and serum glucagon levels.

Differential Diagnosis Pustular psoriasis, mucocutaneous candidiasis, acrodermatitis enteropathica, zinc deficiency, Hailey-Hailey disease (familial pemphigus)

LABORATORY AND SPECIAL EXAMINATIONS

ESR ±Elevated

Chemistry Elevated serum glucagon levels (normal 50 to 250 ng/L). Hyperglycemia, reduced glucose tolerance. Associated findings: severe malabsorption, gross hypoaminoacidemia, low serum zinc.

Dermatopathology Early skin lesions show bandlike upper epidermal necrosis with retention of pyknotic nuclei and pale keratinocyte cytoplasm (electron microscopy shows vacuolar degeneration and lysis of organelles).

CT Scan, Angiography Locates tumor within pancreas

PATHOGENESIS

Most cases are associated with glucagon production by a pancreatic glucagonoma. Isolated cases have been reported of MNE associated with advanced hepatic cirrhosis or bronchial carcinoma.

COURSE AND PROGNOSIS

Depends on the aggressiveness of the glucagonoma. Hepatic metastases often present at time of diagnosis.

TREATMENT

Surgical excision of glucagonoma. Some cases have responded partially to zinc replacement. The alpha-cell inhibitor, streptozocin, has been used successfully to treat nonresectable and metastatic tumors.

SKIN SIGNS OF SYSTEMIC CANCERS

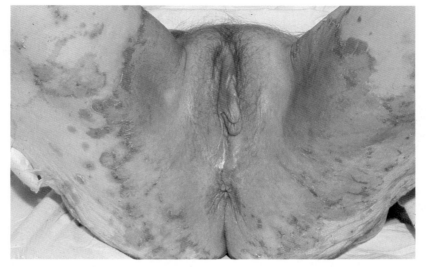

380   Glucagonoma syndrome   *Polycyclic, circinate, arciform, crusted lesions in the anogenital area, thighs, and buttocks. This clinical presentation can be confused with psoriasis, seborrheic dermatitis, impetigo, candidiasis, and zinc deficiency.*

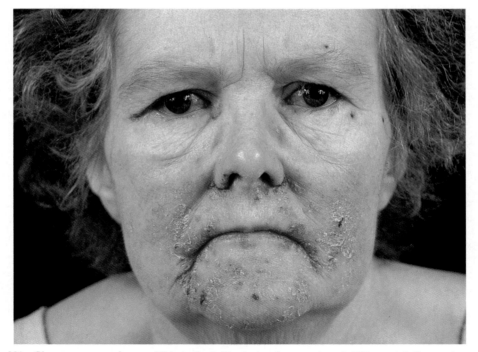

381   Glucagonoma syndrome   *This patient illustrates the angular cheilitis and inflammatory plaques on the cheek and around the nose.*

GLUCAGONOMA SYNDROME   737

This is a familial polyposis characterized by many congenital, small, pigmented macules (lentigines) on the lips and oral mucous membranes (periorificial lentiginosis). There are usually, but not always, multiple hamartomatous polyps in the small bowel, and also in the large bowel and stomach, which cause abdominal symptoms and signs (abdominal pain), occurring usually during childhood or early adulthood.

EPIDEMIOLOGY

Age Lentigines in infants and early childhood, abdominal symptoms appear in late childhood or before age 30

Sex Equal incidence

HISTORY

Duration of Lesions The pigmented macules are congenital or may develop during infancy and early childhood. The macules may disappear over time on the lips, but the pigmentation of the mouth does not disappear and is therefore the *sine qua non* for the diagnosis. *The lentigines occur in some patients who never have abdominal symptoms.*

Systems Review Abdominal symptoms (recurrent attacks of abdominal pain) occur first around age 10 and up to age 30, although rarely are first noted in older adults. Hematemesis and melena are noted with gastric or duodenal polyps.

Family History Autosomal dominant

PHYSICAL EXAMINATION

Skin
TYPE OF LESION Macule
Color Dark brown or black
Size 2.0 to 5.0 mm, the lentigines on the face (Figure 382) are smaller than those on the palms and soles and in the mouth.
SHAPE OF INDIVIDUAL LESION Round or oval
ARRANGEMENT OF MULTIPLE LESIONS The lesions occur on the lips (especially the lower lip) in closely set clusters around the mouth and the bridge of the nose.
DISTRIBUTION OF LESIONS Lips, nose, chin, palms and soles, dorsa of hands

Mucous Membranes These are the *sine qua non*; the lesions are dark brown, black, or bluish-black. They are irregularly distributed on the gums, buccal mucosae (Figure 383), and hard palate.

Nails Pigmented streaks or diffuse involvement of the nail bed (rare)

LABORATORY EXAMINATIONS

Dermatopathology
LIGHT MICROSCOPY *Site* Epidermis
Process Increased melanin synthesis, and in the lentigines of the palms some have noted a block in the melanin transfer to keratinocytes
Cell Types The increased pigmentation occurs in the melanocytes and in the basal cells.
PATHOLOGY OF GI POLYPS Hamartomas, with mixture of glands and smooth muscle
LABORATORY EXAMINATION OF BLOOD Hematologic: Anemia from blood loss may be present.

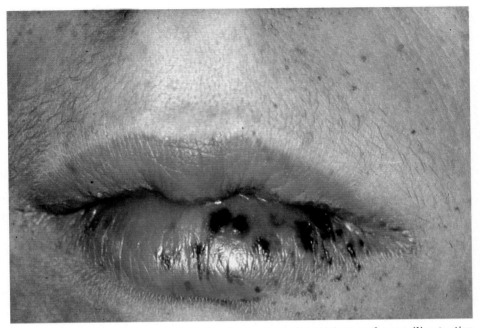

382 Peutz-Jeghers syndrome *Multiple, dark-brown to black lentigines on the vermilion portion of the lip, below the lower lip, and just above the upper lip, occurring in clusters.*

IMAGING

Study of the GI tract is important in patients with the clinical presentation of multiple lentigines of the type noted above.

DIAGNOSIS AND DIFFERENTIAL DIAGNOSIS

In Peutz-Jeghers syndrome the mucosal pigmentation is the constant feature that remains throughout life. The lentigines are much darker than freckles, and they occur in areas not exposed to sunlight (palms). Also the lentigines are not widely distributed as in the multiple lentigines syndrome (LEOPARD syndrome, see page 644); they do not occur on the trunk or extremities but are localized to the central areas of the face, the palms and soles, and dorsa of the hands.

SIGNIFICANCE

It is significant to make the diagnosis of Peutz-Jeghers syndrome in order to manage the bowel polyps.

COURSE AND PROGNOSIS

There is a normal life expectancy unless carcinoma develops in the GI tract and is unrecognized. Malignant neoplasms may be more frequent in the Japanese with this syndrome, and prophylactic colectomy has been recommended for these patients.

SKIN SIGNS OF SYSTEMIC CANCERS

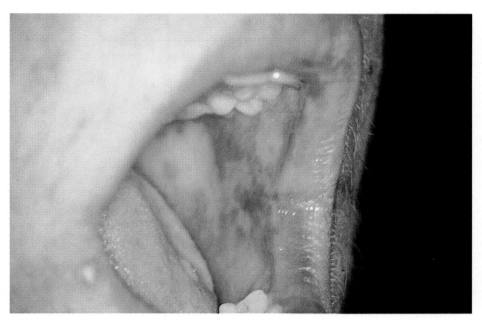

383   Peutz-Jeghers syndrome   *There are clusters of dark-brown macules on the buccal mucosa that are larger than the pigmented lesions on the lips or hands.*

Metastatic cancer to skin is characterized by solitary or multiple dermal or subcutaneous nodules, occurring as cells from a distant noncontiguous primary malignant neoplasm, that are transported to and deposited within the skin or subcutaneous tissue by hematogenous or lymphatic routes, or across the peritoneal cavity.

EPIDEMIOLOGY AND ETIOLOGY

Age Any age but usually older

Incidence 3 to 4% of malignant tumors metastasize to skin.

Etiology Most malignant tumors can produce cutaneous metastases. Most frequent primary sites: breast, stomach, lung, uterus, colon, kidney, prostate, ovary, liver.

HISTORY

Prior history of primary internal cancer. History of chemotherapy for cancer.

PHYSICAL EXAMINATION

Skin Findings

TYPE OF LESION Nodule; raised plaque; thickened fibrotic area. First detected when >5.0 mm. Fibrotic area may resemble morphea; occurring on scalp may produce alopecia.

COLOR May appear inflammatory, i.e., pink-to-red (Figure 384). Metastatic melanoma to dermis: blue to gray-to-black dermal nodules (Figure 385)

PALPATION Firm to indurated

ARRANGEMENT May be solitary, few, or multiple.

DISTRIBUTION OF LESIONS Lung cancer to trunk, scalp. Hypernephroma to scalp, operative scar

Clinical Variants

Breast cancer may spread within lymphatics to skin of involved breast, resulting in inflammatory plaques resembling cellulitis (erysipelas) or firm, flatter, telangiectatic plaques or papules and nodules (Figure 386). With dilatation of lymphatics and superficial hemorrhage, may resemble lymphangioma. With lymph stasis and dermal edema, resembles pigskin or orange peel. May metastasize hematogenously to scalp, forming many subcutaneous nodules with "bag of marbles" feel to scalp.

Lung carcinoma may produce a large number of metastatic nodules within short period. Most commonly, reddish nodules on trunk/scalp (Figure 387), symmetrical, along direction of intercostal vessels.

Hypernephroma can produce solitary lesion. Usually appear vascular ± pulsatile ± pedunculated; can resemble pyogenic granuloma.

Malignant melanoma may spread from primary cutaneous site to distant cutaneous site by lymphatic vessels.

Sister Mary Joseph's nodule is metastatic carcinoma to umbilicus from intraabdominal carcinoma, most commonly stomach, colon, ovary, pancreas; however, primary may be in breast. Easier to detect by palpation than by visual detection. Can be firm to indurated nodules ± fissuring ± ulceration ± vascular ap-

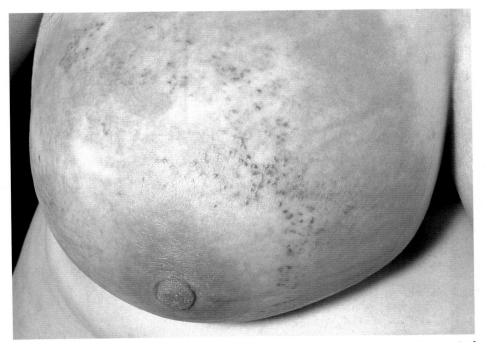

384   Metastatic cancer to the skin   *This inflammatory process represents a lymphatic spread of cancer cells producing an erysipelas-like inflammation.*

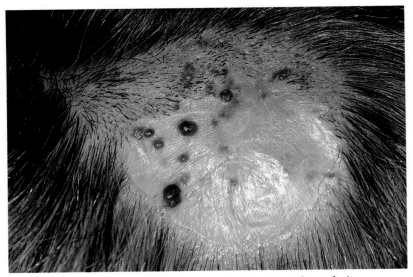

385   Metastatic melanoma   *Metastatic cancer to the skin at the graft site.*

METASTATIC CANCER TO THE SKIN

pearance ± discharge. In 15% may be initial presentation of primary malignancy.

Carcinoma of bladder, ovary can spread contiguously to abdominal and inguinal skin similarly to breast cancer, as described above.

General Examination Look for primary tumor.

DIAGNOSIS AND DIFFERENTIAL DIAGNOSIS

Diagnosis Clinical history of internal cancer suggests diagnosis, confirmed by skin biopsy.

Differential Diagnosis Any type of primary cutaneous or subcutaneous tumor. Cellulitis, lymphangioma, scarring alopecia

LABORATORY AND SPECIAL EXAMINATIONS

Dermatopathology Carcinomatous deposits tend to spread in dermal lymphatic vessels, with resultant "Indian file" appearance of strands of cells. At times cell differentiation sufficient to predict primary site; however, many times cells anaplastic. ±Dilatation of lymphatics secondary to carcinomatous lymphatic obstruction. Hypernephroma produces marked vascular proliferation.

COURSE AND PROGNOSIS

Average survival after detection of cutaneous metastasis only 3 months, except for contiguous spread of breast cancer, which may last for years. Hypernephroma may present with cutaneous metastasis.

TREATMENT

With solitary or few lesions and if patient not terminal, excision may be indicated.

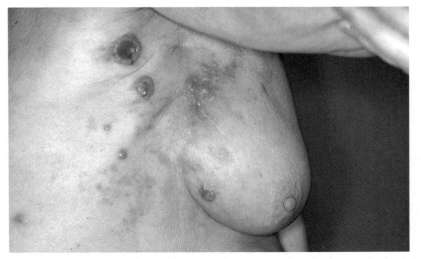

386 Metastatic breast cancer nodules *These nodules represent lymphatic spread of a primary breast cancer to the skin. There are clusters of nodules which were very painful.*

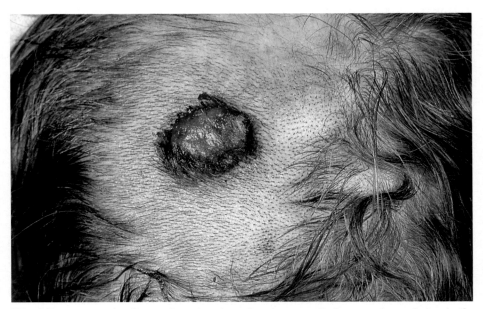

387 Solitary metastatic adenocarcinoma on the scalp *A metastasis from a primary lesion in the lung.*

METASTATIC CANCER TO THE SKIN

This malignant neoplasm unilaterally involves the nipple, or areola, and simulates a chronic eczematous dermatitis.

EPIDEMIOLOGY

Age 30 to 50 years

Sex Females, with rare examples in males

HISTORY

Duration of Lesions Insidious onset over several months or a year

Skin Symptoms Some itching or feeling of discomfort, complaints of soiling of the bra by the exudate

PHYSICAL EXAMINATION

Skin Lesions
TYPE Scaling plaque, rather sharply marginated, and when scale is removed, the surface is moist and oozing (see Figure 388)
COLOR Faintly red
PALPATION In early stages there is no induration, but later, induration and infiltration develop and nodules may be palpated.
SHAPE Oval with irregular borders
DISTRIBUTION *Single lesion localized to one nipple and areola.* May uncommonly occur bilaterally.

Miscellaneous Findings Regional lymph nodes are rarely found unless frank tumor (ulceration) is present in the epidermis. The breast tumor is an intraductal carcinoma.

DIFFERENTIAL DIAGNOSIS

Eczematous dermatitis of the nipples is usually bilateral; it is without any induration and responds rapidly to topical corticosteroids. Nevertheless, be suspicious of Paget's disease if "eczema" persists for longer than a few weeks or is resistant to topical treatment. Bowen's disease, superficial basal cell carcinoma, tinea versicolor.

DERMATOPATHOLOGY

Site Epidermis

Process Neoplastic. Typical large rounded cells with a large nucleus and without intracellular bridges (Paget's cells) which stain much lighter than surrounding keratinocytes

TREATMENT

Surgery

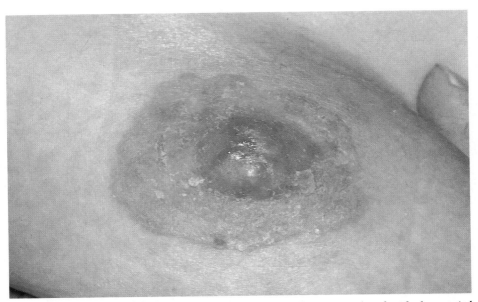

388   Paget's disease of the nipple   *On the nipple and the areola mammae is a sharply demarcated erythematous area with slight scaling and an erosive and moist surface. There is a slight superficial induration. Axillary lymph nodes not palpable.*

Extramammary Paget's disease (EPD) is a neoplasm of the anogenital and axillary skin, histologically and clinically similar to Paget's disease of the breast, and it often represents an intraepidermal extension of a primary adenocarcinoma of underlying secretory glands.

EPIDEMIOLOGY AND ETIOLOGY

Age >40

Sex Women > men

Etiology Unknown

HISTORY

Skin Symptoms ±Itching

PHYSICAL EXAMINATION

Skin Lesions
TYPE Erythematous plaque, ±scaling, ±crusting, ±exudation; eczematous-appearing lesions. Borders sharply defined (Figure 389), geographic configuration.
COLOR Pink to red (Figure 390)
DISTRIBUTION Most commonly vulva, scrotum, penis, perianal (Figure 390), perineal skin; also, axilla, umbilicus, presternal

General Examination Rectum, urethra, cervix should be examined for primary adenocarcinoma. *Proctoscopy.* Careful examination of the anorectum must be performed, to search for a primary tumor.

DIAGNOSIS AND DIFFERENTIAL DIAGNOSIS

Diagnosis Clinical suspicion confirmed by skin biopsy

Differential Diagnosis Eczematous dermatitis, intertriginous *Candida* infection, tinea corporis, erythrasma, Bowen's disease, human papillomaviral-induced intraepithelial neoplasia, (amelanotic) superficial spreading melanoma.

LABORATORY AND SPECIAL EXAMINATIONS

Dermatopathology Characteristic Paget cells are dispersed between keratinocytes, occur in clusters, extend down into adnexal structures (hair follicles, eccrine ducts). Adnexal adenocarcinoma is often found when carefully searched for. Dermis shows chronic inflammatory reaction. In later stages, epidermis may be eroded/atrophic. Paget cells are characterized by clear abundant cytoplasm and do not form intercellular bridges with adjacent keratinocytes. Both the cells and their nuclei are rounded; nuclei are vesicular or hyperchromatic. Cytoplasm PAS positive, diastase-resistant, supporting glandular origin.

PATHOPHYSIOLOGY

The histogenesis of EPD is uncertain. Paget cells in the epidermis may occur as an in situ upward extension of an in situ adenocarcinoma within deeper glands. Alternatively, EPD may have a multifocal primary origin within the epidermis and its related appendages and does not represent an epidermotropic spread or metastasis from an underlying sweat gland carcinoma. Approximately 25% of EPD

SKIN SIGNS OF SYSTEMIC CANCERS

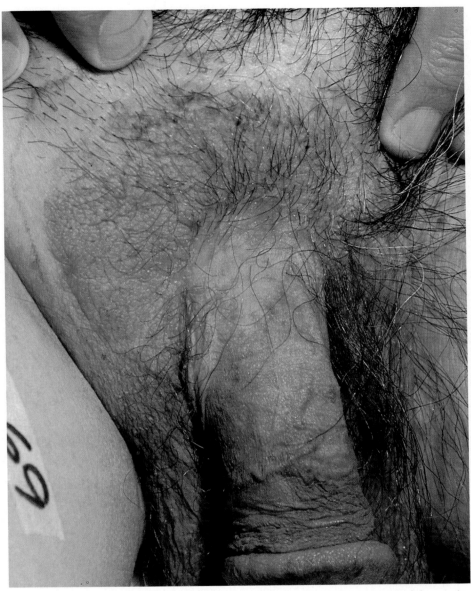

389 **Extramammary Paget's disease** *A sharply demarcated, erythematous lesion which has gradually spread over a period of years from the base of the penis onto the abdomen.*

EXTRAMAMMARY PAGET'S DISEASE

749

can be shown to arise from a primary adenocarcinoma of underlying secretory glands. The primary tumor and Paget cells are usually mucus-secreting. Primary tumors in the anorectum can arise within the rectal mucosa or intramuscular glands.

COURSE AND PROGNOSIS

Prognosis related to existence of underlying adenocarcinoma. When no underlying neoplasm is present, there is a high recurrence rate even after apparently adequate excision; this is due to the multifocal origin within epidermis and adnexal structures.

TREATMENT

EPD is usually much larger than is apparent clinically. Surgical excision must be histologically controlled (Mohs surgery).

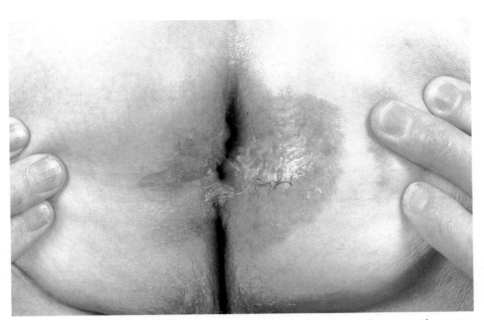

390   Extramammary Paget's disease   *This sharply demarcated, scaling, erythematous plaque surrounds the anus and is in a typical site.*

Skin Signs of Hematologic Diseases

Thrombocytopenic Purpura

Thrombocytopenic purpura is characterized by cutaneous hemorrhages occurring in association with a reduced platelet count. The lesions are clinically usually small (petechiae) but at times larger (ecchymoses) and occur at sites of minor trauma/pressure (platelet count $<40,000/mm^3$) or spontaneously (platelet count $<10,000/mm^3$).

EPIDEMIOLOGY AND ETIOLOGY

Age Acute idiopathic thrombocytopenic purpura (ITP)—children

Sex Females > males, however HIV-associated thrombocytopenic purpura in homosexual men

Etiology *Increased platelet destruction:* immunologic [autoimmune-ITP, drug hypersensitivity (sulfonamides, quinine, quinidine), posttransfusion], nonimmunologic [infection, prosthetic heart valves, disseminated intravascular coagulation, Kasabach-Merritt syndrome (Figure 391*a*), thrombotic thrombocytopenic purpura]. *Decreased platelet formation:* direct injury to bone marrow, replacement of bone marrow, aplastic anemia, vitamin deficiencies, Wiskott-Aldrich syndrome. *Platelet sequestration:* splenomegaly, hypothermia.

HISTORY

Systems Review Usually sudden appearance of asymptomatic hemorrhagic skin and/or mucosal lesions

PHYSICAL EXAMINATION

Skin Findings
TYPE OF LESION *Petechiae*—small (pinpoint to pinhead), red, nonblanching macules (Figures 391*b* and 392). *Ecchymoses*—black-and-blue spots; larger area or hemorrhage. *Vibices*—linear hemorrhages, often due to trauma

COLOR Fresh areas of hemorrhage—red to dark brown. Older lesions—yellowish-green tinge

PALPATION Nonpalpable. Lesions do not blanch with pressure.

ARRANGEMENT OF MULTIPLE LESIONS Possible linear lesions at sites of trauma. May occur in acne lesions. Under blood pressure cuff.

391a Thrombocytopenic purpura: Kasabach-Merritt syndrome *Posterior view of the infant shows a large cavernous hemangioma in which platelets were sequestered and destroyed, resulting in thrombocytopenia.*

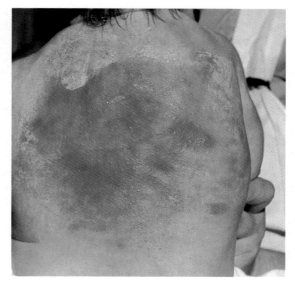

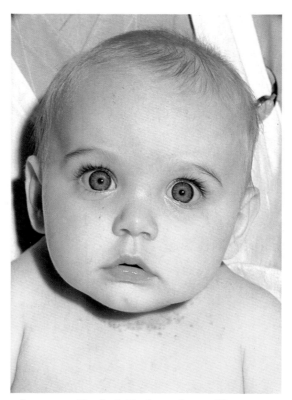

391b Thrombocytopenic purpura: Kasabach-Merritt syndrome *The anterior neck of this infant shows numerous nonblanching petechiae.*

THROMBOCYTOPENIC PURPURA

DISTRIBUTION OF LESIONS   Upper trunk, legs
MUCOUS MEMBRANES   Petechiae, gingival
  bleeding

General Examination   Possible CNS hemorrhage

DIAGNOSIS AND DIFFERENTIAL DIAGNOSIS

Diagnosis   Clinical suspicion confirmed by platelet count

Differential Diagnosis   Must be differentiated from nonhemorrhagic, blanching vascular lesions such as telangiectasia/erythema and palpable nonblanching purpura, i.e., vasculitis. True hemorrhagic lesions: Bateman's (actinic or senile) purpura, purpura of scurvy, progressive pigmentary purpura (Schamberg's disease), purpura following severe Valsalva maneuver (tussive, vomiting/retching), traumatic purpura, factitial or iatrogenic purpura, Gardner-Diamond syndrome (autoerythrocyte sensitization syndrome)

LABORATORY AND SPECIAL EXAMINATIONS

Dermatopathology   May be contraindicated due to postsurgical hemorrhage

PATHOPHYSIOLOGY

Platelet plugs by themselves effectively stop bleeding from capillaries and small blood vessels but are incapable of stopping hemorrhage from larger vessels. Platelet defects produce problems with small-vessel hemostasis, small hemorrhages in the skin or in the central nervous system.

COURSE AND PROGNOSIS

Varies with the etiology

TREATMENT

If platelet counts $<10,000/mm^3$, platelet transfusion may be indicated; bed rest to reduce risk of hemorrhage. For ITP, possible course of oral corticosteroid. Chronic ITP, possible splenectomy.

SKIN SIGNS OF HEMATOLOGIC DISEASES

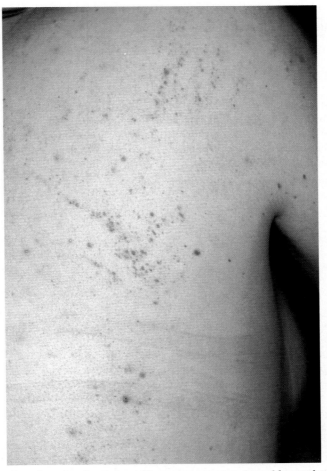

392 Idiopathic thrombocytopenic purpura *There are numerous dermal hemorrhages, manifested by nonblanching, pinpoint-to-pinhead, dusky-red petechiae.*

Disseminated Intravascular Coagulation

Disseminated intravascular coagulation (DIC) is a life-threatening bleeding disorder resulting from widespread blood clotting within blood vessels, associated with a wide range of clinical circumstances (bacterial sepsis, obstetrical complications, disseminated malignancy, massive trauma), and manifested by purpura fulminans (cutaneous infarctions and/or acral gangrene) or bleeding from multiple sites.

Synonyms: purpura fulminans, consumption coagulopathy, defibrination syndrome, coagulation-fibrinolytic syndrome.

EPIDEMIOLOGY AND ETIOLOGY

Age Purpura fulminans most commonly in children

Etiology
EVENTS THAT INITIATE DIC (1) *Massive tissue destruction:* tumor products, crushing trauma, extensive surgery, severe intracranial damage; retained contraception products, placental abruption, amniotic fluid embolism; certain snake bites; hemolytic transfusion reaction; acute promyelocytic leukemia; burn injuries. (2) *Extensive destruction of endothelial surfaces, exposure to foreign surfaces:* vasculitis (Rocky Mountain spotted fever, meningococcemia or, occasionally, gram-negative septicemia); heat stroke, malignant hyperthemia; extensive pump-oxygenation (repair of aortic aneurysm); eclampsia, preeclampsia; giant hemangioma (Kasabach-Merritt syndrome); immune complexes; postvaricella purpura gangrenosa
EVENTS THAT COMPLICATE AND PROPAGATE DIC Shock; complement pathway activation

HISTORY

Duration of Lesions Hours to days; rapid evolution

History Complication developing during or in convalescence from etiologic circumstances. Fever, chills associated with onset of hemorrhagic lesions

PHYSICAL EXAMINATION

Skin Findings
TYPE OF LESION *Hemorrhage* from multiple cutaneous sites, i.e., surgical incisions, venipuncture, or catheter sites. *Preinfarction:* peripheral acrocyanosis. *Infarction (purpura fulminans)* (Figure 393): massive ecchymoses with sharp, irregular ("geographic") borders and erythematous halos ± evolution to hemorrhagic bullae and blue-to-black gangrene; peripheral gangrene on hands, feet, tip of nose with subsequent autoamputation if patient survives.
COLOR Infarctive lesions are deep purple to black.
ARRANGEMENT OF MULTIPLE LESIONS Often symmetrical
DISTRIBUTION OF LESIONS Infarctive lesions: distal extremities; areas of pressure; lips, ears, nose, trunk.
MUCOUS MEMBRANES Hemorrhage from gingiva

General Examination High fever, ±shock. Multitude of findings depending on the associated medical/surgical problem

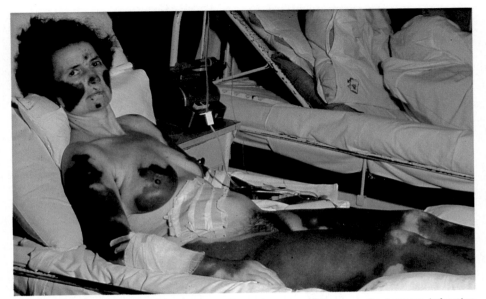

393   Disseminated intravascular coagulation *Extensive geographic areas of cutaneous infarction involving the face, breasts, and extremities.*

DIAGNOSIS AND DIFFERENTIAL DIAGNOSIS

Diagnosis Clinical suspicion confirmed by coagulation studies

Differential Diagnosis Necrosis following initiation of warfarin therapy; heparin necrosis

LABORATORY AND SPECIAL EXAMINATIONS

Dermatopathology Occlusion of arterioles with fibrin thrombi. Dense PMN infiltrate around infarct and massive hemorrhage

Hematologic Studies *CBC:* Schistocytes (fragmented RBC), arising from RBC entrapment and damage within fibrin thrombi, seen on blood smear; platelet count low. *Coagulation studies:* Reduced plasma fibrinogen; elevated fibrin degradation products; prolonged PT, PTT, and thrombin time.

PATHOPHYSIOLOGY

Uncontrolled activation of coagulation results in thrombosis and consumption of platelets/clotting factors II, V, VIII. If the activation occurs slowly, excess activated products produced, predisposing to vascular infarctions/venous thrombosis. If the onset is explosive, the clinical picture is dominated by hemorrhage surrounding wound sites, IV lines/catheters, bleeding into deep tissues.

COURSE AND PROGNOSIS

Mortality rate is high. Surviving patients require skin grafts or amputation for gangrenous tissue. Common complications: severe bleeding, thrombosis, tissue ischemia/necrosis, hemolysis, organ failure

TREATMENT

Correct reversible cause. Control bleeding or thrombosis. Heparin. Prevent recurrence in chronic DIC.

Appendix A: Types of Skin Lesions

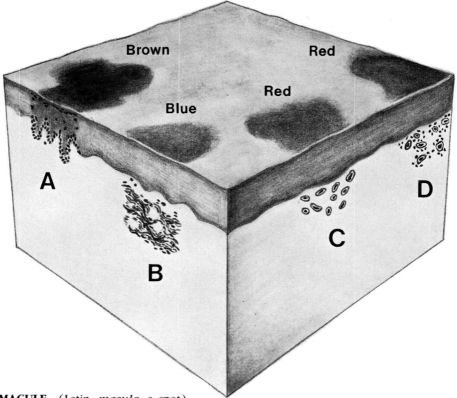

MACULE (Latin, *macula,* a spot)

Figure A-1 A macule is a circumscribed area of change in normal skin color without elevation or depression of the surrounding skin. Lesions may appear as macules but are shown to be elevated (i.e., papular) by oblique lighting. This may be important in pigmented lesions. Macules may be of any size and are the result of (1) hypopigmentation (e.g., vitiligo) or hyperpigmentation—melanin (A) or hemosiderin (B)—such as café-au-lait spots and Mongolian spots (B), (2) permanent vas-cular abnormalities of the skin, as in a capillary hemangioma, or (3) transient capillary dilatation (erythema) (C). Pressure of a glass slide (diascopy) on the border of a red lesion is a simple and reliable method for detecting the extravasation of red blood cells. If the redness remains under pressure from the slide, the lesion may be purpuric (D); if the redness disappears, the lesion is erythematous and is due to vascular dilatation (C).

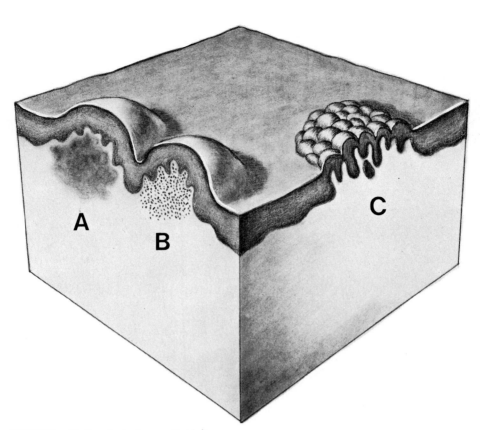

PAPULE (Latin, *papula,* a pimple)

Figure A-2 A papule is a solid lesion, generally considered as less than 0.5 cm in diameter. Most of it is elevated above, rather than deep within, the plane of the surrounding skin. In dermal papules the elevation is caused by metabolic deposits (A) in the dermis or by localized infiltrates (B) in the dermis or by localized hyperplasia of cellular elements (C) in the dermis. Deeper dermal papules resulting from cellular infiltrates have indistinct borders. Papules with distinct borders are seen when the lesion is the result of an increase in the number of epidermal cells (C) or melanocytes. The topography of a papule or plaque may consist of multiple, small, closely packed, projected elevations that are known as a vegetation (C). Confluence of papules leads to the development of larger, usually flat-topped, circumscribed elevations known as plaques (Fr. *plaque,* plate).

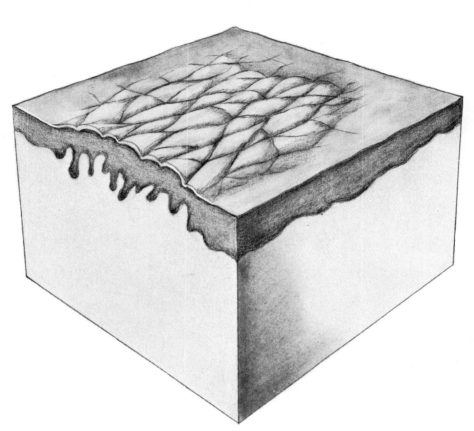

PLAQUE

Figure A-3 A plaque is an elevation above the skin surface that occupies a relatively large surface area in comparison with its height above the skin. Frequently it is formed by a confluence of papules as in psoriasis and mycosis fungoides. Lichenification is a proliferation of keratinocytes and stratum corneum forming a plaquelike structure. The skin appears thickened and the skin markings are accentuated. The process results from repeated rubbing of the skin and frequently develops in persons with atopy. Lichenification occurs typically in eczematous dermatitis but is also found in psoriasis and mycosis fungoides.

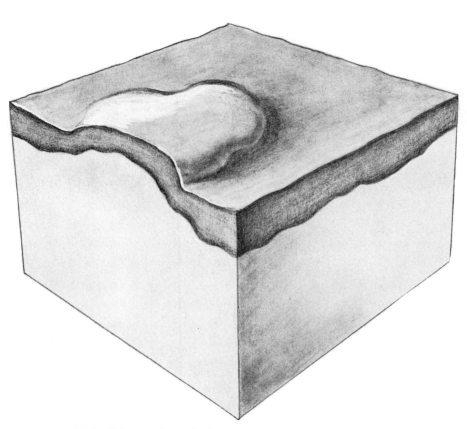

WHEAL (Old English, *weal*, a raised mark on the skin caused by the blow of a rod or lash)

Figure A-4 A wheal is a rounded or flat-topped, pale-red papule or plaque that is characteristically evanescent, disappearing within hours. Wheals may be round, gyrate, or irregular with pseudopods—changing rapidly in size and shape due to shifting edema in the dermis.

> Wheals that do not disappear in 72 hours are typical of *urticarial vasculitis* and a biopsy is indicated.

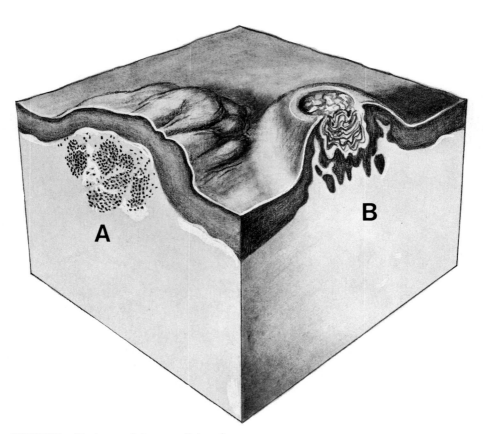

NODULE (Latin, *nodulus,* small knot)

Figure A-5 A nodule is a palpable, solid, round or ellipsoidal lesion deeper than a papule and is in the dermis or subcutaneous tissue (A) or in the epidermis (B). The depth of involvement and the palpability rather than the diameter differentiates a nodule from a papule. Nodules result from infiltrates (A), neoplasms (B), or metabolic deposits in the dermis or subcutaneous tissue and often indicate systemic disease. Tuberculosis, the deep myco- ses, lymphoma, and metastatic neoplasms, for example, can present as cutaneous nodules. Therefore, a biopsy should be performed on unidentified persistent nodules, and a portion of excised tissue should be ground in a sterile mortar and cultured for fungi and bacteria. Nodules can develop as a result of a benign or malignant proliferation of keratinocytes, as in keratoacanthoma (B) and squamous cell and basal cell carcinoma.

> Persistent nontender dermal nodules are important signs of multisystem diseases and biopsy and cutaneous cultures of minced tissue are necessary.

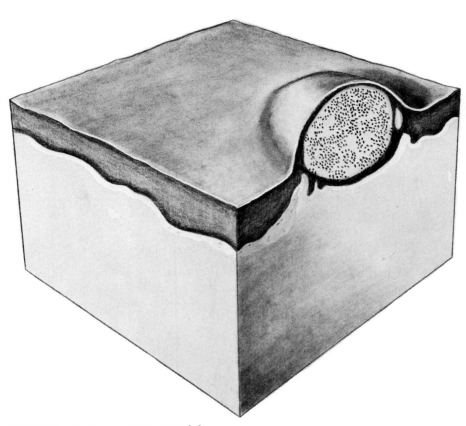

PUSTULE   (Latin, *pustula,* pustule)

Figure A-6   A pustule is a circumscribed elevation of the skin that contains a purulent exudate that may be white, yellow, or greenish yellow. This process may arise in a hair follicle or independently. Pustules may vary in size and shape; follicular pustules, however, are always conical and usually contain a hair in the center. The vesicular lesions of the viral diseases (varicella, variola, vaccinia, herpes simplex, and herpes zoster) may become pustular secondarily.

> A Gram's stain and culture should be done on all pustules for identification of intracellular gram-positive cocci.

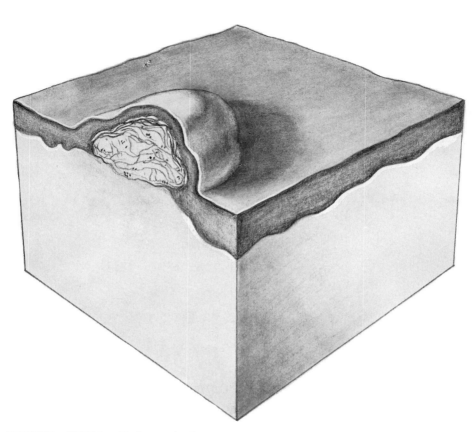

VESICLE—BULLA (Latin, *vesicula,* little bladder; *bulla,* bubble)

Figure A-7 A vesicle (less than 0.5 cm) or a bulla (more than 0.5 cm) is a circumscribed elevated lesion containing fluid. Often the walls are so thin that they are translucent, and the serum, lymph fluid, blood, or extracellular fluid can be seen. Vesicles and bullae arise from a cleavage at various levels of the skin; the cleavage may be within the epidermis (i.e., intraepidermal vesication), or at the epidermal-dermal interface (i.e., subepidermal), as in this figure.

Grouped "herpetiform" vesicles are indications for the Tzanck test and/or viral cultures.

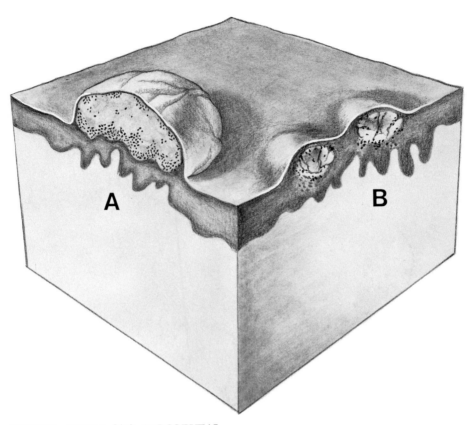

VESICLE—BULLA [(A) SUBCORNEAL, (B) SPONGIOTIC]

Figure A-8 When the cleavage is just beneath the stratum corneum, a subcorneal vesicle or bulla results (A), as in impetigo and subcorneal pustular dermatosis. Intraepidermal vesication may result from intercellular edema, or spongiosis (B), as characteristically seen in delayed-hypersensitivity reactions of the epidermis (e.g., in contact eczematous dermatitis) and in dyshidrotic eczema (B). Spongiotic vesicles may or may not be observed clinically as vesicles.

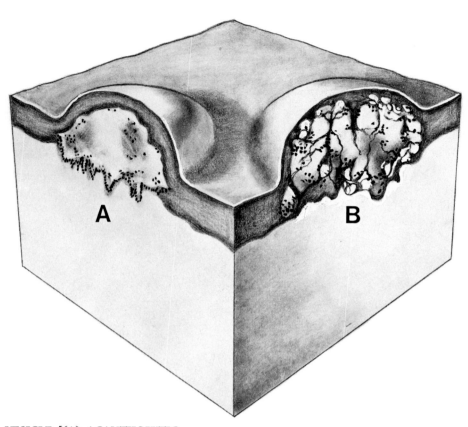

**VESICLE [(A) ACANTHOLYTIC,
(B) VIRAL]**

Figure A-9 Loss of intercellular bridges, or desmosomes, is known as *acantholysis* (A), and this type of intraepidermal vesication is seen in the vesicles or bullae of pemphigus vulgaris; the cleavage is usually just above the basal layer, as in pemphigus vulgaris. Viruses cause a curious "ballooning degeneration" of epidermal cells (B), as in herpes zoster, herpes simplex, variola, and varicella.

> Viral bullae often have a depressed ("umbilicated") center. In older patients with multiple single bullae, a biopsy and immunofluorescence are necessary for diagnosis of pemphigus or pemphigoid.

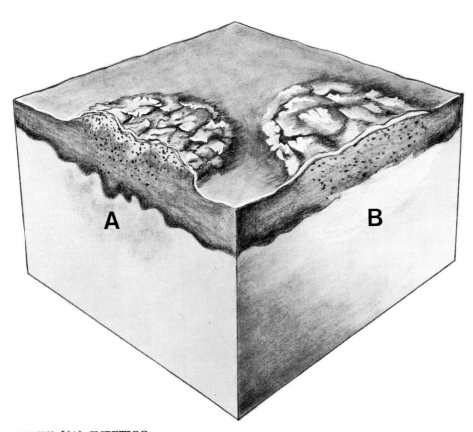

CRUSTS [(A) IMPETIGO, (B) ECTHYMA] (Latin, *crusta,* rind, bark, shell)

Figure A-10 Crusts develop when serum, blood, or purulent exudate dries on the skin surface, are the hallmark of pyogenic infection and cultures are needed. Crusts may be thin, delicate, and friable (A) or thick and adherent (B). Crusts are yellow when formed from dried serum, green or yellow-green when formed from purulent exudate, or brown or dark red when formed from blood. Superficial crusts occur as honey-colored, delicate, glistening particulates on the surface (A) and are typically found in impetigo. When the exudate involves the entire epidermis, the crusts may be thick and adherent, and this condition is known as *ecthyma* (B).

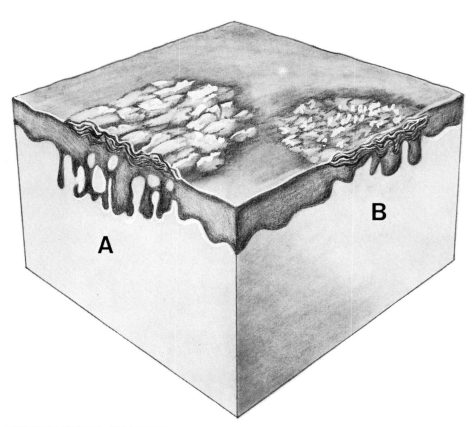

DESQUAMATION (SCALING)
[(A) PSORIASIS, (B) SOLAR
KERATOSIS] (old French, *escale,* shell)

Figure A-11 Epidermal cells are completely replaced every 27 days. The end product of this holocrine process is the stratum corneum. This outermost layer of skin, the stratum corneum, normally does not contain nuclei and is imperceptibly lost. With an increased rate of proliferation of epidermal cells, as in psoriasis, the stratum corneum is not formed normally and the outermost layers of the skin retain the nuclei (parakeratosis). These desquamating layers of skin are seen clinically as scales (A). Densely adherent scales that have a gritty feel (like sandpaper) result from a localized increase in the stratum corneum and are a characteristic of solar keratosis (B).

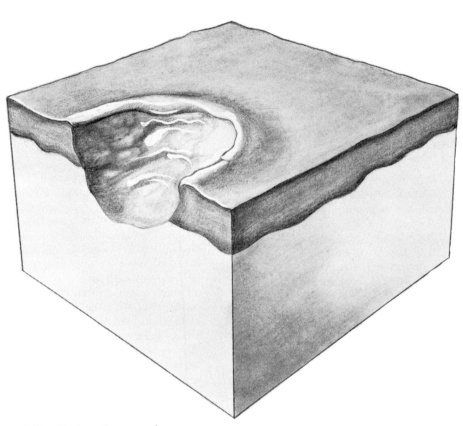

ULCER (Latin, *ulcus,* sore)

Figure A-12 An ulcer is a skin defect in which there has been loss of the epidermis and the upper papillary layer of the dermis. Certain features that are helpful in determining the cause of ulcers include location, borders, base, discharge, and any associated topographic features, such as nodules, excoriations, varicosities, hair distribution, presence or absence of sweating, and pulses.

In any ulcer not related to vascular disease, a wedge biopsy for histology and minced tissue for microbial culture are required.

SPECIAL TECHNIQUES USED IN CLINICAL EXAMINATION

1. *Magnification with hand lens.* To examine lesions for fine morphologic detail, it is necessary to use a magnifier (2× to 7×) or a binocular microscope (5× to 40×). Magnification is especially effective in the diagnosis of lupus erythematosus (follicular plugging), lichen planus (Wickham's striae), carcinomas (translucence and telangiectasia), and malignant melanoma (subtle changes in color, especially gray or blue; this is best visualized following application of a drop of mineral oil). Hand lenses with built-in lighting and a magnification of 10× to 30× are now available which permit observation of lesions covered with a drop of oil (oil immersion effect) and thus allow inspection of deeper layers of the skin (dermoepidermal junction.) This is called *epiluminescence microscopy* and allows the distinction of benign and malignant growth patterns, particularly in pigmented lesions.

2. *Oblique lighting* of the skin lesion, done in a darkened room, is often required to detect slight degrees of elevation or depression, and it is useful in the visualization of the surface configuration of lesions and in estimating the extent of the eruption.

3. *Subdued lighting* in the examining room enhances the contrast between circumscribed hypopigmented or hyperpigmented lesions and normal skin.

4. *Wood's lamp* (ultraviolet long-wave light, "black" light) is valuable in the diagnosis of certain skin and hair diseases and of porphyria. Long-wave ultraviolet radiation can be obtained by fitting a high-pressure mercury lamp with a specially compounded filter made of nickel oxide and silica (Wood's filter); this filter is very opaque to all light except for a band between 320 and 400 nm. The lamp with this filter produces adequate long-wave ultraviolet radiation. When the ultraviolet waves emitted by Wood's lamp (360 nm) impinge on the skin, a visible fluorescence occurs. Wood's lamp is particularly useful in the detection of the fluorescence of dermatophytosis in the hair shaft (green to yellow) and of erythrasma (coral red). A presumptive diagnosis of porphyria can be made if a pinkish-red fluorescence is demonstrated in urine examined with the Wood's lamp; addition of dilute hydrochloric acid intensifies the fluorescence. Wood's lamp also helps to estimate the variation in the lightness of lesions in relation to the normal skin color, in both dark-skinned and fair-skinned peoples; e.g., the lesions seen in tuberous sclerosis and tinea versicolor are hypomelanotic and are not as light as the lesions seen in vitiligo, which are amelanotic. Circumscribed hypermelanosis, such as a freckle and melasma, is much more evident under Wood's lamp. On the other hand, dermal melanin as in a Mongolian sacral spot does not become accentuated under Wood's lamp. Therefore it is possible to localize the site of melanin by use of the Wood's lamp; this, however, does not apply in patients with brown skin.

5. *Diascopy* consists of firmly pressing a microscope slide over a skin lesion. The

examiner will find this procedure of special value in determining whether the red color of a macule or papule is due to capillary dilatation (erythema) or to extravasation of blood (purpura). Diascopy is also useful for the detection of the glassy yellow-brown appearance of papules in sarcoidosis, tuberculosis of the skin, lymphoma, and granuloma annulare.

6. *Acetowhitening* facilitates detection of subclinical penile warts. Ninety to 100% of male partners of HPV-infected females with genital warts are also infected. Gauze saturated with 5% acetic acid (white vinegar) is wrapped around the penis. After 5 to 10 minutes the penis is inspected with a colposcope (dissecting microscope) or a 10× hand lens. Warts appear as small white papules.

CLINICAL TESTS

1. *Darier's sign* is "positive" when a brown macular or a slightly papular lesion of urticaria pigmentosa (mastocytosis) becomes a palpable wheal after being rubbed with the blunt end of an instrument such as a pen. The wheal may not appear for 5 to 10 minutes.

2. *Auspitz's sign* is "positive" when slight scratching or curetting of a scaly lesion reveals punctate bleeding points within the lesion. This suggests psoriasis, but it is not specific.

3. *Patch testing* is used to document and validate a diagnosis of allergic contact sensitization and identify the causative agent. It may also be of value as a screening procedure in some patients with chronic or bizarre eczematous eruptions (e.g., hand and foot dermatoses). It is a unique means of in vivo reproduction of disease in diminutive proportions, for sensitization affects all the skin and may therefore be elicited at any cutaneous site. The patch test is easier and safer than a "use test" with a questionable allergen, for test items can be applied in low concentrations in small areas of skin for short periods of time. See textbooks on contact dermatitis for list of antigens used in patch testing.

4. *Photopatch testing* is a combination of patch testing and UV irradiation of the test site and is used to document photoallergy.

5. *Phototesting* is done to determine the patient's sensitivity to various wavelengths of UV radiation. This is useful in the diagnosis of certain photosensitivities.

MICROSCOPE EXAMINATION OF SCALES, CRUSTS, SERUM, AND HAIR

1. *Gram's stains* and *cultures of exudates and of tissue minces* should be made in lesions suspected of being bacterial or yeast *(Candida albicans)* infections. Ulcers and nodules require a scalpel biopsy in which a wedge of tissue consisting of all three layers of skin is obtained; the biopsy specimen is minced in a sterile mortar and the tissue is then cultured for bacteria (including typical and atypical mycobacteria) and fungi.

2. *Microscope examination* for mycelia should be made of the roofs of vesicles or of the scales (the advancing borders are preferable) or of the hair. The tissue is cleared with 10% KOH and warmed gently (see Figure 51 for illustration of hyphae). Fungal cultures with Sabouraud's medium should be made.

3. *Microscope examination of cells obtained from the base of vesicles* (Tzanck preparation) may reveal the presence of giant epithelial cells and multinucleated giant cells (containing 10 to 12 nuclei) in herpes simplex, herpes zoster, and varicella. Material from the base of a vesicle obtained by gentle curettage

with a scalpel is smeared on a glass slide, stained with Giemsa's or Wright's stain, and examined to determine whether there are giant epithelial cells, which are diagnostic. Cultures of herpes simplex are now easily available.

4. *Laboratory diagnosis of scabies* The diagnosis of scabies is usually immediately considered in a patient with intractable generalized pruritus and with papules and excoriations distributed in characteristic locations—on the flexor aspects of the wrists, in the finger webs, and on the buttocks and genitalia; the diagnosis is established by identification of the mite, or ova or feces, in skin scrapings removed from the papules or burrows (see Figure 80). The burrow, a unique lesion, is a linear or serpiginous elevation of skin in the form of a ridge, 0.5 to 1.0 cm in length. These occur on the anterior surface of the wrists, in the webs of the fingers, or on the ulnar border of the hands. If burrows are not present, select a papule or the roof of a vesicle on the hand. The mineral oil technique is excellent for isolating the mite. Using a sterile scalpel blade on which a drop of sterile mineral oil has been placed, apply oil to the surface of the burrow or papule. Scrape the papule or burrow vigorously (about 6 times) in order to remove the entire top of the papule, tiny flecks of blood will appear in the oil. Transfer the oil to a coverglass and examine for mites, ova, and feces. The mites are 0.2 to 0.4 mm in size and have 4 pairs of legs (see Figure 80).

5. *Dark-field examination of serum from ulcers* on the male or female genitalia (especially the penis, anus, vulva, and cervix) is essential for detection of *Treponema pallidum*. Dark-field examinations are not worthwhile in material obtained from the oral cavity because of the presence of nonpathogenic treponemas indistinguishable from *T.*

pallidum. In this case and after topical treatment of an ulcer with antibiotics, dark-field examination of a lymph node aspirate is made. (A serologic test for syphilis is mandatory for all patients with generalized erythematous and scaling eruptions, including all patients with the presumptive diagnosis of pityriasis rosea.)

BIOPSY OF THE SKIN

Biopsy of the skin is one of the simplest, most rewarding diagnostic techniques in medical practice because of the easy accessibility of the skin and the variety of techniques for study of the excised specimen (e.g., immunofluorescence, electron microscopy).

The selection of the site of the biopsy is based primarily on the stage of the eruption, and early lesions are usually more typical; this is especially important in vesiculobullous eruptions (e.g., pemphigus, herpes simplex) in which the lesion should be no more than 24 hours old. However, older lesions (2 to 6 weeks) are often more characteristic in discoid lupus erythematosus.

A common technique for diagnostic biopsy is the use of a 3.0- to 4.0-mm punch, a small tubular knife much like a corkscrew, which by rotating movements between the thumb and index finger cuts through the epidermis, dermis, and subcutaneous tissue; the base is cut off with scissors. If immunofluorescence is indicated (as, for example, in bullous diseases or lupus erythematosus), a special technique is necessary and the laboratory should be consulted.

For nodules, however, a large wedge should be removed by excision including subcutaneous tissue. Furthermore, all nodules, regardless of size, should be bisected, one half for histology, the other half sent in a sterile container for bacterial and mycotic cultures using a tissue mince.

Specimens for light microscopy should be fixed immediately in buffered neutral formalin. A brief but detailed summary of the clinical history and description of the lesions should accompany the specimen. Biopsy is indicated in *all* skin lesions that are suspected of being neoplasms, in all bullous disorders using immunofluorescence simultaneously, and in all dermatologic disorders in which a specific diagnosis is not possible by clinical examination alone.

Appendix C: Generalized Pruritus without Diagnostic Skin Lesions

Persistent severe pruritus, like pain, is a dominating factor in existence; from day to day it takes over one's life. Intense pruritus may, in fact, be more maddening for the patient than pain because there is no effective medication for the control of pruritus; pain can usually be controlled with analgesics. The physician, therefore, feels somewhat helpless in the management of these unfortunate patients. Pruritus leads to sleepless nights; a state of permanent fatigue ensues that precludes work and confounds and compounds family relationships.

The approach to the patient with generalized pruritus without identifiable skin lesions is to consider this symptom in the same manner as a patient with factitious (i.e., not based on organic disease) dermatosis—*generalized pruritus and factitious dermatosis are both diagnoses of exclusion:* all organic causes must be excluded within reasonable limits.

The differential diagnosis of generalized pruritus is presented in Table C-1. The work-up of these patients is presented in Table C-2.

Table C-1   Differential Diagnosis of Pruritus

METABOLIC AND ENDOCRINE CONDITIONS	MALIGNANT NEOPLASMS	DRUGS INGESTION	INFESTATIONS
Hyperthyroidism	Lymphoma and	Subclinical	Pediculosis
Diabetes	leukemia	drug sensitivities:	corporis
mellitus	Abdominal	aspirin, alcohol,	Scabies*
Hypothyroidism	cancer	dextran, poly-	Hookworm
Hyperparathyroidism	Multiple	myxin B, morphine,	(ancylostomiasis)
secondary to	myeloma	codeine, scopola-	Onchocerciasis
chronic renal		mine, d-tubocura-	Ascariasis
failure		rine	

HEMATOLOGIC DISEASE	HEPATIC DISEASE	PSYCHOGENIC STATES	MISCELLANEOUS CONDITIONS
Polycythemia	Obstructive	Transitory:	Dry skin
vera	biliary disease	Periods of	(xerosis)
Paraproteinemia	(intrahepatic	emotional	"Senile"
Iron deficiency	10%, extrahepatic	stress	pruritus†
	40%)	Persistent:	Pregnancy-
	Pregnancy (intra-	Delusions of	related disorders
	hepatic cho-	parasitosis	Fiberglass exposure
	lestasis)	Psychogenic	Chronic renal
		pruritus	failure (late)
		Neurotic excoriation	

*Diagnostic lesions may or may not be present.

†Unexplained intense pruritus in patients over 70 years without obvious "dry skin" and with no apparent emotional stress.

Table C-2   Approach to the Diagnosis of Generalized Pruritus without Diagnostic Skin Lesions

---

Initial Visit
1. Detailed history of pruritus:
   - Are there any skin lesions that precede the itching?
   - Severity: Does the itching keep the patient awake?
2. History of weight loss, fatigue, fever, malaise
3. Has there been a recent emotional stress situation?
4. History of oral or parenteral medication which can be a cause of generalized pruritus without a rash
5. Examine carefully for subtle primary skin disorders as a cause of the pruritus: xerosis or asteatosis, scabies, pediculosis (nits?)
6. General physical examination including *all* the lymph nodes; rectal examination and stool guaiac in adult patients
7. If pruritus has been present for more than 2 weeks, obtain additional data (see Nos. 1–3 below)
8. Give the patient bath oil, followed by an emollient ointment. No soap; the bath is therapeutic, not for cleansing the skin; shower to clean.
9. Follow-up appointment in two weeks

Subsequent Visit(s)
If no relief from symptomatic treatment given on the first visit, proceed as follows:
1. Obtain chest roentgenogram
2. Detailed review of systems. Refer patient for pelvic examination, Pap smear
3. Laboratory tests: complete blood tests including erythrocyte sedimentation rate, fasting blood sugar, renal function tests, liver function tests, hepatitis antigens, thyroid tests, stool for parasites
4. If the diagnosis has not been established at this point, the patient should be referred to an internist for complete work-up including further imaging (scans, ultrasound, etc.).

The sudden appearance of a rash and fever is frightening for the patient. Medical advice is immediately sought and often in the emergency units of hospitals; about 10% of all patients seeking emergency medical care have a dermatologic problem.

The diagnosis of an acute rash with a fever is a clinical challenge. Rarely do physicians have to "lean" on their eyes as much as when confronted by an acutely ill patient with fever and a skin eruption. If a diagnosis is not established promptly in certain patients (e.g., those having septicemia), life-saving treatment may be delayed.

The cutaneous findings alone may be diagnostic before confirmatory laboratory data are available. As in the problems of the acute abdomen, the results of some laboratory tests, such as microbiologic cultures, may not be immediately available. On the basis of a differential diagnosis, appropriate therapy— whether antibiotics or corticosteroids—may be started. Furthermore, prompt diagnosis and isolation of the patient with a contagious disease, which may have serious consequences, prevents spread to other persons. For example, varicella in adults can rarely be fatal. Contagious diseases presenting with rash and fever as the major findings include *viral infections* (varicella-zoster, herpes simplex, measles, rubella, enterovirus and parvovirus infections) and *bacterial infections* (streptococcal, staphylococcal, meningococcal, typhoid, and syphilis).

The physical diagnosis of skin eruptions is a discipline based on precise identification of the type of skin lesion. The physician must not only identify and classify the *type* of skin lesion but look for additional morphologic clues such as: the *configuration* (annular? iris?) of the individual lesion; the *arrangement* of the lesions (zosteriform? linear?); the *distribution*

pattern (exposed areas? centripetal or centrifugal? mucous membranes?). In the differential diagnosis of exanthems it is important to determine, by history, the *site of first appearance* (the rash of Rocky Mountain spotted fever characteristically appears first on the wrists and ankles), and very important is the *temporal evolution* of the rash (measles spreads from head to toes in a period of 3 days while the rash of rubella spreads rapidly in 24 to 48 hours from head to toes and then sequentially clears—first face, then trunk, and then limbs).

Although there may be some overlap, the differential diagnostic possibilities may be grouped into four main categories according to the type of lesion (see Table D-1).

LABORATORY TESTS AVAILABLE FOR QUICK DIAGNOSIS

The physician should make use of the following laboratory tests immediately or within 8 hours:

1. *Direct smear from the base of a vesicle.* This procedure, known as the *Tzanck test,* is performed by unroofing an intact vesicle, gently scraping the base with a curved scalpel blade, and smearing the contents on a slide. After air drying, the smear is stained with Wright's or Giemsa's stain and examined for multinucleated giant cells. These altered epidermal cells are present in the herpes simplex and herpes zoster-varicella groups.

2. *Viral culture,* especially for herpes simplex.

3. *Gram's stain of aspirates or scraping.* This is essential for proper diagnosis of pustules. Organisms can be seen in the

DISEASES MANIFESTED BY MACULES, PAPULES, NODULES, OR PLAQUES	DISEASES MANIFESTED BY VESICLES, BULLAE, OR PUSTULES	DISEASES MANIFESTED BY PURPURIC MACULES, PURPURIC PAPULES, OR PURPURIC VESICLES	DISEASES MANIFESTED BY WIDESPREAD ERYTHEMA ± EDEMA FOLLOWED BY DESQUAMATION
Drug hypersensitivities	Drug hypersensitivities	Drug hypersensitivities	Drug hypersensitivities
Sweet's syndrome	Allergic contact dermatitis from plants	Bacteremia:*	Scarlet fever
Eosinophilia-myalgia syndrome	Rickettsial pox	Meningococcemia (acute or chronic)	Staphylococcal scalded-skin syndrome
Streptococcal cellulitis	Gonococcemia	Gonococcemia†	Toxic shock syndrome
Erythema migrans of Lyme disease	Varicella (chickenpox)‡	Staphylococcemia	Kawasaki's syndrome
Meningococcemia	Herpes zoster‡	Pseudomonas bacteremia	Toxic epidermal necrolysis
Human immunodeficiency virus, primary infection	Herpes simplex‡	Subacute bacterial endocarditis	Graft-versus-host reaction
Erythema infectiosum (parvovirus B19)	Eczema herpeticum‡	Enterovirus infections (echo and Coxsackie)	von Zumbusch pustular psoriasis
Cytomegalovirus, primary infection	Enterovirus infections (echo and Coxsackie), including hand-foot-and-mouth disease	Rickettsial diseases: Rocky Mountain spotted fever	Erythroderma
Epstein-Barr virus, primary infection	Toxic epidermal necrolysis	Typhus, louse-borne (epidemic)	
Exanthem subitum (human herpesvirus-6)	Staphylococcal scalded-skin syndrome	"Allergic" vasculitis*	
Measles (rubeola)	Erythema multiforme bullosum	Disseminated intravascular coagulation (purpura fulminans‡)	
Measles (rubeola), atypical	Kawasaki's disease		
German measles (rubella)†			
Enterovirus infections (echo and Coxsackie)			
Adenovirus infections			
Typhoid fever			
Secondary syphilis			
Typhus, murine (endemic)			
Rocky Mountain spotted fever (early lesions)†			
Other spotted fevers			
Disseminated deep fungal infection in immunocompromised patients			

DISEASES MANIFESTED BY MACULES, PAPULES, NODULES, OR PLAQUES	DISEASES MANIFESTED BY VESICLES, BULLAE, OR PUSTULES	DISEASES MANIFESTED BY PURPURIC MACULES, PURPURIC PAPULES, OR PURPURIC VESICLES	DISEASES MANIFESTED BY WIDESPREAD ERYTHEMA ± EDEMA FOLLOWED BY DESQUAMATION
Pityriasis rosea (fever, rare)			
Erythema multiforme			
Erythema marginatum			
Systemic lupus erythematosus‡			
Dermatomyositis			
"Serum sickness" (manifested only as wheals and angioedema)			
Urticaria, acute (viral hepatitis)			
Gianotti-Crosti syndrome			

*Often present as infarcts.
†May have arthralgia or musculoskeletal pain.
‡One characteristic lesion of these exanthems is an umbilicated papule or vesicle.

lesions of acute meningococcemia, rarely in the skin lesions of gonococcemia and ecthyma gangrenosum.

4. *Touch preparation.* This is especially helpful in deep fungal infections and leishmaniasis. The dermal part of a skin biopsy specimen is touched repeatedly to a glass slide; the touch preparation is *immediately* fixed in 95% ethyl alcohol. Special stains are then performed and the slide examined for organisms in the cytology laboratory.

5. *Biopsy of the skin lesions.* All purpuric lesions should be biopsied. Inflammatory dermal nodules and most ulcers should be biopsied and a portion of tissue minced and cultured for bacteria and fungi. A 3.0- to 4.0-mm trephine and local anesthesia are used. In many laboratories the biopsy specimen can be processed within 8 hours if necessary.

A histologic diagnosis can be made in instances of Rocky Mountain spotted fever, SLE, erythema multiforme bullosum, toxic epidermal necrolysis, herpes zoster, varicella, allergic vasculitis, secondary syphilis, some bacteremias, and deep fungal infections.

6. *Blood and urine examinations.* Blood culture, rapid serologic test for syphilis and serology for lupus erythematosus require 24 hours. Examination of urine sediment may reveal cell casts in allergic vasculitis.

7. *Dark-field examination.* In the skin lesions of secondary syphilis, repeated examination of papules may show *Treponema pallidum*. The dark-field examination is not reliable in the mouth as nonpathogenic organisms are almost impossible to differentiate from *T. pallidum*.

RECOMMENDATIONS FOR THE MANAGEMENT OF PIGMENTED LESIONS TO FACILITATE EARLY DIAGNOSIS OF MALIGNANT MELANOMA[1]

For the Examining Physician

1. Histologic diagnosis is necessary in all pigmented lesions with the following three physical characteristics—the hallmarks of atypicality in a pigmented lesion:

   a. Irregularity of the borders: with pseudopods, a notch, or even a "maple leaf" configuration (see Figures 340 and 341)

   b. An irregular array of colors: a gradation of red, gray, or blue, admixed with brown or black, displayed in a disorderly, haphazard pigment pattern. *Additional indications:* black nodules with uniform borders, irregularly pigmented lesions with uniform borders

   c. Increases in size

2. All congenital melanocytic nevi should be considered for excision, regardless of size. Lesions should be followed with photography until they can be excised some time before puberty. The timing of excision for small congenital lesions will depend on the clinical characteristics (light brown, uniform color is a sign of benignancy), whether general anesthesia is needed, and on the disability that will result from surgery. All giant nevi should be removed if feasible.

3. Any pigmented lesion striking a physician's eye as "out of the ordinary" should be further evaluated (i.e., excision or referral for same).

4. All patients with a history of melanoma should be thoroughly examined for atypical melanocytic nevi (dysplastic nevi) and for the appearance of new primary melanomas). Patients with dysplastic nevi should be followed at 6-month intervals.

5. All blood relatives of patients with melanoma should be examined for dysplastic nevi and early primary melanoma. (The presence of a family history increases the risk 8- to 13-fold for an individual.)

6. All white patients presenting for any problem should be examined for the presence of large melanocytic nevi (greater than 1.0 cm), for dysplastic nevi, and for nevi on the scalp, mucous membrane, and anogenital area. All black persons should be examined for pigmented lesions of the soles, nail beds, and mucous membranes.

Advice to the Patient

The following advice should be made regarding pigmented lesions.

Seek prompt examination for the following:

All persons with a family history of melanoma

All persons with skin phototype I and II, especially those with a history of intense or prolonged sun exposure

Any pigmented mole that was present at birth

Any newly appearing mole after puberty

[1] Melanoma Cooperative Group (Harvard).

All persons with many (uncountable!) moles >2.0 mm in diameter and/or with any number of moles >5.0 mm in diameter

Any changing mole—in size, color, or border

Any mole that itches or is tender for more than 2 weeks

Any mole that is considered "ugly" because of its size, color, pattern, or borders

Persons with skin phototype I and II should *never* sunbathe. Persons with dysplastic nevi or a melanoma, regardless of skin phototype, should *never* sunbathe or do outdoor work without appropriate clothing. Sunscreens with a sun protection factor (SPF) of >30 should be used in all persons with dysplastic nevi or a previous history of melanoma and in persons with skin phototypes I and II.

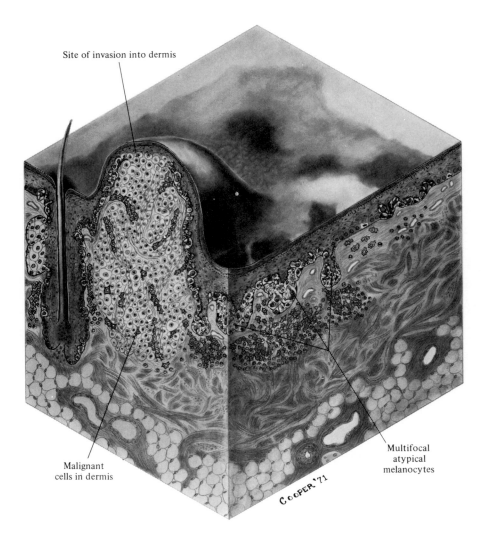

Site of invasion into dermis

Malignant cells in dermis

Multifocal atypical melanocytes

COOPER '71

PRIMARY MELANOMA OF THE SKIN: THREE MAJOR TYPES

Figure E-1 Lentigo maligna melanoma. Illustrated is a large, flat, variegated, freckle-like *macule* (not elevated above the plane of the skin) with irregular borders. These areas show increased numbers of melanocytes, usu- ally atypical and bizarre and distributed along the basal layer; at certain places in the dermis, malignant melanocytes have invaded and formed huge nests. At the left is a large nodule which is comprised of large epithelioid cells in this illustration; the nodules of all three types of melanoma are indistinguishable from each other.

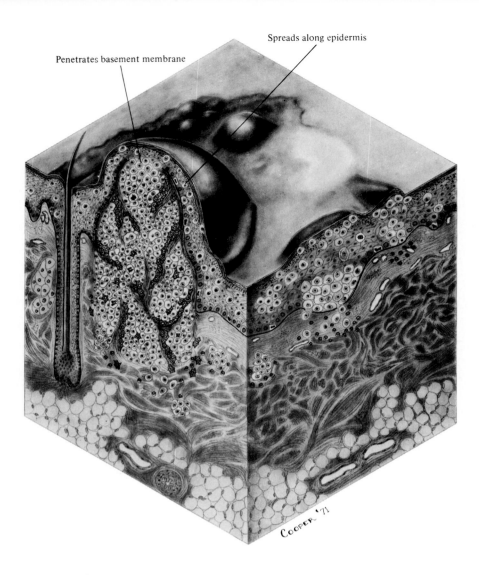

Penetrates basement membrane

Spreads along epidermis

Cooper '71

Figure E-2 Superficial spreading melanoma. The border is irregular and elevated throughout its entirety; biopsy of the area surrounding the large nodule shows a pagetoid distribution of large melanocytes throughout the dermis, occurring singly or in nests, and uniformly atypical. On the left is a large nodule, and scattered throughout the surrounding portion of the nodule are smaller papular and nodular areas. The nodule on the left shows malignant melanocytes that are very large and have an abundance of cytoplasm. The melanocytes often have regularly dispersed fine particles of melanin. The nodules may also show spindle cells or small malignant melanocytes as in lentigo maligna melanoma and nodular melanoma.

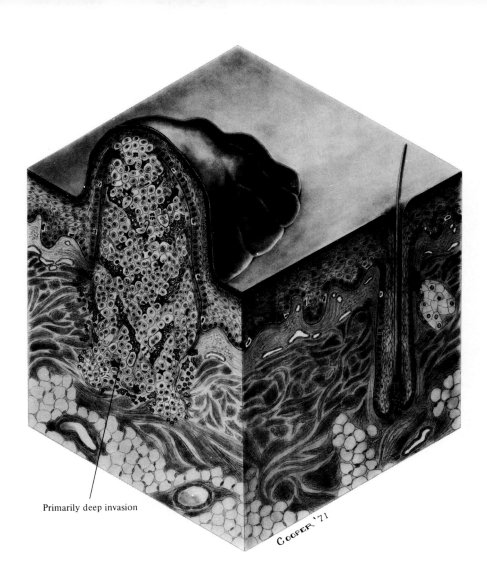

Primarily deep invasion

COOPER '71

Figure E-3 Nodular melanoma. This arises at the dermoepidermal junction and extends laterally in the dermis; intraepidermal growth is present only in a small group of tumor cells that conjointly are also invading the underlying dermis. The epidermis lateral to the areas of this invasion does not demonstrate atypical melanocytes. As in lentigo maligna melanoma and superficial spreading melanoma, the tumor may show large epithelioid cells, spindle cells, small malignant melanocytes, or mixtures of all three.

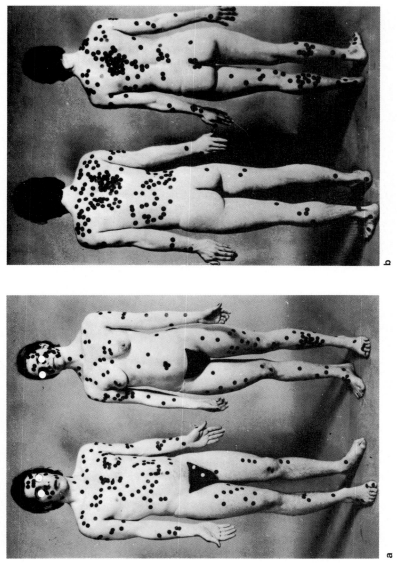

Figure E-4 *Localization of malignant melanoma in 731 males and females.*

SUMMARY DATA ON MALIGNANT MELANOMA OF SKIN

I. **Incidence** (United States, 32,000)   Three percent of all cancers (excluding nonmelanoma skin cancer)

   A. Overall annual crude incidence rates (United States)

     Caucasians   10.4 per 100,000 population per year (1988)

   B. Increasing with time (U.S. whites)

     1. 1970   4.5 per 100,000 population per year

     2. 1975   7.2 per 100,000 population per year

     3. 1980   9.7 per 100,000 population per year

     4. 1985   11.2 per 100,000 population per year

II. **Frequency for Type of Melanoma**

   A. Superficial spreading   70%

   B. Nodular   16%

   C. Lentigo maligna melanoma   5%

   D. Unclassified (includes acral lentiginous type)   9%

III. **Mortality**   Overall deaths (United States, 6500); melanoma represents 1 to 2% percent of all cancer deaths

GUIDELINES FOR BIOPSY, SURGICAL TREATMENT, AND FOLLOW-UP OF PATIENTS WITH MELANOMA

I. **Biopsy**

   A. Total excisional biopsy with narrow margins—optimal biopsy procedure, where possible

   B. Incisional or punch acceptable when total excisional biopsy cannot be performed or when lesion is large, requiring extensive surgery to remove the entire lesion

II. **Lentigo Maligna Melanoma—All Levels**

   1. Excise with a 1-cm or greater margin beyond the clinically visible lesion or biopsy scar provided the flat component does not involve a major organ (e.g., the eye), in which case lesser margins are acceptable.

   2. Excise down to or including the fascia or to the underlying muscle where fascia is absent. Skin flaps or skin grafts may be used for closure.

   3. No node dissection recommended unless nodes are clinically palpable and suspicious for tumor.

III. **Superficial Spreading Melanoma, Nodular Melanoma, and Acral Melanoma**

   A. Thickness <1.0 mm and no clinical or histopathologic evidence of regression

     1. Excise or reexcise with at least a 1.0-cm margin from the lesion edge

     2. Excise down to fascia or underlying muscle where fascia is absent. Direct closure without graft is usually possible.

     3. Node dissection is not recommended unless nodes are clinically suspicious for tumor.

   B. Thickness 1.0 to 4.0 mm

     1. Excise or reexcise 2.0 cm from the edge of the lesion, except on the face.

     2. Excise down to fascia or underlying muscle where fascia is absent. Graft may be required.

     3. Elective nodal dissection is optional and at the discretion of the surgeon. Regional lymph node dissections are done in some centers for melanomas with a thickness of >1.7 mm.

IV. Follow-up (to find second primary melanoma or metastasis)

1. For thin tumors, 1.0 mm or less: the patient should be seen every 6 months for one year, then every year for 10 years. If atypical moles (dysplastic nevus syndrome) are present, follow the patient according to the guidelines for intermediate and thick lesions (see ''2'' below).
2. For intermediate (1.0 to 4.0 mm) and thick (>4.0 mm) lesions *and* patients with dysplastic nevus syndrome and melanoma, patients should be seen every 3 months for two years. Every 6 months for years 3 to 5, and every 6 to 12 months thereafter. A chest x-ray should be obtained yearly.

Table E-1   Eight-Year Survival for Patients with Clinical Stage I Melanoma in the Vertical Growth Phase Based on Single Factor Analysis of Prognostic Variables*

VARIABLE	CATEGORIES	% 8-YEAR SURVIVAL
Mitotic rate/mm^2	0.0	95.1
	0.1–6.0	79.4
	> 6.0	38.2
TILs†	Brisk	88.5
	Nonbrisk	75.0
	Absent	59.3
Thickness	< 0.76 mm	93.2
	0.76–1.69	85.6
	1.70–3.60	59.8
	> 3.60	33.3
Anatomic site	Extremities	87.3
	Head, neck, and trunk	62.4
	Volar or subungual	46.2
Sex	Female	83.8
	Male	56.6
Regression	Absent	77.0
	Present	60.0

*Modified from Clark WH, Jr, et al: Model predicting survival in stage I melanoma based on tumor progression. *JNCI* 81:1893, 1989.
†Tumor-infiltrating lymphocytes

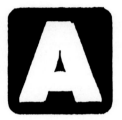

ASYMMETRY in shape—one half unlike the other

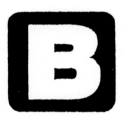

BORDER is irregular—edges irregularly scalloped

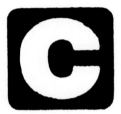

COLOR is mottled—haphazard display of colors: shades of brown, black, gray, and white

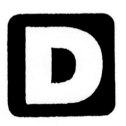

DIAMETER is usually large—greater than the tip of a pencil eraser (6.0 mm)

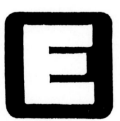

ELEVATION is almost always present—surface distortion, subtle or obvious, assessed by side-lighting. Acral lentiginous lesions may be flat.

Appendix G: Risk Factors of White Adults for Cutaneous Melanoma*

Mortality rates of primary melanoma in white persons for single years from 1975 to 1982 increased at the rate of 3% per year in males. In males living in Connecticut, ages 30 to 49, primary melanoma is the second most prevalent of all cancers—the first being cancer of the testis. Physicians and health care providers are in a unique position to improve the survival rates of melanoma of the skin because not only are the characteristics of early melanoma well delineated (see page 789) and easily detected, but there are now known the characteristics of the population at risk. The following factors list the degree of risk for persons with the risk factor compared with persons without the risk factor. (With a relative risk of 1.0, there is no increased risk.)

	Risk
1. Changing "mole"	Very high

This is seen as a change in color—especially darkening and mottling, in a previously uniformly colored mole. Also, an increase in size (height or diameter) and change in borders (becoming irregular); these are early signs of a mole changing to a melanoma.

2. Large, irregularly shaped, pigmented lesions

A. Clark's dysplastic melanocytic nevi (see page 656):

With a history of melanoma in the family	148 ×
Without a history of melanoma in the family	27 ×
B. Lentigo maligna (see page 664)	10 ×

3. Congenital mole (see page 660)   21 ×

Lesions >1.5 cm are either dysplastic melanocytic nevi or congenital melanocytic nevi

4. Family history of melanoma of the skin in parents, siblings, or children   8 ×

5. Inability to tan normally   3 ×

Skin phototypes I and II (see page 210). There also appears to be increased risk of persons with a history of excessive sun exposure, especially obtained during childhood.

---

*Adapted in part from Rhodes AR et al: Risk factors for cutaneous melanoma. JAMA 258:3146–3154, 1987.

The nails are rarely scrutinized during the physical examination unless there are prominent and obvious abnormalities. It is, therefore, important to carefully examine the nails for signs of multisystem disease.

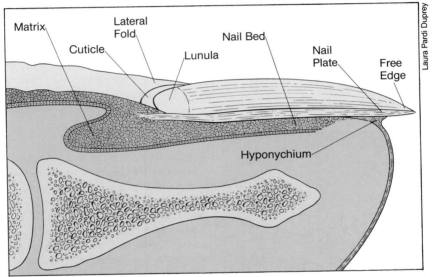

Laura Pardi Duprey

Normal Nail (Figure H-1) The nail has several distinct anatomical areas. The hard nail plate emerges from a matrix of specialized epithelial cells. The matrix begins 7 to 8 mm under the proximal nail fold, and its distal end is the white crescent called the lunula. The richly vascularized nail bed lies directly beneath the plate to provide adherence and support and is the basis of the characteristic pink color. The proximal and lateral nail folds surround the plate on three sides, and the cuticle, an outgrowth of the proximal fold, provides a seal between the fold and the nail plate.

*Modified from Kvedar JC, Fitzpatrick TB: The nails as clues to multisystem disease. *Current Challenges in Dermatology.* Summer, 1990.

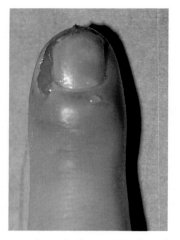

Herpetic Whitlow (Figure H-2) The term *whitlow,* or *felon,* literally refers to infection of the closed space between fascial planes at the terminal phalanx of the finger, but today that term is loosely used to describe herpetic infection of the distal finger. Herpetic whitlow can cause pain—at times severe enough to require morphine—during the period of active infection. The pain, however, usually subsides within 10 to 14 days. In addition to typical herpetiform blisters, clinical signs may include an edematous fingertip, erythematous streaking on the forearm, and enlarged, tender axillary lymph nodes. Visualization of multinucleate giant cells using the Tzanck test will establish the diagnosis. If the Tzanck test is negative, culture for herpes simplex virus should be performed. Antiviral therapy has not yet been proven effective. Because of its low toxicity, oral acyclovir probably should nevertheless be administered. Unfortunately, herpetic whitlow can recur and may be severe; the entire hand and forearm may become edematous.

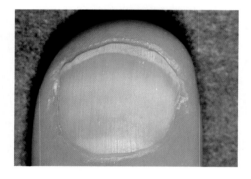

Muehrcke's Nails (Figure H-3) Muehrcke's nails are characterized by paired narrow horizontal white bands, separated by normal color, that remain immobile as the nail grows. Muehrcke's nails are most often seen in patients with hypoalbuminemia associated with nephrotic syndrome, and their presence correlates with low serum albumin levels. The pathogenesis of the nail abnormality is not known.

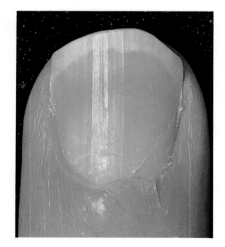

Terry's Nails (Figure H-4) The proximal two-thirds of the nail plate is white, whereas the distal third shows the red color of the nail bed. The dramatic color changes of Terry's nails are rare occurrences, but they may be a manifestation of congestive heart failure or hypoalbuminemia associated with hepatic cirrhosis.

"Half-and-Half" Nail In the classic presentation of the half-and-half nail, the distal half is pink or brown and is sharply demarcated from the proximal half, which is dull and white and obliterates the lunula. The difference between half-and-half and Terry's nails is unclear and debatable. Half-and-half nails are found in 10% of patients with the uremia of chronic renal failure. The color change does not correlate with the severity of renal disease.

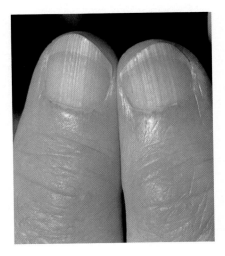

Nail Fold Telangiectasia (Figure H-5) In this condition, the capillary loops of the proximal nail fold become tortuous and dilated, presumably as a result of injury from repeated bouts of microangiitis and immune complex deposition. Nail fold telangiectasia occurs with varying degrees of severity. It is a characteristic feature of dermatomyositis but is also seen in systemic lupus erythematosus and rarely in progressive systemic sclerosis. Some believe a diagnosis of connective tissue disease can reliably be made on the basis of the nail fold abnormality.

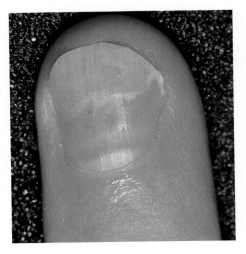

Onycholysis (Figure H-6) Onycholysis, or *Plummer's nail,* is a separation of the nail plate from the nail bed. The separated portion is white and opaque, in contrast to the pink translucence of the attached portion. Plummer's nail may be a sign of hyperthyroidism, especially when it affects only the ring finger. In most cases of hyperthyroidism, the skin of the fingers is warm and moist with a velvety texture and the palm is erythematous. Onycholysis is, however, a very common nail abnormality that also accompanies trauma, chemical exposure, and psoriasis.

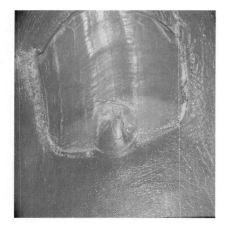

Periungual Fibroma (Figure H-7) The appearance of periungual fibroma in any patient should prompt a careful family history, cutaneous examination, and neurologic workup (including x-rays of the skull) for tuberous sclerosis. This inherited disorder has both cutaneous and neurologic manifestations. The degree of neurologic dysfunction varies, however, and in some patients a minor cutaneous finding such as periungual fibroma may be the only sign of the disease. These fibromas are asymptomatic but can produce a longitudinal groove in the nail plate when located in the proximal nail fold. There is no treatment for tuberous sclerosis; however, it is important to recognize the disease so that the patient and parents can receive genetic counseling.

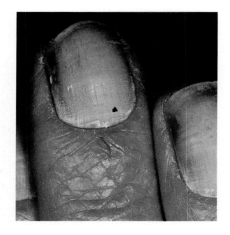

Yellow Nail Syndrome (Figure H-8) A clinical triad characterizes the yellow nail syndrome: opaque yellow and dystrophic nails; lymphatic abnormalities (aplasia, ectasia, lymphedema, lymphangitis); and systemic illness, usually pulmonary disease (bronchiectasis, pleural effusion) or cancer (Hodgkin's lymphoma, endometrial carcinoma, malignant melanoma, lymphoma). Changes include a diffuse yellow-to-green color of the fingernails and toenails, nail thickening, slowed growth, and excessive curvature from side to side. There may be concomitant edema of the fingertips and ankles and on occasion very severe edema of the face. Even when severe, edema may be associated with normal lymph nodes on lymphangiography.

Blue Nails (Figure H-9) Antimalarial drugs, minocycline, hemochromatosis, Wilson's disease, ochronosis, and exposure to silver nitrate may be associated with blue or blue-gray nails. *Wilson's disease* is an autosomal recessive disorder that results in toxic accumulations of copper in the liver, brain, and other organs. The first clinical signs are often neurologic (resting and intention tremors, spasticity, rigidity, chorea), while Kayser-Fleischer rings (deposits of copper in the cornea) and a blue discoloration of the lunulae appear later. *Ochronosis* is an autosomal recessive defect of homogentisic acid metabolism, in which deposits of polymerized homogentisic acid appear as a blue pigmentation of the sclerae, as blue macules on the outer ear, and as a diffuse blue-gray pigmentation of the nail bed. Prolonged ingestion, injection, or mucosal ab-

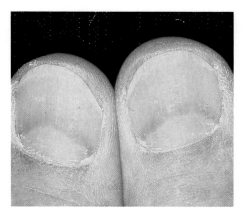

sorption of silver nitrate produces *argyria*—a diffuse gray-blue pigmentation of the skin and bluish discoloration of the lunulae similar to that seen in Wilson's disease.

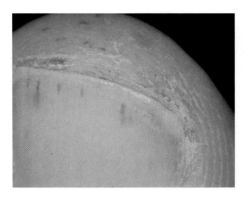

Splinter Hemorrhages (Figure H-10) The brown or red streaks that represent splinter hemorrhages most often result from trauma to the nail. They may, however, be a sign of serious multisystem disease, including trichinosis and subacute bacterial endocarditis. In multisystem disease, splinter hemorrhages develop from infarction of arterioles in the nail bed. The infarction is usually secondary to microembolism.

Beau's Lines (Figure H-11) The horizontal depressions across the nail plate that constitute Beau's lines are caused by a transient arrest in nail growth. A temporary growth arrest can occur during acute stress (e.g., high fever, circulatory shock, myocardial infarction, pulmonary embolism) and will manifest as Beau's lines as the nail grows out. It is, therefore, possible to pinpoint the date of the illness by the distance of the furrow from the proximal nail fold. Depending on the age of the patient, the nail plate takes 3 to 4 months to grow from its base to its distal edge. In a variation of Beau's lines, white transverse bands (Mees' lines) mark the stressful event.

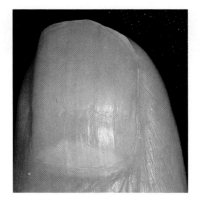

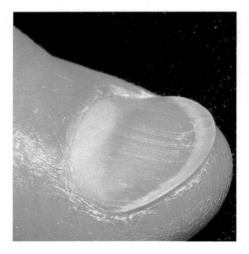

Koilonychia (Figure H-12) Commonly called spoon nails, koilonychia is caused by softening and thinning of the nail plate that results in concave or spoon-shaped nails. Spoon nails are seen in patients with long-standing iron-deficiency anemia or Plummer-Vinson syndrome (a combination of koilonychia, dysphagia, and glossitis that primarily affects middle-aged women). Other causes include Raynaud's syndrome, hemochromatosis, and physical or chemical trauma. Koilonychia also may be inherited as an autosomal dominant disorder.

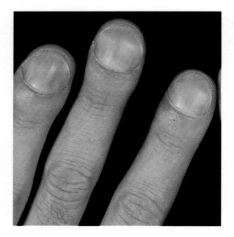

Clubbed Fingers (Figure H-13) Also known as Hippocratic fingers, clubbing appears as a bulbous enlargement and broadening of the fingertips. The angle between the nail plate and proximal nail fold (Lovibond's angle; Figure H-14) is greater than the normal 180° or less. The tissue between the nail and underlying bone has a spongy quality that gives a "floating" sensation when pressure is applied downward and forward at the junction between the plate and proximal fold.

Clubbed fingers are the result of hyperplasia of the fibrovascular tissue between the nail matrix and the bony phalanx. The pathogenesis is unknown, but an increased blood supply to the fingers is seen on arteriography. The hypervascularity is thought to be related to opening of the arteriovenous anastomosis by an unknown humoral vasodilating substance.

Clubbed fingers may be inherited as an autosomal dominant trait and are not associated with systemic disease. When acquired, clubbed fingers are most commonly indicative of cardiac disease (cyanotic heart disease, bacterial endocarditis); pulmonary disease (primary and metastatic cancer, bronchiectasis, lung abscess, mesothelioma); or gastrointestinal disease (regional enteritis, ulcerative colitis, and hepatic cirrhosis).

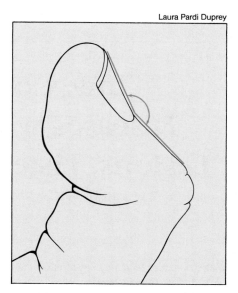
Laura Pardi Duprey

Brown Nails Abnormal pigmentation may affect the nail plate and nail bed individually or together. Brown nails occur in Addison's disease (plate); in hemochromatosis (plate); with gold therapy (plate); with arsenic intoxication (plate); and in malignant melanoma (plate, bed, fold). In white patients with multiple brown nails, important considerations in the differential diagnosis are Addison's disease and Nelson's syndrome (an ACTH-producing pituitary tumor that develops after bilateral adrenalectomy in patients with Cushing's syndrome).

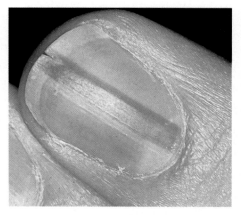

Brown linear bands or streaks are a common and normal finding in black- or brown-skinned persons. In white persons, a single pigmented streak may be a melanocytic nevus (Figure H-15). However, when the proximal nail fold is also involved (Hutchinson's sign; Figure H-16), malignant melanoma must be suspected. Hutchinson's sign may include brown-black discoloration of the proximal and lateral nail folds and brown-black pigmentation of the nail matrix, bed, and plate (obliterating the lunula). The nail plate may also show dystrophic changes.

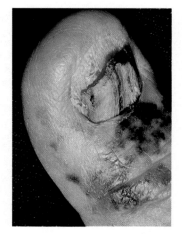

Index of Communicable Diseases with Dermatologic Lesions, Listed by Geographic Area

With the marked increase in international travel in the past decade among all walks of life and all ages, it is necessary to ask a patient with skin lesions where he or she has traveled in recent weeks. The following index* of diseases with skin lesions that can be acquired in various countries is presented to facilitate the diagnosis and, therefore, the appropriate treatment.

Caribbean, Mexico, Central and Tropical South America, Temperate South America, and Andes Mountains

CARIBBEAN ISLANDS	MEXICO	CENTRAL AMERICA AND TROPICAL SOUTH AMERICA	TEMPERATE SOUTH AMERICA	ANDES MOUNTAINS
Dengue	Amebiasis	Amebiasis	Arenavirus	Bartonellosis
Hookworm	Chagas' disease	Anisakiasis	infection:	Brucellosis
	Cysticercosis	Ascariasis	Argentine	Plague
	Dengue	Chagas' disease	hemorrhagic	Tuberculosis
	Hepatitis	Filariasis	fever, Bolivian	Typhus
	Hookworm infec-	Hepatitis	hemorrhagic	
	tion	Hymenolepiasis	fever	
	Leishmaniasis,	Onchocerciasis	Chagas' disease	
	cutaneous	Paracoccidioido-	Hepatitis	
	Leishmaniasis,	mycosis	Typhus	
	visceral	Pinta		
	Leprosy	Relapsing fever		
	Pinta	Sand fly fever		
	Relapsing fever	Schistosomiasis		
	Tuberculosis	Taeniasis		
	Typhus	Tuberculosis		
		Yaws		
		Yellow fever		

* Modified from Warren KS, Mahmoud AAF (eds): *Tropical and Geographical Medicine*, 2d ed. New York, McGraw-Hill, 1990.

APPENDICES

Africa and the Middle East

MIDDLE EAST	NORTH AFRICA	EAST, WEST, AND CENTRAL AFRICA	SOUTH AFRICA
Anthrax	Anthrax	AIDS	Amebiasis
Boutonneuse fever	Boutonneuse fever	Anthrax	Anthrax
Brucellosis	Brucellosis	Boutonneuse fever	Hepatitis
Dracunculiasis	Dracunculiasis	Dracunculiasis	Hookworm infection
Hepatitis	Hepatitis	Hepatitis	Schistosomiasis
Hookworm infection	Hookworm infection	Hookworm infection	Tuberculosis
Hydatid disease	Hydatid disease	Leishmaniasis	
Leishmaniasis	Leishmaniasis	Leprosy	
Plague	Plague	Loiasis	
Schistosomiasis	Relapsing fever	Onchocerciasis	
Tuberculosis	Schistosomiasis	Plague	
	Taeniasis	Rabies	
	Tuberculosis	Schistosomiasis	
		Strongyloidiasis	
		Trichinosis	
		Trypanosomiasis	
		Tuberculosis	
		Typhus	
		Yaws	

Indian Subcontinent and Sri Lanka; Southeast Asia; China and Korea; and the Pacific Islands

INDIAN SUBCONTINENT AND SRI LANKA	SOUTHEAST ASIA	CHINA AND KOREA	PACIFIC ISLANDS
Amebiasis	Anthrax	Ascariasis	Ascariasis
Ascariasis	Ascariasis	Dengue	Dengue
Boutonneuse fever	Dengue	Filariasis	Filariasis
Dengue	Hookworm infection	Hepatitis	Hookworm infection
Filariasis	Leprosy	Hookworm infection	Leprosy
Hepatitis	Malaria	Leishmaniasis,	Scrombroid poisoning
Hookworm infection	Schistosomiasis	visceral	Strongyloidiasis
Leishmaniasis,	Scrub typhus	Leprosy	Trichinosis
cutaneous	Shigellosis	Malaria	Tuberculosis
Leishmaniasis,	Strongyloidiasis	Schistosomiasis	Yaws
visceral	Trichuriasis	Shigellosis	
Leprosy	Tuberculosis	Strongyloidiasis	
Scrub typhus		Trichinosis	
Shigellosis		Tuberculosis	
Strongyloidiasis			
Trichinosis			
Trichuriasis			
Tuberculosis			

NOTE: Anatomic, physiologic, and biochemical factors indigenous to certain areas may account for the localization of skin diseases on the face, perianal area, ear, and other areas. Since a considerable number of skin diseases may be limited to specific regions, the following differential lists of diseases classified by site should prove helpful in narrowing the number of possible diagnoses. The diseases listed below are ones discussed in this book; it is not a complete differential diagnosis of the various body regions.

See also the Subject Index.

SCALP
Macules
Cutaneous lupus erythematosus
Seborrheic dermatitis
Papules or Plaques
Acne
Actinic keratoses
Lichen simplex chronicus
Melanocytic nevi
Psoriasis
Seborrheic keratosis
Nodules or Tumors
Benign neoplasms (melanocytic nevi)
Malignant neoplasms (squamous and basal cell carcinoma)
Metastatic tumor
Nevus sebaceous
Scales
Atopic dermatitis
Lupus erythematosus
Psoriasis
Seborrheic dermatitis
Tinea capitis
Lichenification
Lichen simplex chronicus
Crusts
Acute eczematous dermatitis
Basal cell carcinoma
Pyogenic infections
Seborrheic dermatitis
Tinea capilis
Vesicles or Bullae
Acute eczematous dermatitis
Dermatitis herpetiformis
Herpes zoster

Pustules
Staphylococcal folliculitis

FACE
Macules
ERYTHEMATOUS
Fixed-drug eruption
Lupus erythematosus
Port-wine stain
Seborrheic dermatitis
PIGMENTED
Fixed-drug eruption
Junctional melanocytic nevi
Lentigines, solar
Lentigo maligna
Melanoma
Melasma
Seborrheic keratoses
DEPIGMENTED
Postinflammatory depigmentation
Vitiligo
Papules or Plaques
SKIN-COLORED
Acne
Melanocytic nevi
Molluscum contagiosum
Solar keratosis
Verruca plana
Verruca vulgaris
ERYTHEMATOUS
Acne
Actinic keratosis
Basal cell carcinoma
Chronic eczematous dermatitis

FACE (*Continued*)
>   Dermatomyositis
>   Eosinophilic folliculitis
>   Erysipelas
>   Erythropoietic protoporphyria
>   Hemangioma
>   Hereditary hemmorrhagic telangiecta-
>   sia
>   Lupus erythematosus
>   Pyogenic granuloma
>   Rosacea
>   Sarcoidosis
>   Secondary syphilis
>   Squamous cell carcinoma
>   PIGMENTED
>   Melanocytic nevi
>   Melanoma
>   Peutz-Jeghers syndrome
>   Seborrheic keratosis
> **Nodules or Tumors**
>   SKIN-COLORED
>   Angiofibroma
>   Basal cell carcinoma
>   Dermal melanocytic nevi
>   Squamous cell carcinoma
>   Tricholemmoma (Cowden's disease)
>   ERYTHEMATOUS
>   Lupus erythematosus
>   Pyogenic granuloma
>   Sarcoidosis
>   PIGMENTED
>   Basal cell carcinoma
>   Blue nevus
>   Melanocytic nevi
>   Melanoma
> **Vegetative Lesions**
>   Keratoacanthoma
>   Seborrheic keratosis
>   Verruca vulgaris
> **Wheals**
>   Angioedema
> **Scales**
>   Dermatophytosis
>   Glucagonoma
>   Lupus erythematosus (mostly exposed
>   areas)
>   Seborrheic dermatitis
>   Solar keratosis
>   Subacute eczematous dermatitis
>   Zinc deficiency

Hyperkeratosis
>   Keratoacanthoma
>   Solar keratosis
> **Lichenification**
>   Chronic eczematous dermatitis
> **Crusts**
>   Acute contact eczematous dermatitis
>   Herpes simplex
>   Herpes zoster
>   Impetigo
> **Vesicles or Bullae**
>   Acute contact eczematous dermatitis
>   Bullous impetigo
>   Dermatophytosis
>   Herpes simplex
>   Herpes zoster
>   Pemphigus vulgaris
> **Pustules**
>   Acne
>   Dermatophytosis
>   Impetigo
>   Rosacea
> **Ulcers**
>   Carcinoma
>   Factitial
>   Melanoma
> **Excoriations**
>   Neurotic excoriations

EYELIDS
> **Papules**
>   Carcinoma
>   Kaposi's sarcoma
>   Molluscum contagiosum
>   Seborrheic keratosis
>   Xanthelasma
> **Wheals or Edema**
>   Angioedema
>   Contact dermatitis
> **Vegetative Lesions**
>   Basal cell carcinoma
>   Verruca vulgaris
> **Nodules or Tumors**
>   Dermal or compound melanocytic
>   nevus
>   Sarcoidosis
> **Scales**
>   Seborrheic dermatitis
>   Subactue eczematous dermatitis

EYELIDS (*Continued*)
Lichenification
Chronic eczematous dermatitis
Crusts
Acute eczematous dermatitis
Any vesicular dermatosis
Impetigo

EARS
Plaques
Psoriasis
Nodules or Tumors
Carcinoma
Lyme borreliosis
Melanocytic nevi
Scales
Psoriasis
Seborrheic dermatitis
Subacute eczematous dermatitis
Hyperkeratosis
Solar keratosis
Seborrheic keratosis
Lichenification
Chronic eczematous dermatitis

MOUTH
Plaques
Candidiasis
Hairy leukoplakia
Leukoplakia
Lichen planus
Nodules
Carcinoma
Pyogenic granuloma
Hyperkeratosis
Hairy leukoplakia
Leukoplakia
Vesicles or Bullae
Erythema multiforme
Herpes simplex, primary
Herpes zoster
Pemphigus vulgaris
Ulcers
Carcinoma
Histoplasmosis
Lupus erythematosus
Syphilitic chancre

Oral and Ocular Lesions
Erythema multiforme
Herpes simplex
Herpes zoster
Oral and Cutaneous Lesions
Candidiasis
Erythema multiforme
Herpes simplex
Lichen planus
Lupus erythematosus
Pemphigus vulgaris
Secondary syphilis

TRUNK
Macules
ERYTHEMATOUS
Drug eruption
Pityriasis rosea
Seborrheic dermatitis
Secondary syphilis
Tinea corporis
PIGMENTED
Café-au-lait (neurofibromatosis)
Tinea versicolor
DEPIGMENTED
Leprosy
Tinea versicolor
Tuberous sclerosis
Vitiligo
Papules or Plaques
SKIN-COLORED
Dermal nevus
Molluscum contagiosum
Neurofibromatosis
ERYTHEMATOUS
Acne
Chronic eczematous dermatitis
Dermatitis herpetiformis
Erythema migrans
Lichen planus
Papular urticaria
Papulosquamous drug eruption
Pityriasis rosea
Psoriasis
Secondary syphilis
Urticaria pigmentosa
PIGMENTED
Melanocytic nevi
Melanoma

TRUNK (*Continued*)
    Pigmented basal cell carcinoma
    Seborrheic keratosis
    Urticaria pigmentosa
Wheals
  Drug eruptions
  Insect bites
  Urticaria
Nodules
  SKIN-COLORED
    Cancer, metastatic
    Neurofibromatosis
  ERYTHEMATOUS
    Acne conglobata
    Cancer, metastatic
    Dermal melanocytic nevi
    Gumma
    Leprosy
    Mycosis fungoides
    Sarcoid
  PIGMENTED
    Fixed drug eruption
    Kaposi's sarcoma
    Melanocytic nevi
    Melanoma
    Seborrheic keratosis
Scales
  Papulosquamous drug eruption
  Parapsoriasis en plaque
  Pityriasis rosea
  Psoriasis
  Seborrheic dermatitis
  Secondary syphilis
  Subacute eczematous dermatitis
  Tinea corporis
  Tinea versicolor
Vesicles or Bullae
  Acute eczematous dermatitis
  Bullous pemphigoid
  Dermatitis herpetiformis
  Drug eruptions
  Herpes zoster
  Pemphigus vulgaris
  Scabies
  Tinea corporis
  Varicella
Pustules
  Acne
  Acne conglobata
  Drug eruptions

  Impetigo
  Psoriasis pustulosa (von Zumbusch)
  Scabies
  Tinea corporis

AXILLAE
Macules
  Ephelides (small, brown frecklelike)
  Fixed drug eruption (reddish brown)
  Intertrigo (erythematous)
  LEOPARD syndrome
  Vitiligo vulgaris (white)
  von Recklinghausen's neurofibromatosis
Papules or Plaques
  Acanthosis nigricans (velvety, brown
    pigmented)
  Acrochordon
  Candidiasis
  Contact eczematous dermatitis (deodor-
    ant, antiperspirant)
  Psoriasis
  Seborrheic dermatitis
  Tinea corporis (rare)
Lichenification
  Lichen simplex chronicus
Nodules
  Hidradenitis suppurativa (tender, red)
  Scabies
Scales
  Candidiasis
  Contact eczematous dermatitis
  Psoriasis
  Seborrheic dermatitis
  Tinea corporis (rare)
Vesicles or Bullae
  Acute contact dermatitis
  Bullous impetigo
  Pemphigus vulgaris
  Scabies (anterior axillary fold)
Erosions
  Bullous pemphigoid
  Pemphigus vulgaris

FEMALE BREAST
Papules or Plaques
  Chronic eczematous dermatitis
  Paget's disease of the nipple
  Scabies
  Seborrheic keratosis

FEMALE BREAST (*Continued*)
Nodules
  Neurofibromas of the areolae
Lichenification
  Chronic eczematous dermatitis
  Lichen simplex
Crusts
  Any vesicular, bullous, excoriated,
    eroded, or ulcerated dermatosis
Scales
  Eczematous dermatitis
  Tinea corporis
Vesicles
  Acute contact eczematous dermatitis
  Paget's disease of the nipple
  Scabies
Ulcers
  Syphilitic chancre

INGUINAL REGIONS
Macules
  Seborrheic dermatitis
  Tinea cruris (scaling)
Papules or Plaques
  Candidiasis
  Chronic eczematous dermatitis
  Psoriasis
Scales
  Candidiasis
  Psoriasis
  Seborrheic dermatitis
  Subacute eczematous dermatitis
  Tinea cruris
Crusts
  Eczematous dermatitis
Vesicles or Bullae
  Acute contact eczematous dermatitis
  Impetigo
  Pemphigus vulgaris
Pustules
  Candidiasis
  Furunculosis
Erosions
  Impetigo
  Moniliasis
  Pemphigus vulgaris
Lichenification
  Chronic eczematous dermatitis

PUBIC AREA
Macules
  Macula cerulea (pediculosis pubis)
  Seborrheic dermatitis (scaling)
Papules or Plaques
  Lichen simplex chronicus
  Psoriasis
  Seborrheic dermatitis
Scales
  Psoriasis
  Seborrheic dermatitis
  Subacute eczematous dermatitis
  Tinea corporis
Lichenification
  Chronic eczematous dermatitis
  Lichen simplex
Crusts
  Any vesicular, eroded, excoriated, or
    ulcerated dermatitis
Excoriations
  Pediculisis pubis
Vesicles
  Acute eczematous dermatitis
  Herpes zoster
  Scabies
Ulcers
  Syphilitic chancre

GENITALIA (MALE AND FEMALE)
Macules
  Seborrheic dermatitis
  Secondary syphilis
  Vitiligo
Papules or Plaques
  Bowenoid papulisis
  Chronic eczematous dermatitis
  Condylomata acuminata
  Lichen planus
  Melanoma
  Psoriasis
  Scabies
  Secondary syphilis
Nodules or Tumors
  Melanoma
  Scabies (scrotum and penis)
  Squamous cell carcinoma
Vegetative Lesions
  Condylomata acuminata
  Condylomata lata
  Squamous cell carcinoma

GENITALIA (MALE AND FEMALE)
(*Continued*)
Lichenification
Chronic eczematous dermatitis
Scales
Candidiasis
Psoriasis
Seborrheic dermatitis
Secondary syphilis
Tinea cruris
Crusts (*see* Erosions; Ulcers; Vesicles)
Vesicles or Bullae
Acute eczematous dermatitis
Erythema multiforme
Herpes simplex
Scabies
Pustules
Candidiasis
Scabies
Erosions
Herpes simplex
Syphilitic chancre
Ulcers
Squamous cell carcinoma
Syphilitic chancre
Excoriations
Scabies

BUTTOCKS
Macules
Fixed-drug eruption
Papules
Acne
Scabies
Wheals
Insect bites
Vesicles
Contact
Herpes simplex
Scabies
Tinea corporis
Pustules
Acne
Candidiasis
Folliculitis
Scabies
Tinea corporis
Scales
Psoriasis
Tinea corporis

PERIANAL REGION
Macules
Psoriasis
Seborrheic dermatitis
Tinea corporis
Vitiligo
Papules or Plaques
Chronic eczematous dermatitis
Condylomata acuminata
Condylomata lata
Psoriasis
Secondary syphilis
Vegetative Lesions
Condylomata acuminata
Condylomata lata (syphilis)
Scales
Candidiasis
Psoriasis
Subacute eczematous dermatitis
Tinea corporis
Lichenification
Chronic eczematous dermatitis (pruritus ani)
Vesicles
Acute eczematous dermatitis
Erosions
Candidiasis
Moniliasis
Syphilitic chancre
Fissures
Chronic eczematous dermatitis
Psoriasis
Ulcers
Syphilitic chancre

ARMS AND FOREARMS
Papules or Plaques
Chronic eczematous dermatitis
Lichen planus
Lupus erythematosus
Melanocytic nevi
Psoriasis
Nodules
Carcinoma, squamous cell
Granuloma annulare
Melanoma
Hyperkeratosis
Keratosis pilaris
Solar keratosis

ARMS AND FOREARMS (*Continued*)
  Scales
    Lupus erythematosus
    Psoriasis
    Subacute or chronic eczematous dermatitis
    Tinea corporis
  Lichenification
    Chronic eczematous dermatitis
  Crusts
    Ecthyma

HANDS
  Macules
    Erythema multiforme
    Lentigo, solar (dorsum)
    Lupus erythematosus (dorsum)
    Secondary syphilis
    Vitiligo (dorsum)
  Papules or Plaques
    Erysipeloid
    Erythema multiforme (palm and dorsum)
    Granuloma annulare
    Lichen planus
    Lupus erythematosus (dorsum)
    Psoriasis
    Pyogenic granuloma (around nails)
    Scabies
    Solar keratosis (dorsum)
    Subacute or chronic eczematous dermatitis
    Verruca plana
    Verruca vulgaris
  Nodules or Tumors
    SKIN-COLORED
      Keratoacanthoma
      Squamous cell carcinoma
      Verruca vulgaris
    ERYTHEMATOUS
      Granuloma annulare
      Pyogenic granuloma
    PIGMENTED
      Melanoma
  Vegetative Lesions
    Keratoacanthoma
    Squamous cell carcinoma
    Verruca vulgaris

  Scales
    Lupus erythematosus (dorsum)
    Psoriasis
    Secondary syphilis
    Subactue or chronic eczematous dermatitis
    Tinea manus
  Hyperkeratosis
    Keratoacanthoma (dorsum)
    Solar keratosis (dorsum)
    X-ray dermatitis
  Lichenification
    Chronic eczematous dermatitis
  Burrows
    Scabies (between digits)
  Vesicles or Bullae
    Acute eczematous dermatitis
    Dermatophytosis
    Dyshydrotic dermatitis
    Erythema multiforme
    Herpes simplex
    Porphyria (exposed areas)
    Scabies
  Pustules
    Dermatophytosis
    Eczematous dermatitis
    Palmoplantar pustulosis
    Pustular psoriasis (palm)
    Scabies
  Erosions
    Moniliasis (webs of fingers)
    Porphyria cutanea tarda
  Ulcers
    Carcinoma, squamous cell
    Melanoma
    Syphilitic chancre
    X-ray dermatitis
  Scars
    Porphyria cutanea tarda (discrete, pink; on exposed areas)

FEET
  Papules
    Secondary syphilis (plantar surface)
    Subacute or chronic eczematous dermatitis
    Verruca vulgaris (plantar region)
  Nodules or Tumors
    Carcinoma, squamous cell
    Melanoma

FEET (*Continued*)
Scales
Psoriasis
Subacute or chronic eczematous dermatitis
Tinea pedis (intertriginous areas particularly)
Vesicles
Dyshidrotic eczema
Eczematous dermatitis
Tinea pedis
Lichenification
Chronic eczematous dermatitis
Vesicles or Bullae
Acute eczematous dermatitis
Tinea pedis
Pustules
Pustular psoriasis
Scabies
Lichenification
Chronic eczematous dermatitis
Erosions
Tinea pedis

LEGS
Papules or Plaques
Ichthyosis
Lichen planus
Psoriasis
Melanocytic nevi
Solar keratosis
Squamous cell carcinoma
Subacute or chronic eczematous dermatitis
Vesicles or Bullae
Eczematous dermatitis
Insect bites
Wheals
Insect bites
Edema
Stasis dermatitis (varicose veins, cardiac failure)
Nodules
ERYTHEMATOUS
Carcinoma, squamous cell
Erythema nodosum
PIGMENTED
Melanoma

Vegetative Lesions
Verruca vulgaris
Hyperkeratosis
Solar keratosis
Scales
Dermatophytosis
Ichthyosis
Psoriasis
Lichenification
Chronic eczematous dermatitis
Crusts
Ecthyma
Ulcers
Carcinoma, squamous cell
Stasis dermatitis with ulcer

GENERALIZED DISTRIBUTION INCLUDING CHARACTERISTIC PATTERNS
Macules
Drug eruption
Lupus erythematosus
Pityriasis rosea
Seborrheic dermatitis
Syphilis (secondary)
Vitiligo
Vesicles and Bullae
Bullous pemphigoid
Dermatitis herpetiformis
Drug eruption
Eczematous dermatitis, atopic
Eczematous dermatitis, contact
Erythema multiforme
Herpes simplex
Herpes zoster
Pemphigus vulgaris
Scabies
Pustules
Drug eruption
Generalized pustular psoriasis syndrome (von Zumbusch)
Papules
Atopic dermatitis
Drug eruption
Erythema multiforme
Lichen planus
Lupus erythematosus
Mycosis fungoides
Psoriasis
Secondary syphilis

**GENERALIZED DISTRIBUTION
   INCLUDING CHARACTERISTIC
   PATTERNS** (*Continued*)
Scales
   Drug eruption
   Ichthyosis vulgaris
   Mycosis fungoides (Sézary's syndrome)
Wheals
   Insect bites
   Urticaria

Nodules
   Mycosis fungoides
   Neurofibromatosis
Lichenification
   Atopic dermatitis

Chancre, 390–393
Chancroid, 390–393
Cherry angioma, 164–165
Cherry hemangioma, 164–165
Chickenpox, 306–309
China, communicable diseases with derma-
  tologic lesions in, 799
Chloasma, 640–642
Cholesterol embolism, 552–553
Cholinergic urticaria, 452, 454
Chronic discoid lupus erythematosus, 486,
  492
Circinate balanitis in Reiter's syndrome,
  528–529
Clark melanocytic nevus, 656–659
Clinical aids in diagnosis, 772–773
  clinical tests and, 773
  special techniques and, 772–773
Clubbed fingers, 796–797
Coagulation, disseminated intravascular,
  756–758
Coagulation-fibrinolytic syndrome, 756–758
Coagulopathy, consumption, 756–758
Coccidioidomycosis, 324–325
Cold sore, 70–73
Cold urticaria, 452
Communicable diseases with dermatologic
  lesions, index of, by geographic area,
  798–799
Complement-mediated urticaria, 452
Condyloma acuminatum, 402–405
Condyloma latum, 382
Conjunctivitis in Reiter's syndrome, 528,
  531
Consumption coagulopathy, 756–758
Contact dermatitis, 16–21
  caused by Balsam of Peru, 17
  caused by nickel, 19
  caused by shoes, 21
  textile, 20
Cowden's syndrome, 734–735
Crab dermatitis, 96–97
Crab lice, 128–131
Cradle cap, 54, 56–57
Cranial arteritis, 518–521
Creeping eruption, 142–143
Crusts:
  ecthyma, 769
  impetigo, 769
Cryoglobulinemia, 524–527

Cryptococcosis, 326–327
Culture:
  of exudates and tissue minces, 773
  viral, 778
Cushing's syndrome, 558–559
Cutaneous T-cell lymphoma, 712–717
  classification of, 716
  Sézary's syndrome and, 718–719
  staging system for, 716
Cyst:
  digital mucoid (digital myxoid), 186–187
  epidermal (epidermoid; infundibular; seba-
    ceous), 180–181
    inclusion (traumatic epidermoid), 184–
    185
  retention, 186–187
  tricholemmal (isthmus catagen; pilar; se-
    baceous), 182–183

Darier's sign, 773
Dark-field examination, syphilis, 780
  of serum from ulcers, 774
Defibrination syndrome, 756–758
Dermatitis:
  berloque, 224
  chronic superficial, 260
  crab, 96–97
  eczematous
    adult-type atopic, 26–27
    asteatotic (eczema craquelatum), 38–39
    atopic, 22–23
    childhood-type atopic, 26
    contact, 16–21
    dyshidrotic, 32–35
    infantile atopic, 24–25
    lichen simplex chronicus, 28–29
    nummular (discoid) eczematous, 30–31
    stasis dermatitis with ulcer, 36–37
  gonococcal arthritis-dermatitis syndrome
    and, 270–272
  herpetiformis, 462–465
  perioral, 14–15
  pustular, contagious, 78–81
  radiation, 686–689
  rosacea-like, 14–15
  seborrheic, 54–57
Dermatofibroma, 174–175
Dermatoheliosis, 208, 214–217
Dermatomyositis, 466–469

Nails (*Continued*)
nail fold telangiectasia and, 793
normal, 791
ochronosis and, 795
onycholysis and (Plummer's nail), 793
periungual fibroma of, 794
splinter hemorrhages of, 795
Terry's, 792–793
yellow nail syndrome and, 794
Necrobiosis lipoidica diabeticorum, 548–550
Necrolysis, toxic epidermal, 314–315
Necrosis, due to warfarin, 604–606
Necrotizing vasculitis, 506–509
Nelson's syndrome, 648–649
Neoplasia, intraepithelial:
penile, 406–409
squamous, 406–409
vulvar, 406–409
Neoplasms and hyperplasias, benign, 144–187
Neurofibromatosis, 584–587
Neuronevus, blue, 156–157
Neurosyphilis, 388
Neutrophilic dermatosis, acute febrile, 542–543
Nevomelanocytic nevus, congenital, 660–663
malignant melanoma arising in, 680–681
Nevus:
angiomatous, 160–161
araneus, 168–169
basal cell (*see* Basal cell nevus syndrome)
blue
cellular, 156
combined blue nevus-nevomelanocytic nevus, 156
common, 156–157
blue rubber bleb, 162
flammeus, 158–159
nuchae, 158
halo nevomelanocytic, 154–155
melanocytic, Clark (dysplastic), 656–659
melanocytic nevocellular, 150–153
compound, 150, 152–153
dermal, 150, 152–153
junctional, 150–151
nevomelanocytic, congenital, 660–663
spider, 168–169
strawberry, 160–161
Nodular melanoma, 676–677, 785, 787–788

Nodule, 764
Nodulus cutaneus, 174–175
Nonlipid reticuloepitheliosis (*see* Langerhans cell histiocytosis)
North American blastomycosis, 321–323
Norwegian scabies, 134
Nummular eczema, 30–31
Nutritional diseases, 548–595

Ochronosis, nails in, 795
Ohio Valley disease, 328–329
Onycholysis, 793
Onychomycosis, 104–105
Oral leukoplakia, 682–684
viral (hairy), HIV-associated, 420–421
Oriental/Allepo sore, 354–358
Osler-Weber-Rendu disease, 554–557

Pacific Islands, communicable diseases with dermatologic lesions in, 799
Paget's disease:
extramammary, 748–751
mammary, 746–747
Palmoplantar pustulosis, 52–53
Panarteritis nodosa, 510–513
Pancreatic panniculitis, 572–573
Panniculitis, pancreatic, 572–573
Papilloma, cutaneous, 178–179
Papular urticaria, 138–139
Papule, 761
Papulosis, bowenoid, 406–409
Parapemphigus, 540–541
Parapsoriasis, 260–261
large-plaque, 260–261
small-plaque, 260
Paravaccinia, 78–81
Paronychia, candidal, 118, 121
Patch testing, 773
Pediculosis capitis, 126–127
Pediculosis pubis, 128–132
Pellagra, 628–629
Pemphigoid, bullous, 540–541
Pemphigus:
Brazilian, 538
drug-induced, 538
erythematosus, 538
foliaceus, 538
neonatorum, 294–297

Rash (*Continued*)
  fever and, 262–320
  photosensitivity and, 208
Raynaud's disease, 502–505
Raynaud's phenomenon, 502–505
Reiter's syndrome, 528–531
Retention cyst, 186–187
Reticuloendotheliosis, nonlipid (*see* Langerhans cell histiocytosis)
Rheumatic diseases:
  skin signs of, 448–547
  (*See also specific diseases*)
Ringworm, 98, 108–109
  of beard, 98, 114–115
  "black dot," 112
  of face, 98, 110–111
  "gray patch," 112–113
Ritter's disease, 294–297
Rocky Mountain spotted fever, 282–285
  abdominal syndrome of, 284
  "spotless," 284
  thrombotic thrombocytopenic purpura and, 284
Rodent ulcer basal cell carcinoma, 690–691
Rosacea, 10–13
Rosacea-like dermatitis, 14–15
Rubella, 286–289
Rubeola, 290–293

San Joachin Valley fever, 324–325
Sarcoidosis, 544–547
Sarcoma:
  hemorrhagic, multiple idiopathic, 432–437
  Kaposi's, epidemic, 432–437
Scabies, 132–137
  animal, 134
  "crusted," 134
  geriatric, 134
  laboratory diagnosis of, 774
  nodular, 134
  Norwegian, 134
Scalded-skin syndrome, staphylococcal, 294–297
Scaling eruptions of unknown etiology, 54–61
Scarlet fever, 298–301
Scars:
  hypertrophic, 176
  keloidal, 176–177

Scleroderma, 498–501
  guttate, 252–255
  localized (circumscribed), 248–251
  systemic, 498–501
Sclerosing hemangioma, 174–175
Sclerosis:
  progressive systemic (systemic), 498–501
  tuberous, 578–583
Scrofuloderma, 340, 342, 344, 347
Scurvy, 564–567
Sebaceous cyst (*see* Cyst, epidermal; Cyst, tricholemmal)
Seborrheic dermatitis, 54–57
Seborrheic keratosis, 144–147
Senear-Usher syndrome, 538
Senile angioma, 164–165
Senile keratosis, 220–223
Serum sickness, 597
Sexually transmitted diseases, 376–413
Sézary's syndrome, 718–719
Shulman's syndrome, 470–472
Sister Mary Joseph's nodule, 742, 744
Skin tag, 178–179
Sneddon's syndrome, 484
Solar keratosis, 220–223
  desquamation in, 770
Solar lentigo, 218–219
Solar urticaria, 238–241, 452, 454
South America, communicable diseases with dermatologic lesions in, 798
Southeast Asia, communicable diseases with dermatologic lesions in, 799
Spider, vascular (arterial), 168–169
Spider angioma, 168–169
Spider hemangioma, 168–169
Spider nevus, 168–169
Spider telangiectasia, 168–169
Spoon nails, 795
Sporotrichosis, 330–333
  chronic lymphangitic (sporotrichoid), 330–331
  fixed cutaneous, 330, 333
  local cutaneous (chancriform), 330
Squamous cell carcinoma, 682, 700–705
  arsenical keratoses and, 702, 705
  Bowen's disease and, 701–704
  erythroplasia of Queyrat and, 701–704
Sri Lanka, communicable diseases with dermatologic lesions in, 799
Staphylococcal impetigo, 84–85

SUBJECT INDEX

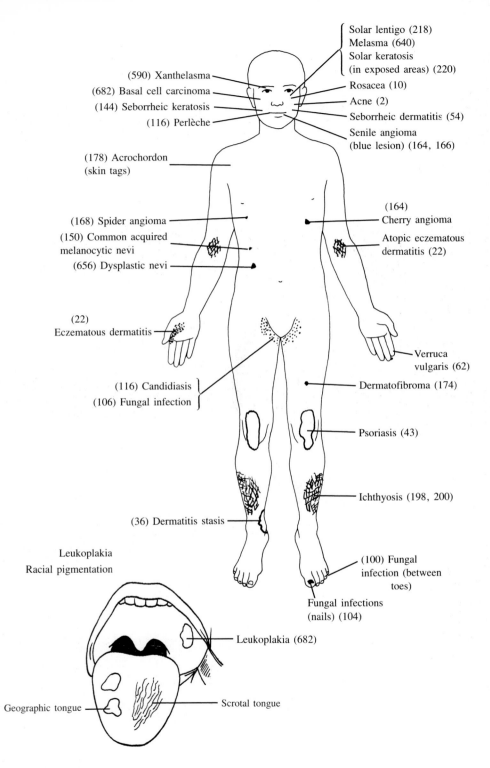

Solar lentigo (218)
Melasma (640)
Solar keratosis
(in exposed areas) (220)

(590) Xanthelasma

(682) Basal cell carcinoma

(144) Seborrheic keratosis

(116) Perlèche

Rosacea (10)

Acne (2)

Seborrheic dermatitis (54)

Senile angioma
(blue lesion) (164, 166)

(178) Acrochordon
(skin tags)

(164)
Cherry angioma

(168) Spider angioma

(150) Common acquired
melanocytic nevi

(656) Dysplastic nevi

Atopic eczematous
dermatitis (22)

(22)
Eczematous dermatitis

Verruca
vulgaris (62)

(116) Candidiasis

(106) Fungal infection

Dermatofibroma (174)

Psoriasis (43)

Ichthyosis (198, 200)

(36) Dermatitis stasis

Leukoplakia
Racial pigmentation

(100) Fungal
infection (between
toes)

Fungal infections
(nails) (104)

Leukoplakia (682)

Geographic tongue

Scrotal tongue

NOTE: Numbers in parentheses refer to pages where disorder in discussed.